Principles of
Clinical Toxicology
Third Edition

Principles of
Clinical Toxicology
Third Edition

Thomas A. Gossel, Ph.D.
Professor of Pharmacology and Toxicology
Department of Pharmacology
Dean, College of Pharmacy
Ohio Northern University
Ada, Ohio

J. Douglas Bricker, Ph.D.
Associate Professor of Pharmacology and Toxicology
Chairman, Department of Pharmacology and Toxicology
School of Pharmacy
Duquesne University
Pittsburgh, Pennsylvania

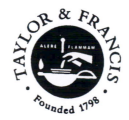

Reprinted 2001, 2002 by Taylor & Francis
11 New Fetter Lane, London EC4P 4EE

Transferred to Digital Printing 2003

Taylor & Francis is an imprint of the Taylor & Francis Group

© 2001 Taylor & Francis

Library of Congress Cataloging-in-Publication Data
Gossel, Thomas A.
    Principles of clinical toxicology / Thomas A. Gossel, J. Douglas Bricker —
3rd ed.
      p. cm.
    Includes bibliographical references and index.
    ISBN 0-7817-0125-2
    1. Toxicology I. Bricker, J. Douglas. II. Title.
    [DNLM: 1. Poisoning. 2. Poisoning—drug
therapy. 3. Poisons. 4. Antidotes. QV 600 G6785p 1994]
    RA1211.G6 1994
    615.9—dc20
    DNLM/DLC
    for Library of Congress   93-37532

Printed by Biddles Short Run Books, King's Lynn

9 8 7 6 5 4 3 2 1

Contents

Acknowledgments

To all individuals who supported our work, offered valuable suggestions, helped with various stages of manuscript preparation, or reviewed previous editions of this textbook, we extend our heartfelt thanks. A special and sincere thanks to our wives, Phyllis Gossel and Lillian Bricker, who gave unselfish understanding and patience; our children and grandchildren, for providing us with countless reasons to secure our own homes against poisoning; our mentors, who planted the original seeds that grew into a love for toxicology; and numerous other colleagues, who aided our work with support and suggestions, and provided critical analysis of various chapters in this book.

We extend special thanks to Stewart Graham and Linda Graham for preparation of artwork, and to the staff at Raven Press for their careful attention to all phases of manuscript preparation.

Finally, to those who have taught us much more than we could ever hope to teach them, we thank our students for their own personal quest for learning. We dedicate this book to them.

Preface to the Second Edition

This second edition of *Principles of Clinical Toxicology* emphasizes the same goal as the First Edition. It is a textbook for students of pharmacy and the health sciences to help them learn the principles of clinical toxicology. Principles are rules of action or reasons why certain procedures are undertaken; they are also the foundation of a science. This book adheres to its title in that it is neither reference book nor laboratory manual; rather, it attempts to explain fundamental principles. By understanding the basis for events that occur and the reasons why a certain treatment is used or perhaps not used, we should then be able to approach any toxic emergency with few reservations.

Since publication of the First Edition, we received a number of suggestions for change and have incorporated those that strengthen the book as a text. This Second Edition has been updated, and many portions revised in format and content to reflect contemporary toxicology. For example, anticholinergics, phenothiazines, and tricyclic antidepressants have been combined into one chapter. Topics such as toxicokinetics and cardiovascular drugs have been added. Case studies following each chapter have been expanded.

T. A. Gossel
J. D. Bricker
1989

Preface

Since publication of the second edition of *Principles of Clinical Toxicology*, there have been many changes in protocols for managing various toxic ingestions. New antidotes have been added. Flumazenil, a specific antagonist for benzodiazepine derivitives, is one example. Succimer, a chelating agent for lead, is another. Particular treatments have changed; for example, physostigmine is not now recommended for routine use in anticholinergic drug poisoning.

The third edition of *Principles of Clinical Toxicology* maintains the same goal as the previous editions. It is a textbook for students of pharmacy and the health sciences to help them learn basic principles of clinical toxicology.

Selected topics have been expanded, others added where necessary, and still others have been deleted. We welcome your suggestions and criticism.

T. A. Gossel
J. D. Bricker

Principles of
Clinical Toxicology
Third Edition

1 ‖ Toxicology in Perspective

INTRODUCTION TO TOXICOLOGY

Toxicology is a science that has evolved over the last several years. New concepts and theories are being developed and implemented into clinical practice. However, there is one basic concept that does remain fairly constant: certain principles of toxicology do not change. Principles are rules for action, basic concepts, or reasons why certain procedures are undertaken. Principles also form the foundation of a science.

Toxicology is not an easy term to define. The word is derived from Greek and Latin origins (L. *toxicum* = poison; Gr. *toxicom* = arrow poison; L. *logia* = science or study) and literally means a study of poisons on living organisms. A *toxicologist* may be described as an individual who studies or works in the area of toxicology, but toxicology is not restricted to such a narrow definition, and toxicologists do much more than simply work with poisons. In its broadest sense, the science of toxicology involves all aspects of the adverse effects of chemicals on biologic systems, including their mechanisms of harmful effects, conditions under which these harmful effects occur, socioeconomic considerations, and legal ramifications.

HISTORICAL PERSPECTIVES

Toxicology is a relatively new discipline. It has slowly developed over the years, beginning with an essence of observation and reaching its current status as an analytical science. This development is exciting to study, but an in-depth consideration is beyond the scope of this chapter. Interested students should consult Holmstedt and Liljestrand (6) or Casarett and Bruce (2) for specific details. There is one individual, however, who deserves to be cited. He, more than anyone else, established toxicology as an absolute science.

The father of modern toxicology was Mathieu Joseph Bonaventura Orfila (1787–1853). Orfila was a Spaniard who served as attending physician to Louis XVIII of France and taught at the University of Paris. During his early professional life, Orfila quickly realized the inadequacy of toxicology as a science. So, in 1815 he wrote the first book on general toxicology that was devoted to adverse effects of chemicals (21). Before that time, toxicology had been largely descriptive, leaving wide gaps of information open for broad and often erroneous interpretation. Intuitive hunches often served as the sole basis for determining the cause of a poisoning incident.

Orfila, concerned with legal implications of poisoning, pointed out the importance of chemical analysis in establishing a definitive cause of poisoning. He then devised analytical procedures, many of which are still in use today, for detecting specific chemicals in body fluids and tissues. Orfila's text established the basis for future experimental and forensic toxicologic evaluations and subsequently was translated into several languages. He eventually supplemented his book with numerous

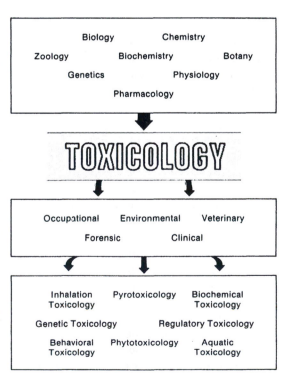

FIG. 1.1. The evolution of toxicology with its numerous applications.

monographs that discussed additional toxicologic information in detail.

During the developmental years, many principles and techniques from various basic biologic and chemical sciences were incorporated into this new science called toxicology. Figure 1.1 illustrates the progression of information received by the student of toxicology and the basic sciences upon which toxicology is founded. The basic sciences are followed at another level by specific subdisciplines of toxicology that have evolved over the years and some of the specialty areas within these disciplines. These specialty areas will be discussed briefly to define the limits of each and to promote an appreciation of modern toxicology, which has developed into a meaningful and necessary science.

DIVERSITY OF TOXICOLOGY

Occupational (industrial) toxicology grew out of a need to protect workers from toxic substances, making their working environment safe. The objective is to prevent impairment of the health of individuals while on the job. Occupational diseases caused by industrial chemicals account for an estimated 50,000 to 70,000 deaths and 350,000 new cases of illness each year in the United States (29).

The industrial toxicologist is responsible for defining permissible concentrations of potentially toxic agents that are safe and do not produce adverse acute symptoms of chronic diseases. As a result of the need for workers to be protected, the Occupational Safety and Health Act (OSHA) of 1970 was passed. Under the Secretary of Labor, OSHA was established to assure that no employees will suffer diminished health or functional capacity or limited life expectancy as a result of their work experiences.

Two agencies are particularly critical to the operation of OSHA. One is its sister agency, the National Institute for Occupational Safety and Health (NIOSH). This federal body is charged with developing safety and health standards and is involved in the research aspect of occupational toxicology. It publishes *Criteria Documents* on specific chemicals, giving pertinent toxicity and safety information. For example, NIOSH lists 8-hr/day exposure limits for chemicals [threshold limit values (TLVs)], the immediate first aid procedures in case of skin or eye exposure, and so forth (29).

The other agency is the American Conference of Governmental Industrial Hygienists (ACGIH), which is devoted to setting safety standards for chemicals in the working environment. The research undertaken by this group results in useful data, such as threshold limit values and maximum allowable concentrations (MACs) of chemicals. *Environmental toxicology* is a broad discipline that encompasses the study of chemicals that are contaminants of food, water, soil, or the atmosphere. It was Dr. Harvey Wiley, of the Food and Drug Administration (FDA), who first noted the potential health problems of food additives (chemical preservatives and dyes), the deplorable conditions of the meat-packing industry, and the many "cure-all" claims for worthless medicines that, in many cases, probably were direct or indirect causes of death (26). Today, specific information must be supplied to the FDA concerning the use of any substance, such as a food additive, before the food is released for consumption. The list of safe food additives is referred to as the GRAS list (generally recommended as safe).

Environmental toxicology is also concerned with toxic substances that enter the lakes, streams, rivers, and oceans. The most common environmental toxicology problems are waterborne viruses and bacteria, waste heat from electrical plants, radioactive wastes, sewage eutrophication, and industrial pollutants. *Forensic toxicology* is the discipline that combines analytical chemistry with essential toxicologic principles to deal with the medicolegal aspects of the toxic effects of drugs and chemicals on humans. The role of forensic toxicology is to help establish cause and effect relationships between exposure to a drug or chemical and the toxic or lethal effects that result. To confirm a cause and effect relationship unequivocally, the forensic toxicologist relies on specific, highly sensitive analytical methods that can efficiently isolate, identify, and quantitatively determine the toxic compound in question from biologic fluids and tissues. *Clinical toxicology,* as might be expected, is involved with specific pathophysiologic changes caused by toxic agents and the management of these events. Clinical toxicology encompasses the study of chemicals originating from all sources. It is concerned with all aspects of the interaction between these chemicals and humans. *Veterinary toxicology* is the animal aspect of clinical toxicology. Cattle, sheep, and other farm animals and household pets are frequently poisoned by plants and chemicals. Toxicologists who are trained in veterinary medicine or animal husbandry tend to them.

TOXICITY: WHEN DOES IT START?

When considering the term *toxic* or *toxicity,* one of the first images that may come to mind is the traditionally pictured "skull and crossbones." This image of death and destruction is automatically associated with toxicity. But what is a toxic substance? Do all toxic chemicals cause death and destruction? What about the converse? Are chemicals that are usually considered nontoxic always safe?

TOXIC SUBSTANCES

A poisonous or toxic substance is any chemical that is capable of producing detrimental actions on a living organism. As a result of damage, there is an alteration of structural components or functional processes which may produce injury or even death. An important principle to remember is that any chemical may be poisonous at a given dose and route of administration. Breathing too much pure oxygen, drinking excessive amounts of water, or ingesting too much salt can cause poisoning or even death (22). On the other hand, even the classic "toxic"

chemicals may be ingested in subtoxic quantities and not cause symptoms of toxicity (17). We cannot truthfully segregate those compounds that are generally considered to be toxic (e.g., cyanide, arsenic, and lye) from those assumed to be nontoxic. All chemicals are potentially toxic under the proper conditions.

Many people assume that signs and symptoms of poisoning start the moment exposure occurs. Although this is true in some cases, it is an incorrect assumption for many toxic exposures. In some instances, the onset of toxic effects is delayed hours or days. Certain pesticides, heavy metals, and timed-release dosage forms of pharmaceuticals illustrate a delayed onset. Although people are exposed to a wide variety of toxic substances each day, they often do not display any symptoms of toxicity.

An important principle is illustrated by considering the hazard factor of chemical substances. The hazard factor describes a substance's packaging, formulation, access, and other components of availability (14). An extremely toxic substance may be packaged with a child-resistant safety closure or in a container with a tiny aperture. It would be difficult for a child to gain access to it; thus, it has a low hazard factor. Another extremely toxic substance may be rarely encountered around the home. It, too, would have a low hazard factor. And, in a third case, substances with mild to moderate toxicities may be readily available to children or adults. These would be considered to have a much higher hazard factor because of availability, even though the chance of serious poisoning is minimal.

Toxicity Values

People often ask when a chemical is considered to be toxic or how much of a substance must be ingested to cause symptoms of toxicity? Chemicals produce toxic effects on a biologic system whenever they reach a critical concentration in the target tissues. Overall, the toxicity of a substance is routinely expressed

TABLE 1.1. *Approximate LD$_{50}$ of a selected variety of chemical agents*

Agent	Animal	Route[a]	LD$_{50}$ (mg/kg)
Ethyl alcohol	Mouse	p.o.	10,000
Sodium chloride	Mouse	i.p.	4,000
Ferrous sulfate	Rat	p.o.	1,500
Morphine sulfate	Rat	p.o.	900
Phenobarbital, sodium	Rat	p.o.	150
DDT[b]	Rat	p.o.	100
Picrotoxin	Rat	s.c.	5
Strychnine sulfate	Rat	i.p.	2
Nicotine	Rat	i.v.	1
d-Tubocurarine	Rat	i.v.	0.5
Hemicholinium-3	Rat	i.v.	0.2
Tetrodotoxin	Rat	i.v.	0.10
Dioxin	Guinea pig	i.v.	0.001
Botulinus toxin	Rat	i.v.	0.00001

From ref. 15.
[a] i.p., intraperitoneal; i.v., intravenous; p.o., per os (oral); s.c., subcutaneous.
[b] DDT, dichlorodiphenyltrichloroethane.

by an LD$_{50}$ value, or the dose of a chemical required to produce death in 50% of the organisms exposed to it. An LD$_{50}$ determination is used to categorize the potential toxicity of chemical compounds to humans.

Determinations of LD$_{50}$ are plagued with variations. Species variations, interlaboratory differences in values, and the fact that it is very difficult to correlate these data directly to known exposures are a few of the variables that make an LD$_{50}$ value only an estimate. These values, then, are said to "estimate" the relative degree of toxicity for a given compound.

Table 1.1 illustrates the wide range of doses of different chemicals that induce lethal effects in animals. As can be seen from the table, some chemicals cause death in microgram quantities; these can, therefore, be described as *extremely toxic*. Other chemicals may be relatively harmless in doses in excess of several grams. A toxicity rating scale for chemicals is used to approximate their potential toxicity. Table 1.2 illustrates this rating scale, which lists the categories of toxicity based on their probable lethal oral dose in humans. Another application of a LD$_{50}$ determination is to compare the value with the ED$_{50}$, the dose of a chemical that is therapeutically effective in 50% of the subjects receiving it. From this comparison, a therapeutic index or margin of safety can be calculated.

The therapeutic index (TI) is defined as the ratio of the LD$_{50}$ to the ED$_{50}$ (TI = LD$_{50}$/ED$_{50}$). Figure 1.2 illustrates hypothetical dose-response curves for the therapeutic effect and lethal effect of a given compound. As the LD$_{50}$ curve shifts to the left, the TI value becomes smaller and, thus, the compound has a reduced margin of safety. (It is more toxic.) An even more critical technique with which to evaluate a compound for the potential to produce toxic-

TABLE 1.2. *Toxicity rating chart for chemicals in general*

Rating	Dose	Probable oral lethal dose for average 150-pound adult
Practically nontoxic	>15 g/kg	More than 1 quart
Slightly toxic	5–15 g/kg	Between 1 pint and 1 quart
Moderately toxic	0.5–5 g/kg	Between 1 ounce and 1 pint
Very toxic	50–500 mg/kg	Between 1 teaspoonful and 1 ounce
Extremely toxic	5–50 mg/kg	Between 7 drops and 1 teaspoonful
Super toxic	<5 mg/kg	A taste (<7 drops)

From ref. 3.

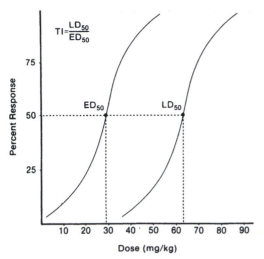

FIG. 1.2. Hypothetical dose-response curves illustrate the therapeutic effect (ED_{50}) and the lethal effect (LD_{50}) of a given chemical.

ity relative to its margin of safety is to calculate the ratio of the LD_1 to the ED_{99}.

Some compounds are considered relatively harmless because large quantities would need to be ingested to produce toxic or lethal action (Table 1.2). Table 1.3 shows that not all substances found around the home are toxic. These items have been reported to be involved in household poisonings, but these usually can be regarded as nontoxic ingestions. Unless unusually large quantities are ingested, no serious toxic effects should result. Knowing when emergency treatment is not needed is just as vital as knowing when it is required (5,19).

POISONING

Accidental and intentional poisonings constitute a major cause of morbidity and mortality in the United States. There is no way to determine accurately the exact incidence of poisoning, since not all poisonings are reported. Although it is reported that at least 5,000 to 10,000 Americans die from poisoning each year (28), it is quite possible that there is another group of victims, in number equal to or exceeding 5,000 to 10,000, who die each year from unreported poisonings. For exam-

ple, in an automobile fatality, the victim may have taken a medication, such as an antihistamine, which caused drowsiness while driving. The cause of death in this case would probably be reported as a vehicular accident rather than as a drug-induced incident. Or the victim may have been at work in a closed area where an internal combustion engine was running and have inhaled a large quantity of carbon monoxide. Shortly after leaving the area, the victim may have collapsed of an apparent "heart attack." If the blood was never analyzed for carbon monoxide, the death may have been reported as due to natural causes rather than acute carbon monoxide poisoning.

There is also another way to consider the data. It is very possible that a majority of reported "poisonings" should, more accurately, be classified as "ingestions" because the quantities ingested were much too low to cause toxic symptoms (25). The bottom line is that the actual number of true poisonings in the United States or in any other country is not known.

The American Association of Poison Control Centers began collecting data in 1983 and has continued to monitor the incidence, frequency, severity, and management of accidental and intentional poisonings reported by participating poison control centers. Some of these data will be presented, but the reader is advised to consult the September issues of the *American Journal of Emergency Medicine* for annual data.

Categories of Substances Frequently Involved with Poisoning

The leading incidences of poisoning exposures in children under six years of age are listed in Table 1.4. At the top of the list are cosmetics and personal care products. Some of the items in this category include perfume, cologne, aftershave fragrances, soaps, hair shampoos, deodorants, creams, lotions, and makeup.

The second category includes various cleaning substances, such as bleaches, ammo-

TABLE 1.3. *Partial listing of substances that are usually not toxic[a]*

Antacids	Lipstick
Antibiotics	Lubricant
Baby product cosmetics	Lubricating oils
Ballpoint pen inks	Magic Markers
Bath oil (castor oil and perfume)	Makeup (eye, liquid, facial)
Bathtub floating toys	Matches
Bleach (less than 5% sodium hypochlorite)	Mineral oil
Body conditioners	Motor oil
Bubble bath soaps	Newspaper
Calamine lotion (without phenol)	Paint (indoor or latex)
Candles (beeswax or paraffin)	Pencil (lead-graphite)
Caps (toy pistol) (potassium chlorate)	Perfumes
Chalk (calcium carbonate)	Petroleum jelly
Cigarettes or cigars (small amounts of	Phenolphthalein laxatives
nicotine)	Play-Doh
Clay (modeling)	Polaroid picture coating fluid
Contraceptives	Porous tip ink marking pens
Cosmetics	Putty (less than 2 ounces)
Crayons (marked A.P., C.P.)	Rouge
Dehumidifying packets (silica or charcoal)	Rubber cement[b]
Deodorants	Sachets (essential oils, powder)
Deodorizers (spray and refrigerator)	Shampoos (regular, not treated)
Detergents (phosphate type, anionic)	Shaving creams and lotions
Elmer's glue	Soap and soap products (hand soaps)
Etch-A-Sketch	Spacles
Fabric softeners	Spackling compound
Fertilizer (if no insecticides added)	Suntan preparations
Fish bowl additives	Sweetening agents (saccharin, aspartame)
Glues and pastes	Teething rings (water)
Golf ball (core may cause injury)	Thermometers (mercury)[c]
Greases	Thyroid tablets, 3 g
Hair products (dyes, sprays, tonics)	Toilet water
Hand lotions and creams	Toothpaste
Hydrogen peroxide (medicated, 3%)	Vitamins (without fluoride or iron)
Indelible markers	Water colors
Laxatives (small amounts)	Zinc oxide

From ref. 19.
[a] If large quantities of any of these substances are ingested, consult a poison control center.
[b] May cause acute poisoning if inhaled in a closed area.
[c] Broken glass may induce injury.

nia, household disinfectants and deodorizers, laundry detergents, fabric softeners, oven cleaners, toilet bowl cleaners, and automatic dishwasher detergents. As a group, household cleaning agents do not exhibit a high toxicity hazard, since many produce little more than minor gastrointestinal intolerance after ingestion. The exceptions to this, of course, include products containing strong acids and alkali.

The third highest ranking category of toxic exposures involves plants. This should not surprise anyone in view of the current popularity of cultivating indoor and outdoor varieties of plants. Furthermore, many plants bear attractive fruit or berries that appear enticing to inquisitive children. Few people who cultivate plants understand the potentially toxic effects that may occur after their ingestion. They fail to warn children of the danger and take no precautionary measures to avoid the poisoning. Approximately 30% of all reported toxic exposures are caused by substances contained in the first three categories.

On a more positive side, however, most plant ingestions do not cause serious toxicity, and only simple supportive and palliative measures are usually necessary. There are exceptions, of course, and some plants can be deadly if ingested. Plant poisoning is discussed in chapter 11).

TABLE 1.4. *Major poison exposures*[a]

Substance	Total pediatric exposures (1985–89)	Number of major effects	Number of deaths
Cosmetics and personal care	395,985	57	3
Cleaning substances	386,052	205	4
Plants	375,649	33	1
Analgesics	325,539	119	8
Cough/cold preparations	249,038	72	4
Topicals	175,378	55	2
Foreign bodies, toys	163,722	21	0
Vitamins	145,872	33	1
Hydrocarbons	129,024	168	5
Antimicrobials	122,686	28	3
Insecticides/pesticides	100,105	122	6
Gastrointestinal preparations	99,636	48	3
Chemicals	87,463	72	3
Arts/crafts/office supplies	80,494	3	0
Alcohols	80,443	46	5
Hormones	63,157	1	1

From ref. 14.

[a] Total reported exposures in children younger than six years from 1985 through 1989 was 3,852,618.

Pharmaceuticals comprise the majority of the remaining categories in Table 1.4. The highest incidence involves analgesics, such as acetaminophen, aspirin, and ibuprofen, which are followed by cough and cold preparations. In pediatric fatalities, the most frequently encountered ingested substances are iron supplements.

There has been a significant decline in the number of poisoning fatalities in children (12,18,25). This is largely due to child-resistant safety closures, product reformulation, parental awareness of poisoning potential, and intervention by poison centers and other health professionals. However, toxic drugs that cause poisoning are more often out of their usual storage location and in non-child-resistant prescription packaging or in no container (7).

Proper management of the poisoned patient can prevent serious damage and save lives. It is estimated that over three-fourths of all calls to poison control centers can be handled adequately over the telephone if sufficient, accurate information is given (16). Generally, all that is required is reassurance, not treatment (Fig. 1.3). It is, therefore, extremely important that health professionals understand basic principles of clinical toxicology and know how these principles apply to the poisoned patient.

Who Is Poisoned? Why Do Poisonings Occur?

Statistics indicate that the majority (approximately 70%) of poisonings occur in children under age 5 (19). A study of nearly 2,000 potentially toxic ingestions in children under 6 years of age revealed that 30.1% of the poisoned victims had experienced a prior poison exposure (Table 1.5) (13). Children older than 5 years constitute the next group (approximately 15%), and adults comprise the rest. Although the number of poisonings in children younger than 5 years is high, overall morbidity and mortality are remarkably low except for certain classes of poisons that are invariably fatal (16).

The reasons why children younger than 5 years constitute the largest poisoning group are many and varied. No study of basic principles of toxicology can be complete without indicating some of those causes.

A toddler's immediate environment includes areas around the home about which adults are generally not concerned. Adults

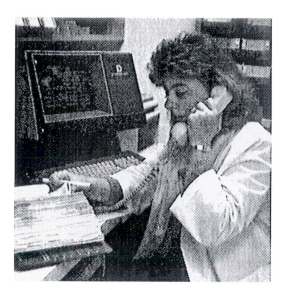

FIG. 1.3. A pharmacist answers a question from a concerned caller regarding a possible poisoning. (Photograph courtesy of Miami Valley Hospital, Dayton, OH.)

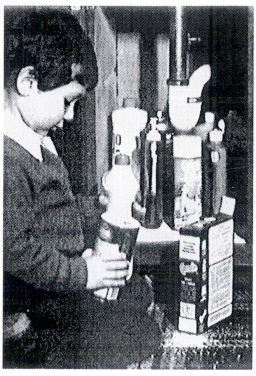

FIG. 1.4. A curious child and his environment.

take few precautions to keep these areas secure and free from poisons. The space under the kitchen sink, for example, is out of the immediate sight of most adults. To view this area thoroughly, an adult must stoop low, bend the knees, or actually kneel or sit on the floor. To a child, however, this area is in direct line of sight, affording an entirely new world to conquer (Fig. 1.4).

Another example is mothballs that may have fallen from a closet shelf onto a dark

corner on the closet floor. They are probably not seen by an adult but are quickly detected by an inquisitive toddler who believes that they are candy meant to be devoured.

Children are curious and investigative. A closed cabinet door or even a high shelf quickly becomes a major challenge to the child to see what is behind that door or on

TABLE 1.5. *Effect of age on repeater rates*

Patient age (years)	Number of repeaters (%)[a]	Number of first exposures (%)[a]	Number in total sample (%)[b]
<1	34 (12.0)	244 (86.2)	283 (14.6)
1	141 (23.9)	445 (75.4)	590 (30.4)
2	242 (37.0)	409 (62.5)	654 (33.7)
3	106 (44.2)	133 (55.4)	240 (12.4)
4	42 (34.7)	79 (65.3)	121 (6.2)
5	20 (43.5)	26 (56.5)	46 (2.4)
Unknown	0 (0.0)	1 (11.1)	9 (0.5)
Total	585 (30.1)	1,337 (68.8)	1,993 (100.0)

From ref. 13.
[a] Percentages shown are for each age.
[b] Includes 21 patients where repeater status is unknown.

that shelf. A youngster may quickly open the door or stack books or boxes to get to the shelf. There are numerous reports of youngsters building elaborate raised platforms to gain access to the top of the bathroom sink, which then allows fairly easy access to drugs in the medicine cabinet. In many instances, these climbing aids were constructed in a few minutes while the parent was out of sight. Remember: *Children act fast . . . so do poisons!*

Many household products are marketed in attractive packages or contain enchanting labels that are intended to catch the eye of potential purchasers. These labels that picture spring meadows layered with colorful flowers, dancing maidens or fairies, musical notes, or fresh citrus fruits may also catch the roving eye and challenge the inquisitiveness of a young child. The bright red berries on the evergreen shrubbery outside the house may appear to a child to be the same as the red berries in last night's dessert, and so into the mouth they go.

The natural tendency of children is to place anything and everything into their mouths. That the substance may bear no resemblance to food and perhaps does not even taste good is purely irrelevant to a youngster. A young child may be unable to distinguish between good and bad tastes. Every parent is aware that young children will often accept and consume foods at the dinner table without thinking about their taste or appearance, until an older (and wiser!) brother or sister "teaches" them that they are not supposed to like the taste of certain vegetables and other foods. Taste discrimination is a trait that is learned later. For example, a mothball, which an adult would immediately spit out, may remain in a child's mouth for a sufficient time to allow a significant amount of the chemical to be absorbed.

Parents foster poisonings because they take medication in the presence of their children. The old adage, "If I see it, I can do it," is especially meaningful in young children. In some instances, parents administer candy-flavored medications or multiple vitamins to

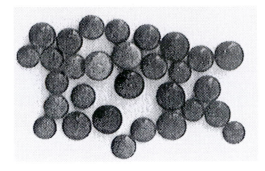

FIG. 1.5. Iron and vitamin tablets appear much the same as pieces of candy. Can you distinguish between them?

children. Because of the substance's desirable flavor, an unattended child may return to that same container for more "candy." Too often, prenatal vitamins and iron tablets resemble candy confection products (Fig. 1.5).

McCormick et al. (17) presented an interesting example that illustrated the extent of poisoning of infants during diaper changing. In 138 cases of poisoning during this procedure, 19% of the infants were directly handed the harmful material to keep them occupied. The authors also admitted that the actual number of parent-aided poisonings was probably even greater than reported. The case histories "Nonaccidental Poisoning in a Child" and "Overdose Partly as a Result of a 'Large' Teaspoon" at the end of this chapter describe how a grandparent caused poisoning in a 2-month-old child in one case and how an overly large teaspoon measure resulted in an overdose in the other.

Dosing errors due to the administration of liquid medication in inappropriate dosing cups or improper household spoons are quite common (11). During an 8-day surveillance period of 99 poison control centers, 34 cases of poisoning were reported by 16 of the centers. Twenty-nine of these incidences occurred during the surveillance period. Thirty of the 34 cases involved children 10 years of age or younger. Four were adults. All reports involved the ingestion of more than the recommended dose of medication; most subjects took two to three times the recommended

TABLE 1.6. *Reasons for dosing error*

Reason	%
Teaspoonful confused with tablespoonful	47
Assumed cup was unit of measure	18
Assumed recommended dose was one cupful	12
Unintentional pediatric ingestion	6
Miscellaneous/other/unknown	18

From ref. 12.

dose. Recurring reasons for the dosing errors are listed in Table 1.6.

A brief look around most homes should convince anyone that poisons are often left in easy view and, thus, are readily accessible to the unsuspecting. Count the number of unlabeled containers around a home that are filled with some poisonous liquid or solid substance. Also, observe where these items are stored. They are often found in unlocked cabinets, suitcases, or purses; on open shelves; in the bathroom; under the kitchen or bathroom sink; on the bedroom dresser; or in the garage or basement. Too often an item that is normally kept in a secured area will be removed from that site for use and then remain within easy reach of some toddler's investigative fingers. It may even remain there for many days, weeks, or months. Studies have shown that poisonings have occurred while the substance was in use or after recent use before return to its storage site (8,20).

Poisonings also occur because of the public's general lack of concern or apathetic denial that a potential problem always exists. For example, cleaning aids, paint strippers and thinners, gasoline, and other highly noxious products are used in unvented areas. People may work on an automobile, motorcycle, lawn mower, or other internal combustion engine while it is running in an unvented garage, allowing the accumulation of toxic concentrations of carbon monoxide.

New products are continually being introduced into the market. Frequently, the toxic potential of the products has not been evaluated completely. Seldom has the toxic potential been evaluated in persons of various ages, with certain disease states, or consuming alternate diets. Also, when newer products replace older ones, there may be significant differences in toxicity potential, especially if the new product is used incorrectly. Many products on the market exist in concentrated form. A product label may indicate that the product is "slightly alkaline" and, thus, would be expected to cause minimal skin irritation. But the alkalinity of the product may refer to the diluted substance and, when the concentrate comes into contact with the skin, it may produce severe burns.

Manufacturers often change product formulations. A toilet bowl cleaner that at one time may have been highly alkaline may now be an acidic product. The switch in ingredients could have been made subtly. An individual who is familiar with the older, alkaline product may not even consider that the new product may be completely different, especially if the name has not changed. Even though both products are corrosive, their compatibility with other cleaning agents would be different, possibly causing toxic exposure.

Another problem common in acute poisonings occurs because the complete name of the product may not be given to the health professional who is trying to assess the toxicity of the compound. The name given may not be descriptive of the constituents. Clorox, for example, is the name of a bleaching product that contains sodium hypochlorite, whereas Clorox-2 contains sodium carbonate. Drano granules consist of sodium hydroxide (54%), an alkali, and Drano liquid drain cleaner contains sodium hydroxide and 1,1,1-trichloroethane, a moderately toxic hydrocarbon. Thus, an important principle is always to make sure that the product name to which the victim refers is actually descriptive of the ingredients.

The correct diagnosis of a symptomatic patient may be overlooked because a health care provider failed to identify the contents of a product as the source of poisoning. The second case study at the end of this chapter, "The Missed Diagnosis," illustrates the unfamiliarity of some health care professionals with the names of ingredients of products and the fact that many of these ingredients may undergo metabolic conversion to toxic substances. In this case the physician was unaware that the paint thinner contained methylene chloride. Repeated exposures led to an increase in morbidity and subsequent death.

A disturbing cause of poisoning is that some product labels contain inaccurate or inappropriate treatment information. Previously, using a salt solution to induce vomiting was considered appropriate. It is now recognized that giving salt to a poisoned patient may be more toxic than the actual poisoning event per se, and its use has been the cause of some deaths (see chapter 3). Although labels on newly manufactured products no longer include such statements, containers that may have been purchased 10 or more years ago can still be found around the home. The parent who is instructed by one of these older labels to administer a salt solution may be subjecting a poisoned victim to even more serious intoxication.

Consider yet another example of erroneous information. In this instance, a toddler swallowed some lye. First aid information on the label instructed that, in case of ingestion, vinegar should be administered as an antidote. A vinegar solution was, therefore, given to the child, but serious problems resulted. The mild acid actually increased the toxic effects of the lye because of an explosive exothermic (heat release) reaction, causing severe gastrointestinal damage that could have been avoided (1). The extent of such inaccurate label information has been reduced in recent years.

Sources of inaccurate information go be-yond product labels. Johnson and Welch showed that even the scientific literature contains numerous ambiguities that can lead to inaccurate treatment of poisoning (9). Table 1.7 illustrates their point. It lists equivalence values for methyl salicylate (a liquid) to a number of aspirin tablets or a quantity of aspirin. The authors compared values listed in various literature sources to actual values. The extent of false values for the examples listed in Table 1.7 ranged from approximately 2% to 61% error. The values differ greatly and could result in mistakes in treating an ingestion of methyl salicylate. Thus, using only one reference source may not provide all the answers.

Where Do Poisonings Occur?

Poisonings may occur anywhere, including around the home, in the workplace or school, or while traveling, and by any route of exposure. Most accidental and suicidal poisonings occur through oral ingestion, whereas most industrial and agricultural toxic reactions follow pulmonary or dermal exposure (10).

At home, most poisonings happen in the kitchen, followed (in order of frequency) by the bathroom, bedroom, and garage. It is not uncommon for a mother to report that her youngster got into some household cleaning agent found under the kitchen sink or into a toilet cleaning aid or container of medicine from the medicine chest in the bathroom, or

TABLE 1.7. *Equivalence statements for salicylate from various reference sources*

Statement	Calculated equivalence	Potential for error
"One mL of 98% methyl salicylate is equivalent to 1.4 g of ASA[a] in salicylate potency." (1,400 mg)	1,370 mg	Insignificant
"One teaspoonful (5 mL) is equivalent to about 21 aspirin tablets (325 mg each)." (6,825 mg)	6,849 mg	Insignificant
"One teaspoonful is equivalent to 12 standard tablets of aspirin." (3,900 mg)	6,849 mg	Undertreat
"One-and-a-half teaspconful (8 mL) of oil of wintergreen will provide a quantity of salicylate equivalent to thirteen regular adult aspirin tablets." (4,225 mg)	10,957 mg	Undertreat

From ref. 9.
[a] ASA, acetylsalicylic acid.

into a bottle or cosmetic package on the nightstand in the bedroom. Likewise, numerous reports describe a person drinking a liquid from a soda bottle found in the garage. The liquid was apparently believed to be a palatable beverage but was actually gasoline, antifreeze, insecticide, or paint thinner.

In the field, herbicides and insecticides serve as repeated sources of poisoning through inhalation and skin contact. There are also many reports in the literature of persons being intoxicated because they drank water that was transported in containers previously filled with insecticides or herbicides. Occasionally, a farmer who is cleaning liquid manure tanks is exposed to toxic fumes of hydrogen sulfide, collapses, and dies after inhaling only a few breaths.

Another incidence of agriculture-related toxic exposure occurs during fertilization of the fields. In such incidences, application of liquid ammonia produces a cloud of ammonia gas which, if blown across the field onto an adjoining area where people are enjoying the evening on the patio, may cause coughing, severe respiratory distress, or even death.

At the workplace, literally thousands of chemicals may be accidentally ingested through contamination of food or water or absorbed through the skin. Situations have been documented in which factory workers have taken chemicals home, apparently thinking they were nontoxic. However, when these chemicals were used at home, they resulted in serious toxicity. In one instance, a family of three died when each of them ingested soup that had been seasoned with a lethal quantity of sodium nitrite. The sodium nitrite was thought to have been placed in the salt container by an unsuspecting worker who brought

---

TABLE 1.8. *Useful tips on reducing the incidence of poisoning*

Store all medications in their original containers and a locked cabinet, out of the reach of children. Replace them immediately after use. Use child-resistant containers. Periodically discard medications no longer used. Flush them down the toilet, rinse containers, and discard.

Discard household cleaning aids or other products that are no longer being used. Flush them down the toilet, rinse containers well, and discard.

Store toxic household and garden products in their original containers in cabinets fitted with safety latches or locks. When in use, always make sure an adult is present. Put the product away immediately after use.

Work with household chemicals in a well-ventilated area; do not mix chemicals (e.g., bleach and toilet bowl cleaner) unless specifically directed to do so.

Keep all items in their original containers. Never store toxic substances such as gasoline or insecticides in soda bottles or cups or in any other unmarked or unapproved container. Use child-resistant containers, and keep the caps securely shut between uses.

Never equate medicines with candy when administering drugs to children.

If you are interrupted while trying to administer a medicine, take it with you. Children could consume a medicine while you are out of the room.

Never take medicines in front of small children, or joke or make light of taking any medication to a child.

Never take medicines in the dark or if you are not fully awake. If you normally wear eyeglasses, put them on before taking the medication.

Keep poisonous plants away from children or others likely to ingest them. There is no reason, for example, to cultivate castor bushes, which produce deadly and enticing castor beans, around a household with small children.

Educate children about the dangers of poisons in the home. Teach them never to put anything into their mouths unless a parent or guardian has given it to them.

Use adhesive stickers showing Mr. Yuk or similar characters to help children identify dangerous substances.

In older houses, check for peeling paint or loose plaster, both of which can be significant sources of lead poisoning.

Never run fuel-consuming engines, kerosene heaters, and so forth in a poorly ventilated area.

Formulate and rehearse a plan of action in case a poisoning should occur. Right now, look up important phone numbers (doctor, pharmacist, emergency rescue squad, poison control center, etc.) and record these by the phone.

Make sure an up-to-date antidote chart is available. If in doubt about the validity of the one you have, bring it to a pharmacist or doctor to check.

Stock emergency antidotes (activated charcoal and syrup of ipecac), and know how to use them.

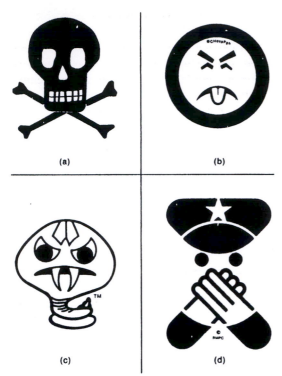

FIG. 1.6. Poison prevention symbols: **a,** traditional skull and crossbones; **b,** Mr. Yuk; **c,** SIOP; **d,** Officer Ugg.

these literature reports was from clothing stamped with laundry ink containing an aniline dye.

In the final analysis, it is easy to see that the potential for poisoning exists *everywhere*. And that is the answer to the question, "Where do poisonings occur?"

Will We Ever Stop Poisonings?

Earlier in this chapter the question, "When does toxicity end?" was proposed. The answer may well be that it never ends. The possibility for toxic reactions to chemicals will always exist. However, the incidence and consequences of toxic exposure can be reduced.

The frequency of toxic exposures may be reduced in many ways. It is impossible to re-

some home from his place of employment, apparently thinking it was table salt, sodium chloride.

Many more examples demonstrate where unexpected toxic exposures to a variety of chemicals may occur. Schoolchildren, through negligence or perhaps even by mischievous intent, may become careless with various chemicals they obtain from their chemistry laboratories, and their careless use of these ultimately may lead to some toxic episode. The fascination for metallic mercury has caused numerous toxicities, not through swallowing the mercury but by chronically inhaling its vapors after it is spilled on a living room carpet and dispersed into small globules with the vacuum cleaner. Another example is unexpected toxic exposure to aniline-containing products. Aniline dyes are easily absorbed through the skin and can cause methemoglobinemia. The route of exposure in

TABLE 1.9. *Examples of information about poisoning for the general public[a]*

Your Child and Household Safety; Chemical Specialties Manufacturers Association, Inc., 1913 Eye Street, N.W., Washington, DC 20006

Home Safe Home; The Soap and Detergent Association, 475 Park Avenue South at 32nd Street, New York, NY 10016

Preventing Accidental Poisonings; National Safety Council, 444 North Michigan Avenue, Chicago, IL 60611

Babysitter's Checklist; Council on Family Health, 225 Park Avenue South, Suite 1700, New York, NY 10003

Emergency First Aid for Children; Poison Prevention Week Council, PO Box 1543, Washington, DC 20013

Plants that Poison; Bronson Hospital Poison Prevention, 252 E. Lovell (Attn: Nancy), Kalamazoo, MI 49007

First Aid for Poisoning Chart; American Academy of Pediatrics, Publications Department, PO Box 927, Elk Grove Village, IL 60009

National Poison Prevention Week Packet; Secretary, Poison Prevention Week Council, PO Box 1543, Washington, DC 20013

"Locked up Poisons"; Secretary, Poison Prevention Week Council, PO Box 1543, Washington, DC 20013

A General Approach to the Emergency Management of Poisonings; ACEP Distribution Center, PO Box 619911, Dallas, TX 75261

[a] Generally, these are free of charge. Interested persons should contact the source for further information.

move all toxic substances from the home. However, there are three major considerations that may reduce this problem. First, the home should be made poison-proof. We can make the public aware of the kinds of substances and situations that lend themselves to a poisoning episode. All unused chemicals and medications should be discarded, and all potentially toxic substances should be placed out of the reach of children. Table 1.8 lists some useful ideas that may help reduce the risk of household poisonings. Feel free to pass these on to anyone willing to accept them.

Second, proper use of stickers that depict a deterring symbol, such as Mr. Yuk, increases public awareness of toxic substances. A variety of symbols have been developed to replace the typical "skull and crossbones" (Fig. 1.6). Many people have become calloused to the skull and crossbones because it has been used indiscriminately. Often, children associate the skull and crossbones with pirates and adventure and perhaps even with a popular breakfast cereal. Using Mr. Yuk is a learning process for parent and child. The parent must be aware of which items should receive the sticker to avoid indiscriminate use. The child must be taught that Mr. Yuk means "No! Stay away!"

The third phase concerns the question of what to do in case of a poisoning. Call a poison control center. It has been estimated that most incidents precipitating calls to poison control centers can be managed at home. There should be a bottle of ipecac in every home, especially those with young children.

If the general public is well aware of these three points, there will be a considerable decrease in the incidence and severity of household poisonings. National Poison Prevention Week is the third week of March each year. The motto for many years has been "Children act fast . . . So do poisons!" During this time of the year health professionals should make a special effort to increase public awareness of the potential for accidental poisoning around the home and of how to react to a poisoning situation. Table 1.9 lists the types of information that can be used to educate the general public about poisoning.

SUMMARY

An understanding of what is toxic, of who is poisoned, and of why, where, and how poisonings occur is essential to the study of clinical toxicology. This chapter forms the basis for the remainder of the textbook.

Case Studies

CASE STUDY: POISONING BY RAT POISON—A CLASSIC EXAMPLE

History

A 24-month-old girl was hospitalized after her mother discovered her vomiting. Nearby was an empty container of rat poison. The child had found the package in a low-lying cabinet and emptied its contents into her cereal, which she had then consumed. The rat poison was not packaged in a child-resistant container. The substance resembled cereal and smelled like peanuts, so the reason for the child's behavior was obvious.

The victim was treated with syrup of ipecac and a cathartic and was held for 2 days for observation, during which time she received a vitamin supplement as her only other medication. She was released at the end of the second day without further complications.

Manufacturing of the product had been discontinued approximately 2 years earlier because of its visual similarity to food; numerous poisonings with the product had been reported in previous years. No packages were recalled from retail shelves, and the item may still be found in some areas.

This classic example illustrates many of the principles discussed earlier in this chapter. The package of rat poison was found in a location generally inaccessible to adults but easily noticed by the child. The product itself looked and smelled good and was apparently not repulsive to the taste. It was not packaged to prevent access by a child and had no graphic poison identification on the label. Manufacture of the product had long been discontinued, although the product remained available for sale and, in this instance, was found in the home. Furthermore, although a poisoning occurred, the victim was not seriously harmed. (See ref. 23.)

Discussion

1. Outline the specific steps that could have been undertaken to prevent this poisoning. How should the child's parents guard against recurrence?
2. What kinds of questions should you ask parents if they call you for advice on poisoning in a child?

CASE STUDY: THE MISSED DIAGNOSIS

History

A retired man became ill after working 3 hr in his basement workshop. He had been using a commercial paint and varnish remover to strip a piece of furniture. The product contained methylene chloride. On admission to the hospital, he complained of chest pain and discomfort. He also brought the can of paint and varnish remover with him.

The attending physician found that the victim had experienced an anterior wall myocardial infarction. The physician noted the name of the ingredient in the stripping product; the label did indicate that the product should be used only in a well-ventilated area. However, the physician did not associate the victim's symptoms with the use of the product.

The patient returned home 2 weeks later and resumed his project. Shortly, he experienced severe chest pains and was readmitted. This time his diagnosis stated severe myocardial infarction complicated by cardiogenic shock.

Six months after recovery, the man again attempted to complete his task. He entered his workshop and, although he worked slowly and without unnecessary effort, soon collapsed and died.

This case illustrates that an uninformed health care provider failed to recognize the potential harm from a commercial product containing methylene chloride. The physician did not understand that methylene chloride is metabolized to carbon monoxide. The resulting carboxyhemoglobin placed considerable stress on the victim's cardiovascular system, with each subsequent exposure causing increased damage. It is unfortunate that the symptoms that necessitated admission to the hospital on both occasions were not associated with the paint and varnish remover. The victim could have been warned not to use these products again, especially in a closed environment. His life may have been spared. (See ref. 27.)

Discussion

1. Who was at fault for this tragedy—the product's manufacturer, the physician, or the patient? Or was it the seller of the product?
2. What steps can be taken to prevent such poisonings from recurring?

CASE STUDY: DISHWASHER EFFLUENT BURNS ON AN INFANT

History

A 6-month-old boy was being bathed in the kitchen sink while the dishwasher was running. He was sitting on a sponge ring that was occluded with a plunger-type drain cover. He started to cry loudly and suddenly and was quickly lifted from the sink. It was noted that dishwasher effluent was backing into the sink. The child was admitted to a hospital with deep burns on his perineum and thighs. Four weeks were required for the burns to heal.

The dishwasher drain entered the top of a garbage disposal unit that was mounted immediately below the sink's drain (Fig. 1.7). The child's parents noted, after the accident, that when the garbage disposal was not completely

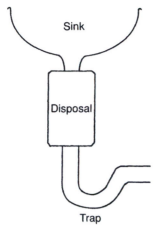

FIG. 1.7. Arrangement of disposal and trap in relation to kitchen sink. (From ref. 24.)

empty hot water from the dishwasher entered the sink during the drain cycle. (See ref. 24.)

Discussion

1. This case study illustrates that accidents (and poisonings) can happen when they are least expected. Contact with water at 160°F (71°C) for 1 sec will cause a full thickness burn in an adult. Is it probable that this infant's burns were caused solely by the hot water effluent from the dishwasher? At what temperatures do dishwasher units operate? What, if anything, did the dishwashing granules contribute to this child's distress? (Hint: see chapter 10.)
2. How could the plumbing shown in Fig. 1.7 be modified to prevent future mishaps?

CASE STUDY: NONACCIDENTAL POISONING IN A CHILD

History

The victim was the 2-month-old son of a 15-year-old, unwed mother who left him in the care of his maternal grandmother. The boy was well until he was 17 days old. The evening before admission to a hospital, he was irritable and cried intermittently. The next morning he was lethargic and had a swollen abdomen. He had not vomited, and stools were normal.

On presentation at the emergency department, the boy's pulse was 165 beats/min. His abdomen was distended with absent bowel sounds. The child was admitted to the intensive care unit and treated with ampicillin and gentamicin for 7 days. Symptoms declined over the next 2 days, and he was discharged back to his grandmother after 10 days.

At about 7 weeks of age, the grandmother brought the infant back to the hospital. The child had again been fussy and irritable the night before. On the morning of admission, the child was lethargic, limp, and unresponsive to stimuli. On arrival, the child's heart rate was slow (value not stated), and his respiration was labored. His blood pressure was not detectable.

The child was resuscitated, at which time his pulse rate increased to 173 beats/min. Pupils were dilated, mucous membranes dry, and abdomen distended. Urine and gastric aspirate were evaluated for chemical contents and revealed the presence of amitriptyline. The child continued to recover, and 2 days later was awake, alert, and active.

The grandmother denied giving amitriptyline to the child. Finally, however, she did admit to having some "pills" around which she occasionally took for her "nerves." The medication was identified as amitriptyline, and the prescription had been filled just 2 days before the first episode.

It was unclear why the grandmother gave this medication to the child. Amitriptyline tablets are small, and she may have believed the tablets were "too small to be harmful." Regardless, she was the direct cause of poisoning. (See ref. 9.)

Discussion

1. Based upon your knowledge of pharmacology, what type of drug is amitriptyline?
2. Were all symptoms displayed by this child

consistent with those that are classically reported for the drug?

3. Why do you suppose antibiotics were given to this child on the first hospital admission?

CASE STUDY: OVERDOSE PARTLY AS A RESULT OF A "LARGE" TEASPOON

History

For itching, a pediatrician prescribed tripelennamine citrate 37.5 mg [25 mg of the hydrochloride (HCl) salt] to be taken every 4 hr by a 5-year-old girl with chicken pox. After the third dose the child began to hallucinate, stating that she saw "elves running around the house and insects flying at her."

She was taken to an emergency facility. Examination was unremarkable except for mildly dilated pupils. The mother was instructed to discontinue the medication. The child returned 4 days later with continuing symptoms. A toxicology screen for drugs was negative. Laboratory values were normal. A neurologist and a psychiatrist concluded that she was neurologically and psychologically sound. After 3 days of hospitalization, hallucinations disappeared.

An investigation later revealed the cause of this child's symptoms. The teaspoon that was used to administer the medication held 7 mL. It was calculated that the mother had administered three doses of 6.33 mL instead of 5 mL each, as intended. The child's physician had actually prescribed 1.5 times the recommended dose for this child. This error was compounded by the fact that the teaspoon was extra large. Overall, the child received approximately twice the recommended dose for a period of 12 hr. (See ref. 4.)

Discussion

1. This overdose was modest but sizable enough for this child to develop symptoms of toxicity. What specific measures should

health care providers take to reduce the incidence of errors such as this?

2. How is tripelennamine citrate classed pharmacologically?

Review Questions

1. When the LD_{50} curve shifts to the left, how does this affect the therapeutic index (TI) for a drug?
   A. The TI increases.
   B. The TI decreases.
   C. Only the toxic dose increases.
   D. Both the toxic and the therapeutic doses increase.

2. The majority of all poisonings occur in which of the following age groups?
   A. Under the age of 5 years
   B. 5 to 11 years
   C. 12 to 20 years
   D. 20 years and older

3. Which of the following toxicology subdisciplines is most closely associated with the medicolegal aspects of the toxic activity of chemicals on humans?
   A. Occupational toxicology
   B. Environmental toxicology
   C. Forensic toxicology
   D. Veterinary toxicology

4. In children under 5 years of age, which of the following is the leading cause of all reported poisonings in the United States?
   A. Plants
   B. Soaps, cleaners
   C. Cosmetics and personal care items
   D. Aspirin

5. Most household poisonings occur at which of the following sites?
   A. Kitchen
   B. Bedroom
   C. Bathroom
   D. Garage

6. National Poison Prevention Week is celebrated each year during the third week of:
   A. January
   B. March
   C. June
   D. September

7. Cite ten important steps that may be taken to reduce the incidence of poisoning around the home.

8. Why is it important for consumers to know where most household poisonings occur?

9. Define the meaning of the term *poison*. What is meant by the statement that "all chemicals must be assumed to be toxic?"

10. What is an LD_{50} value? How does it relate to human toxicity?

11. Explain why the young boy depicted in Fig. 1.4 is especially vulnerable to accidental poisoning.

References

1. Anonymous. Home-poison menace: inaccurate first-aid labels. *Med World News* 1977;(Mar 21).
2. Casarett LJ, Bruce MC. Origin and scope of toxicology. In: Klaassen CD, Amdur MO, Doull J, eds. *Toxicology—the basic science of poisons.* 3rd ed. New York: Macmillan; 1986:3–10.
3. Gosselin RE, Smith RP, Hodge HC. *Clinical toxicology of commercial products.* 5th ed. Baltimore: Williams and Wilkins; 1984.
4. Hays DP, Johnson BF, Perry R. Prolonged hallucinations following a modest overdose of tripelennamine. *Clin Toxicol* 1980;16:331–333.
5. Henry J, Wiseman H. Non-poisons. *Br Med J* 1984;289:240–241.
6. Holmstedt B, Liljestrand G, eds. *Readings in pharmacology.* New York: Raven Press; 1981.
7. Jacobson BL, Rock AR, Cohn MS, Litovitz T. Accidental ingestions of oral prescription drugs: a multicenter survey. *Am J Public Health* 1989;79:853–856.
8. Jensen GD, Wilson WW. Preventive implications of a study of 100 poisonings in children. *Pediatrics* 1960;25:490–495.
9. Johnson PN, Welch DW. Methyl salicylate/aspirin equivalence: who do you trust? *Vet Hum Toxicol* 1984;26:317–318.
10. Klaassen CD, Doull J. Evaluation of safety: toxicologic evaluation. In: Doull J, Klaassen CD, Amdur MO, eds. *Toxicology—the basic science of poisons.* 2nd ed. New York: Macmillan; 1980:11–27.
11. Krenzelok EP, Dunmire SM. Acute poisoning emergencies: resolving the gastric decontamination controversy. *Postgrad Med* 1992;91:179–186.
12. Litovitz T. Implication of dispensing cups in dosing errors and pediatric poisonings: a report from the American Association of Poison Control Centers. *Anal Pharmacother* 1992;26:917–918.
13. Litovitz TL, Flagler SL, Manoguerra AS, Veltri JC, Wright L. Recurrent poisonings among paediatric poisoning victims. *Med Toxicol Adverse Drug Exp* 1989;4:381–386.
14. Litovitz T, Manoguerra A. Comparison of pediatric poisoning hazards: an analysis of 3.8 million exposure incidents. *Pediatrics* 1992;89:999–1006.
15. Loomis TA. *Essentials of toxicology.* 3rd ed. Philadelphia: Lea and Febiger; 1978.
16. Lovejoy FH, Berenberg W. Poisoning in children under age 5. *Postgrad Med* 1978;63:79–89.
17. McCormick MA, Lacouture PG, Gandreault P, Lovejoy FH. Hazards associated with diaper changing. *JAMA* 1982;248:2159–2160.
18. McIntire MS, Angle CR. Trends in childhood poisonings: a collaborative study 1970, 1975, 1980. *Clin Toxicol* 1984;21:321–331.
19. Mofenson HC, Greensher J, Caraccio TR. Ingestions considered nontoxic. *Clin Lab Med* 1984;4:587–602.
20. O'Connor PJ. Epidemiology of accidental poisoning in children. *Med J Aust* 1983;2:181–183.
21. Orfila MJB. *Traite des poisons tires mineral, vegetal et animal on toxicologie generale sous le rapports de la pathologie et de la medicine legale.* Paris: Crochard; 1815.
22. Rendell M, McGrane D, Cuesta M. Fatal compulsive water drinking. *JAMA* 1978;240:2557–2559.
23. Schum TR, Lachman BS. Effect of packaging and appearance on childhood poisoning. *Clin Pediatr* 1982;21:282–285.
24. Sheridan RL, Sheridan MG, Tompkins RG. Dishwasher effluent burns in infants. *Pediatrics* 1993;91:142–143.
25. Sibert JR, Routledge PA. Accidental poisoning in children: can we admit fewer children with safety? *Arch Dis Child* 1991;66:263–266.
26. Sonnedecker G. *History of pharmacy.* Philadelphia: JB Lippincott; 1963.
27. Steward RD, Hake CL. Paint-remover hazard. *JAMA* 1976;235:398–401.
28. Veltri JC, McElwee NE, Schumacher MC. Interpretation and uses of data collected in poison control centers in the United States. *Med Toxicol* 1987;2:389–397.
29. Zien GE, Castleman BI. Threshold limit values: historical perspectives and current practice. *J Occup Med* 1989;31:910–918.

2 ‖ Factors That Influence Toxicity

SIGNIFICANCE OF UNDERSTANDING THE FACTORS

The presentations of poisoning episodes do not always follow traditional "textbook" descriptions commonly listed for them. Signs and symptoms that are often said to be pathognomonic (characteristic) for a particular toxic episode may or may not be evident with each case of poisoning. Victims may even display behavior totally unexpected and largely unpredictable. An experimentally determined acute oral toxicity expression, such as an LD_{50} value, is not an absolute description of the compound's toxicity in every individual. It neither assesses the inherent capacity of the compound to produce injury nor reflects the victim's ability to respond in a manner other than predicted.

An important principle in evaluating a victim's response to a toxic agent is that numerous factors may modify the reaction to a particular toxic agent. Frequently, health care professionals are faced with a difficult and confusing dilemma. There may be strong suspicion that a patient has been subjected to a toxic exposure of a particular substance; the decision may be to wait until the onset of certain symptoms before treatment is initiated. Meanwhile, the victim is not presenting in the expected manner.

The factors that influence toxicity are essentially the same as those that determine many of the pharmacologic actions of a drug. These factors will be reviewed to emphasize their importance in altering a toxic response.

COMPOSITION OF THE TOXIC AGENT

When examining a toxic episode, a basic fallacy is to view the responsible poison as a "pure" substance. This implies that there are no contaminants present—that the vehicle, various adjuvants and excipients, and formulation ingredients are innocuous (17,18); the victim has not taken any drugs previously; and there is no batch-to-batch variation in the substance or product. These criteria are rarely observed in the "real world" of poisoning. The possibility that the toxic exposure may be the result of more than one toxic agent is important (12). An excellent example is the toxic exposures that have resulted from the presence of the toxic impurity, dioxin, in the herbicide 2,4,5-trichlorophenoxyacetic acid (2,4,5-T) (see chapter 8).

The physicochemical composition of the toxic agent can sometimes be helpful in predicting the risk involved in exposure to a particular compound. In general, solids are less easily swallowed than are liquids, and bulky, high-density solids are more difficult to consume than are light, more fluffy compounds, especially for a small child. Thus, poisoning from the ingestion of bulky solids is less likely than is poisoning from liquids and small particles. These solid dosage forms can lodge in the oral cavity to cause local effects, however. An example that will be discussed in chapter 10 concerns the toxic action of sodium hydroxide pellets upon the oral mucosa. These pellets are not easily swallowed, and they stick to the moist mucosal tissue, whereas a solution of sodium hydroxide is easily swallowed.

The particulate size of the toxic agent is especially important in exposure by inhalation. Only particles with a small diameter (1 μm or less) will effectively reach the alveoli and be available for pulmonary absorption. Larger particles may be deposited on the walls of the throat and trachea to produce irritation or local injury to those tissues.

The pH of the compound is another factor to consider. If the chemical is a strongly corrosive acid or alkali, obvious deleterious effects will occur with limited exposure of any tissue to the compound. On the other hand, the ingestion of mildly acidic or alkaline substances may cause little more than localized irritation.

Another factor that can modify the toxicity of an agent is its chemical stability. Are breakdown products formed during storage? Will the compound remain active in a definite concentration? When added to water, does the chemical composition change? These are important questions that need to be answered when establishing a compound's toxicity potential.

Sometimes a compound that was pure when packaged may have undergone a chemical change to produce an entirely different species capable of causing symptoms of toxicity that are unrelated to those expected from the original chemical. Paraldehyde, a liquid hypnotic, is an example. Overdoses of paraldehyde are characterized by central nervous system (CNS) depression. If paraldehyde is exposed to light and air, it may partially decompose to acetaldehyde. When pure acetaldehyde is ingested, nausea, severe reddening of the skin, coughing, and pulmonary edema are characteristically noted. A patient who ingested a large quantity of impure paraldehyde solution theoretically could be described as having symptoms more characteristic of acetaldehyde poisoning.

To emphasize the importance of knowing the composition of the product, assume that a caller explains that a victim has swallowed a particular substance identified on the label as an insecticide. The victim's parent reads the name of the insecticide from the label and describes the victim's behavior. You realize that the observed symptoms do not match those expected for the particular insecticide. What is wrong? Did the bottle contain a different substance than the label stated? Was an insignificant amount ingested so that the onset of the expected symptoms may be delayed or may not even occur?

In the above case the victim experienced nausea, coughing, gagging, and mild CNS depression. The product involved was a pediculicide intended to kill head and pubic lice. The active ingredient was pyrethrum, which alone does not produce significant toxicity to humans. In this case, symptoms were characteristic of the solvent, a petroleum distillate, that is used in the formulation of the product, rather than of pyrethrum. If emergency personnel had thought that the victim's symptoms would quickly dissipate because of the relatively nontoxic nature of pyrethrum and had not assessed the victim for "solvent" toxicity, a disastrous outcome may have resulted.

Each poisoning occurrence must be assessed individually by carefully examining all facts, rather than simply making an assumption or casually looking at laboratory data and then proceeding with treatment. And, remember, the accuracy of toxicologic testing varies greatly by drug class and analytical methods used (36).

The first rule in the identification of a potentially toxic substance is to examine the label carefully. Determine which substances in the product are potentially toxic and which are probably not toxic. Then proceed accordingly.

DOSE AND CONCENTRATION

One of the major factors influencing the potential toxicity of a chemical is the dose administered or the exposure concentration. Nearly anything can be toxic at a given dose and route of administration. Conversely, even the most toxic substances may not be harmful at extremely low concentrations. The intravenous LD_{50} of distilled water in the mouse is 44 mL/kg and that of isotonic saline is 68 mL/kg (1). Neither distilled water nor isotonic saline is considered toxic; at a high enough volume or dose, however, toxicity becomes evident (30).

Doses are normally calculated according to body weight, and larger doses usually imply a greater chance for a toxic response. When a child accidentally ingests adult aspirin tablets (325 mg), as opposed to children's aspirin tablets (81 mg), there is greater risk for toxicity. It will obviously take fewer adult aspirin to produce significant toxicity in a child (see chapter 12).

Ingestion of a dilute solution of a potentially toxic compound generally results in greater chance for toxicity to occur than if the same quantity of a concentrated solution was ingested. Diluted forms are more quickly absorbed and available for distribution to susceptible tissues.

ROUTES OF ADMINISTRATION

The manner in which a potentially toxic substance enters the body can influence time of onset, intensity, and duration of toxic effects. The route of administration may also predict the degree of toxicity and possibly the target systems that will most readily be affected. A toxic chemical injected by the intravenous route would be expected to result in the most rapid onset of toxicity and the greatest potential for multiple organ exposure. When administered by other routes, the approximate descending order of toxicity is inhalation > intraperitoneal > subcutaneous > intramuscular > intradermal > oral > topical (24).

Oral

Eighty percent of acute toxic episodes result from accidental or intentional ingestion of a toxic agent (25). The basic parameters governing drug absorption also apply to toxic substances. There is potential for a compound to be absorbed throughout the entire gastrointestinal (GI) tract, including the buccal cavity and rectum. Absorption is dependent largely on lipid solubility and the amount of nonionized form available. Gastric absorption of most toxic substances is usually limited, but intestinal absorption is extensive because of its large surface area.

Several important factors may significantly modify absorption of solid drug dosage forms and chemicals after ingestion. Dissolution of a solid is a major consideration in absorption of the drug or chemical. This is not a major concern with liquids, but for solid dosage forms absorption is dependent on dissolution rate. This also raises a concern for the treatment of a poisoned patient. Many treatment protocols suggest that ingested poisons should first be diluted. There may be instances where dilution could produce adverse effects by increasing the rate of absorption and/or by producing heat. This will be discussed further in chapters 3 and 10.

Another problem experienced with the ingestion of large quantities of solid dosage forms is the formation of concretions (bezoars, gastric pharmacobezoars) in the stomach (6,20,23). These clumps of unabsorbed drug may be difficult to remove by emesis or lavage. Lavage until the return solution is "clear" can give a false sense of security. It may be assumed that all of the stomach contents were removed (including the solid dosage form) but, in fact, particles too large to fit through the opening of the lavage tube may still be present. This mass of tablets or capsules may now act like a repository of drugs or a sustained-release dosage form. Case studies at the end of this chapter illustrate this point.

The type of food previously ingested may modify the rate of absorption of the toxic agent. A meal rich in protein or fat usually delays absorption. Carbonated beverages increase the rate of intestinal absorption by shortening gastric emptying time because of the liberation of carbon dioxide in the stomach. Ingestion of a concentrated chemical frequently causes decreased absorption because of gastric irritation and constriction of the pyloric sphincter. On the other hand, if the substance is an irritant or corrosive, exposure to a diluted solution may cause less toxicity (1).

On a positive side, the oral route of intoxication may give the body a chance to metabolize and detoxify the ingested toxic agent. The portal circulation transports all chemical substances absorbed from the GI tract directly to the liver, the major organ of detoxification. This is especially beneficial for toxic compounds that undergo a significant first-pass effect. At the same time, as will be explained shortly, some compounds are activated by the liver to a more toxic form (24).

Inhalation

The lung is a large target organ that constantly undergoes multiple insults from air pollutants, dusts, fibers, and other irritants. Serious toxic effects may follow from pulmonary absorption of vapors and aerosols. The pulmonary route can greatly accentuate the expected onset of toxicity for a given compound because the lung has a rich blood supply, is in close proximity (10 μm) to alveolar air, and has a large surface area (50 to 100 m^2). Toxic agents that are absorbed by the lung fall into two categories: vapors and aerosols.

Vapors of toxicologic significance consist of gases, such as carbon monoxide, hydrogen sulfide, sulfur oxides, and nitrogen oxides. Vapor fumes from volatile liquids include chloroform, benzene, and carbon tetrachloride, and fumes from solids include mercury vapor, among others. Transport of vapors across the alveolar membrane occurs by simple diffusion. Blood concentrations of the toxic chemical will depend on its solubility, since blood equilibrates with alveolar gases almost instantaneously. In the case of hydrogen sulfide, which is very soluble, inhalation of vapors of high concentrations of the gas may be all that is necessary to cause death.

Since aerosols are suspensions of particulate matter, the chief limiting factor in determining pulmonary absorption is the size of the particle. As stated earlier, only particles with a mean aerodynamic diameter of 1 μm or less will be transported into the alveolar region to be available for absorption into the blood. Pulmonary absorption of soluble particles can occur by either the lipid-soluble diffusion or the water-soluble filtration process.

Dermal

Percutaneous absorption involves the transport of a compound through various layers of skin into the systemic circulation. Entry of a toxic agent through sebaceous or sweat glands or hair follicles is possible but relatively uncommon. Skin is the organ most readily accessible to all forms of toxic substances. It is also an efficient barrier to most environmental toxicants. Penetration by a chemical is time dependent and a function of its lipid solubility and concentration gradient.

Most toxic skin exposures occur accidentally. The degree of toxicity is influenced by the compound involved, length of exposure, and condition of the skin. Cuts or abrasions

on the skin's surface allow the toxic agent to bypass the first layers of defense, keratin and epidermis, and permit substances that would generally not penetrate the epidermis to pass easily into the deeper strata and into the circulation.

Industrial accidents often involve dermal exposure due to the handling of extremely toxic solvents. If a worker is heavily clothed and comes in contact with a chemical, the clothing may keep the toxic chemical localized to an area and extend contact time with the skin. The type of chemical is also an important factor; for example, corrosive acids and alkali will alter skin permeability by their destruction of the stratum corneum (see chapter 10).

METABOLISM OF THE TOXIC AGENT

Metabolism of a toxic compound is usually the primary mechanism of detoxification. The metabolite produced is generally a more polar compound that can be readily excreted by the kidney. Unfortunately, this is not always the

TABLE 2.1. *Representative examples of chemicals that are metabolized to more toxic substances*

Acetaminophen
Acetanilid
Aniline
Arsenicals, pentavalent
Benzene
Carbon tetrachloride
Chloral hydrate
Chloroform
Codeine
Cyclophosphamide
Dimethylnitrosamide
Ethylene glycol
Heptachlor
Imipramine
Isopropanol
Methanol
2-Naphthylamine
Parathion
Pyridine
Schradan
Sulfanilamide
Tri-*o*-cresyl phosphate

situation. Some chemicals are metabolized to compounds that are equally as active or sometimes even more active. Methanol is an example of such a chemical; it must first be oxidized to its intermediate metabolites, formaldehyde and formic acid, before it produces its most toxic effects (see chapter 4). A partial list of chemicals known to be converted to more toxic compounds is presented in Table 2.1.

STATE OF HEALTH

Most descriptions of poisoning and its management are based on how healthy individuals are affected. However, healthy persons are not the only ones poisoned. The presence of hepatic or renal disease may significantly affect the pharmacokinetics and outcome of exposure to a particular toxicant (4). Acidosis, from any cause, potentiates the action of tubocurarine and decreases the activity of insulin. Hypertensive patients may respond more intensely to chemicals that have sympathomimetic activity. Opioids and other respiratory depressants have greater toxicity potential in patients with head injuries. Psychotomimetics may provoke the recurrence of mental diseases in patients with histories of psychiatric disease. Disease states that cause diarrhea or constipation may decrease or increase the time of contact between chemical and absorptive sites and, thus, reduce or enhance absorption. Stress-mediated changes in hormone concentrations (e.g., hyperthyroidism) may alter the toxic effects of certain chemicals (9).

AGE AND MATURITY

The patient's age must be considered as the extent of toxicity is assessed (13). Most anticipated toxic effects and reported prognoses are based on individuals who are neither too young nor too old. Unfortunately, not all victims of poisoning fall within this age group. The majority of accidental poisonings in fact occur in persons less than 5 years of age, and

toxicity among the geriatric population is increasing.

Age as a major influence in determining extent of toxicity may be illustrated by considering the classic chloramphenicol-induced gray baby syndrome. In the early 1960s, it was a popular practice to administer chloramphenicol prophylactically to premature infants. It became apparent after several years that a number of infants receiving this antibiotic were showing signs of intoxication. Within days of treatment initiation, signs and symptoms of aplastic anemia—the "gray baby" appearance, surfaced (11,22). Chloramphenicol is normally metabolized and excreted largely as a glucuronide conjugate. There had been no reports of aplastic anemia from chloramphenicol in adults. It was discovered later that infants were unable to metabolize chloramphenicol because their hepatic microsomal enzyme system was not fully developed. Consequently, toxic concentrations of chloramphenicol were reached after only a few doses. Once an infant developed an adequate liver microsomal enzyme system, chloramphenicol could be metabolized normally and the incidence of aplastic anemia decreased proportionately. In geriatric patients the toxic effects of drugs and chemicals may be complicated by decreased hepatic and renal function. These factors may alter the metabolism or excretion of toxic agents.

NUTRITIONAL STATE AND DIETARY FACTORS

Certain nutritional factors, such as food or liquid contents of the stomach (e.g., acidic or alkaline, hot or cold, high fat or lean, high or low volume, and viscosity), are important to the absorption characteristics of many chemicals. In general, higher blood concentrations are achieved when drugs are taken on an empty as opposed to a full stomach (3). Certain foods may significantly increase or decrease drug absorption. For example, calcium may bind to tetracycline and reduce its absorption (31). Fatty foods, on the other hand, enhance griseofulvin absorption (32).

TABLE 2.2. *Tyramine content of various foods*

Food/beverage	Tyramine content (μg/g)
Cheese	
Cheddar	120–1,500
Camembert	20–2,000
Emmenthaler	225–1,000
Stilton	466–2,160
Processed	25–30
Brie	0–200
Gruyere	516
Gouda	20
Brick, natural	524
Mozzarella	410
Roquefort	27–520
Parmesan	4–290
Romano	238
Provolone	38
Cottage	5
Fish	
Salted, dried	0–470
Pickled herring	3,000
Meat	
Meat extracts	95–304
Beef liver (stored)	274
Chicken liver	1,000
Vegetable	
Avocado	23
Fruit	
Banana	7
Alcoholic beverage	
Beer and ale	2–12
Wine	
Chianti	25.4
Sherry	3.6

Some foods may antagonize drug effects. Foods rich in pyridoxine can significantly attenuate the pharmacologic action of levodopa (8).

Nutritional effects on absorption are not limited to drugs. Heavy metal absorption, to illustrate, is influenced by diet. Calcium, iron, fat, and protein are all reported to enhance lead absorption (2). Deficiency of calcium, iron, or protein, on the other hand, enhances cadmium absorption.

Some foods can actually increase the toxicity of certain drugs by means other than influencing their absorption. An excellent example are those foods that are rich in the pressor amine, tyramine (Table 2.2). If one of these foods in ingested while an individual is taking a monoamine oxidase-inhibiting drug (for ex-

ample, pargyline, phenelzine), severe symptoms of hypertensive crisis and even death may occur. Tyramine-containing foods are ordinarily metabolized to a nontoxic substance by monoamine oxidase, which is located within the cells lining the GI tract. Therefore, only a small amount of tyramine is absorbed. When monoamine oxidase is inhibited, tyramine is not metabolized but absorbed into the blood, where it causes toxic pressor activity.

Individuals on starvation diets or those with low protein intake may have lower-than-normal plasma levels of albumin (35). This may leave a proportionately greater amount of highly protein-bound drug in its free form. Since it is the free form of a drug (versus that which is protein bound) which causes toxicity, the drug will produce a greater degree of toxicity. Also, a low dietary protein intake may result in a decreased level of hepatic microsomal enzymes, resulting in decreased drug metabolism.

GENETICS

The term *pharmacogenetics* (or *toxicogenetics*) has entered the toxicologist's vocabulary in recent years (19). While sometimes used interchangeably with the term *idiosyncrasy*, pharmacogenetics describes the differences in an individual's response to drugs and chemicals that are related to hereditary influences (29).

It is commonly recognized that, if a population of men is sampled and their body weight

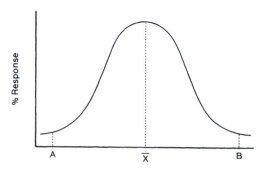

FIG. 2.1. A normal distribution curve.

measured, the results would distribute graphically as shown in Fig. 2.1. The majority of men would weigh close to the arithmetic mean of the group. A few would weigh much less (area A in Fig. 2.1), whereas others would weigh much more (area B in Fig. 2.1). The graph would assume the shape of a normal distribution curve, which is also characteristic of numerous other factors that can be measured within a population (e.g., height, blood pressure, intelligence). Each of these values is determined by a multiplicity of variables which are largely inherited. However, occasionally a bimodal (Fig. 2.2) or even trimodal curve results when some responses are measured, and an entirely different variable then becomes important.

To illustrate the importance of pharmacogenetics as it relates to drug toxicity, consider the polymorphic expression of several enzymes that are linked to the metabolism of several compounds. Succinylcholine is a skeletal muscle relaxant that is often administered by infusion during the induction of general anesthesia. All skeletal muscle activity, including that of respiration, is depressed. Ordinarily the metabolism of succinylcholine proceeds as shown in Fig. 2.3. Most people quickly inactivate the drug by hydrolysis via plasma pseudocholinesterase to its first inactive metabolite, succinylmonocholine. The initial step proceeds rapidly and activity is lost within minutes. Once intravenous infusion is discontinued, skeletal muscle tone begins to increase and the patient's normal respiration is restored. Metabolism is later completed by

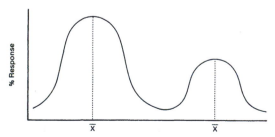

FIG. 2.2. A bimodal distribution curve showing two population groups.

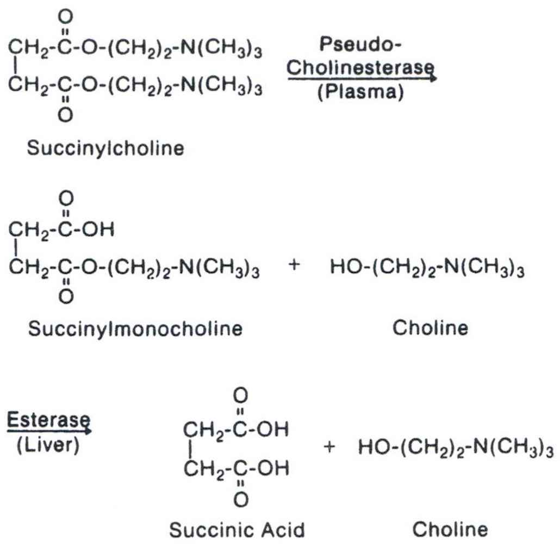

$$CH_2\text{-}\overset{O}{\overset{\|}{C}}\text{-O-}(CH_2)_2\text{-N}(CH_3)_3$$
$$CH_2\text{-}\underset{O}{\overset{\|}{C}}\text{-O-}(CH_2)_2\text{-N}(CH_3)_3 \quad \xrightarrow{\text{Pseudo-}\atop\text{Cholinesterase}\atop\text{(Plasma)}}$$

Succinylcholine

$$CH_2\text{-}\overset{O}{\overset{\|}{C}}\text{-OH}$$
$$CH_2\text{-}\underset{O}{\overset{\|}{C}}\text{-O-}(CH_2)_2\text{-N}(CH_3)_3 \quad + \quad HO\text{-}(CH_2)_2\text{-N}(CH_3)_3$$

Succinylmonocholine   Choline

$$\xrightarrow[\text{(Liver)}]{\text{Esterase}} \quad \begin{array}{l} CH_2\text{-}\overset{O}{\overset{\|}{C}}\text{-OH} \\ CH_2\text{-}\underset{O}{\overset{\|}{C}}\text{-OH} \end{array} \quad + \quad HO\text{-}(CH_2)_2\text{-N}(CH_3)_3$$

Succinic Acid   Choline

FIG. 2.3. Biochemical transformation of succinylcholine.

liver enzymes, resulting in succinic acid and choline.

The toxicologic problem arises because there is a segment of the population which exhibits unusual susceptibility to the effects of succinylcholine (5,16). The presence of an atypical pseudocholinesterase predisposes them to a prolonged and life-threatening paralysis of respiratory muscles because the initial detoxifying step in succinylcholine metabolism is hampered. Metabolism of succinylcholine in these individuals is slower, resulting in prolonged apnea and skeletal muscle relaxation that may last for several hours, even after discontinuation of infusion. Figure 2.4 illustrates the rate of hydrolysis of succinylcholine by normal and atypical plasma pseudocholinesterase. It can readily be seen that the atypical enzyme hydrolyzes succinylcholine very slowly. A review of the literature suggests that succinylcholine is 4 to 7 times as potent in persons with genetically determined low plasma pseudocholinesterase compared with normal individuals (34). The incidence of this toxicogenetic problem is about one person in 2,800 (5).

Naphthalene (a component in some mothballs) is another compound that can be more toxic in certain people depending on their genetic background. Naphthalene exposures oc-

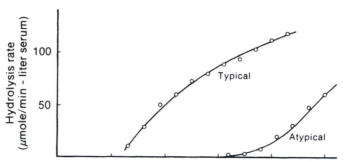

FIG. 2.4. Rate of hydrolysis of succinylcholine in the presence and absence of the normal enzyme. (From ref. 24.)

cur more frequently during the spring and fall when winter clothing is packed and unpacked. Mothballs containing naphthalene are occasionally placed around young plants in gardens and lawns to repel pets and other animals.

para-Dichlorobenzene, another moth repellent that is much less toxic, is now more commonly used to repel moths than naphthalene. It is also used as a toilet bowl and diaper pail deodorizer.

At special risk of toxicity to naphthalene are individuals with erythrocytic glucose 6-phosphate dehydrogenase (G6PD) deficiency (14). About 200 million people are estimated to be deficient in this enzyme (7). Glucose 6-phosphate dehydrogenase is involved in regulation of the pentose phosphate pathway (hexose monophosphate shunt), which is especially important in energy production for red blood cells (RBCs). This pathway is required for erythrocytes to maintain viability. Older erythrocytes obtain their energy via glucose metabolism, since they are unable to synthesize proteins. Glucose metabolism via the pentose phosphate pathway, using G6PD, generates reduced nicotinamide adenine dinucleotide phosphate (NADPH). Formation of NADPH offers protection to RBCs by providing for reduction of methemoglobin (Fe^{+3}) and maintaining glutathione in its reduced form, GSH.

Reduced glutathione acts as a reducing agent. When RBCs are exposed to oxidizing agents, such as naphthalene, aminoquinolines, and sulfonamides, GSH protects them from cellular injury and hemolysis. Regeneration of glutathione to its reduced form (GSH) again requires NADPH and glutathione reductase. Obviously, when G6PD is deficient, RBCs are unable to generate NADPH and, therefore, GSH function is impaired. Consequently, when exposure to oxidizing agents occurs in individuals with G6PD deficiency, erythrocytes are not protected and cellular injury results in hemolysis. The genetic deficiency finds full expression in male subjects, usually of dark-skinned races (7,10). Naphthalene toxicity may also be reported in girls and in persons of light-skinned races. Ijiri et al. (21) reported the death of a 2-month-old Japanese boy who was given two naphthalene mothballs (approximately 5 g) with milk by his mother. Melzer-Lange and Walsh-Kelly (27) described hemolysis after the accidental ingestion of an unstated quantity of naphthalene by a 20-month-old black girl. In both instances, a fatty substance (milk, cooking oil) was given soon after ingestion. Because naphthalene is extremely lipid soluble, this probably hastened absorption and, thus, toxicity.

One of the better known genetic metabolic polymorphisms is the ability to acetylate certain drugs. Acetylation is a metabolic process catalyzed by *N*-acetyltransferase. Some drugs and carcinogens have been shown to be substrates for this enzyme, including isoniazid (INH) (19). Slow acetylators are more prone to peripheral neuropathy from INH, systemic lupus erythematous from hydralazine and procainamide, and bladder cancer from exposure to beta-naphthalene.

TABLE 2.3. *Examples of pharmacogenetics-related differences in reponse to selected drugs*

Genetic abnormality	Drug/chemical	Response
Atypical pseudocholinesterase	Succinylcholine	Prolonged skeletal muscle relaxation; apnea
Deficient NADH[a] methemoglobin reductase	Nitrates Chlorates Oxidizing agents	Abnormally high and prolonged methemoglobin levels
Deficient hepatic acetyltransferase	Isoniazid Hydralazine Phenelzine Procainamide Sulfonamides	Enhanced toxicity, qualitatively and quantitatively
Deficient glucose-6-phosphate dehydrogenase	Acetylsalicylic acid Doxorubicin Nalidixic acid Primaquine Quinine Nitrofurantoin Naphthalene Fava beans	Hemolytic anemia
Increased δ-aminolevulinic acid synthetase activity	Barbiturates	Hepatic porphyria
Presence of atropine esterase (rabbits)	Atropine	Atropine resistance
Increased hepatic enzymes	Warfarin	Warfarin resistance

[a] NADH, reduced nicotinamide adenine dinucleotide.

A case study entitled ''Theophylline Toxicity as a Result of Altered Metabolism'' is presented at the end of chapter 16. It illustrates what can happen in a patient when theophylline, which is normally metabolized by first-order kinetics, is metabolized by zero-order kinetics.

Most genetically controlled differences in reactions to drugs and chemicals are due to differences in rates of metabolism. However, the same consideration should be extended to variations in absorption, distribution, and excretion. A partial list of important genetically controlled conditions in which individuals display altered responses to drugs and chemicals is presented in Table 2.3.

SEX

Toxicologists are beginning to understand the differences in drug and chemical responses between men and women. Although significant quantitative differences in pharmacologic responses have been experimentally shown in animals, such a definitive statement on the expected toxicity of drugs and chemicals in humans has not been established.

For example, some studies report a sex-related difference in absorption of erythromycin, resulting in less drug being absorbed by women after oral administration (26,28). Women were also reported to have lower serum phenytoin levels than did men because of an increased metabolic rate (33).

Bioavailability of ethanol is greater in women than in men. This is associated with decreased gastric alcohol dehydrogenase activity in women, which contributes to reduced gastric oxidation of ethanol. This in turn may contribute to the enhanced vulnerability of women to acute and chronic complications of ethanol (15). Although the pharmacologic activity and onset, as well as the severity of adverse reactions (e.g., nausea and vomiting), for these drugs may differ among the sexes, there is still little evidence that an *acute toxic dose* of either will produce significantly different toxic manifestations between men and women.

Several other important differences should be considered. Men traditionally weigh more and have a greater blood volume and tissue mass than do women. Therefore, a given dose in a man would be expected to produce lower blood and tissue concentrations than the same dose taken by a woman. For substances injected intramuscularly, lower blood levels can be expected in individuals (usually men) with greater muscle mass. Also, drugs with a high lipid coefficient may produce different toxicologic responses in different sexes, based on the individual's ratio of body fat to total weight.

Admittedly, many of these factors are of more theoretical and experimental interest than clinical importance. However, they illustrate the extent of variability that a chemical may produce in different people. Most studies that report sex-related differences in drug action are conducted with pharmacologic, rather than toxicologic, doses of the drug.

ENVIRONMENTAL FACTORS

Temperature

The response of a biologic system to a toxic agent generally decreases as environmental temperature is lowered, but the duration of overall response may be prolonged. This is related to a decreased rate of absorption and a lowered rate of metabolic degradation and excretion in colder environments.

Additionally, some drugs are more toxic in certain environmental temperatures. Atropine-like compounds may inhibit sweating and prevent cooling of the body. Anticholinergics may, therefore, produce significantly greater toxicity in a warm environment than in a colder one.

Alternatively, drugs such as reserpine and chlorpromazine, which suppress the body's thermal regulatory center, may be more toxic at certain temperatures. These drugs permit the body temperature to assume that of the environment. An individual's body temperature will tend to rise in a warmer climate and decrease in a colder climate.

Occupation

Persons working in industries where organic compounds, such as chlorinated hydrocarbon pesticides or volatile substances, are used may have an enhanced ability to metabolize drugs and chemicals. The reason for this is that the chemical's presence in the environment may have caused the induction of liver microsomal enzyme activity. The expected reaction to a toxic agent that is normally detoxified by the liver microsomal enzyme system would be reduced. Of course, the reaction would be greater than normal for those substances listed in Table 2.1 that are metabolized to more toxic forms.

Living Conditions

The final factor under consideration in this chapter is a person's living conditions. We should remember that the potential relevance of this factor is based on animal studies, and its relation to humans can only be surmised. The amphetamine-aggregation toxicity test can be used to illustrate this factor.

The LD_{50} value for amphetamine is determined for mice placed individually in containers (such as coffee cans). If the number of animals placed in each container is increased, the LD_{50} decreases (i.e., the drug becomes more toxic). There seems to be a crowding factor related to living conditions that significantly affects the toxic dose of amphetamine.

More work is needed to ascertain whether this response in mice is significant in humans and, if so, for what chemicals. If this response is valid in humans, it may at least partially explain differences in toxicity of a chemical in persons living in scantily populated rural areas versus crowded urban settings. At present, factors such as crowding, noise, and social pressures are important areas for research but are difficult to quantify.

SUMMARY

An understanding of what may modify the effects of a toxic agent in the body will be enhanced if we realize that most factors are based on firm pharmacologic principles and common sense. Any individual factor discussed in this chapter is not *a priori* more important than the others. Indeed, the factors included in this chapter illustrate the importance of the topic in general and were not selected because of greater relevance than others.

As will be demonstrated throughout this book, victims of poisoning frequently respond in an unpredictable, nontextbook manner. Understanding why their responses may vary from the "normal" will greatly aid in the management of these patients.

Case Studies

CASE STUDIES: PROLONGED POISONING CAUSED BY A GASTRIC CONCRETION

History: Case 1

The patient was obtunded (dull, lifeless) when brought to an emergency facility. It was learned that he was 43 years old and had a long history of intravenous amphetamine and heroin abuse. He had been previously hospitalized for shoe polish ingestion, insulin-dependent diabetes mellitus, and a chronic seizure disorder. Two months previous to this admission, he had been hospitalized at a different facility for pulmonary tuberculosis. He was taking the following medications: INH, rifampin, phenobarbital, insulin, and pyridoxine.

On this admission, he appeared critically ill and cachexic. Vital signs included blood pressure, 90/56 mm Hg; heart rate, 78 beats/min; respirations, 24/min; and temperature, 36.4°C. He had evidence of icteric sclera, and his lungs had bilateral coarse rhonchi; heart and bowel sounds were normal. Neurologically, the patient was obtunded, but all four extremities responded to painful stimuli. Deep tendon reflexes were absent.

Laboratory values showed an elevated serum chloride concentration. A toxicology screen ordered on the 2nd day disclosed a bromide concentration of 140 mg/L. The patient

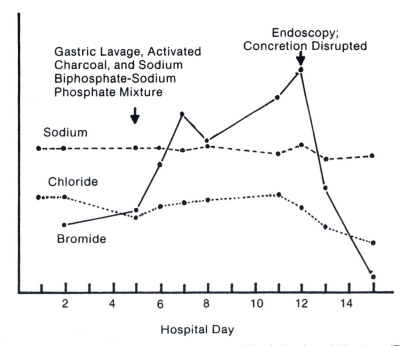

FIG. 2.5. Relative levels of sodium, chloride, and bromide during hospitalization. (From ref. 20.)

received furosemide and saline to hasten its elimination.

By day 5 the bromide concentration was 160 mg/L (Fig. 2.5). Because it was believed that the patient was experiencing prolonged gastrointestinal absorption of bromide, gastric lavage was followed by the administration of activated charcoal and a mixture of sodium biphosphate-sodium phosphate (Phospho-Soda). Serum bromide and chloride concentrations remained elevated.

On day 12, the possibility of a gastrointestinal concretion was raised. Subsequent endoscopy revealed a mass with identifiable pill fragments within the stomach. The mass was broken up, and lavage with saline solution was performed. The gastric aspirate contained high concentrations of bromide.

Over the next several days, the patient's serum bromide and chloride concentrations returned to normal. After the concretion was disrupted and its fragments were removed, the patient's neurologic status returned to nearly normal (20).

History: Case 2

This second case shows a more serious outcome. After gastric lavage and the administration of activated charcoal and a cathartic, symptoms of acute toxicity cleared, but the patient died 8 hr after discharge from the hospital.

The victim was a 54-year-old woman who was brought to the hospital with a chief complaint of having taken large amounts of theophylline (Theo-Dur) and ibuprofen (Motrin) along with some alcohol in a suicide attempt. The time of ingestion was never established. In the ambulance the patient remained alert; blood pressure was 110 mm Hg; pulse, 176 beats/min; respirations, 28/min. Five minutes later, systemic blood pressure was 100 mm Hg; pulse, 150 beats/min; and respirations, 30/min. She vomited once during transport.

Upon admission she was described as lethargic and "somewhat somnolent." She was given oxygen by nasal prongs, and normal saline was started intravenously. An Ewald tube was placed nasally, and lavage of her stomach with normal saline was continued until the return was clear. No pill fragments were seen. Fifty grams of activated charcoal followed by magnesium citrate was given, after which the tube was removed. Serum theophylline concentration was 31.1 mg/L; her toxicology screen was negative for ethanol, methanol, isopropanol, salicylates, benzodiazepines, and barbiturates.

Two hours after arrival the patient was alert, oriented, and in no distress. Vital signs at that time were blood pressure, 122/66 mm Hg; heart rate, 98 beats/min; and respirations, 16/min. She was transferred to a psychiatric section of the emergency department (ED). While there, she vomited once. She was discharged home after approximately 1 hr.

Her family later reported that she vomited repeatedly for the next 8 hr and then she suddenly collapsed. Any additional ingestion was denied. She was in cardiac arrest when emergency medical technicians arrived, and resuscitation was unsuccessful.

At autopsy, the patient's serum theophylline concentration was 190.1 mg/L. A white, waxy mass mixed with charcoal and weighing 318.8 g was found in her stomach. Toxicologic analysis of the mass revealed a content of theophylline estimated to be 29 g. No additional toxins were found on forensic toxicologic screening, and the autopsy was otherwise unremarkable. (6)

Discussion

1. Case 1 illustrates that a concretion formed of fragments of tablets containing a bromide (CNS sedative) can form in the stomach. The patient's prolonged high blood bromide concentrations showed that concretions of solid dosage units can significantly alter the toxicity profile. Based upon your knowledge of renal physiology, why was saline solution administered when it was realized that this patient was poisoned by bromide?

2. Which of the preadmission medications of patient 1 most likely potentiated the bromide-induced CNS depression?
3. The authors of case 2 reported that the incidence of gastric concretion formation may be underestimated because of the difficulty in diagnosing the disorder. Do you agree, or were the authors trying to cover a misdiagnosis?
4. Neither bromides nor theophylline are radiopaque; thus, how can their presence as gastric concretions be identified? How can they be removed?
5. What characteristics of an ingested dosage form may suggest that a gastric concretion can form?

CASE STUDY: SUCCINYLCHOLINE-INDUCED PROLONGED APNEA

History

A 3-week-old male newborn was admitted for pylorotomy (surgical incision of the pylorus, a fairly common procedure in newborn boys). Vital signs and laboratory values were normal. The family history was negative for anesthetic complications. Anesthesia was induced with thiopental and maintained with halothane in nitrous oxide. Six milligrams of succinylcholine were given intravenously. The operation was successfully completed 45 min after the induction of anesthesia, and halothane and nitrous oxide were discontinued. During the entire procedure no abnormalities were noted.

At the end of the procedure, the child remained apneic and flaccid. Controlled ventilation was continued. He was tested for residual neuromuscular block without response even to supramaximal nerve stimulation. One hour later he still showed no change.

Serum cholinesterase P Behring, equivalent to the plasma cholinesterase activity of 200 mL of adult human plasma, was then given. Serum cholinesterase P Behring is a concentrate of the highly purified enzyme. Recovery of neuromuscular function and spontaneous

breathing was observed within a few minutes after the administration of the plasma cholinesterase. The patient did well postoperatively and showed no clinical signs of residual muscle weakness (5).

Discussion

1. Explain pharmacologically how succinylcholine induces neuromuscular blockade. Describe how it is normally removed from the body?
2. Were you surprised that this hospital would have serum cholinesterase P Behring on hand? (Hint: When case 2 was published, the product was available for use only in Germany, Switzerland, and Austria. The surgical procedure was undertaken in Austria.)

CASE STUDIES: NAPHTHALENE POISONING

History: Case 1

A 2-month-old boy was brought to a hospital by his mother. He was dead on arrival. Two days earlier his mother, described as neurotic, had given him a small dose of desiccant and some pebbles because the boy had cried through the night. The following day, he was also given two sewing needles and, shortly thereafter, two mothballs, each weighing 6 g, broken into small pieces and mixed with milk. His face turned pale within 30 min of ingesting the naphthalene.

An autopsy performed 18 hr after death revealed no marks of trauma on the external surface of the body. Three pieces of naphthalene (45, 120, and 182 mg), two sewing needles, and three pebbles were found in the stomach. Two pieces of naphthalene (17 and 36 mg) were found in the jejunal contents. No other changes were noted on gross examination of other organs.

Microscopic features showed congestion, edema, and partial hemorrhage of the lungs, mild fatty change of the liver cells, and a cloudy swelling of tubular epithelial cells of the kidney. The concentrations of naphthalene in the blood, liver, and kidney were estimated at 0.55 μg/mL, 0.12 μg/g, and 0.03 μg/g, respectively. Hematocrit was 41.5%. None of the metabolites of naphthalene was detected, suggesting that the boy's death must have occurred shortly after naphthalene ingestion (21).

History: Case 2

A 20-month-old black girl was brought to a hospital after a syncopal episode 3 to 4 min in duration. There was no seizure activity and no bladder or bowel incontinence.

Two days before admission, the girl had ingested two or three naphthalene mothballs. Family members gave her cooking oil and milk to induce emesis, but without success. Medical attention was not sought.

The day before admission, the child was noted to have dark orange urine in her diapers. She was taking no drugs or vitamins with iron. The family history was positive for sickle cell disease and trait.

Physical examination was largely unremarkable. She displayed mucosal and nail bed pallor and scleral icterus. Vitals included: temperature, 37.8°C; pulse, 124 beats/min; respirations, 24/min; and blood pressure, 84/44 mm Hg. A complete blood cell count showed the following: hemoglobin, 7.0 g/dL; hematocrit, 20.9%; red blood cell count, 2.25 million/mm^3; white blood cell count, 9.6 million/mm^3; mean cell volume (MCV), 82 μm^3; and platelets, 443,000/mm^3.

Treatment consisted of magnesium sulfate administered orally to increase the gastric transit time of naphthalene, intravenous fluids, and close monitoring of urine output.

During her hospitalization, the girl had no further syncopal episodes and remained alert and active. Her hemoglobin declined to a low of 62 g/dL on the 3rd hospital day. Occult blood testing of stools was negative. A glucose 6-phosphate dehydrogenase assay

yielded 83.1 U/dL (laboratory normal, 150 to 215 U/dL). Plasma hemoglobin was 11.3 mg/dL (normal, 0 to 3.0), consistent with hemolysis.

The patient was observed for several additional days (the case study did not indicate the length of her hospital stay) and then released. Six months after admission, she was reported to be well but did not return to her primary care physician for follow-up examination or repeat blood counts (27).

Discussion

1. What effect on the rate of absorption of naphthalene would milk have in patient 1 and cooking oil and milk have in patient 2?
2. The usual cause of death due to naphthalene is hemolysis. Speculate why the hematocrit remained so high (41.5%) in patient 1 at the time of his death.
3. Of what possible significance was patient 2's positive genetic history for sickle cell disease?

Review Questions

1. Which of the following is a true statement?
   A. In general, chemicals are absorbed more rapidly when food is present in the stomach.
   B. Foods rich in ascorbic acid may significantly reduce the pharmacologic effect of levodopa.
   C. Calcium, iron, and fat all enhance lead absorption.
   D. Tyramine-containing foods may induce a hypotensive crisis.
2. The usual effect of succinylcholine in a person who has a toxicogenetic related reaction is:
   A. Increased onset of action due to enhanced absorption.
   B. Increased onset of action due to sensitized receptors.

C. Increased duration of action due to decreased renal excretory mechanisms.

D. Increased duration of action due to decreased hepatic metabolism to less active form.

E. None of the above

3. A deficiency of methemoglobin reductase will most likely cause an adverse reaction with ingestion of which of the following?
    A. Atropine
    B. Succinylcholine
    C. Nitrate
    D. Isoniazid

4. Succinylcholine is initially detoxified by enzymes found in the:
    A. Lung
    B. Plasma
    C. Liver
    D. Kidney

5. Most poisons are pure substances.
    A. True
    B. False

6. Hepatic porphyria results from barbiturate administration to a person who has:
    A. Atypical pseudocholinesterase
    B. Deficient glucose 6-phosphate dehydrogenase
    C. Deficient hepatic acetyl transferase
    D. Sensitive delta-aminolevulinic acid synthetase

7. Concentrated forms of most chemicals are more quickly absorbed than diluted forms.
    A. True
    B. False

8. Absorption is favored when an orally ingested chemical is in which form?
    A. Ionized
    B. Nonionized

9. Carbonated beverages shorten gastric emptying time.
    A. True
    B. False

10. All of the following substances are metabolized to more toxic compounds except:
    A. Acetaminophen
    B. Carbon tetrachloride
    C. Phenytoin
    D. Parathion

11. Which of the following is an expected toxic response from an overdose of paraldehyde?
    A. CNS depression due to paraldehyde
    B. Severe nausea due to acetone
    C. CNS depression due to metaldehyde
    D. Retinal damage due to paraldehyde

12. Hydrazine is a potentially toxic metabolite produced by which of the following substances?
    A. Paraldehyde
    B. Methanol
    C. Imipramine
    D. Isoniazid

13. Which of the following must be used with caution by a person known as a *slow acetylator:* phenelzine (I), hydralazine (II), or primaquine (III)?
    A. II only
    B. III only
    C. I and II only
    D. II and III only
    E. I, II, and III

14. Which of the following should be used with extreme caution by persons with deficient hepatic acetyltransferase enzyme activity: hydralazine (I), primaquine (II), or quinine (III)?
    A. I only
    B. II only
    C. III only
    D. I and II only
    E. I and III only
    F. II and III only
    G. I, II, and III

15. Pharmacogenetic differences in individuals' response to a given drug are primarily related to what specific kinetic parameter?
    A. Absorption
    B. Distribution
    C. Metabolism
    D. Excretion

16. Which drug is *least* likely to induce hemolytic anemia in an individual deficient in glucose 6-phosphate dehydrogenase?
    A. Quinine
    B. Primaquine
    C. Nitroglycerin
    D. Nitrofurantoin

17. What is the term applied to a sign or symptom that is so unique to and/or highly characteristic of a particular disease that its presence allows a positive diagnosis of that disease?
    A. Etiologic
    B. Idiosyncratic
    C. Pharmacogenetic
    D. Pathognomonic

18. What term(s) refer(s) to a mass of swallowed foreign material that may cause gastric obstruction?
    A. Concretion
    B. Bougienage
    C. Bezoar
    D. All of the above
    E. Only two of the above

19. Naphthalene is more toxic than *p*-dichlorobenzene.
    A. True
    B. False

20. Elderly people often show a different response to a toxic chemical than do younger adults. Cite various factors that influence this difference in response.

21. What happens when an ingested solid dosage form develops into a concretion? What are the limitations to using a gastric lavage tube to remove these poisons?

22. Discuss why the most significant toxic response from ingested methanol may be delayed for many hours after ingestion.

References

1. Balazs T. Measurement of acute toxicity. In: Paget GE, ed. *Methods in toxicology*. Philadelphia: FA Davis; 1970:10–15.
2. Barltrop D, Khoo HE. The influence of nutritional factors on lead absorption. *Postgrad Med J* 1975;51:795–800.
3. Benet LZ, Sheiner LB. Pharmacokinetics: the dynamics of drug absorption, distribution, and elimination. In: Gilman AG, Goodman LS, Rall TW, Murad F, eds. *The pharmacological basis of therapeutics*. 7th ed. New York: Macmillan; 1985:3–34.
4. Bennett WM, Singer I, Coggins CJ. A guide to drug therapy in renal failure. *JAMA* 1974;230:1544–1553.
5. Benzer A, Luz G, Oswald E, et al. Succinylcholine-induced prolonged apnea in a 3-week-old newborn: treatment with human plasma cholinesterase. *Anesth Analg* 1992;74:137–138.
6. Bernstein G, Jehle D, Bernaski E, Braen GR. Failure of gastric emptying and charcoal administration in fatal sustained-release theophylline overdose: pharmacobezoar formation. *Ann Emerg Med* 1992;21:1388–1390.
7. Beutler E. Glucose-6-phosphate dehydrogenase deficiency. *N Engl J Med* 1991;324:169–174.
8. Bianchine JR. Drugs for Parkinson's disease: spasticity, and acute muscle spasms. In: Gilman AG, Goodman LS, Rall TW, Murad F, eds. *The pharmacological basis of therapeutics*. 7th ed. New York: Macmillan; 1985:473–490.
9. Boyd EM. *Predictive toxicometrics*. Bristol, England: Scientechnia; 1972.
10. Brewer GJ, Tarlov AR, Alving AS. The methemoglobin reduction test for primaquine-type sensitivity of erythrocytes. *JAMA* 1962;180:386–388.
11. Burns LE, Hoggman JE, Cass AB. Fatal circulatory collapse in premature infants receiving chloramphenicol. *N Engl J Med* 1958;261:1318–1321.
12. Cartright AC. Toxicology of impurities in organic synthetic drugs. *Int Pharm J* 1990;4:146–150.
13. Crome P. The elderly. *Br Med J* 1984;289:546–548.
14. Doull J. Factors influencing toxicity. In: Doull J, Klaassen CD, Amdur MO, eds. *Toxicology: the basic science of poisons*. 2nd ed. New York: Macmillan; 1980:70–83.
15. Frezza M, DiPadova C, Pozzato G, et al. High blood alcohol levels in women. *N Engl J Med* 1990;322:95–99.
16. Goldstein A, Aronow L, Kalman SM. *Principles of drug action*. 2nd ed. New York: Harper and Row; 1974.
17. Golightly LK, Smolinske SS, Bennett MS, et al. Adverse effects associated with inactive ingredients in drug products (part I). *Med Toxicol* 1988;3:128–165.
18. Golightly LK, Smolinske SS, Bennett MS, et al. Adverse effects associated with inactive ingredients in drug products (part II). *Med Toxicol* 1988;3:209–240.
19. Guttendorf RJ, Wedlund RJ. Genetic aspects of drug disposition and therapeutics. *J Clin Pharmacol* 1992;32:107–117.
20. Iberti TJ, Patterson BK, Fisher CJ. Prolonged bromide intoxication resulting from a gastric bezoar. *Arch Intern Med* 1984;144:402–403.
21. Ijiri I, Shimosato K, Ohmae M, Tomita M. A case report of death from naphthalene poisoning. *Jpn J Legal Med* 1987;41:52–55.
22. Iossifides IA, Smith I, Keitel HG. Chloramphenicol-bilirubin interaction in premature babies. *J Pediatr* 1963;62:735–741.
23. Jenis EH, Payne RJ, Goldbaum LR. Acute meprobamate poisoning: a fatal case following a lucid interval. *JAMA* 1969;207:361–362.
24. Klaassen CD. Principles of toxicology. In: Klaassen CD, Amdur MO, Doull J, eds. *Toxicology: the basic science of poisons*. 3rd ed. New York: Macmillan; 1986:11–32.
25. Krenzelok EP, Dunmire SM. Acute poisoning emergencies: resolving the gastric decontamination controversy. *Postgrad Med* 1992;91:179–186.
26. Lake B, Besll SM. Variations in absorption of erythromycin. *Med J Aust* 1969;1:449–450.
27. Melzer-Lange M, Walsh-Kelly C. Naphthalene-induced hemolysis in a black female toddler deficient

in glucose-6-phosphate dehydrogenase. *Pediatr Emerg Care* 1989;5:24–26.

28. Philipson A, Sabath LD, Charles D. Erythromycin and clindamycin absorption and elimination in pregnant women. *Clin Pharmacol Ther* 1976;19:63–77.

29. Preisig R. Pharmacogenetics. *Pharm Int* 1983;4:314–317.

30. Rendell M, McGrave D, Cuesta M. Fatal compulsive water drinking. *JAMA* 1978;240:2557–2559.

31. Sande MA, Mandell GL. Tetracyclines, chloramphenicol, erythromycin, and miscellaneous antibacterial agents. In: Gilman AG, Goodman LS, Rall TW, Murad F, eds. *The pharmacological basis of therapeutics.* 7th ed. New York: Macmillan; 1985:1170–1198.

32. Sande MA, Mandell GL. Antifungal and antiviral agents. In: Gilman AG, Goodman LS, Rall TW, Murad F, eds. *The pharmacological basis of therapeutics.* 7th ed. New York: Macmillan; 1985:1219–1239.

33. Sherwin AL. Effects of age, sex, obesity and pregnancy on plasma diphenylhydantoin levels. *Epilepsia* 1974;15:507.

34. Smith CE, Lewis G, Donati F, Bevan DR. Dose-response relationship for succinylcholine in a patient with genetically determined low plasma cholinesterase activity. *Anesthesiology* 1989;70:156–158.

35. Welling PG. Influence of food and diet on gastrointestinal drug absorption: a review. *J Pharmacokinet Biopharm* 1977;5:291–334.

36. Wiley JF. Difficult diagnosis in toxicology. *Pediatr Clin North Am* 1991;38:725–737.

3 ‖ Principles in Management of the Poisoned Patient

GENERAL CONSIDERATIONS

One of the most important aspects in management of poisoning or of a toxic exposure is knowing what to do and in what order to do it! This chapter explains the fundamental principles of managing acute poisonings. These include specific methods to reduce absorption of the toxic agent or to increase its elimination from the body. The chapter also discusses more specific antidotes that can be used to counteract the effects of selective toxic agents.

Throughout history, numerous procedures have been advocated to treat the toxic effects of chemicals. These have ranged from car-rying talismans (charms) and chanting prayers to making incisions in the body and blood-letting with leeches. These were primitive methods, and some of the unfortunate victims of poisoning might have been better off if nothing had been done! Although the art of treating acute exposures to toxic agents has advanced tremendously over the years, it was not too long ago when the normal protocol for treatment of poison ingestion included salt solutions, burnt toast, copper sulfate, and, of course, the "universal antidote."

Today, such items have been replaced by more effective treatments and some have even been condemned. In some cases, standard pro-

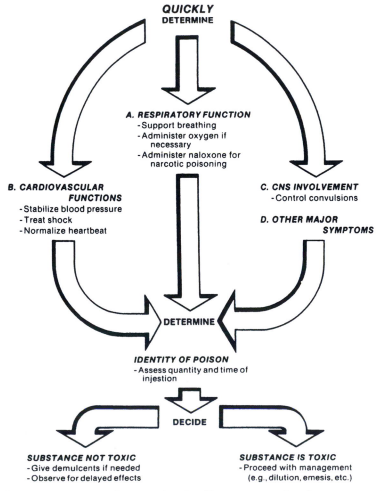

FIG. 3.1. The flow chart illustrates the steps involved in assessment and management of a poisoned patient.

tocols have been established for management of some poisons. For other treatments, many currently recommended procedures remain in the formative stages and are controversial in the scientific literature. Several of these will be explored throughout this textbook.

Successful management of a poisoning victim can generally be accomplished as outlined in Fig. 3.1. Overriding all other considerations must be the realization that care of the *PATIENT* is the first priority. The familiar adage, "Treat the patient, not the poison!" must always be followed. It is of little value to make heroic attempts at removing an ingested poison from the victim's stomach if breathing has stopped or blood pressure has plummeted.

The first step is to assess the patient's condition and to follow whatever treatment is necessary to stabilize the vital signs. Attention to the airway, breathing, and circulation (the "ABCs") take precedent (26). Once the patient's condition is stabilized, attempts can be made to identify the toxic agent, route of administration, quantity, and time since exposure. After this information has been obtained, general and specific methods for treatment may be considered.

Several questions may arise, and their answers can alter treatment. For example: Is the amount or composition of the substance involved considered toxic or nontoxic? Can the toxic agent be easily removed, neutralized, or eliminated? Is there a specific antidote available for the toxic substance involved? If the substance is considered toxic and a long period has elapsed from the time of ingestion: (a) Will removal still be effective? (b) Will a specific antidote still be useful? (c) Can elimination of the toxic agent be enhanced? If the ingested substance is determined to be of minimal toxic potential, is its removal from the stomach still necessary? If the ingested substance is considered toxic or potentially toxic but no significant signs or symptoms of toxicity are apparent: (a) Should the toxic substance be removed? (b) If appropriate, should the specific antidote still be administered? (c) Should treatment be delayed until classic signs or symptoms appear?

CLINICAL EVALUATION OF THE POISONED PATIENT

A victim of poisoning must be carefully evaluated for extent of poisoning before a management plan can be initiated (32,64,82). The first step is to provide the patient with good supportive care. Is the patient breathing? Health care personnel may need to administer oxygen or start mechanical ventilation. Is the patient's blood pressure stabilized? Shock is best treated with a fluid challenge and, if necessary, vasopressor agents. Is there normal sinus rhythm? Is the patient experiencing seizures or tremors? Is the patient comatose? Are there any other underlying medical problems, such as liver or renal disease? If so, the patient may require more aggressive therapy. After cardiorespiratory functions are supported, the next step is to obtain a history of the poisoning.

History of Poisoning

An accurate history should include identification of the poison, amount and time of ingestion or length of contact, emergency first aid treatment already administered, and the patient's psychologic profile. Obtaining the history is often difficult because the poisoned individual may be unconscious, unresponsive, or confused. Frequently, an accurate history may be impossible to obtain. Information obtained from relatives or friends is often (but not always) questionable. Symptoms may suggest one cause of poisoning, but the circumstances of poisoning may strongly indicate an entirely different cause. As a result, emergency medical personnel must make quick decisions about what to do and where to start in treating many victims.

Clinical Assessment

Some poisons produce clinical characteristics that strongly suggest the involvement of a particular drug or chemical (Table 3.1). For example, with cholinesterase-inhibiting or-

TABLE 3.1. *Characteristic manifestations of poisoning*

Signs or symptoms	Possible cause
Ataxia	Alcohol, barbiturates, bromides, hallucinogens, heavy metals, phenytoin, solvents (organic)
Breath odor	Acetone: isopropanol, nail polish remover, salicylates, lacquer, alcohol, ketoacidosis
	Alcohol: ethyl alcohol
	Ammoniacal: uremia
	Bitter almonds: cyanide
	Coal gas (stove gas): carbon monoxide (odorless but associated with coal gas)
	Disinfectants: phenol, creosote
	Eggs (rotten): hydrogen sulfide, mercaptans, disulfiram
	Fish or raw liver (musty): hepatic failure, zinc phosphide
	Fruitlike: amyl nitrite, ethanol, isopropyl alcohol
	Garlic: arsenic, organophosphate compounds, phosphorus, dimethyl sulfoxide (DMSO), thallium
	Mothballs: camphor-containing products
	Pearlike (acrid): chloral hydrate, paraldehyde
	Pungent: ethchlorvynol
	Shoe polish: nitrobenzene
	Tobacco (stale): nicotine
	Violets: turpentine
	Wintergreen: methyl salicylate
	Others (characteristic): ammonia, gasoline, kerosene, petroleum distillates, phenol, mothballs
Coma; drowsiness	Alcohol, antihistamines, antipsychotics, antidepressants, barbiturates and other sedatives, opioids, salicylates
Fasciculations; convulsions[a]	Alcohol, amphetamines, antihistamines, barbiturate withdrawal, chlorinated hydrocarbons, cyanide, isoniazid, lead, organophosphorous insecticides, methaqualone, plants (some), salicylates, strychnine, tricyclic antidepressants, phenothiazines
Gastrointestinal	
Emesis (often bloody)	Boric acid, caffeine, corrosives, heavy metals, phenol, salicylates, theophylline
Abdominal colic	Arsenic, lead, organophosphorous compounds, mushrooms, opioid withdrawal
Diarrhea	Arsenic, boric acid, iron, mushrooms, organophosphorous compounds
Constipation	Lead, opioids
Hallucinations	Alcohol, cocaine, LSD, mescaline, PCP
Heart rate	
Bradycardia	Cholinergics digitalis, opioids, sedatives
Tachycardia	Amphetamines, atropine, cocaine
Mouth	
Dry	Amphetamine, atropine, antihistamines, opioids
Salivation	Mushrooms, organophosphorous compounds, mercury, arsenic, corrosives, strychnine
Gum discoloration	Lead and other heavy metals
Paralysis	Botulism, heavy metals
Pupils	
Miosis	Mushrooms (muscarinic type), opioids, organophosphorous compounds
Mydriasis[b]	Amphetamine, antihistamines, atropine, barbiturate (coma), cocaine, glutethimide, LSD,[c] opiate withdrawal, tricyclic antidepressants
Nystagmus	Barbiturates, phenytoin, sedatives, PCP[d]
Vision disturbance	Botulism, methanol, organophosphates
Respiration	
Rapid rate	Amphetamines, barbiturates (early), methanol, petroleum distillates, salicylates
Slow rate	Alcohol, barbiturates (late), opioids
Paralysis	Botulism, organophosphorous compounds
Wheezing; pulmonary edema	Opioids, organophosphorous compounds, petroleum distillates

TABLE 3.1. *Continued.*

Signs or symptoms	Possible cause
Skin	
Cyanosis	Nitrites, strychnine
Red, flushed	Alcohol, antihistamines, atropine, carbon monoxide, boric acid
Purpura	Salicylates, snake and spider bites
Jaundice	Acetaminophen (delayed), arsenic, carbon tetrachloride, castor bean, mushroom (delayed)
Sweating	Amphetamine, barbiturates, cocaine, LSD, mushrooms, organophosphorous compounds
Needle marks	Amphetamine, opioids, PCP
Bullae	Barbiturates, carbon monoxide

From refs. 27, 60, and 89.
[a] May be caused by any substance that causes hypoxia.
[b] May indicate severe stage of opioid poisoning, caused by hypoxia.
[c] LSD, lysergic acid diethylamide.
[d] PCP, phencyclidine.

ganophosphorous insecticides, cholinergic effects such as miosis, excessive salivation, and gastrointestinal hyperactivity will predominate. In tricyclic antidepressant overdose, anticholinergic effects, such as mydriasis, loss of consciousness, absent bowel sounds, and cardiac arrhythmias, will dominate the clinical picture.

Clinical assessment generally begins with recording of vital signs, such as blood pressure, heart rate, respirations, and body temperature. Assessment of neurologic function and level of consciousness is the next priority. A typical scoring system for coma and hyperactivity is given in Table 3.2. These classifications are often used in initial assessment of

the poisoned patient, as well as in evaluation of the progress of treatment.

Once emergency procedures have been performed and the poisoned patient is stabilized or at least is out of immediate danger, additional steps can be taken to remove the poison, prevent or delay absorption, enhance excretion, or administer a specific antidote.

Another point to stress is the value in using blood, urine, and vomitus for toxicologic analysis. Qualitative and quantitative assays can quickly identify a toxic substance. The results of these tests can be used to aid diagnosis of the poisoned patient, evaluate the progress of treatment, and predict outcomes of therapy (55,80). But, as was indicated in chapter 2,

TABLE 3.2. *Neurologic status*

CNS[a] depression or excitation	Symptoms
Depression	
Stage 0	Asleep; drowsy but accountable; responds to verbal commands
Stage 1	Corneal, gag, and deep tendon reflexes present; responds to pain
Stage 2	Deep tendon reflexes present; gag reflex present; no response to pain
Stage 3	Deep tendon reflexes absent; no response to pain; may have decorticate or decerebrate rigidity
Stage 4	Stage 3 symptoms plus cardiovascular and respiratory compromise; convulsions may be present
Excitation	
Stage 1	Restlessness; insomnia; tachycardia; flushed face; mydriasis
Stage 2	Stage 1 symptoms plus convulsions and mild pyrexia
Stage 3	Arrhythmia; delirium and mania; hypertension; hyperpyrexia
Stage 4	Stage 3 symptoms plus convulsions and/or coma

From ref. 81.
[a] CNS, central nervous system.

TABLE 3.3. *Comparison of toxicokinetics and pharmacokinetics*

Parameter	Pharmacokinetics	Toxicokinetics
Dose	Known, low	Unknown, high
Effect	Therapeutic	Toxic
Steady state	Usually	No
Corroborating human data	Frequently	Generally not complete
Other drugs with similar or antagonistic effects	Generally not	Usually, especially in adult patients ·
Known concentration effects	Yes	Generally not as well defined

From ref. 95.

the accuracy of toxicologic testing varies widely by drug class and analytical methods used (98).

TOXICOKINETIC CONSIDERATIONS

Toxicokinetics is a discipline that can be described as the toxicologist's use of clinical pharmacokinetics, the quantitative study of absorption, distribution, metabolism (biotransformation), and elimination of drugs in biologic systems (58) (Table 3.3). Mathematical descriptions of these processes allow predictions to be made of body burdens of a drug or chemical, of half-life, of duration in the body after exposure has been terminated, and of rate of elimination. Knowledge of the toxicokinetics of a specific poison is beneficial when formulating the proper management protocol, especially if forced diuresis, hemodialysis, or hemoperfusion is indicated.

It is important to note at the onset that pharmacokinetic data available from reference tables may not apply to overdoses of the same drug. Kinetic parameters often change with large or toxic doses. To illustrate, the amount and rate of absorption may be increased or decreased, distribution patterns may be different, and rates of metabolism and excretion may be increased or decreased. If the major route of elimination is via hepatic metabolism, enzymes may become saturated and thereby allow plasma drug concentrations to increase.

Most drugs are absorbed, distributed, and eliminated by *first-order* kinetics, or exponential/logarithmic relationships. The rates of these processes are directly proportional to

concentration or amount of chemical present at a particular time. The rate-limiting factor is the amount of drug or chemical in the body; half-life ($t_{1/2}$) is independent of dose. *Half-life* is defined as the time required to eliminate 50% of the chemical from the body. For chemicals exhibiting first-order kinetics, half-life can be calculated from the following equation:

$$t_{1/2} = 0.693/K_{el}$$

Half-life can also be determined by plotting concentration versus time, obtained at three or more time intervals on semi-log graph paper. The slope of the line represents the apparent first-order elimination rate constant (K_{el}), which can be used in the previous equation to calculate the $t_{1/2}$.

Some drugs follow *zero-order* kinetics. The rates of these processes remain constant and are independent of concentration or amount of chemical present in the body. The biologic system is the rate-limiting factor, and metabolizing enzymes are rapidly saturated. For chemicals metabolized by zero-order kinetics, $t_{1/2}$ increases with dose. An excellent example of a compound eliminated by zero-order kinetics is ethanol. This will be discussed in chapter 4.

Some chemicals follow first-order kinetics at low or therapeutic doses but revert to zero-order or saturation kinetics at higher doses or overdoses. Consequently, determining the half-life during the course of poisoning is a valuable approach to formulating a management plan. The overdose $t_{1/2}$ (OD $t_{1/2}$) would determine the rate at which chemical concentrations approach therapeutic or nontoxic range. For a chemical whose OD $t_{1/2}$ is increased, management should be directed at measures to increase elimination (e.g., forced diuresis, dialysis) and, therefore, reduce the chemical half-life. Two examples serve to illustrate this point. Refer to the salicylate text commentary in chapter 12 and a theophylline case study in chapter 16. In both instances, drug $t_{1/2}$ values can be significantly prolonged.

Volume of distribution (V_d) is the relationship of plasma chemical concentration and the amount of chemical distributed throughout the body. This is not a real volume in the true sense but an apparent (mathematical) volume that can be estimated by:

$$V_d = \frac{D}{C_0}$$

where D = dose administered and C_0 = plasma concentration at time zero.

Clearance (Cl) is the volume of blood/plasma which is cleared of chemical by elimination per unit of time. This is an important kinetic parameter that is an index of chemical elimination regardless of the amount that needs to be cleared. Direct measurement of clearance is not possible, but it may be estimated by the following equations:

$$Cl = (K_{el})(V_d) \quad \text{or} \quad K_{el} = \frac{0.693}{t_{1/2}}$$

It is sometimes beneficial to use these kinetic equations to predict the severity of an overdose. The data obtained would be more significant than relying on LD_{50} values or single chemical concentrations. For example, if a 20-kg child ingested three pentobarbital capsules (300 mg total) and the V_d for pentobarbital is approximately 2 L/kg, then the estimated pentobarbital blood concentration would be approximately 7.5 μg/mL (0.75 mg%), which is in the toxic range (see appendix table 3).

METHODS TO REDUCE OR PREVENT ABSORPTION: GASTROINTESTINAL DECONTAMINATION

Once the patient is stabilized, attention should be directed to removing any unab-

sorbed poison from the GI tract and other sites such as the skin. Severity of intoxication in many instances will be proportional to the length of time an unabsorbed toxic agent remains in the body.

Gastric decontamination methods (emesis, gastric lavage, catharsis, and adsorption with activated charcoal) are undergoing critical scrutiny (26). Many time-honored procedures have changed drastically during the past 5 years, and others will probably change over the next several years.

Dilution

The initial procedure often recommended whenever ingestion of a poison is suspected is dilution with water. The amount recommended is generally 1 to 2 cupfuls for a child and 2 to 3 cupfuls for an adult. However, fluids should never be forced. Offer the patient a quantity that can be comfortably swallowed. Excessive liquid may distend the stomach wall, causing premature evacuation of its contents into the duodenum and making it more difficult to remove the poison.

A general rule is that nothing should be administered orally to an unconscious patient or if the gag reflex is absent. In cases of ingestion of solid dosage forms, such as tablets or capsules, dilution is not universally recommended (11). In this case dilution can promote dissolution of the medication, which favors absorption. Most chemicals and household products, such as cleaning agents, are best managed by dilution.

Dilution with water accomplishes at least two functions. First, it helps reduce the gastric irritation induced by many ingested poisons. Second and more importantly, it adds bulk to the stomach that may be needed later for emesis. Ipecac-induced emesis is more effective if there is fluid or bulk present in the stomach.

There is still some controversy over the use of milk as a diluent and demulcent with ipecac. Previously, a study involving adult volunteers demonstrated that milk delayed the onset of emesis when given with ipecac (93). More

TABLE 3.4. *Conditions in which emesis should not be attempted*

Do not induce vomiting if the ingested substance is a:
  convulsant
  hydrocarbon
  corrosive acid or alkali
  sharp object (e.g., needle, pin, razor blade)
  nontoxic substance
Do not induce vomiting if the patient:
  is unconscious or comatose
  has a diminished gag reflex
  has severe cardiovascular disease or emphysema or extremely weakened blood vessels
  has recently undergone surgery
  is expected to deteriorate rapidly
  has a hemorrhagic diathesis (e.g., cirrhosis, varices, thrombocytopenia)
  has vomited significantly before this moment
  is under 6 months of age

recently, studies have demonstrated that milk does not interfere significantly with the onset of emesis when given with ipecac (33,36).

Emesis

For many years emesis has been a mainstay for treating the ingestion of toxic agents. Emetics have been used since earliest recorded history. Chemically induced emesis is generally accepted to be a first-line procedure in the management of poisonings because it can be easily done at home. The American Academy of Pediatrics recommends that ipecac syrup be available in all homes with young children to be used only after consultation with a poison information specialist or a physician (26).

Certain precautions and contraindications for emesis are listed in Table 3.4. If the victim is unconscious, there is danger that vomitus may be aspirated into the lung and cause chemical pneumonitis. If the poison is a convulsant, forced emesis may precipitate seizures.

In alert, conscious patients who have swallowed liquid hydrocarbons such as petroleum distillates (gasoline, etc.), the recommendation to induce emesis is dependent on the amount ingested and the relative toxicity of

the hydrocarbon, as outlined in chapter 7. Petroleum or pine distillates, for example, have a low viscosity and surface tension. These substances can be readily aspirated into the lungs during emesis (Fig. 3.2) to cause chemical pneumonitis.

If the ingested poison is corrosive, emesis should be avoided because it may cause further damage to the esophagus and oral mucosa as the substance is brought up. The tissue damage induced by these substances is related, in part, to contact time between poison and tissue.

Children under 6 months of age should not receive syrup of ipecac unless supervised by a physician. Their gag reflex is poorly developed, and emetics may cause choking with aspiration. For children under 6 months, lavage is preferred.

Emetics should be used with care in patients

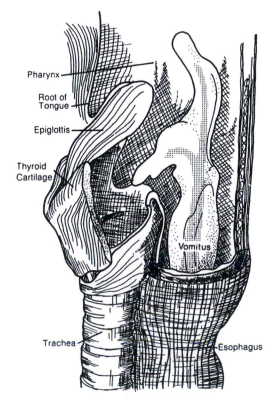

FIG. 3.2. Graphic representation illustrating the manner in which vomitus can easily be aspirated into the trachea.

with severe cardiovascular disease, aneurysms, severe emphysema, or other conditions where blood vessels are weakened and there is risk of hemorrhage.

Vomiting should be induced only if there is sufficient bulk (fluid) in the stomach to serve as a carrier for the ingested poison. Adequate dilution with water increases the efficacy of emetics, as was stated earlier.

Syrup of Ipecac

Use of ipecac was first mentioned in the *Natural History of Brazil* (1648). Ipecac root was brought to Europe in 1672 as a "cure" for dysentery. Its popularity was limited because recommended doses were excessive and caused numerous undesirable effects. These problems were eventually resolved.

As recently as 1964, syrup of ipecac required a prescription for purchase. In 1965 it was listed by several references as an alternative to sodium chloride, powdered mustard, or mechanical stimulation of the pharynx as a method to induce vomiting. Its action was described as being generally slow, with vomiting occurring after 30 to 60 min. It was also considered to be toxic if too much were given. Much of the reported toxicity was due to the use of the fluid extract form of ipecac, which is 14 times more potent than the syrup (see the case study, "Ipecac Misuse," Case 4, at the end of this chapter).

Ipecac is derived from the root of *Cephaelis ipecacuanha* or *C. acuminata*. The principal active alkaloids are emetine and cephaeline. Ipecac causes emesis through both early and late phases of vomiting (50). Early vomiting usually occurs within 30 min and is due to direct stimulant action on the GI tract. A second phase occurs after 30 min, resulting from direct stimulant action on the chemoreceptor trigger zone that activates the vomiting center located in the reticular formation. This effectuates coordinated somatic and visceral motor activity to produce vomiting (88). Therefore, if vomiting does not occur within the first 15 to 20 min, the drug should not be discounted as ineffective.

Effectiveness of syrup of ipecac as an emetic has been variously described as poor to excellent. Some studies indicate that a significant number of people will not vomit with ipecac. Most investigations have definitely established that syrup of ipecac is effective, even for poisons (such as phenothiazines) that have antiemetic activity.

Monoguerra and Krenzelok (51) reported that 81% of 232 patients given a single dose of syrup of ipecac vomited; an additional 15% vomited when the dose was repeated. The average time from ipecac administration to vomiting was 24 min. Of 63 patients who swallowed drugs with antiemetic properties, 81% vomited after the first dose and an additional 14% required a second dose.

There is a practical way to look at the issue. It can be assumed that, even if a poisoned victim vomited only a portion (perhaps one-fourth or one-half) of the ingested substance before it was absorbed, this could be sufficient to change the prognosis from "critical" to a point where there was a greater chance for survival or there was less chance for serious damage.

The usual doses of syrup of ipecac are listed in Table 3.5. A second dose may be given if the patient fails to vomit within 20 to 30 min. The success rate and onset of ipecac-induced emesis seem to be dose related. The overall success rate approaches 100%, with an average time to emesis of 24 min (26,37,46,51).

In a recent prospective study, 30 mL was more effective than 15 mL in inducing emesis in children (38). Also, the failure rate for 30 mL of syrup of ipecac is only 0.5%, compared to 8.8% for 15 mL (37).

Toxicity of Ipecac

Syrup of ipecac is generally safe and well tolerated, and toxicity is rarely seen in doses

TABLE 3.5. *Recommended doses of syrup of ipecac*

Age	Quantity
6–12 months	5–10 mL
1–12 years	15 mL
Adults	30 mL

recommended (26). Some of its adverse effects may include protracted vomiting, diarrhea, lethargy, diaphoresis, and fever. The toxic component of ipecac is emetine, a cardiotoxin (50). Chronic abuse of ipecac in patients with anorexia nervosa or bulimia has resulted in peripheral myopathies and sometimes fatal cardiomyopathies (9,29). There are reports of serious adverse effects associated with long-term abuse of syrup of ipecac (35). (See the case studies at the end of this chapter.) These cases demonstrate that significant cumulative toxicity can result from repeated ingestion of a substance that is ordinarily not toxic in doses normally ingested acutely. There is no evidence that routinely associates therapeutic doses of ipecac with cardiovascular or neurotoxicity.

General Considerations for Using Syrup of Ipecac

Ipecac can be given at home by parents after they receive proper instructions from a qualified health professional. Because it may take approximately 20 to 30 min after administration for vomiting to begin, early administration is essential. Emergency medical vehicles usually stock syrup of ipecac. If it takes 10 min for the vehicle to reach a home, plus another 20 to 30 min to induce vomiting, serious poisoning may occur within this latent period. Worse, if treatment is not instituted until the victim arrives at the hospital, even more valuable time will be lost and the potential for damage accentuated. Therefore, parents of small children should be strongly urged to keep syrup of ipecac on hand at all times but use it only when directed by the poison control center.

There is another advantage to giving ipecac at home, followed by an automobile ride to a hospital or physician's office. The physical jostling due to riding in a vehicle (especially with the windows closed and heater on) may help promote more rapid emesis.

Another reason for early use of syrup of ipecac in poisonings is that induced emesis

is generally less traumatic to the patient than gastric lavage. The insertion of a lavage tube is unpleasant to most people, especially children, and must be undertaken only by qualified personnel. Lavage is slow, is relatively inefficient, and may result in forcing material out of the stomach into the intestine, where it cannot be easily recovered. Chemical emetics can also recover particles of material that are too large to pass through the opening of a lavage tube.

Apomorphine

Apomorphine is a morphine derivative that produces rapid emesis, usually within 3 to 5 min, through direct stimulation of the chemoreceptor trigger zone. Onset of emesis is more rapid, but recovery of gastric contents is essentially the same as with ipecac (15,48). It is no longer recommended.

Soap Solution

When rapid emesis is indicated and syrup of ipecac is not available, one alternative is to administer a dish-washing liquid detergent (30). Two to three tablespoonfuls should be mixed with 6 to 8 ounces of water. Detergents are believed to produce emesis by direct stimulation of the gastrointestinal mucosa.

In one study, the mean time to emesis was less than 10 min, compared to 15 to 20 min for syrup of ipecac (30). The solution is difficult to swallow, so this method usually has poor patient acceptance.

Liquid detergents should not be confused with laundry detergents or electric dishwasher granular products. The latter are corrosive and may cause injury.

Mechanical Stimulation

Stimulation of the back of the tongue or pharynx has been recommended as a means to evoke emesis. This involves placing the victim in a spanking position and gently stroking the area with a blunt object such as a spoon or tongue depressor. Fingers are not advised, since the victim may reflexively bite down as he or she is gagged, causing injury to the individual's finger.

The advantage of this procedure is its availability. Its major disadvantage is lack of effectiveness; gagging is not the same as vomiting. In a study of 30 poisoned children, only 2 children vomited after mechanical stimulation, and the volume was insignificant (2 mL and 4 mL, respectively). All victims had previously been given 6 to 8 ounces of fluid (18). Consequently, mechanical stimulation is *not* recommended to induce vomiting.

Outmoded Emetics

Numerous substances have been advocated over the years as emetics. *Potassium and antimony tartrate* (tartar emetic), *copper sulfate,* and *zinc sulfate* were once considered outstanding emetics. Because of erratic, slow action and possible toxicity if absorbed, they should no longer be recommended (87). *Mustard powder* mixed into a slurry in water was formerly advocated. It is unreliable as an emetic, and few households actually have it available. It also produces an extremely gritty, bitter taste in the mouth. Valuable minutes may be wasted in first trying to locate the powder and then attempting to coax an unwilling child to ingest it. Therefore, mustard powder is no longer recommended as an emetic. Condiment (spice) mustard does not possess emetic value.

Numerous reference books and first aid charts and some package labels until recently advocated the induction of vomiting with a *salt solution.* Today this measure is considered potentially dangerous; it should never be undertaken (4,20,75). To illustrate this change in thinking, several points must be considered.

First, differences in measuring a tablespoonful and feelings that "if one tablespoonful of salt is a good emetic, then two will be even better" can result in extremely large, toxic doses being administered to a child. In

some cases reported in the literature, children have received more than 4 heaping tablespoonfuls of salt given repeatedly, two to three times.

When salt solution is administered and emesis does not occur, the salt is absorbed. As the sodium concentration rises, increased tonicity of extracellular fluid (blood) results. Intracellular fluids move outward, resulting in crenation (shrinking) of cells. At the same time, there is increased intracranial pressure.

The first cells to be affected are those within the CNS. The shrunken cells cannot perform their normal activities. The combination of damaged brain cells with disturbed metabolic functions, along with distension of intracranial blood vessels, leads to severe intraventricular hemorrhage and thrombosis throughout the brain. When this occurs, death is imminent.

Lavage

Lavage (Fr. *laver* = to wash) is a process of washing out the stomach with solutions, including water, saline, sodium bicarbonate, calcium salts, tannic acid, and potassium permanganate. Lavage is sometimes indicated when poisons must be quickly removed from the stomach or when emesis is contraindicated (Table 3.6).

The patient's airway should be protected by intubation, using a cuffed endotracheal or nasotracheal tube (39). Intubation should precede gastric lavage in the unconscious or convulsing patient. Any patient who can tolerate intubation without trauma should be intubated (76,78). Indications for intubation of poisoned patients are listed in Table 3.7.

The patient is placed in the left lateral decubitus position to permit pooling of gastric contents and to reduce the risk of aspiration of gastric contents into the lungs (Fig. 3.3) (82). Also, the patient's head should be slightly lower than the rest of the body. To remove the stomach contents effectively, one should use the largest diameter tube. A 32 French to 40 French or Ewald orogastric tube is recommended for adults and a 16 F to 26 F tube for children.

TABLE 3.6. *Gastric lavage*

Indications
  Semiconsciousness
  Unconscious child or adult
  Loss of gag reflex
  Ipecac-induced emesis is ineffective or
    contraindicated
  Conscious patient ingesting large quantity of
    highly toxic substance, repeated charcoal
    administration is useful
Contraindications
  Corrosives
  Petroleum distillates: awake patient, unless
    distillate is vehicle for toxic substance
  Seizures
Complications/hazards
  Aspiration pneumonia secondary to emesis with
    unprotected airway
  Laryngospasm with cyanosis
Factors determining effectiveness
  Physical characteristics of toxic agent (e.g.,
    plants, capsules, tablets, liquids)
  Rate of absorption of toxic agent
  Diameter of lavage tube
  Volume and rate of instillation of lavage solution

From refs. 76 and 78.

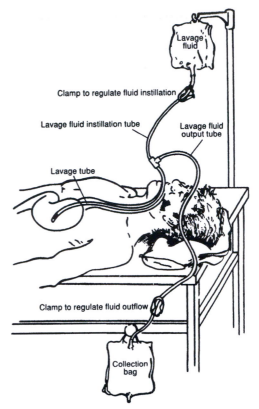

FIG. 3.3. Correct positioning of a patient for performing gastric lavage.

A large-volume reservoir is attached to the gastric hose (Fig. 3.4). In some instances, aspiration of stomach contents with a syringe will remove large amounts of solid dosage forms. The aspirate should be saved for toxicologic analysis.

Lavage is usually initiated using aliquots of tap water or normal saline. Saline is recommended in children to prevent electrolyte imbalance (67,76). Aliquots of 50 to 100 mL in children and 200 to 300 mL in adults should be instilled, allowed to mix, and then drained into a collection bag positioned below the pa-

TABLE 3.7. *Indications for intubation of poisoned patients*

Respiratory insufficiency
Decreased level of consciousness with
  accompanying danger of aspiration
Combativeness to degree that performance of
  therapeutic measures is inhibited
Intoxication with substances that result in rapid
  clinical deterioration (e.g., tricyclic
  antidepressants, calcium channel blockers,
  clonidine)

From ref. 39.

tient. A minimum of 2 L are required to wash out most of the stomach contents.

The consensus is to lavage the stomach until returned fluid is clear (i.e., keep introducing lavage solution into the stomach and withdrawing it until the return solution is clear). Caution must be exercised! There is always the possibility that, even though lavage was performed until the returned fluid was clear, there may still be particles or clumps of chemicals [concretions (see chapter 2)] remaining in the stomach. This point will be illustrated in later chapters.

Lavage is not always a procedure of first choice for removing ingested poisons (43) and may be associated with numerous risks and complications (see Table 3.6). For example, the tube may be accidentally inserted into the

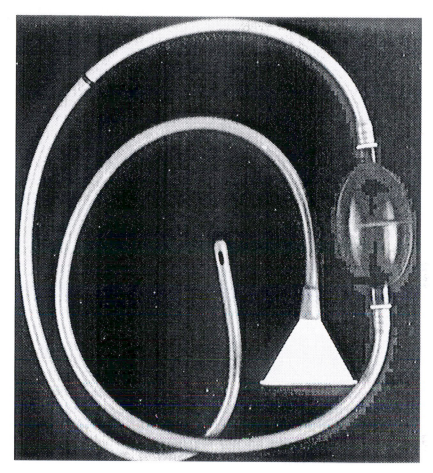

FIG. 3.4. Stomach tube for performing gastric lavage. (Photograph courtesy of Davol Inc.)

trachea. Improperly used lavage can create a greater risk for pulmonary aspiration, esophageal perforation, or hastened gastric emptying time into the intestine. If a cool lavage solution is used too rapidly, the body's core temperature may be dangerously lowered. Gastric lavage is contraindicated for the ingestion of most hydrocarbons, acids, alkali, and sharp objects (26).

Early animal and human studies suggested that gastric lavage was less effective than ipecac in removing ingested poisons (77). Later studies, using larger tube sizes and fluid volumes, clearly demonstrated the procedure's effectiveness (10,13,39). There is still controversy over the value of lavage more than 2 hr

after ingestion. Gastric lavage was shown to be effective in removing some drugs as long as 9 and 27 hr postingestion (53,79). For most toxic ingestions, significant delays impair effectiveness because the stomach empties itself into the small intestine, making retrieval of the toxic agent more difficult.

Adsorbents

Another means to reduce absorption of an ingested poison is by use of an adsorbent. Although several adsorptive substances, including kaolin, Fuller's earth, cholestyramine, pectin, and attapulgite are occasionally recommended, they are not always effective binders of ingested chemicals. Activated charcoal is used for routine adsorption of gastrointestinal poisons. Others are useful with selected poisons. Fuller's earth, for example, has a high affinity for the herbicide paraquat.

Activated Charcoal

Activated charcoal used in the treatment of poisoning can be traced to the time of Hippocrates. The first person specifically to demonstrate its adsorbent activity and usefulness in reducing the absorption of poisonous substances was the French chemist Bertrand. He publicly demonstrated its efficacy in 1813 by swallowing 5 g of arsenic trioxide mixed with activated charcoal. Bertrand suffered no untoward symptoms of toxicity.

A few years later, in 1831, the French pharmacist Touery conducted an even more impressive demonstration. Touery swallowed 10 times the lethal dose of strychnine, which had been mixed with activated charcoal. He stood before members of the French Academy of Medicine for several hours awaiting symptoms of strychnine toxicity, which he was confident would never occur. Luckily, he was correct (22). Although this demonstration must have been dramatic, there is little written evidence today to suggest that it had any significant influence on French medical practice. In fact, it would be another 5 years before the academy formally mentioned it.

Until the past couple of decades, activated charcoal did not receive high praises as an adsorbent (22,63). Few studies demonstrated its absolute role in adsorbing poisons from the GI tract. Prior to this time, it was also common to mix activated charcoal with tannic acid and magnesium oxide to form the traditional "universal antidote," which, for so many years, dominated all other "antidotes" as being the "best method" for treating many cases of ingested poisons. By the mid-1960s, toxicologists had developed renewed interest in activated charcoal and began looking at it more critically. It has been a topic of much research

ever since. Today, activated charcoal has become the most frequently used and most effective agent for gastric decontamination (26).

It can be speculated that there are many reasons why activated charcoal was neglected until recently. Its physical characteristics make it undesirable to force upon a poisoned patient. In some cases it has been used indiscriminately, leading to numerous negative reports of adsorptive value. Many early studies with activated charcoal were conducted with animals or in vitro models, and few attempts were made to correlate these findings with clinical efficacy. Many of the clinical studies were not particularly useful because they analyzed extremely small doses of drugs or poisons that were far below those encountered in most actual poison situations. Many other studies used doses of activated charcoal that were too small to show beneficial action.

Perhaps the greatest deterrent to serious consideration of activated charcoal until recent times relates to the notoriety of the "universal antidote." This mixture (1 part tannic acid, 1 part magnesium oxide, and 2 parts activated charcoal) was popularized years ago as a first-line treatment for poisoning by a variety of substances. Experimental evidence subsequently showed that it was not the effective measure originally promoted. Although it may still be available, the "universal antidote" should not be used (2).

We now know that the activated charcoal component of the "universal antidote" adsorbs part of the magnesium oxide and/or tannic acid (19). This reduces its overall adsorptive property. Some studies have also shown that tannic acid can be hepatotoxic.

Composition

Activated charcoal is a finely divided, black powder that is sparingly soluble in water. It is prepared by pyrolysis of organic materials, such as wood pulp. The activation process occurs when charcoal fragments are exposed to an oxidizing gas composed of steam or oxygen at temperatures of 600° to 900°C (66).

The result is an increased surface area of about 1,000 M^2/g (26) for most charcoals; superactivated charcoals with a surface area of up to 3,500 M^2/g have been manufactured (22). These were recently taken off the market because of detected impurities (26). Not all activated charcoal preparations have the same binding capacity (17,66,94). Although increasing the surface area of activated charcoal should increase its effectiveness, no differences among current formulations are apparent (56).

Commercial activated charcoal tablets and capsules and coal products intended for other purposes, such as water filtration units and fish tanks, are ineffective (72). Also, burnt toast scrapings and crushed coal are unacceptable substitutes for activated charcoal.

Activated charcoal reduces absorption of a wide variety of poisons but has little or no effect on others (Table 3.8). In the stomach and intestine, poisons diffuse through the numerous pores on its surface to form tight chemical bonds. This charcoal-chemical complex then passes through the intestinal tract to reduce the chance of the chemical being absorbed. Effectiveness of adsorption is dependent on the quality of activated charcoal used and the time between ingestion and charcoal administration.

Administration

Activated charcoal is unsightly and readily adsorbs materials from the air and water when mixed and allowed to stand. Therefore, it should be mixed immediately before use with sufficient water, preferably in a dark container to keep youngsters from viewing it! Several commercial products contain a premeasured quantity in a tightly closed, opaque (nontransparent) plastic bottle. Water is added to the powder, the bottle is shaken vigorously, and the mixture is then administered directly from its container. Other preparations are ready-to-use with sorbital added.

Activated charcoal leaves a gritty sensation in the mouth, temporarily discolors the gums

TABLE 3.8. *Properties of activated charcoal*

Dose
  Adult, 50–100 g
  Child, 25–50 g
  Infant, 1 g/kg
Factors affecting efficacy
  Time since ingestion
  Charcoal:drug ratio
  Drug dose
  Stomach contents (pH, composition)
Binds poorly to:
  Elemental metals (lead, lithium, boron, mercury)
  Boric acid
  Cyanide
  Electrolytes
  Ferrous sulfate
  Pesticides (malathion, DDT,[a] N-methylcarbamate)
  Petroleum distillates
  Ethanol
  Methanol
  Mineral acids, alkali
Multiple oral doses useful with:
  Carbamazepine
  Dapsone
  Digitoxin
  Nadolol
  Phenobarbital
  Phenylbutazone
  Theophylline

[a] DDT, dichlorodiphenyltrichloroethane.

and mouth to some extent, and sticks to the throat. For these reasons, children may refuse to drink it. Studies have shown that activated charcoal slurry is tolerated by most children. Liquid activated charcoal slurry preparations that are commercially available should be acceptable to children.

Various flavoring and thickening agents have been added to increase the palatability of activated charcoal (21,44,54,100). These include sodium alginate, carboxymethylcellulose, carrageenin, bentonite, gelatin, ice cream and sherbet, jams and jellies, cocoa powder, fruit syrups, saccharin sodium, and sorbitol.

Caution is advised before any such substance is added. Levy et al. (44) demonstrated that aspirin adsorption onto activated charcoal was reduced by nearly 25% when melted ice cream was mixed with the charcoal. Addition of sorbitol to activated charcoal results in a product with a sweet taste that enhances patient compliance. Sorbitol produces catharsis, which enhances transit time of the activated charcoal-complex through the intestinal tract (61).

Dose

The optimal dose of activated charcoal is uncertain (65). The usual recommended dose is 50 to 100 g for an adult, 25 to 50 g for a child, and 1 g/kg for infants (39). Animal studies suggest that activated charcoal should be given in a relative dose ratio of at least 10:1, charcoal to drug (26,66). This ratio might be unrealistic in a child, however, because activated charcoal is such a fine, light powder, and it is often difficult to estimate the quantity ingested (Fig. 3.5). The important point to remember is that a large enough dose must be given to be effective.

Activated charcoal is pharmacologically inert and not absorbed systemically. Large doses cause occasional constipation but may be used safely. Activated charcoal is contraindicated if there is gastrointestinal obstruction (26).

The use of multiple doses of 1 g of activated charcoal per kg every 2 to 4 hr has been reported to enhance elimination of certain drugs, including aspirin, carbamazepine, cyclosporine, dextropropoxyphene, nadolol, phenobarbital, phenytoin, piroxicam, theophylline, digoxin, digitoxin, and tricyclic antidepressants (5,31,63,65,68,70,90,92). Proposed mechanisms for this effect include interruption of enterohepatic recirculation, adsorption of drug secreted across gastric membranes into the bowel lumen, or continued adsorption of depot-forms of orally administered drug within the GI tract (76). A single dose of sorbitol is often given with the first dose of charcoal, although sorbitol is sometimes given with each dose. The single-dose regimen is preferred.

Minor adverse effects of activated charcoal include nausea and constipation. If sorbitol is added, diarrhea may occur. Serious adverse effects are rare, but multiple doses of activated charcoal have been associated with intestinal obstruction (47,96).

Time Interval and Efficacy

For maximal effectiveness, activated charcoal should be administered within 30 min of poison ingestion. However, when used to adsorb drugs that slow gastric emptying (e.g., anticholinergics and sedatives), beneficial results have been obtained when activated charcoal was given 6 to 8 hr after poison ingestion. Following aspirin ingestion, a 9- to 10-hr interval between ingestion of drug and charcoal has still produced beneficial results.

Two studies illustrate that charcoal effectively reduces the quantity of various drugs and chemicals in the GI tract. In the first investigation subjects received a dose of phenobarbital alone or with charcoal concurrently, at various time intervals (62). Activated charcoal was effective even when administered 10 to 48 hr after drug ingestion (Fig. 3.6).

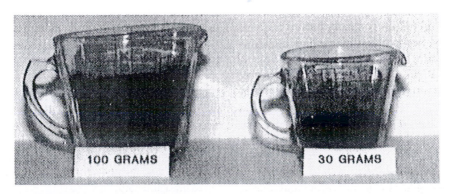

FIG. 3.5. Graphic illustration showing the bulkiness of 30 g and 100 g of activated charcoal.

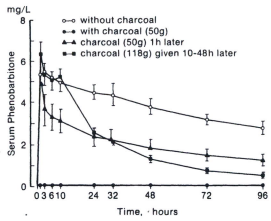

FIG. 3.6. Effect of activated charcoal on serum phenobarbitone (phenobarbital) concentration. Subjects received 200 mg phenobarbitone with or without activated charcoal. (From ref. 62.)

In another study (Fig. 3.7), volunteers were given nortriptyline followed by a single dose of activated charcoal 30 min later or multiple doses ranging over the next 6 hr (16). The results clearly indicate that repeated administration of the adsorbent reduced absorption of nortriptyline better than did a single dose.

Kulig et al. (43) evaluated the efficacy of gastric decontamination in 592 acute oral drug overdose patients. The effect of activated charcoal alone on clinical outcome was compared to that of syrup of ipecac or gastric lavage followed by activated charcoal. Results demonstrated that patients receiving activated charcoal alone did just as well as the comparison group. The investigators noted that use of

syrup of ipecac delayed administration of the charcoal by more than 2 hr. Also, the value of gastric lavage was questionable if performed more than 1 hr postingestion.

Use of Activated Charcoal with Ipecac or N-Acetylcysteine

It has been stated that activated charcoal should not be given within 30 min of syrup of ipecac unless the victim has already vomited (25). If both substances are to be administered, ipecac should precede the charcoal. This is important to remember because emetine and cephaeline, which comprise over 90% of the active emetic alkaloids of ipecac (14), are adsorbed onto activated charcoal, thus negating their pharmacologic action.

More recent investigation suggests that the two substances can be given within 10 min of each other (28). In one study, emesis was successfully induced in patients given 60 mL of syrup of ipecac followed 5 min later by activated charcoal (40).

Although activated charcoal has been shown to bind acetaminophen effectively, it is not recommended for concurrent use when *N*-acetylcysteine is indicated as the antidote for acute acetaminophen poisoning (34) (see chapter 12). A recent study reported no significant difference in *N*-acetylcysteine serum concentrations, peak concentrations, or half-life after *N*-acetylcysteine alone or *N*-acetylcysteine plus activated charcoal (73).

Cathartics

Saline cathartics are preferred by most experts when catharsis is desired to remove toxic substances from the GI tract, although there have been few studies to evaluate their effectiveness. A rule of thumb is that, whenever contact time between the poison and absorption sites is reduced, the potential for toxicity will likewise be lessened (88). Commonly used cathartics and recommended doses are listed in Table 3.9.

Catharsis should not be attempted when the

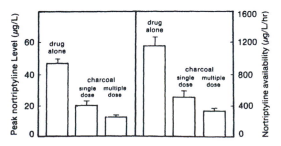

FIG. 3.7. Effect of activated charcoal on peak plasma nortriptyline levels and nortriptyline availability. (From ref. 16.)

TABLE 3.9. *Cathartics used in poison treatment*

Cathartic	Dose	
	Child	Adult
Magnesium sulfate 10% (epsom salts)	250 mg/kg	5–10 g
Magnesium citrate (Citrate of Magnesia)	4 mL/kg	250–300 mL
Sodium sulfate 10%	250 mg/kg	15–20 g
Sodium sulfate/sodium phosphate (Fleet Phosphosoda)	20 mL[a]	40 mL[a]
Sorbitol	1.5 g/kg[b]	1.5 g/kg (50 mL)

[a] Diluted with water.
[b] Use with caution.

poison is strongly corrosive, the patient has electrolyte disturbance, or bowel sounds are absent. Aside from a few exceptions, including castor oil for phenol intoxication and mineral oil for fat-soluble vitamin overdoses, no stimulant or lubricant cathartic or laxative other than saline catharsis should be recommended. Additionally, magnesium-containing cathartics should not be given to persons with compromised renal function because of the possibility of causing CNS depression due to accumulation of high concentrations of magnesium in the serum. Sodium-containing cathartics are, likewise, best avoided by persons with congestive heart failure or other conditions where fluid retention would pose significant danger (83). Use of concentrated disodium phosphate enema (Fleet Phospho-Soda) has led to hypernatremia, hyperphosphatemia, and hypocalcemia (7,52,74). Multiple-dose cathartic therapy has resulted in severe hypermagnesemia even in patients with good renal function (86). Metabolic disturbances are the most common consequences of acute cathartic use (83).

The efficacy of saline cathartics to decrease drug absorption has been evaluated by many investigators (23,41,85). Evacuation action of saline cathartics inconsistently decreases drug absorption and may require several hours (12,88). In another study, examining the effect of saline cathartics on the efficacy of activated charcoal showed that addition of a saline cathartic to the regimen of a patient receiving activated charcoal does not enhance the effect of charcoal alone (85).

The use of sorbitol at doses of 1 to 1.5 g/ kg as a cathartic has recently been advocated over other osmotically active drugs. It may be a superior cathartic to both magnesium and sodium sulfate (39) and may become the cathartic of choice when such activity is desired. Moreover, it is associated with the fewest electrolyte abnormalities and has the shortest gastrointestinal transit time (26).

Whole Bowel Irrigation

A new therapy that looks promising for gastric decontamination is whole bowel irrigation (26). The procedure is also used to cleanse the entire gastrointestinal tract before surgery. The solution most commonly used is a sodium sulfate and polyethylene glycol electrolyte solution (e.g., Golytely, Colyte) that is not absorbed and does not lead to fluid or electrolyte imbalance.

Experimental studies have shown decreased absorption for salicylates, lithium, and ampicillin. Whole bowel irrigation has also been used in overdoses of iron and zinc sulfate and in removing ingestions of cocaine packets. Whole bowel irrigation seems to be safe in children.

Demulcents

Occasionally a demulcent is all that is needed to treat a poisoning. Many plants and chemicals cause oral and gastric mucosal irritation but no serious toxicity. Management of these acute ingestions may include ice cream, milk, or another soothing demulcent to reduce irritation. Egg whites (up to a dozen for an adult), which serve as a source of readily available protein, have been given for corrosive intoxications and can be unofficially classed as a demulcent.

Demulcents are also of benefit when treatment is not needed but it is obvious that the patient or parent demands that "something be done!" Thus, a demulcent frequently serves as important placebo or palliative therapy.

Topical Decontamination

Numerous lipid-soluble chemicals can be absorbed through the skin and cause systemic toxicity within minutes. After dermal exposures, all contaminated clothing should be removed. Skin should be thoroughly flushed with water and washed with mild soap. Some recommend that tincture of green soap (soft soap liniment, which contains 30% alcohol) be used to clean the area, as its alcohol content will solubilize some poisons. Few homes have tincture of green soap available, and valuable time may be lost while trying to locate it. Ordinary soap is adequate for most routine procedures.

No creams, ointments, or occlusive bandages should be placed over the contaminated area. These would have to be removed before a physician could treat the area.

The eye poses a special problem with spilled or splashed chemicals. Many substances are absorbed within minutes through the cornea, causing permanent damage, including loss of eyesight. When ocular contamination occurs, irrigation with lukewarm water must be immediately instituted and continued for at least 15 to 20 min. Contact lenses, if present, should be removed and the eyes held directly under a softly flowing stream of water. Medicine droppers or irrigation syringes are inadequate for rinsing the eyes because they do not hold a sufficient reservoir of water. The victim should seek medical attention immediately after irrigation.

METHODS TO INCREASE ELIMINATION OF TOXIC AGENTS

It was previously stated that repeated dosing with activated charcoal can reduce blood levels of certain drugs. Other methods of enhancing the elimination of a toxic agent include forced diuresis and pH alteration, peritoneal dialysis, hemodialysis, hemoperfusion, and the use of specific antibodies. After gastric decontamination, the next logical step in the management of a poisoned patient is to address methods for eliminating the toxic agent that has been absorbed into the blood. The factors listed in Table 3.10 are useful in determining when methods to enhance elimination will be applicable.

Forced Diuresis and pH Alteration

Forced diuresis was once recommended to help remove chemicals and drugs from blood. It is useful when compounds or active metabolites are eliminated by the kidney and diuresis enhances their excretion. Although many diuretic agents have been recommended over the years, either mannitol or furosemide was generally used. The use of these drugs in overdoses was fraught with complications, such as pulmonary and cerebral edema. This method of enhanced renal elimination is no longer recommended. At best, forced diuresis may increase excretion of a chemical twofold.

Many toxic compounds are weak acids or

TABLE 3.10. *Indications for use of methods to enhance elimination of a toxic agent*

Patient presents with overt signs and symptoms of toxicity.
Patient's status deteriorates despite good supportive care.
Amount of toxic agent ingested is likely to produce significant toxicity or death.
Blood concentration of the toxic agent absorbed is likely to produce significant toxicity or death.
Normal routes of detoxification and elimination of the toxic agent are impaired.
Patient ingested significant quantity of an agent that is metabolized to a toxic metabolite.

weak bases and in solution become ionized. The degree of ionization depends upon the dissociation constant (Ka) of the compound and the pH of the medium; the ratio of ionized to nonionized form of the compound is governed by the Henderson-Hasselbach equation. At physiologic pH, most drugs are partially ionized. The pKa of a particular compound is 50% ionized (polar) and 50% nonionized (nonpolar). Weak acids have a pKa between 3.0 and 7.5, and the pKa of weak bases ranges from 7.5 to 10.5.

Nonionized (nonpolar) compounds move easily across cell membranes, whereas ionized (polar) compounds are much less diffusible. The goal of urinary pH manipulation is to enhance renal excretion of a compound by increasing the amount of the ionized (polar) form in the kidney. As toxic agents pass through the kidney, they are filtered, secreted, and reabsorbed across the tubular membrane. The ionized (polar) form is trapped in the renal tubule and excreted; the nonionized form is reabsorbed in the blood. The purpose of pH manipulation is to present to the kidney the compound in its ionized (polar) form so that renal elimination of that compound is enhanced. Ideally, increased elimination of weak acids will occur when urinary pH is more alkaline. Conversely, enhanced elimination of weak bases will occur when urinary pH is nonacidic.

Alkaline diuresis is achieved by administration of sodium bicarbonate, 1 to 2 mEq/kg every 3 to 4 hr. The objective is to increase urinary pH to between 7 and 8. This will be virtually impossible unless any potassium chloride deficiency has been corrected. The potential uses of urine alkalinization have been with weak acids, such as salicylates, phenobarbital, and 2,4-dichlorophenoxyacetic acid (2,4-D) (45,59,71).

Acid diuresis is possible by using ammonium chloride, 75 mg/kg/24 hr. The endpoint for acidification is a urinary pH between 5.5 and 6.0. At one time, acid diuresis was favored to increase the elimination of weak bases, such as amphetamines, phencyclidine, and quinidine. However, because of complications of using acid diuresis and its questionable effectiveness, it is no longer recommended.

Dialysis and Hemoperfusion

The following procedures are limited in scope and not routinely performed for every toxic ingestion. They are used as adjuncts to management of severely intoxicated patients.

The frequency and severity of complications that may develop after drug overdoses increase with the length of time the patient remains unconscious (3,6). It is desirable to reduce this time by any means available. Even though the concentration of toxic agent in the blood has decreased and the victim has awakened, irreversible damage may have occurred. To illustrate, a patient who ingested approximately 100 mL of carbon tetrachloride (an otherwise lethal dose) awoke after 7 hr of hemoperfusion, but irreversible pulmonary insufficiency and hepatic damage appeared weeks later (99).

Dialysis and perfusion methods should never replace the use of more specific treatment or antidotes. A patient with an acute opioid overdose, for example, is best treated with naloxone, the specific antidote. These procedures would be of little value in treating acute ingestion of cytotoxic poisons, such as cyanide, which produce toxic effects very rapidly, often within minutes. Furthermore, if the ingested drug has a high therapeutic index, these procedures would have questionable value.

Dialysis is governed by the laws of osmosis (69). A diffusible chemical dissolved in water partitions across a semipermeable membrane, and the solution moves from an area of higher concentration (i.e., the blood) to one of lower concentration (i.e., a dialyzing solution). The utility of dialysis in treating drug and chemical intoxications has expanded over the past decade. The literature now documents numerous studies that compare the efficacy of different dialytic procedures for removing toxic substances.

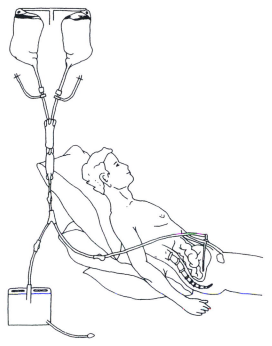

FIG. 3.8. Procedure for peritoneal dialysis.

Peritoneal Dialysis

Peritoneal dialysis is the most easily performed method and is associated with the lowest risk for complications. However, it is also the least effective method for removing most poisons.

The procedure is undertaken by inserting a tube through a small incision made in the midabdominal area into the peritoneum (Fig. 3.8). The peritoneal membrane serves as the semipermeable (dialyzing) membrane. In this way, the dialyzable chemical diffuses from blood across the peritoneal membrane into the dialyzing fluid (moves from an area of higher to lower concentration). A warmed sterile dialyzing solution (up to 2 L for adults and 1 L for children) is introduced into the peritoneal cavity over a period of 15 to 20 min. The fluid is left in place for 45 to 60 min for equilibration to occur and then removed. A fresh solution is reintroduced and the process repeated. Up to 30 L or more of dialysis fluid may be used.

The dialysis solution normally consists of a balanced electrolyte solution, although various solutions from different manufacturers vary in composition. The osmotic pressure of the fluid is maintained above that of extracellular fluid with dextrose. By making the dialysis fluid hypertonic, there should be an increased recovery of water-soluble chemicals. For chemicals that are highly protein-bound, addition of albumin to the dialyzing solution may be helpful to increase recovery. The dialysis solution may also be modified by adjusting its pH. In acute phenobarbital ingestion, for example, using an alkaline solution may considerably increase total drug recovery. Some dialysis procedures use lipids such as peanut oil to attract such chemicals as glutethimide, which are highly lipid soluble.

In general, peritoneal dialysis is 5 to 10 times less efficient than hemodialysis (8,84). It is not the procedure of choice when rapid removal of a toxic substance is needed. On the other hand, peritoneal dialysis does not require elaborate equipment and needs little medical supervision.

Complications of peritoneal dialysis include abdominal pain; intraperitoneal bleeding; intestinal, bladder, liver, or spleen perforation; peritonitis; water and electrolyte imbalance; and protein loss.

Hemodialysis

The same basic principles apply to hemodialysis (extracorporeal dialysis). For peritoneal dialysis, an *in vivo* (peritoneal) membrane is utilized; in hemodialysis, however, a cellophane bag (artificial kidney) forms the semipermeable membrane.

Two catheters are inserted into the patient's femoral vein, about 2 inches apart. Blood is pumped from one catheter through the dialysis unit, across the semipermeable membrane, and back through the other catheter. The procedure is usually continued for 6 to 8 hr. The solubilized chemical diffuses across the semipermeable membrane into the dialysis solution. Clearance of the toxic agent is based on differences in osmotic and concentration gradients.

If a chemical is to be effectively removed by dialysis, it must have a low molecular weight and small molecular size to diffuse passively across the dialyzing membrane. Usually, chemicals with molecular weights greater than 500 daltons do not cross the membrane. Since only free chemical diffuses from blood into the dialysis solution (proteins are too large to pass through the membrane), hemodialysis is less effective for drugs that are highly protein-bound.

The effectiveness of hemodialysis is determined by the rate of clearance, plasma concentration, and duration of dialysis. This means that certain pharmacokinetic parameters may be helpful in estimating whether a particular chemical can be dialyzed. For example, if the volume of distribution (V_d) is greater than 250 to 300 L, less chemical per unit of blood is available for elimination by dialysis. Chemicals such as salicylates, which have a small volume of distribution, are more readily removed by dialysis because the plasma concentrations are greater in relation to the total amount of drug in the body. Additionally, there is a high concentration gradient between the blood and dialysis solution. Hemodialysis is virtually useless for chemicals that are extensively taken up by tissues because, at steady state, they circulate only at very small concentrations. Also, unless the overall clearance of a chemical with dialysis is much greater than the total body clearance rate, the elimination half-life of the drug is not significantly shortened.

Complications include clotting and seepage of blood from around connections, hypoten-

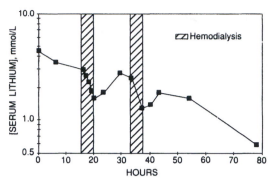

FIG. 3.9. Serum concentrations of lithium in a patient who took an intentional overdose. Blood samples were taken before, during, and after two hemodialyses. (From ref. 69.)

sion, convulsions, arrhythmias, infection, and hematologic defects.

Figure 3.9 illustrates the effectiveness of hemodialysis. Serum concentrations of lithium are shown to decrease appreciably during the procedure. For other examples, see the case studies at the end of this chapter and chapter 4.

Hemoperfusion

Hemoperfusion is significantly more effective than peritoneal dialysis and hemodialysis (Table 3.11) for removing intoxicating compounds, particularly those that are lipid soluble or protein bound or those that, for other reasons, are poorly dialyzable. A list of common poisonous substances that are easily removed by hemoperfusion is shown in Table 3.12.

TABLE 3.11. *Comparison of hemodialysis with hemoperfusion*

Chemical	Hemodialysis[a]	Charcoal hemoperfusion[a]	Resin hemoperfusion[a]
Phenobarbital	0.27	0.5	0.8−0.9
Amobarbital	0.26	0.3	0.9
Paraquat	0.5	0.6	0.9
Carbromal	0.25−0.4	0.5−0.6	1
Digoxin	0.15	0.3−0.6	0.4
Glutethimide	0.16	0.6−0.7	0.8
Methaqualone	0.13	0.4−1	0.5−1

From ref. 99.
[a] Expressed as plasma extraction ratio: PER = inlet concentration − outlet concentration/inlet concentration.

TABLE 3.12. *Partial list of poisonous substances removed by hemoperfusion*

Barbiturates
  Amobarbital
  Butabarbital
  Carbromal
  Pentobarbital
  Phenobarbital
  Secobarbital
Nonbarbiturate sedatives
  Ethchlorvynol
  Glutethimide
  Methyprylon
  Methaqualone
  Diazepam
  Chloral hydrate
  Chlorpromazine
  Promazine
  Meprobamate
Analgesics
  Aspirin
  Methyl salicylate
  Acetaminophen
Antidepressants
  Amitriptyline
  Desipramine
Cardiovascular agents
  Digoxin
  Procainamide
Miscellaneous
  Amanita phalloides (poisonous mushrooms)
  Carbamazepine
  Carbon tetrachloride
  Ethylene glycol
  Organochlorine insecticides
  Ethylene oxide
  Lithium
  Methotrexate
  Paraquat
  Polychlorinated biphenyls
  Selected organophosphate insecticides
  Theophylline

From refs. 69 and 99.

The ability of activated charcoal to adsorb toxic substances has been recognized for many years. Numerous analytical procedures have used anion exchange resins, as well as nonionic resins, such as Amberite XAD-2, to separate drugs. Consequently, either of the resins may be used.

Regardless of the type of adsorbent used, blood is withdrawn via an arteriovenous or venovenous shunt (Fig. 3.10) and passed directly over the adsorbing material contained in sterile columns (Fig. 3.11). The procedure is simple, and columns are commercially available.

Indications for hemoperfusion in severe intoxications are evaluated by two important criteria. The first consideration is whether the adsorbent will eliminate the chemical from the blood. Second, the volume of distribution must be small and the half-life of the intoxicant relatively long, so that the drug can continue to be drawn from the tissues to the blood and consequently removed.

Primary complications include trapping of white blood cells and platelets and microembolization. These problems have largely been eliminated with newer systems. When thrombocytopenia (decreased platelets) does occur, it seldom poses a significant problem in treating overdoses.

SPECIFIC ANTIDOTES

Although there are some specific antidotes based on their pharmacologic activities, relatively few are actually used for treatment of poisoning. Specific antidotes are explained only briefly in this chapter but are discussed in more detail in appropriate chapters as they are applicable for specific poisonings. A list of common antidotes and formulations and their recommended uses is given in Table 3.13.

Classification of Specific Antidotes

Specific antidotes may be classified into one of four categories: chemical, receptor, dispositional, and functional. *Chemical antidotes* react with the poisonous chemical to produce a compound of lesser toxicity or one that is absorbed to lesser degree than the parent compound. In oxalic acid poisoning, absorption produces renal damage. Calcium salts react with oxalic acid to yield a poorly soluble compound, calcium oxalate, which passes through the intestines without being absorbed.

Antidotes such as dimercaprol [British antilewisite (BAL)], deferoxamine (Desferal), and succimer (Chemet) form chemical chelates with heavy metals. Chelated complexes are water soluble and readily excreted by the kidney.

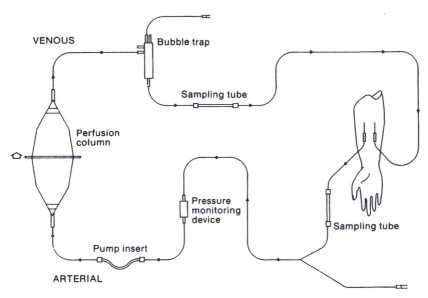

FIG. 3.10. Diagram illustrating hemoperfusion technique for removing poisonous compounds from the blood.

Receptor antidotes compete with the poison for receptor sites. Examples include naloxone reversal of morphine-induced respiratory depression and cholinergic blockade by atropine.

For atropine or other anticholinergic poisons, physostigmine is a specific antidote. Physostigmine is a reversible cholinesterase inhibitor. Although it does not directly block atropine's effects by competing with it for muscarinic receptor sites, it inhibits the activity of plasma pseudocholinesterase. This inhibition results in increased acetylcholine levels, which then compete with atropine for its receptor sites.

Dispositional antagonism involves alteration of absorption, metabolism, distribution, or excretion of toxic agents to reduce the amount available to tissues. In acetaminophen overdose, for example, a toxic metabolite causes hepatotoxicity. Conversion of this toxic intermediate to a nontoxic form proceeds by conjugation with glutathione, a sulfhydryl (-SH) group donor. When glutathione reserves are depleted, as occurs after massive overdoses of acetaminophen, toxic manifestations appear. *N*-Acetylcysteine is also a source of sulfhydryl groups, which serve the same function as endogenous glutathione. Acetamino-phen and its toxic metabolite are therefore detoxified with *N*-acetylcysteine administration, and the liver cells are not subjected to prolonged toxicity.

A *functional (physiologic) antagonist* acts on one biochemical system to produce effects that are opposite from those produced on another system. For example, during an anaphylactic reaction after administration of a drug, the individual experiences severe breathing difficulties, due in part to intense bronchoconstriction. Epinephrine reverses this effect, and breathing is normalized.

SUMMARY

Common sense is the dictum that governs most procedures discussed in this chapter. Successful management of acute poisonings requires a systematic plan. Management of poisoned patients is based largely on clinical experience rather than tested methods.

Before proceeding to the next chapter, review the procedures outlined for management of acute poisonings. Take special effort to understand when a treatment should be used and when treatment would be considered detrimental to the patient.

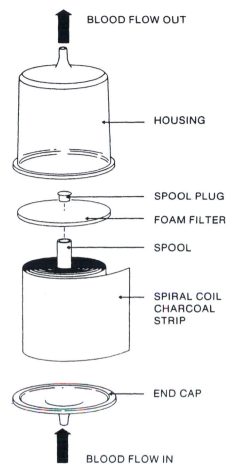

FIG. 3.11. Illustration showing the components of a hemoperfusion cartridge.

Case Studies

CASE STUDY: FATAL POISONING FROM A SALT EMETIC

History

A 3-year-old boy was given an unmeasured quantity of salt in water to induce emesis after his mother discovered that he had ingested 36 baby aspirin tablets (81 mg each). The boy did not vomit, and so he was taken to the hospital. Three hours after receiving the salt solution at home, he underwent lavage with saline solution. Shortly, he lost consciousness. Approximately 3 hr after the lavage proce-

dure, he experienced a tonic-clonic convulsion. Although convulsions were managed with anticonvulsant therapy, he died 2 days later of cardiac arrest.

During his hospitalization, the victim's serum sodium concentration was approximately 180 mEq/L; it remained elevated throughout the period. His heart rate had increased to 220 beats/min. There were no murmurs or signs of cardiac enlargement and no history of congestive heart failure. Toward the end he developed respiratory arrest and required mechanical ventilation. Two separate electroencephalograms, taken 24 hr apart, showed no evidence of electrical activity. Symptoms of aspirin intoxication were present but not severe, and aspirin was not considered to be a major factor in his death.

Autopsy permission was not given. All sequelae were consistent with CNS abnormalities caused by hypernatremia. (See ref. 4.)

Discussion

1. Explain how hypernatremia could lead to CNS abnormalities and cause this child's death. Why do you suppose he died from cardiac failure?
2. Was lavage with saline (approximately 3 hr after the victim was first given the salt solution) wise or unwise?
3. It has been calculated that a level tablespoonful of salt contains at least 250 mEq sodium. This is a sufficient quantity to raise the serum sodium concentration in a 3-year-old child, if all is retained, by 25 mEq/L. (The child's mother did not recall how much salt she had given the boy; we can only guess it was excessive.) Knowing that this sodium level is inconsistent with life, what conclusions can you draw about recommending salt solution for emesis?

CASE STUDIES: IPECAC MISUSE

History: Case 1

Ipecac syrup was prescribed for a 23-month-old girl after she swallowed an un-

TABLE 3.13. *Selected antidotes and formulations for treating poisoning*

Antidote/formulation	Use(s) or application in poisoning
N-Acetylcysteine	Acetaminophen
Activated charcoal	General adsorbent
α- and β-Adrenergic blockers	Sympathomimetic
Atropine	Cholinesterase inhibitors, β-adrenergic blockers, bradycardia to digitalis, certain mushrooms
Bicarbonate, sodium	Aspirin, tricyclic antidepressants
Botulism antitoxin	*Clostridium botulinum*
Calcium	Oxalates, fluorides, ethylene glycol, calcium channel blockers
Calcium gluconate	Hydrofluoric acid burns
Chlorpromazine	Amphetamine
Cyanide antidote kit (nitrites and sodium thiosulfate)	Cyanide
Deferoxamine	Iron salts
Dextrose in water 50%	Hypoglycemic agents, altered mental status
Diazepam	CNS stimulants
Digoxin Fab antibody fragments	Digoxin, digitoxin
Dimercaprol (BAL)[a]	Arsenic, other selected metals
Dopamine HCl[b]	Hypotension
Edrophonium chloride	Anticholinergic agents
EDTA[c]	Lead
Epinephrine	Anaphylactic reactions
Ethanol	Methanol, ethylene glycol
Flumazenil	Benzodiazepines
Folinic acid (leucovorin)	Methotrexate
Fuller's earth	Paraquat
Glucagon	β-Adrenergic blockers, calcium channel blockers, oral hypoglycemics
Ipecac syrup	General-use emetic
Magnesium citrate	General (oral cathartic)
Magnesium sulfate (Epsom salts)	General (oral cathartic)
Mannitol	Osmotic diuretic, cerebral edema, rhabdomyolysis, myoglobinuria
Methylene blue	Methemoglobinemia
Naloxone	Opioids
Nitroprusside	Hypertension
Norepinephrine	Hypotension
Oxygen	Carbon monoxide, cyanide, methemoglobinemia
Penicillamine	Copper, other selected metals
Phenytoin	Seizures
Physostigmine	Anticholinergic agents
Pralidoxime	Organophosphorous insecticides
Protamine sulfate	Heparin
Pyridoxine HCl	Isoniazid
Snake antivenom	Snake bites (coral and pit viper)
Sorbitol	Cathartic
Starch	Iodine
Succimer	Lead
Sympathomimetics	α- and β-Adrenergic blocking drugs, antihypertensives
Thiamine HCl	Thiamine deficiency, ethylene glycol
Vitamin K$_1$	Oral anticoagulants

From refs. 32, 42, and 91.
[a] BAL, British antilewisite.
[b] HCl, hydrochloride.
[c] EDTA, ethylenediaminetetraacetic acid.

known number of tablets of an antiemetic preparation (no longer marketed). A physician instructed the child's baby-sitter to give the child 1 teaspoonful every 5 min until she vomited, and a 120 mL bottle of syrup of ipecac was dispensed.

Two hours later, the baby-sitter was worried because the baby had become very drowsy and still had not vomited. It was estimated that 90 mL of syrup of ipecac had been given to the child by this time.

On admission to the emergency department, the child was extremely drowsy but responsive to stimuli. Her pupils were constricted; blood pressure was 95/65 mm Hg; respirations, 20/min; and pulse, 120 beats/min. Gastric lavage was performed, followed by a dose of magnesium sulfate.

The next morning she began to exhibit cardiac arrhythmias but was alert about 6 hr after admission. She recovered uneventfully. (See ref. 1.)

History: Case 2

A 26-year-old woman presented to the emergency department with palpitations, chest tightness, exertional dyspnea, and extreme fatigue that had been persistent for the past 10 days. Medications included oral contraceptives (discontinued 1 month before admission) and amphetamines (discontinued 10 days before admission). To lose weight she had been consuming three to four 1-ounce bottles of syrup of ipecac daily, after meals, for 3 months.

On admission, her blood pressure was 75/60 mm Hg; pulse, 150 beats/min; respirations, 20/min; and temperature, 36.7°C. Electrocardiogram recordings showed supraventricular tachycardia (150 beats/min). The patient became severely hypotensive and dyspneic and steadily worsened. Despite intensive medical treatment, she died of ventricular arrhythmias. (See ref. 9.)

History: Case 3

An 18-year-old woman had suffered with anorexia nervosa for several years. Her ado-

lescent desire to decrease food intake gradually turned into periods of starvation and bulimia (constant craving for food; abnormal eating binges). Her obsession with dieting was probably due to some deeply rooted emotional process. To increase weight loss, she began to use indiscriminately about 60 Ex-Lax tablets (phenolphthalein—a stimulant cathartic) per day. Over a period of 2.5 years, the patient lost approximately 35% of her original body weight (71 kg).

For the next 5 months, she used syrup of ipecac for its emetic effects. On a weekly basis, she probably ingested close to 300 mL in doses up to 85 mL each. This made her extremely weak, and she was constantly fatigued.

She was finally admitted to a hospital by her family physician because of tiredness, slurred speech, dysphagia, and weight loss. On admission she weighed 54.5 kg. Her blood pressure was 80/44 mm Hg (supine); pulse was 76 beats/min. She displayed severe skeletal muscular weakness. Laboratory results were unremarkable except for mild neutropenia, lymphocytosis, transient increase in serum glutamate oxaloacetate transaminase (SGOT), and increase in creatinine phosphokinase (CPK) and uric acid. Her electrocardiogram (ECG) showed some minor T-wave changes and sinus arrhythmias.

Treatment of this individual consisted of psychotherapy and discontinuing the use of the laxative and ipecac. She improved considerably by 5 months. (See ref. 49.)

History: Case 4

A 3-year-old boy was admitted to an emergency facility with status epilepticus of unknown cause. The previous evening the child had ingested three 100-mg tablets of propoxyphene napsylate, and his mother promptly notified a poison control center. Her instructions were to obtain a bottle of syrup of ipecac, give the child 1 tablespoonful followed by water, and repeat the dose only once if vomiting did not occur within 15 to 20 min.

Following these instructions, she sent a nephew to the local pharmacy. The pharmacist was unable to find any small bottles of syrup of ipecac, but he did find an old, half-filled bottle in the back room labeled "ipecac." He dispensed this preparation to the boy. The substance was eventually identified as fluid extract of ipecac.

The victim was given 1 tablespoonful of this preparation. Twenty minutes later, the mother tried unsuccessfully to give him another tablespoonful, since he had not vomited with the initial dose. He soon began to vomit and continued for the next 12 hr. Six hours before his hospital admission, he had an episode of profuse watery diarrhea. Also, opisthotonic generalized convulsions occurred about an hour before he was brought to the hospital.

On admission the child presented with tachypnea. Pulse was 140 beats/min; respirations, 35/min; blood pressure, 110/80 mm Hg; and temperature, 101.7°F. There was generalized abdominal tenderness, and bowel sounds were normal. Watery diarrhea persisted for several days. Electrocardiogram monitoring revealed T-wave inversion, and the child had extreme muscular weakness.

The child was treated with phenobarbital to control seizures and was given glucose intravenously. He remained in the hospital for 2 weeks and was given supportive and symptomatic care. Follow-up examination revealed normal growth, development, and hematologic profiles. (See ref. 57.)

Discussion

1. In all cases, cardiac arrhythmias were present. Why did they occur?
2. In case 2, how many milliliters of syrup of ipecac did the patient ingest per day? How does this compare to case 3? Syrup of ipecac contains approximately 0.17 mg of emetine per mL. What was the dose of emetine per day of the patient in case 2?
3. How many equivalent teaspoonfuls of syrup of ipecac did the victim in case 4

receive with 1 tablespoonful of fluid extract of ipecac?
4. How does syrup of ipecac induce vomiting? What is the most logical explanation for why it did not induce vomiting in case 1?
5. There are many lessons to be learned from these case studies. For example, in case 1, what specific instructions on dosing syrup of ipecac should the physician and pharmacist have told the baby-sitter? In case 4, what could the pharmacist who dispensed the fluid extract product have done to prevent this poisoning from ever happening?

CASE STUDY: EFFECTIVENESS OF CHARCOAL HEMOPERFUSION

History

A 48-year-old woman was brought to the emergency department 2 hr after ingesting 50 200-mg aminophylline tablets (10 g aminophylline containing 8.5 g theophylline) prescribed for an asthmatic condition. On admission, she was lethargic and confused but coherent. Her blood pressure had "bottomed-out" (50/0 mm Hg), and cardiac arrhythmias were present.

Initial treatment consisted of lavage, followed by activated charcoal and a saline cathartic (magnesium citrate). Lidocaine was given to control the arrhythmias. She was in severe metabolic acidosis with an arterial pH of 6.59. She became nonresponsive and anuric and had a grand mal seizure. Serum theophylline concentration was 190 μg/mL (50 μg/mL is frequently associated with seizures, hypotension, and arrhythmias), and her prognosis was grave.

At this point, approximately 9 hr after admission, she was placed on charcoal hemoperfusion. Within 1 hr, blood pressure and urine output improved, as well as all other signs of theophylline toxicity. Charcoal hemoperfusion was continued for 5 additional hours. She recovered with some residual neurologic deficiency due to the cerebral anoxia. (See ref. 24.)

Discussion

1. Explain the meaning of the patient's blood pressure, described as "bottomed-out." What caused this to occur?
2. Explain how the anuric state and metabolic acidosis are related to theophylline overdose.
3. Compare the rate of elimination of serum theophylline before, during, and after charcoal hemoperfusion. Are you convinced hemoperfusion was of benefit? If so, what specific event(s) led you to your decision?

CASE STUDY: MULTIPLE-DOSE ACTIVATED CHARCOAL AS ADJUNCT THERAPY AFTER CHRONIC PHENYTOIN INTOXICATION

History

The patient was a 67-year-old, thin woman whose history included alcohol abuse, hepatic cirrhosis, hepatic encephalopathy, and a seizure disorder. She was admitted to the hospital because of altered mental status. Four months previously she had been admitted because of phenytoin toxicity.

On this admission she was lethargic and ataxic but arousable. Her speech was dysarthric, and she had decreased movements of the right upper and lower extremities. The remainder of her physical examination was unremarkable.

Laboratory data included prothrombin time, 19.8 sec (control, 10.2 to 11.7 sec); activated partial thromboplastin time, 48 sec (control, 22 to 31 sec); serum albumin concentration, 30g/dL (normal, 3.5 to 5 g/L); total bilirubin concentration, 1.4 mg/dL (normal, 0.1 to 1 mg/dL); and serum phenytoin concentration, less than 0.5 mg/L (usual therapeutic range, 10 to 20 mg/L). A computed tomographic (CT) scan of the head showed cortical and cerebellar atrophy but no evidence of acute hemorrhage. Cerebrovascular fluid was unremarkable. She received 100 mg of thiamine hydrochloride, 50 mL of 50% dextrose solution, and 0.4 mg of naloxone hydrochloride without improvement in her mental status. Because of her seizure disorder, phenytoin was prescribed, 300 mg orally twice a day. Over the next 3 days her mental status improved, and her neurologic examination became nonfocal.

On hospital day 3 the patient's serum phenytoin concentration was 11.7 mg/L. Phenytoin therapy was continued. By day 7 her mental status had deteriorated. She was incoherent and agitated, with slurred speech, and was oriented only to person. Her serum phenytoin concentration was 44.4 mg/L. Phenytoin therapy was discontinued; however, the patient's mental status did not improve over the next 2 days. Her serum phenytoin concentration on day 9 was 45.2 mg/dL. A repeat CT scan of the head was unchanged. Her serum glucose concentration was normal.

Treatment consisted of 30 g activated charcoal mixed in 70% sorbitol solution given by nasogastric tube every 4 hr beginning on day 9 of hospitalization. Lactulose was given every 4 hr. The following day the patient was slightly improved; serum phenytoin concentration was 40.0 mg/L. Therapy with activated charcoal/sorbitol was continued. By the following day there was substantial improvement in mental status; the serum phenytoin concentration was 16.6 mg/L. Activated charcoal/sorbitol was discontinued after the third dose on day 11 (Table 3.14). The patient remained awake, alert, and oriented. She was discharged 4 days later.

Records from a prior admission for phenytoin toxicity showed that her phenytoin concentration decreased from 42.5 to 27.5 mg/L over a 4-day period with no specific therapy, and the patient was discharged.

It is safe to say that, during the recent admission, multiple doses of activated charcoal increased the clearance of phenytoin. (See ref. 97.)

Discussion

1. What was the purpose for administering thiamine, naloxone, and dextrose upon admission?

TABLE 3.14. *Phenytoin and charcoal dosing history*

Day	Phenytoin daily dosage (mg/day)	Phenytoin concentration (mg/L)	Times[a] of activated charcoal doses (hr)
1	600		
2	600		
3	600	11.8	
4	600		
5	600		
6	600		
7	300	44.4	
8		39.5	
9		45.2	2300
10		40.0	0400, 0800, 1200, 1600, 2000, 2400
11		16.6	0400, 1200, 1600
12		11.4	
13			
14			
15		10.2	
16			

From ref. 97.

[a] The patient refused the 0800 dose on day 11.

2. The laboratory results (prothrombin time, etc.) mentioned earlier were reported by the authors of this case study to make a point. What was it?
3. The sorbitol mixed with activated charcoal served a function. Explain it. Also, discuss a possible alternative dosing schedule for sorbitol for use with multiple charcoal doses.
4. The patient was determined to have a severely impaired ability to metabolize phenytoin (approximately 10% of normal). List the factors, based on her previous history, which may have attributed to this.
5. Comment on the dose of activated charcoal used. Would a smaller dose have been effective, and would a larger dose have been appreciably better?
6. Recall that the activated charcoal enhanced phenytoin clearance; it did not prevent its original absorption. How do you suppose it accomplished this? (Hint: Phenytoin has a small volume of distribution, along with modest biliary secretion.)

CASE STUDIES: POISONING FROM AN ENEMA

History: Case 1

An 81-year-old man with a history of arteriosclerotic cardiovascular disease was admitted to the hospital for control of rapid atrial fibrillation. Physical examination was unremarkable except for atrial fibrillation that soon converted to normal rhythm with administration of digoxin. Laboratory data included white blood cell count, 5,900/mm^3; hemoglobin, 11.0 g/L; sodium, 135 mEq/L; potassium, 4.7 mEq/L; chloride, 96 mEq/L; bicarbonate, 26 mEq/L; blood urea nitrogen, 31 mg/dL; creatinine, 2.7 mg/dL; calcium, 9.3 mg/dL; phosphorus, 3.2 mg/dL; and magnesium, 2.0 mg/dL.

The next day he complained of constipation and was given suppositories and stool softeners (identity not stated). These brought no relief. He was then given 135 mL of a sodium phosphate enema containing 16 g sodium biphosphate and 6 g sodium phosphate. He retained nearly all of the enema, passing very little stool during the next 24 hours. He soon developed abdominal pain, distension, nausea, and vomiting and became confused and lethargic. Blood analysis was remarkable for calcium, 5.4 mg/dL; phosphorus, 18.0 mg/dL; blood urea nitrogen, 49 mg/dL; and creatinine, 3.4 mg/dL. Electrocardiography showed Q-T interval prolongation. Rectal examination revealed a large fecal mass.

The patient received calcium gluconate. Digital disimpaction was performed and was followed by copious amounts of loose stool. Physical symptoms and laboratory abnormalities resolved over the next several days, and he was discharged home. (See ref. 7.)

History: Case 2

The patient was a 11-month-old, 8.9-kg male infant admitted to the hospital to correct an imperforate anus. The child was given 800 mL orally of a gastrointestinal lavage solution (Golytely) containing polyethylene glycol, 60 g/L; sodium chloride, 1.46 g/L; and sodium sulfate, 5.68 g/L. This was followed by four adult-sized sodium phosphate enemas each containing 118 mL of solution consisting of sodium biphosphate, 143 g/L, and sodium monophosphate, 53 g/L. Profuse return of clear solution followed.

Two and a half hours after the enemas were given, the patient underwent cardiac arrest. Laboratory values included serum calcium, 5.4 mg/dL, and serum phosphorus, 63.3 mg/dL. A 6-hour resuscitation that included calcium administration, fluid expansion, phosphate-binding resins, and peritoneal dialysis was unsuccessful. The child died (52).

Discussion

1. Both case studies show that a common hypertonic enema can cause toxicity, even death. Outline the events of both cases that led to the toxic outcomes.
2. Explain the relationship between blood calcium and phosphorus concentrations. Why did the calcium concentration decrease when phosphorus increased?
3. Calculate the total quantity of sodium biphosphate and sodium phosphate received by patient 2.
4. Arterial pH values were not reported in either case. Speculate what probably happened, if anything (acidosis or alkalosis), and tell why.

Review Questions

1. A patient presenting with deep tendon reflexes but without response to painful stimuli is in which of the following stages of CNS depression?
   A. Stage 1
   B. Stage 2
   C. Stage 3
   D. Stage 4
2. Tannic acid has been shown to cause toxic problems in which of the following systems?
   A. Heart
   B. Brain
   C. Liver
   D. Blood
3. Which of the following is a true statement about activated charcoal?
   A. It should be administered in adult dosages of 10 to 20 g.
   B. The best grade is manufactured from powdered coal.
   C. It is a better treatment than the "universal antidote."
   D. For best overall activity it should be taken in dry form.
4. All of the following statements about syrup of ipecac are true *except:*
   A. It is 14 times stronger than fluid extract of ipecac.
   B. It causes emetic action by direct stimulation of the GI tract.
   C. If given along with activated charcoal, it should precede the latter by at least 30 min.
   D. Ipecac has been shown to cause cardiac toxicity.
5. In which type of poisoning is a chelating agent used?
   A. Insecticide
   B. Heavy metal
   C. Digitalis
   D. Acetaminophen
6. A first aid measure for eye contamination is to:
   A. Instill eye drops containing a sympathomimetic amine

B. Cover the eye(s) with gauze bandages

C. Irrigate the eye(s) with water for at least 15 to 20 min

D. Attempt to remove particulate matter with tweezers

7. Which of the following is a true statement?

   I. Generally, a concentrated solution of a chemical is absorbed more quickly from the stomach than is a diluted solution of the same chemical.

   II. Ipecac-induced emesis is more intense if the victim is supine and calm versus upright and active.

   III. Once a substance has passed from the stomach into the intestine, it can no longer be retrieved by emesis.

   A. I only

   B. II only

   C. III only

   D. I and II only

   E. I and III only

   F. II and III only

   G. I, II, and III

8. Which of the following statements is true?

   A. When ipecac syrup is to be given in a poison case, emesis must be induced before activated charcoal is administered.

   B. Universal antidote is superior to activated charcoal for treating poisonings.

   C. All brands of activated charcoal are interchangeable because they are standardized to assure they exert the same binding activity.

   D. To enhance its activity, activated charcoal should be given as a dry powder, not mixed with liquids.

9. For which of the following ingestions should emesis not be considered?

   A. Diazepam

   B. Ethanol

   C. Acids

   D. Camphor

10. Emesis ordinarily should be recommended for all of the following poison ingestions *except:*

   A. Aspirin

   B. Barbiturates

   C. Hydrocarbons

   D. Insecticides

11. First aid for dermal exposure to poisons is to:

   A. Flush the affected area with cool water for at least 10 min

   B. Apply antibiotic ointments

   C. Wrap the wound in bandages

   D. Soak the affected area in ethanol

12. An order to administer sodium bicarbonate to treat an overdose of an acidic drug would increase excretion of the toxic drug because the:

   A. Alkaline urine decreases the quantity of ionized drug.

   B. Alkaline urine increases the quantity of ionized drug.

   C. Acid urine decreases the quantity of ionized drug.

   D. Acid urine increases the quantity of ionized drug.

13. Activated charcoal is used in the treatment of poisonings to:

   A. Provide a bulk laxative effect

   B. Induce emesis

   C. Coat the GI tract

   D. Adsorb toxic agents in the GI tract

14. In which of the following intoxications is naloxone hydrochloride employed?

   A. Quinidine

   B. Opioids

   C. Acetaminophen

   D. Salicylates

15. The average adult dose of activated charcoal is closest to:

   A. 10 g

   B. 30 g

   C. 100 g

   D. 300 g

16. The goal of demulcent therapy is to:

   A. Chelate the poison with calcium, which is present in most dairy products

   B. Induce emesis

   C. Hasten the movement of the toxicant through the GI tract

   D. Minimize abdominal discomfort by soothing and coating the GI tract

17. Fuller's earth is an adsorbent of choice for which of the following?
    A. Cyanide
    B. Carbon monoxide
    C. Paraquat
    D. Isopropyl alcohol
18. Which of the following should be addressed only *after* the other four considerations have been assessed satisfactorily?
    A. Ensuring respiratory function
    B. Determining the identity of suspected poison
    C. Normalization of heart beat
    D. Control of convulsions
    E. Stabilization of blood pressure
19. All of the following chemicals are poorly adsorbed by activated charcoal *except:*
    A. Boric acid
    B. Salicylic acid
    C. Ferrous sulfate
    D. Lithium salts
    E. Mineral acids
20. When the elimination of a drug can be enhanced by changing the pH of the urine, the half-life will become dependent upon the pH of the urine and the urinary flow rate.
    A. True
    B. False
21. For peritoneal dialysis (PD), hemodialysis (HD) and hemoperfusion (HP), which of the following is correctly ranked in *increasing* order of clinical effectiveness for enhancing the elimination of a poison?
    A. PD < HD < HP
    B. PD < HP < HD
    C. HD < HP < PD
    D. HP < HD < PD
22. When a cathartic is indicated to treat a poisoning, Epsom salts may be the item of choice. Which of the following best describes this cathartic?
    A. Sodium sulfate
    B. Sodium phosphate
    C. Magnesium citrate
    D. Magnesium sulfate
23. When a cathartic is indicated to decontaminate the GI tract, unless otherwise stated, the cathartic should be a:

    A. Lubricant product
    B. Stool-softening agent
    C. Saline cathartic
    D. Bulk-former laxative
    E. Stimulant cathartic
24. What advice should be given to a mother who asks about how much water should be given to her child to dilute an ingested poison? Comment on the use of (a) milk and (b) carbonated beverages for use in diluting a poison.
25. State the pros and cons of giving syrup of ipecac to treat an ingestion of a substance that has antiemetic action.
26. Discuss the mechanism of action of syrup of ipecac. Why might a second dose given within 20 to 30 min be considered of little additional value over the first dose?
27. Discuss the role of demulcents in treating an ingested poison (e.g., their validity and limitations).
28. Cite several risks associated with gastric lavage.

References

1. Adler AG, Walinsky P, Krall RA, Cho SY. Death resulting from ipecac syrup poisoning. *JAMA* 1980;243:1927–1928.
2. American Association of Poison Control Centers and American Academy of Clinical Toxicology Policy Statement. Universal antidote. *J Toxicol Clin Toxicol* 1982;19:527–529.
3. Arieff AI, Friedman EA. Coma following non-narcotic drug overdose: management of 208 adult patients. *Am J Med Sci* 1973;66:405–426.
4. Barer J, Hill LL, Hill RM, Martinez WM. Fatal poisoning from salt used as an emetic. *Am J Dis Child* 1973;125:889–890.
5. Berg MJ, Berlinger WG, Goldberg MJ, et al. Acceleration of the body clearance of phenobarbital by oral activated charcoal. *N Engl J Med* 1982;307:642–644.
6. Berman JB. The art and science of clinical toxicology. *JAMA* 1978;240:265–267.
7. Biberstein M, Parker BA. Enema-induced hyperphosphatemia. *Am J Med* 1985;79:645–646.
8. Boen ST. Kinetics of peritoneal dialysis. *Medicine (Baltimore)* 1961;40:243–287.
9. Brotman MC, Forbath N, Garfinkel PE, Humphrey JG. Myopathy due to ipecac syrup poisoning in a patient with anorexia nervosa. *Can Med Assoc J* 1981;125:453–454.
10. Burke M. Gastric lavage and emesis in the treatment

of ingested poisons—a review and clinical study of lavage in ten adults. *Resuscitation* 1972;1:91–105.

11. Chin L. Gastrointestinal dilution of poisons with water—an irrational and potentially harmful procedure. *Am J Hosp Pharm* 1971;28:712–714.

12. Chin L, Picchioni AL, Gillespie T. Saline cathartics and saline cathartics plus activated charcoal as antidotal treatments. *Clin Toxicol* 1981;18:865–871.

13. Comstock EG, Faulkner TP, Boisaubin EV, et al. Studies on the efficacy of gastric lavage as practiced in a large metropolitan hospital. *Clin Toxicol* 1981;18:581–597.

14. Cooney DO. *In vitro* evidence for ipecac inactivation by activated charcoal. *J Pharm Sci* 1978; 67:426–427.

15. Corby DG, Decker WJ, Moran MJ, et al. Clinical comparison of pharmacologic emetics in children. *Pediatrics* 1968;42:361–364.

16. Crome P, Dawling S, Braithwaite RA, et al. Effect of activated charcoal on absorption of nortriptyline. *Lancet* 1977;2:1204.

17. Curd-Sneed CD, McNutt LE, Stewart JJ. Absorption of sodium pentobarbital by three types of activated charcoal. *Vet Hum Toxicol* 1986;28:524–526.

18. Dabbous IA, Bergman AB, Robertson WO. The ineffectiveness of mechanically induced vomiting. *J Pediatr* 1965;66:952–954.

19. Daly JS, Cooney DO. Interference by tannic acid with the effectiveness of activated charcoal in "universal antidote." *Clin Toxicol* 1978;12:515–522.

20. DeGenaro F, Nyhan WL. Salt: a dangerous antidote. *J Pediatr* 1971;78:1048–1049.

21. DeNeve R. Antidotal efficacy of activated charcoal in presence of jam, starch and milk. *Am J Hosp Pharm* 1976;33:965–966.

22. Derlet RW, Albertson TE. Activated charcoal—past, present and future. *West J Med* 1986;145:493–496.

23. Easom JM, Caraccio TR, Lovejoy FH. Evaluation of activated charcoal and magnesium citrate in the prevention of aspirin absorption in humans. *Clin Pharmacol* 1982;1:154–156.

24. Ehlers SM, Zasko DE, Sawchuk RJ. Massive theophylline overdose. *JAMA* 1978;240:474–475.

25. Fane LR, Maetz HM, Decker WJ. Concurrent use of activated charcoal and ipecac in the treatment of poisoning. *Clin Toxicol Bull* 1971;2:4–5.

26. Fine JS, Goldfrank LR. Update in medical toxicology. *Pediatr Clin North Am* 1992;39:1031–1051.

27. Flomenbaum N, Goldfrank L, Roberts JR. Toxicologic evaluation and management by clinical presentation. In: Schwartz GR, Cayten CG, Mangelsen MA, Mayer TA, Hanke BK, eds. *Principles and practice of emergency medicine.* Philadelphia: Lea and Febiger; 1992:2951–2963.

28. Freedman GE, Pasternak S, Krenzelok EP. A clinical trial using syrup of ipecac and activated charcoal concurrently. *Ann Emerg Med* 1987;16:164–166.

29. Friedman EJ. Death from ipecac intoxication in a patient with anorexia nervosa. *Am J Psychiatry* 1984;141:702–703.

30. Gieseker DB, Troutman WG. Emergency induction of emesis using liquid detergent products: a report of 15 cases. *Clin Toxicol* 1981;18:277–282.

31. Goldberg MJ, Berlinger WG. Treatment of pheno-

barbital overdose with activated charcoal. *JAMA* 1982;247:2400–2401.

32. Goldberg MJ, Spector R, Park GD, Roberts RJ. An approach to the management of the poisoned patient. *Arch Intern Med* 1986;146:1381–1385.

33. Grybeich PA, LaCoutre PG, Lewander WJ, Lovejoy FH Jr. Effect of milk on ipecac-induced emesis. *J Pediatr* 1987;110:973–975.

34. Jackson JE, Picchioni AL, Chin L. Contraindications for activated charcoal use. *Ann Emerg Med* 1980;9:599.

35. Johnson JE, Carpenter BLM, Benton J, et al. Hemorrhagic colitis and pseudomelanosis coli in ipecac ingestion by proxy. *J Pediatr Gastroenterol Nutr* 1992;12:501–506.

36. Klein-Schwartz W, Litovitz T, Oderda GM, Bailey KM, Kuba A. The effect of milk on ipecac-induced emesis. *Clin Toxicol* 1991;29:505–511.

37. Krenzelok EP, Dean BS. Syrup of ipecac failures—a two year review of 4,306 cases. *Vet Hum Toxicol* 1985;28:317.

38. Krenzelok EP, Dean BS. Effectiveness of 15-mL versus 30-mL doses of syrup of ipecac in children. *Clin Pharm* 1987;6:715–717.

39. Krenzelok EP, Dunmire SM. Acute poisoning emergencies: resolving the gastric decontamination controversy. *Postgrad Med* 1992;91:179–186.

40. Krenzelok EP, Freeman GE, Pasternak S. Preserving the emetic effect of syrup of ipecac with concurrent activated charcoal administration—a preliminary study. *J Toxicol Clin Toxicol* 1986;24:159–166.

41. Krenzelok EP, Keller R, Stewart RD. Gastrointestinal transit times of cathartics combined with charcoal. *Ann Emerg Med* 1985;14:1152–1155.

42. Kulig K. Initial management of ingestions of toxic substances. *N Engl J Med* 1992;326:1677–1684.

43. Kulig K, Bar-Or D, Cantrill SV, et al. Management of acutely poisoned patients without gastric emptying. *Ann Emerg Med* 1985;14:562–567.

44. Levy G, Soda DM, Lampman TA. Inhibition by ice cream of the antidotal efficacy of activated charcoal. *Am J Hosp Pharm* 1975;32:289–291.

45. Linton AL, Luke RG, Briggs JD. Methods of forced diuresis and its application in barbiturate poisoning. *Lancet* 1967;2:377–379.

46. Litovitz TL, Klein-Schwartz W, Oderda GM, et al. Ipecac administration in children under one year of age. *Pediatrics* 1985;76:761–764.

47. Longdon P, Henderson A. Intestinal pseudo-obstruction following the use of enteral charcoal and sorbitol and mechanical ventilation with papaveretum sedation for theophylline poisoning. *Drug Safety* 1992;7:74–77.

48. MacLean WC. A comparison of syrup of ipecac and apomorphine in the immediate treatment of ingestions of poisons. *J Pediatr* 1973;82:121–124.

49. MacLeod J. Ipecac intoxication—use of a cardiac pacemaker in management. *N Engl J Med* 1963; 268:146–147.

50. Manno BR, Manno JE. Toxicology of ipecac: a review. *Clin Toxicol* 1977;10:221–242.

51. Manoguerra AS, Krenzelok EP. Rapid emesis from high dose ipecac syrup in adults and children intoxicated with antiemetics or other drugs. *Am J Hosp Pharm* 1978;35:1–6.

52. Martin RR, Lisehora GR, Braxton M, Barcia PJ. Fatal poisoning from sodium phosphate enema. *JAMA* 1987;257:2190–2192.

53. Matthew H, Mackintosh TF, Tompsett SL, et al. Gastric aspiration and lavage in acute poisoning. *Br Med J* 1966;1:1333–1337.

54. Mayersohn M, Perrier D, Picchioni AL. Evaluation of a charcoal-sorbitol mixture as an antidote for oral aspirin overdose. *Clin Toxicol* 1977;11:561–567.

55. McCarron MM. The role of the laboratory in treatment of the poisoned patient: clinical perspective. *J Anal Toxicol* 1983;7:142–145.

56. McFarland AK, Chyka P. Selection of activated charcoal products for the treatment of poisonings. *Ann Pharmacother* 1993;27:358–361.

57. Miser JS, Robertson WO. Ipecac poisoning. *West J Med* 1978;128:440–443.

58. Mofenson HC, Caraccio TR. Toxicologic evaluation and management by specific poisonings: quick reference guide to initial treatment of common poisonings. In: Schwartz GR, Cayten CG, Mangelsen MA, Mayer TA, Hanke BK, eds. *Principles and practice of emergency medicine*. Philadelphia: Lea and Febiger; 1992:2972.

59. Morgan AG, Polak A. The excretion of salicylate in salicylate poisoning. *Clin Sci* 1971;41:475–484.

60. Morrelli HF. Rational therapy of poisoning. In: Melmon KL, Morrelli HF, eds. *Clinical pharmacology—basic principles in therapeutics*. New York: Macmillan; 1978:1028–1051.

61. Navarro RP, Krenzelok EP. Relative efficacy and palatability of three activated charcoal mixtures. *Vet Hum Toxicol* 1980;22:6–10.

62. Neuvonen PJ, Elonen E. Effect of activated charcoal on absorption and elimination of phenobarbitone, carbamazepine and phenylbutazone in man. *Eur J Clin Pharmacol* 1980;17:51–57.

63. Neuvonen PJ, Olkkola KT. Oral activated charcoal in the treatment of intoxications. *Med Toxicol* 1988;3:33–58.

64. Olson KR, Pentel PR, Kelley MT. Physical assessment and differential diagnosis of the poisoned patient. *Med Toxicol* 1987;2:52–81.

65. Palatnick W, Tenenbein M. Activated charcoal in the treatment of drug overdose. *Drug Safety* 1992;7:3–7.

66. Park R, Pector R, Goldberg MJ, Johnson GF. Expanded role of charcoal therapy in the poisoned and overdosed patient. *Arch Intern Med* 1986;146:969–973.

67. Peterson CD. Electrolyte depletion following emergency stomach evacuation. *Am J Hosp Pharm* 1979;36:1366–1369.

68. Pond SM. Role of repeated oral doses of activated charcoal in clinical toxicology. *Med Toxicol* 1986;1:3–11.

69. Pond SM. Extracorporeal techniques in the treatment of poisoned patients. *Med J Aust* 1991;154:617–622.

70. Pond SM, Jacobs M, Marks J, et al. Treatment of digitoxin overdose with oral activated charcoal. *Lancet* 1981;2:1177–1178.

71. Prescott L, Park J, Darrien T. Treatment of severe 2,4-D and mecoprop intoxication with alkaline diuresis. *J Clin Pharmacol* 1979;7:111–116.

72. Remmert HP, Olling M, Slob W, et al. Comparative antidotal efficacy of activated charcoal tablets, capsules and suspension in healthy volunteers. *Eur J Clin Pharmacol* 1990;39:501–505.

73. Renyi FP, Donovan JW, Martin TG, et al. Concomitant use of activated charcoal and N-acetylcysteine. *Ann Emerg Med* 1985;14:568–572.

74. Riegel JM, Becker CE. Use of cathartics in toxic ingestions. *Ann Emerg Med* 1982;10:254–258.

75. Robertson WO. A further warning on the use of salt as an emetic agent. *J Pediatr* 1971;79:877.

76. Rodgers GC, Matyunus NJ. Gastrointestinal decontamination for acute poisoning. *Pediatr Clin North Am* 1986;33:261–285.

77. Rumack BH. Management of acute poisoning and overdose. In: Rumack BH, Temple AR, eds. *Management of the poisoned patient*. Princeton: Science Press; 1977:250–280.

78. Rumack BH. Poisoning—prevention of absorption. In: Bayer MJ, Rumack BH, eds. *Poisoning and overdose*. Rockville, MD: Aspen; 1983:13–18.

79. Rumack BH, Temple AR. Lomotil poisoning. *Pediatrics* 1974;53:495–500.

80. Rygnestad T, Berg KJ. Evaluation of benefits of drug analysis in the routine clinical management of acute self poisoning. *Clin Toxicol* 1984;22:51–61.

81. Saxena K, Kingston R. Acute poisoning—management protocol. *Postgrad Med* 1982;71:67–77.

82. Schwartz GR. Emergency management of the toxicologic patient. In: Schwartz GR et al., eds. *Principles and practice of emergency medicine*. 2nd ed. Philadelphia: WB Saunders; 1986:1671–1684.

83. Shannon M, Fish SS, Lovejoy FH. Cathartics and laxatives. Do they still have a place in management of the poisoned patient? *Med Toxicol* 1986;1:247–252.

84. Simon NM, Krumlovsky FA. The role of dialysis in the treatment of poisonings. *Ration Drug Ther* 1971;3:1–7.

85. Sketris IS, Moury JB, Czajka PA, et al. Saline catharsis: effect on aspirin bioavailability in combination with activated charcoal. *J Clin Pharmacol* 1982;22:59–64.

86. Smilkstein MJ, Smolinske SC, Kulig KW, Rumack BH. Severe hypermagnesemia due to multiple-dose cathartic therapy. *West J Med* 1988;148:208–211.

87. Stein RS, Jenkins D, Korns ME. Death after use of cupric sulfate as emetic. *JAMA* 1976;235:801.

88. Stewart JJ. Effects of emetic and cathartic agents on the gastrointestinal tract and the treatment of toxic ingestion. *J Toxicol Clin Toxicol* 1983;20:199–253.

89. Sullivan JB. Drug overdose and poisoning-management update. *Drug Therapy* 1991;21:15–25.

90. Swartz CM, Sherman A. The treatment of tricyclic antidepressant overdose with repeated charcoal. *J Clin Psychopharmacol* 1984;4:336–340.

91. Thoman M. Antidote and formulary list. *Vet Hum Toxicol* 1988;30:267–268.

92. True RJ, Berman JM, Mahutte CK. Treatment of theophylline toxicity with oral activated charcoal. *Crit Care Med* 1984;12:113–114.

93. Varipapa RJ, Oderda GM. Effect of milk on ipecac-induced emesis. *J Am Pharm Assoc* 1977;17:510.

94. Watson WA. Factors influencing the clinical effi-

cacy of activated charcoal. *Drug Intell Clin Pharm* 1987;21:160–166.

95. Watson WA. Toxicokinetics and management of the poisoned patient. *US Pharm* 1990;15(10):H1–H23.

96. Watson WA, Crewer KK, Chapman JA. Gastrointestinal obstruction associated with multiple dose activated charcoal. *J Emerg Med* 1986;4:401–407.

97. Weidle PJ, Skiest DJ, Forrest A. Multiple-dose activated charcoal as adjunct therapy after chronic phenytoin intoxication. *Clin Pharm* 1991;10:711–714.

98. Wiley JF. Difficult diagnosis in toxicology. *Pediatr Clin North Am* 1991;38:725–737.

99. Winchester JF, Gelfand MC, Tilstone WJ. Hemoperfusion in drug intoxication: clinical and laboratory aspects. *Drug Metab Rev* 1978;8:69–104.

100. Yancy RE, O'Barr TB, Corby DG. *In vitro* and *in vivo* evaluation of the effect of cherry flavoring on the adsorptive capacity of activated charcoal for salicylic acid. *Vet Hum Toxicol* 1977;19:163–165.

4 ‖ Alcohols, Glycols, and Aldehydes

Alcohols are hydroxy derivatives of straight or branched chain aliphatic hydrocarbons. The more common alcohols may include up to three hydroxyl groups with no more than one on each carbon. Lesser common alcohols may contain more than one hydroxyl group per carbon atom. Those alcohols that are the most common causes of toxicity include ethanol (ethyl alcohol; alcohol), methanol (methyl alcohol), and isopropanol (isopropyl alcohol). In general, the longer the carbon chain, the greater the toxicity. The exception to this rule is methanol, which is more toxic than ethanol.

Dihydroxy alcohols are called glycols (*glyc-* or *glyco-* from the Greek stem word meaning sweet), referring to their sweet taste. Dihydroxyethane is better known as ethylene glycol, the simplest glycol. It is commonly referred to as permanent antifreeze and is a fairly frequent cause of poisoning. Another glycol is dihydroxypropane (propylene glycol), a constituent of numerous pharmaceutical products. For the most part, propylene glycol is not toxic.

Alcohols and glycols are discussed together in this chapter for several reasons. First, they are chemically similar. They also share many common characteristics of acute poisoning, and their acute toxicities are treated similarly. However, each of the compounds in this chapter has its own specific characteristics.

ETHANOL

Ethanol is the only alcohol that has widespread intentional internal human use. Ethanol is one of the oldest drugs and is the primary alcohol present in fermented and distilled beverages. It is also the most commonly used psychoactive drug in the world (1).

Ethanol is a clear, colorless liquid that imparts a burning sensation to the mouth and throat when swallowed. Pure ethanol has a slightly pleasant odor. Ethanol is a powerful CNS depressant that acts primarily on the reticular activating system in the brain. In fact, its actions are qualitatively similar to those of general anesthetics. It has a relatively low order of toxicity compared to methanol or isopropanol.

Ethanol is discussed first because it is the most frequently reported cause of alcohol toxicity and because an understanding of certain aspects of its metabolic pathway and toxic actions is necessary to understand the mechanism of toxicity and management of overdoses involving methanol and ethylene glycol. As with all alcohols and glycols discussed in this chapter, only acute toxicologic considerations will be presented.

Mechanism of Toxicity

The exact mechanisms by which ethanol produces its pharmacologic and toxicologic actions are not completely understood and have been investigated for many years. The CNS is selectively affected. Ethanol is thought to act directly on neuronal membranes and not on synapses. At the membrane, it may involve ion transport and biogenic amines.

The effect of ethanol on the CNS is directly proportional to its blood concentration (47). The first region affected is the reticular activating system, resulting in disruption of the motor and thought processes. Suppressing the cerebral cortex causes a variety of behavioral changes. Which specific behaviors will be suppressed and which will be released from inhibition depend on the individual. In general, complex, abstract, and poorly learned behaviors are disrupted at low alcohol concentrations.

Ethanol depresses the CNS in a descending order from the cortex to the medulla. Table 4.1 illustrates the correlation between blood alcohol concentration (BAC) and the area of the brain affected. Also, subjective feelings are noted based on blood alcohol concentration and the area of the brain where ethanol produces its effect.

Toxicokinetics of Ingestion

Absorption

The physicochemical properties of ethanol are such that it is slightly polar and has a weak

TABLE 4.1. *Range of toxicity of ethanol*

Clinical description/ symptoms	Blood alcohol concentration (w/v)	Part of brain
Mild	0.05−0.10% (50−100 mg/dL)	Frontal lobe
Decreased inhibitions		
Slight visual impairment		
Slowing or reaction time		
Increased confidence		
Moderate	0.15−0.30% (150−300 mg/dL)	Parietal lobe
Ataxia		
Slurred speech		
Decreased motor skills		
Decreased attention		Occipital lobe
Diplopia		
Altered perception		Cerebellum
Altered equilibrium		
Severe	0.3−0.5% (300−500 mg/dL)	
Vision impairment		Occipital lobe
Equilibrium		Cerebellum
Stupor		Diencephalon
Coma		
Respiratory failure	>0.5% (>500 mg/dL)	Medulla

electronic charge and low molecular weight. Ethanol is miscible in water and lipid soluble. Therefore, it is easily absorbed and can pass through cell membranes by simple diffusion.

The most common route of exposure to ethanol is ingestion, but it also can be absorbed by inhalation of vaporized ethanol or through the skin. Ethanol absorption after ingestion begins in the stomach, but only a small percentage of the amount ingested is absorbed directly into the blood through the stomach wall. The rate of absorption is much greater in the small intestine. Since absorption through the stomach wall is minimal and rapid absorption occurs in the small intestine, any factor that delays or enhances gastric emptying will influence the rate of absorption of alcohol into the blood.

Several factors govern gastric emptying. Food has a significant effect. When food, especially food rich in fat, is present in the stomach, gastric emptying time is slower and absorption of ethanol is delayed. On an empty stomach, complete absorption will take place in about 1 to 2 hr. On a full stomach, complete absorption may be delayed up to 6 hr.

Other factors that affect ethanol absorption include the amount, concentration, and composition of the alcoholic beverage. Absorption is fastest from beverages containing 20% to 30% ethanol. Higher concentrations (e.g., straight whiskey) cause gastric irritation and pylorospasm, which delays gastric emptying. Lower concentrations of ethanol, such as beer, are absorbed more slowly because of their low alcohol content. Carbonated beverages, such as sparkling wines and champagnes, are absorbed faster because the presence of carbon dioxide promotes evacuation of the stomach.

Distribution

After absorption, alcohol is uniformly distributed throughout all tissues and body fluids. The distribution pattern parallels the water content and blood supply of each organ. Equilibrium is rapidly established between alcohol in the blood and in the tissue compartments. Distribution of alcohol between alveolar air and blood depends on the speed of diffusion, its vapor pressure, and the concentration of alcohol in the lung capillaries. The distribution ratio between alveolar air and blood is 1:2,100. This consideration is utilized in determination of blood alcohol concentrations by breath analysis methods.

Metabolism

Understanding the metabolism of ethanol is useful in predicting and managing the consequences of its ingestion. Between 90% and 98% of absorbed ethanol is removed from the body by enzymatic oxidation. Normally, about 2% to 10% is excreted unchanged, mainly through the lungs and kidneys. Small amounts can be detected in sweat, tears, bile, gastric juice, saliva, and other secretions. Enzymatic oxidation of ethanol occurs primarily in the liver and to a smaller extent in the kidney. The metabolic process involves three enzymatic reactions, as shown in Fig. 4.1. During the first step, ethanol is oxidized to acetaldehyde by alcohol dehydrogenase, which requires nicotinamide adenine dinucleotide (NAD) as a cofactor. This is the rate-limiting step in dissipation of alcohol from the body. Hepatic alcohol dehydrogenase is a nonspecific enzyme that also catalyzes conversion of other primary alcohols and aldehydes, as well as secondary alcohols and ketones.

Acetaldehyde, in the second step, is then converted by aldehyde dehydrogenase, in the presence of NAD, to acetic acid. Acetic acid is available for the formation of acetyl coenzyme A (CoA). Acetyl CoA enters the Krebs cycle, where it is eventually metabolized to CO_2 and water.

The metabolism of ethanol involves utilization of NAD and accumulation of its reduced form, $NADH_2$, as shown in Figs. 4.1 and 4.2. This results in a significant decrease in the NAD/$NADH_2$ ratio in the liver and is responsible for some of the metabolic effects of ethanol intoxication. Although the metabolic consequences of ethanol ingestion are complex, it is thought that they are partly due to inhibition of gluconeogenesis by ethanol as a result of depletion of NAD. This can be easily understood if all of the reactions in Fig. 4.2 that require NAD are located. Since NAD is depleted during ethanol metabolism, these reactions will proceed in the direction of the *open arrows*. Consequently, amino acids that normally enter the glycolysis pathway and tricarboxylic acid (TCA; Krebs) cycle are shunted into other pathways. There is a decrease in oxaloacetate and pyruvate and an accumulation of lactate and glycerol, resulting in accumulation of fat in the liver. Also, significant hypoglycemia can occur after acute and chronic intoxication with ethanol (54). This can sometimes be extremely critical, especially in children, and is often ignored.

Elimination

First-order elimination kinetics is the general rule for most drugs. That is, most are eliminated from the body at a rate that depends on the amount of drug present in the body, and the amount of drug remaining at any given time in the body decreases exponentially to zero. For ethanol, first-order elimination occurs only for very low, clinically insignificant BAC levels of less than 20 mg/dL or 0.02%.

Studies have established the K_m, or Michaelis-Menten dissociation constant, for alcohol dehydrogenase to be 9.7 mg/dL (range of 8 to 14 mg/dL) and the V_{max}, or the maximum velocity, to be 23.3 mg/dL (range of 22 to 24 mg/dL) (60,63). When the substrate (ethanol) concentration is less than the K_m, the rate of elimination is first order. However, when the substrate concentration is much greater than the K_m (i.e., the rate approaches the V_{max} or maximum velocity for the enzymatic reaction), the rate of elimination is constant, regardless of concentration, and is referred to as zero-order kinetics.

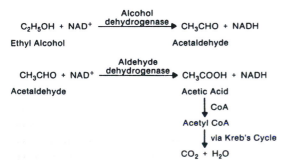

FIG. 4.1. Biochemical pathway for ethanol metabolism.

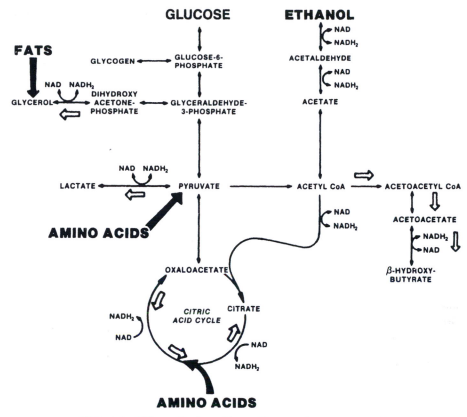

FIG. 4.2. Effect of ethanol ingestion on gluconeogenesis.

To apply these principles to acute ethanol ingestion, refer to Fig. 4.3. Plasma concentrations of ethanol that are commonly encountered with alcohol intoxication are at least 100 mg/dL, which is about 10 times greater than the K_m. Therefore, the rate of elimination, or dissipation rate, for ethanol follows zero-order kinetics and is constant at 100 mg/kg/hr. For a man weighing 150 pounds, approximately 7 g of ethanol (approximately 10 mL of 100% ethanol) will be eliminated every hour. In terms of the BAC, the dissipation rate will average about 18 mg/dL/hr (0.018% per hr) and is referred to as the Widmark B factor in Fig. 4.4. From this information, the approximate length of time required to eliminate enough alcohol to be considered sober or out of danger can be calculated. To achieve a BAC of 100 mg/dL (0.1%), a 150-pound individual needs to ingest 55 mL of absolute ethanol. In a practical setting, this requires the ingestion of 120 mL or about 4 ounces of gin, whiskey, or vodka, but the maximum quantity that can be oxidized in the liver is 10 mL/hr. Consequently, it will take about 5 hr to eliminate the amount of alcohol ingested [55

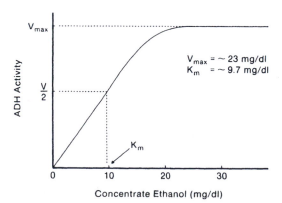

$V_{max} = \sim 23$ mg/dl
$K_m = \sim 9.7$ mg/dl

Concentrate Ethanol (mg/dl)

FIG. 4.3. The rate of enzymatic activity for alcohol dehydrogenase using ethanol as the substrate.

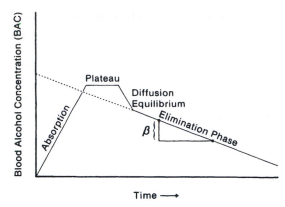

FIG. 4.4. Depiction of the pharmacokinetic profile of ethanol. The average rate of elimination of ethanol is 0.018% per hr, with a range of 0.015 to 0.020% per hr.

mL of absolute (or 100%) 200-proof ethanol or 120 mL of 50- to 60-proof (25 to 30%) ethanol]. Therefore, there is some validity to the suggestion that a safe ''maintenance'' dose of ethanol would be 10 mL of absolute ethanol per hr, which translates into one shot of liquor (25 to 30 mL) per hour.

Estimation of Blood Alcohol Concentration (BAC)

The Swedish scientist Widmark developed a formula for estimating the amount of alcohol needed to produce a given blood alcohol concentration. Conversely, the formula can be used to estimate the BAC that will result from ingestion of a stated quantity of alcohol in an individual with a known body weight.

The Widmark formula is expressed as:

$$A = \frac{WrCT}{0.8}$$

where:

A = ethanol (mL) ingested
W = body weight (g)
r = distribution ratio of ethanol
CT = blood alcohol concentration (decimal equivalent)
0.8 = specific gravity of ethanol

The Widmark r factor is based on the distribution of alcohol in the blood to that of the whole group, i.e.,

$$r = \frac{\% \text{ alcohol in body}}{\% \text{ alcohol in blood}}$$

For men $r = 0.68$ and for women $r = 0.55$ because women usually have less body water and a greater proportion of adipose tissue. To predict the BAC of an individual, consider the following example.

A man weighing 150 pounds who consumes 1 ounce (approximately 30 mL) of 100-proof (50% ethanol v/v) whiskey or other distilled spirit or one 12-ounce can of beer (5% ethanol v/v) will obtain, after complete absorption, a blood alcohol concentration of 0.025% (25 mg/dL), i.e.,

$$A = \frac{WrCT}{0.8}$$

$$A = \frac{68,100 \times 0.68 \times 0.025\%}{0.8}$$

$$A = \frac{11.58}{0.8}$$

A = approximately 15 mL, or 1/2 ounce of pure ethanol, or 1 ounce of 50% ethanol

If we rearrange the equation, the BAC for a stated volume ingested can easily be estimated. For a man weighing more or less than 150 pounds or if the alcoholic content of the beverage is different than 50%, the BAC would be proportionately altered. In any case, the estimated BAC can be calculated by the following formula:

$$\frac{150}{\text{Body weight}} \times \frac{\% \text{ EtOH}}{50}$$

$$\times \text{ Number of ounces ingested} \times 0.025\%$$

$$= \text{Maximum BAC}$$

In acute ethanol overdoses, the intoxicated patient may present with a variety of signs and symptoms. In many cases the degree of intoxication would correspond to the drinking history of the patient. However, consider the situation where a 200-pound man presents to the emergency department in a semicomatose state with severe hypotension and decreased respirations. Friends of the patient said he passed out after drinking two 12-ounce beers. Using the above equations, the BAC resulting from complete absorption of two 12-ounce beers (4% EtOH) in a 200-pound individual would be approximately 0.04%. A BAC of 0.04% is not sufficient to produce such a profound state of CNS depression. Therefore, either the history is incorrect or the patient ingested other CNS depressant drugs in addition to the alcohol. For a comprehensive study of the toxicokinetics of alcohols, consult the excellent reference by Walgreen (61).

Characteristics of Acute Toxicity

Clinical manifestations of ethanol intoxication include a wide variety of signs and symptoms that range from ataxia to coma (see Table 4.1). Typically, the acutely intoxicated patient is 20 to 30 years old and has ingested a large volume of an alcoholic beverage. The patient may have vomited previously and complained of nausea. The patient may appear stuporous or dazed with cold, clammy, and dry skin as a result of dehydration; hypothermia may or may not be obvious. The breath smells of alcohol. Respirations may be decreased, and there may be an increase in heart rate.

At concentrations less than 100 mg/dL, the frontal lobe shows selective impairment. Subjective effects include decreased inhibitions, mild euphoria, increased confidence, altered judgment, and decreased attention span. As the blood alcohol concentration rises from 100 mg/dL (0.10%) to 200 mg/dL (0.20%), the parietal lobe is affected. At these concentrations, there is decreased motor skill and sensory response, impairment of memory and comprehension, loss of critical judgment, emotional instability, slurred speech, tremor, and ataxia. Blood alcohol concentrations reaching 300 mg/dL (0.3%) affect the cerebellum, as well as the occipital lobe of the cere-

bral hemisphere. Alcoholic coma usually occurs when the BAC exceeds 300 mg/dL. These areas of the brain respond to alcohol by additionally causing altered equilibrium, muscular incoordination, staggered gait, decreased pain perception, disorientation, mental confusion, and dizziness. When the blood alcohol concentration reaches the LD_{50} value (450 to 500 mg/dL; about 0.45% to 0.50%), impaired consciousness is usually evident with marked respiratory depression, peripheral vascular collapse, and coma. At this point the medulla has been affected, and the outcome may be fatal. Death results from respiratory failure.

In alcoholic ketoacidosis, lactate, pyruvate, beta-hydroxybutyrate, acetone, and acetoacetate concentrations are increased, but not to the same extent as seen in diabetic patients. Glucose may be normal or slightly elevated. Insulin levels are low. Growth hormone, catecholamines, cortisol, glucagon, and free fatty acids are elevated (41). Alcoholic ketoacidosis must always be suspected in chronic alcoholism, especially in an alcoholic who has not been eating properly (56).

Management of Acute Toxicity

Severe, acute ethanol toxicity in nontolerant patients generally responds well to good supportive care. Particular attention needs to be directed to protection of the airway from aspiration and intubation of the patient if necessary. Analeptics (stimulants) are not recommended and, in fact, should be avoided. Blood glucose should be monitored to determine if hypoglycemia is present. Potassium and magnesium deficiencies may need to be corrected. In alcoholic ketoacidosis, the mainstay of treatment is glucose and saline to correct the ketosis and volume depletion (37,41). In the alcoholic patient, nutritional deficiencies may need to be corrected, using magnesium, thiamine, pyridoxine, and vitamins K and C. Hemodialysis may be indicated if symptoms are severe and the patient's BAC exceeds 450 mg/dL (0.45%) or if there is significant decrease in hepatic function.

Usually, specific therapy is not required for acute alcoholic intoxication. The patient is treated symptomatically and monitored carefully until the ingested alcohol is metabolized.

METHANOL

Methanol (wood alcohol, methyl alcohol, Columbian spirits, colonial spirit, wood naphtha) is the alcohol with the simplest structure. Numerous studies over the years have investigated its toxicity potential, as well as the most beneficial means for treating acute toxicity.

Methanol is widely used in industry and around the home as a general solvent, paint thinner, antifreeze, fluid for desk "spirit" duplicating machines, and source of heat for fondue burners (e.g., Sterno). Occasionally, at concentrations up to 5%, methanol is used as a denaturant for ethanol that is not intended for human consumption. It is called "wood" alcohol because, formerly, its primary source was from distillation of wood.

Most reports of methanol toxicity relate to ingesting methanol itself or a methanol-containing product, although poisonings have been reported after absorption through the skin and inhalation of air that contained as little as 0.2%. Since yeast fermentation does not produce even trace quantities of methanol, pure "moonshine" liquor does not contain methanol. Occasionally, reported cases of severe intoxication from "shine" fail to mention that the actual cause of poisoning was methanol that was added to increase the quantity of product to be sold.

Methanol poisoning continues to be a worldwide (although regional) problem associated with high mortality and morbidity. Massive outbreaks of intoxication have been reported, especially during wartime, ethanol shortages, and prohibition (53). Because new uses for methanol, such as an alternate fuel source, are currently being proposed, the problem will undoubtedly become more significant in future years.

Accidental ingestions also occur because methanol closely resembles ethanol in appearance and odor, is readily available, is tax-free (thus cheaper), and, in general, is not considered by the public to be more dangerous than ethanol (48). The lethal dose is reported to range from 30 to 240 mL. A reasonable lethal dose in a man is 1 g/kg (22,23).

Toxicokinetics of Ingestion

Absorption and Distribution

Methanol is absorbed from the gastrointestinal tract very easily. Peak blood methanol concentrations occur 30 to 90 minutes after ingestion (5). Methanol, like ethanol, is distributed throughout the body in proportion to the water content of various tissues. The volume of distribution (Vd) of methanol is 0.6 to 0.7 L/kg.

Metabolism and Elimination

Methanol is metabolized by the same hepatic enzymes as ethanol, alcohol dehydrogenase and aldehyde dehydrogenase (Fig. 4.5). It is oxidized to formaldehyde by alcohol dehydrogenase, which is rapidly converted to formic acid by aldehyde dehydrogenase. Formic acid is further oxidized to carbon dioxide by an enzymatic pathway dependent on folate (35). The alcohol dehydrogenase and folate-dependent oxidative pathways proceed at a much slower rate than does aldehyde dehydrogenase; therefore, formic acid accumulates in tissues. In acute methanol toxicity, elimination follows zero-order kinetics (concentration independent).

Although methanol and ethanol share the same metabolic pathways, their affinity for alcohol dehydrogenase is different. Methanol is metabolized at a much slower rate than ethanol (about $\frac{1}{7}$th the rate); therefore, when both alcohols are present, ethanol will be metabolized preferentially.

Metabolic conversion is not the sole means for elimination. A significant amount may be excreted unchanged through the lung and

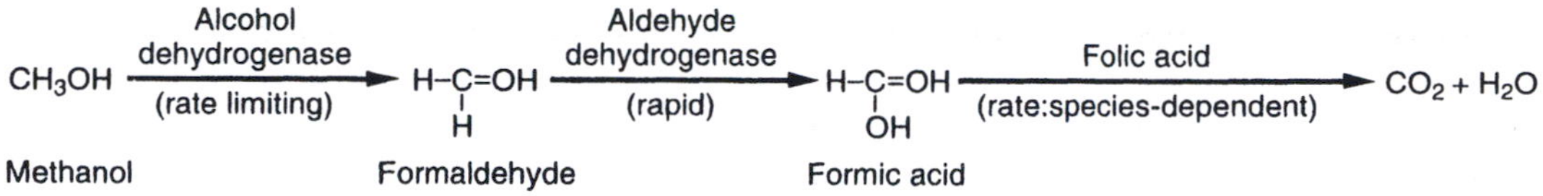

$$CH_3OH \xrightarrow[\text{(rate limiting)}]{\text{Alcohol dehydrogenase}} H-\underset{H}{\overset{}{C}}=OH \xrightarrow[\text{(rapid)}]{\text{Aldehyde dehydrogenase}} H-\underset{OH}{\overset{}{C}}=OH \xrightarrow[\text{(rate:species-dependent)}]{\text{Folic acid}} CO_2 + H_2O$$

Methanol   Formaldehyde   Formic acid

FIG. 4.5. Biochemical pathway for methanol metabolism.

kidney. However, metabolism is the major reaction.

Mechanism of Toxicity

The major toxicologic concerns following acute methanol exposure are severe metabolic acidosis, visual disturbances, and permanent blindness. Although these toxicologic consequences were once thought to be caused by the formation of formaldehyde and formic acid (27–29), recent animal data reveal that formaldehyde does not play a major role in methanol toxicity. Rather, the *rapid* formation and accumulation of formic acid has been shown to be most responsible for producing metabolic acidosis in the early stages and is implicated as a factor in ocular toxicity as well (22). Ocular damage is of special concern. Ingestion of as little as 4 mL of methanol has caused blindness. In fact, 6% of all blindness in the U.S. armed forces during World War II is reported to have been caused by methanol consumption (18).

Lactate accumulates in the later stages of methanol poisoning. Some explanations have included formate inhibition of mitochondrial respiration, tissue hypoxia, and altered lactate metabolism due to an increased NADH/NAD ratio (23). When methanol is oxidized to formaldehyde and formic acid, there is increased conversion of NAD^+ to NADH. Excess NADH favors reduction of pyruvate to lactate. Thus, metabolic acidosis associated with methanol poisoning is related to the formation and accumulation of both formic acid and lactic acid and to the decrease in serum bicarbonate concentration (9). Consequently, there is an increased anion gap (difference between total cations and total anions). The normal anion gap is 18 mEq/L (calculated as $[Na^+ +$ $K^+] - [Cl^- + HCO_3^{-1}])$. This value may be two or more times above normal after methanol intoxication.

Characteristics of Acute Toxicity

Characteristics of methanol intoxication are qualitatively similar, regardless of the quantity ingested. However, they vary widely from person to person. Because of the slow rate of metabolism of methanol to formic acid, the onset of symptoms other than CNS depression is often delayed 12 to 24 hours. Central nervous effects may include euphoria, muscle weakness, suppression of inhibitions, and, in severe cases, coma and convulsions. Inebriation per se is usually not a significant problem, except when larger quantities are consumed or ethanol has been concurrently ingested.

As should be expected, in cases of concomitant ethanol and methanol ingestion, initial symptoms of toxicity are predominantly those of ethanol. In persons suspected of concurrent consumption, an analytical method of analysis for determining ethanol and methanol must be performed as soon as possible. This should be done even in the absence of immediate symptoms, since, as stated above, the toxic actions of methanol are frequently delayed.

After an asymptomatic latent interval, there is abrupt onset of nausea with vomiting, dizziness, headache, delirium, intense gastrointestinal pain, and perhaps diarrhea, back pain, and cold and clammy extremities.

Ocular toxicity may include blurred vision, decreased visual acuity, hyperemia of the optic disc, retinal edema, fixed and dilated pupils with absence of light reflex, and even blindness. In severe methanol poisoning, respiration and heart rate are depressed, and such depression signals a grave prognosis.

Laboratory findings that may be indicative of methanol poisoning include alterations in blood gases, metabolic acidosis with elevated anionic gap, and increased serum osmolality (high osmolal gap).

Management of Toxicity

In acute ingestion of a large quantity of methanol, attention should be directed to evacuation of the stomach by emesis or lavage, depending on the time lapse since ingestion. A wide variety of treatment regimens for methanol poisoning have been proposed over the years. The major focus should involve correcting the acidosis because it may be life-threatening (22). Severity of ocular damage is also somewhat dependent on the rapidity and completeness of acidosis reversal. Therefore, infusion of sodium bicarbonate should be started immediately and maintained until urinary pH is normal. Also, formate elimination may be pH dependent, and aggressive treatment of the acidosis may increase its elimination (24).

Ethanol is a specific antidote for methanol toxicity. Since ethanol has a greater affinity for alcohol dehydrogenase than does methanol, it preferentially serves as the substrate for this enzyme. Ethanol treatment should be initiated orally or by intravenous injection as soon as possible. A loading dose of 0.6 to 0.8 g/kg, followed by a maintenance dose of 125 to 130 mg/kg/hr, is typically used so that the blood ethanol level remains approximately 100 mg/dL (0.1%) (44). As stated earlier, metabolism of alcohols proceeds independently of blood concentration. Consequently, this amount of ethanol is sufficient to slow the rate of methanol metabolism to its more toxic metabolites and thus reduce overall toxicity. In addition, by decreasing the formation of formic acid, the source of acidosis also will be reduced.

Hemodialysis will effectively hasten methanol elimination (16). Dialysis should be initiated if the blood methanol concentration is greater than 25 mg/dL and should be continued until blood methanol concentrations are negative and acidosis is reversed. Since ethanol will be removed along with methanol, it is imperative that the ethanol infusion rate be adjusted throughout the dialysis period (44). Peritoneal dialysis, hemoperfusion, or forced diuresis have not been shown to be effective in enhancing elimination of methanol.

Alternative therapeutic measures have been suggested to overcome deficiencies of ethanol therapy. Leucovorin calcium, a folate analog, is reasoned to provide beneficial action because it enhances metabolism of formic acid to carbon dioxide via folate-dependent enzyme systems (38). 4-Methylpyrazole (4-MP), a potent inhibitor of alcohol dehydrogenase in animals, has also been suggested for use in humans (29,36). At this time, more clinical studies are needed.

ISOPROPANOL

Isopropanol (isopropyl alcohol) is used as a solvent and disinfectant. It is a constituent of many perfumes, colognes, and personal grooming products. Reports of ingestion have been rare; most victims have a history of alcohol abuse (26). The fatal dose of isopropanol is reported to be 4 to 8 ounces, although as little as 20 mL may cause symptoms (17).

The toxicity as well as the disposition of isopropanol remains controversial (42). Initial CNS actions of isopropanol are similar to those of ethanol intoxication but are reported to be at least twice as severe (47). Its duration of action is also longer than that of ethanol because it is oxidized by alcohol dehydrogenase at a slower rate. Approximately 80% of ingested isopropanol is converted to acetone, which may be responsible for many of the symptoms of isopropanol poisoning, including CNS depression (30).

Isopropanol absorption from the stomach is rapid and complete within 15 to 30 min (42). Intoxication can be observed within 30 to 60 min postingestion. The severely intoxicated patient may exhibit respiratory depression, grade 3 to 4 coma, severe hypotension, mild acidosis, acetonemia, and acetonuria. Also, isopropanol will produce hypoglycemia and a slight increase in serum osmolality and anion gap. Ingestions of isopropanol may initially appear solely as an ethanol ingestion, but the hallmark of isopropanol intoxication is acetonemia (30).

Treatment of acute isopropanol ingestions should consist of gastric evacuation, maintenance of blood pressure with fluids and possibly pressor amines, correction of electrolyte imbalance and dehydration with glucose and sodium bicarbonate, and hemodialysis (13,49). Hemodialysis is indicated particularly when isopropanol blood concentrations exceed 400 mg/dL, which is generally associated with severe hypotension and coma (30).

ETHYLENE GLYCOL

Numerous glycols are used in many industrial applications: as hydraulic fluids and heat exchangers, in chemical syntheses, and as components of cosmetics, inks, lacquers, and various pharmaceuticals. Only ethylene glycol is of current toxicologic interest. Its magnitude of toxicity ranges between the extremely toxic diethylene glycol and the relatively nontoxic propylene glycol.

Diethylene glycol (Fig. 4.6) was the cause of more than 100 deaths in 1937 when it was inadvertently used as a solvent for sulfanilamide in a pharmaceutical preparation (14,52). After 2 to 5 days of consuming this "elixir," which contained 72% diethylene glycol, patients complained of nausea with vomiting, intense gastrointestinal cramping

and diarrhea, and back pain referred to the kidney area. These symptoms soon led to progressive liver necrosis, renal tubular degeneration, and death. Although today diethylene glycol is not a significant cause of toxicity, it is still used in several industrial processes and must be handled with special precaution.

Ethylene glycol is most generally encountered around the home as "permanent" automotive antifreeze. It is a colorless, nonvolatile liquid having a sweet taste. Antifreeze products are usually artificially colored. Ethylene glycol is a commonly ingested poison because of its sweet taste and availability to inquisitive children from carelessly stored containers of antifreeze in the garage. Also, it is consumed by adults for the purpose of inebriation which, in its early stages, closely resembles the effects of ethanol. Ethylene glycol can produce extremely serious symptoms, even death, with toxic doses for adults reported at approximately 100 mL (22).

Mechanism of Toxicity

Ethylene glycol, like methanol and isopropanol, is converted to metabolites that are more toxic than the parent compound. As with ethanol, methanol, and isopropanol, the same enzyme system, alcohol dehydrogenase, is involved. Not all metabolites have been identified, but Fig. 4.7 illustrates possible intermediates. These toxic intermediates are responsible for producing tissue destruction and severe metabolic acidosis.

Aldehyde production forms the first group of metabolites and has been shown to inhibit oxidative phosphorylation, cell respiration, glucose metabolism, and protein and nucleic acid synthesis (43,59). Also, the prominent cerebral symptoms that occur during the first stage correspond to aldehyde production, which has been shown to decrease central serotonin metabolism and alter central amine levels (3,43). Tissue damage results from deposition of calcium oxalate crystals. Acidosis results from accumulation of lactic acid (due to the increased alcohol dehydrogenase activ-

FIG. 4.6. Chemical structures for glycols shown in order of increasing toxicity. **a**, propylene glycol; **b**, ethylene glycol; **c**, diethylene glycol.

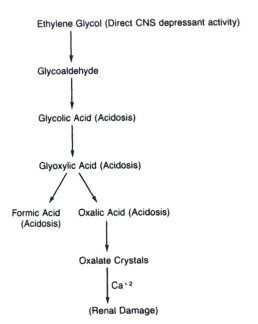

Ethylene Glycol (Direct CNS depressant activity)

Glycoaldehyde

Glycolic Acid (Acidosis)

Glyoxylic Acid (Acidosis)

Formic Acid (Acidosis)   Oxalic Acid (Acidosis)

Oxalate Crystals

Ca^{+2}

(Renal Damage)

FIG. 4.7. Biochemical pathway for ethylene glycol metabolism.

ity and NADH/NAD ratio), glycolic acid, glyoxylic acid, formic acid, and oxalic acid (22,43,59).

Characteristics of Toxicity

Characteristics of ethylene glycol toxicity are outlined in Table 4.2. Signs and symptoms of toxicity result from direct toxic actions of ethylene glycol or its metabolites on the CNS, cardiorespiratory, and renal systems.

Initial CNS depression may be as severe as with ethanol and may persist for 12 or more hours. The patient may appear to be inebriated but lacks the characteristic odor of ethanol on the breath (33,57). Other CNS effects include muscle paralysis, decreased tendon reflexes, convulsions, and tetany due to hypocalcemia. These are usually accompanied by nausea and vomiting, ataxia, stupor, and, depending on the amount ingested, coma and death. If death occurs during the early phase of poisoning, it is due to respiratory and/or cardiac failure.

If the patient survives the initial effects, pulmonary edema (enhanced by CNS depression), congestive heart failure, tachycardia, and renal failure may develop as a result of calcium oxalate deposition. The kidney is especially susceptible to deposition of calcium oxalate crystals in the renal tubules, producing tubular epithelial necrosis with fat inclusion (21). Glomeruli develop thickened basement membranes and granule deposits.

Other distinguishing characteristics of ethylene glycol toxicity include a large anion gap acidosis with Kussmaul respirations, an osmolal gap, hypocalcemia, and the presence of calcium oxalate crystals in the urine.

TABLE 4.2. Characteristics of ethylene glycol toxicity

Phase	Time (postingestion)	Symptoms
Stage 1	30 min–12 hr	Patient appears "drunk" without odor of ethanol on breath Nausea, vomiting Metabolic acidosis Muscle paralysis Decreased tendon reflexes Convulsions and coma
Stage 2	12–24 hr	Tachycardia; mild hypertension Tachypnea Congestive heart failure Pulmonary edema Renal failure
Stage 3	24–72 hr	Flank pain Costovertebral angle tenderness Acute tubular necrosis

From refs. 6, 58, and 59.

Management of Toxicity

The principal goal in management of ethylene glycol poisoning is to correct acidosis with sodium bicarbonate, enhance elimination using hemodialysis, and inhibit metabolism by providing ethanol as a competitive substrate for alcohol dehydrogenase (45). Ethanol inhibits ethylene glycol metabolism, thus reducing its toxicity potential after ingestion (17,22,57). Ethanol should be given within 8 hr of ethylene glycol ingestion and continued for at least 5 days. The dosing is the same as described previously for treatment of methanol toxicity.

Calcium salts are recommended to replace calcium, which is lost from the blood through combining with oxalate. Generally, hemodialysis is reserved for patients who have renal failure. Short-term dialysis has been shown to be effective in children before the onset of renal failure in acute ethylene glycol poisoning (50).

Recently, 4-MP, the alcohol dehydrogenase inhibitor mentioned earlier, has been used in treatment of ethylene glycol poisoning. It was successful when administered early, before coma, seizures, or renal failure (4,8,29).

PROPYLENE GLYCOL

Propylene glycol is generally reported to have a low order of systemic toxicity and, in fact, is widely used as a solvent for pharmaceutical products and cosmetics and in foods. However, the literature suggests that propylene glycol may be toxic if it is used inappropriately (2,34). In a few susceptible children, ingesting a propylene glycol-based product for long periods has caused seizures, tachypnea, diaphoresis, and unconsciousness. Such reports are rare.

FORMALDEHYDE

Recently, there has been renewed interest in accidental poisoning caused by formaldehyde (3). Most of this interest has centered on the release of formaldehyde into the air from insulation composed of urea formaldehyde (10,20). Formaldehyde may also cause contact urticaria in susceptible individuals, and it is a suspected carcinogen and mutagen (31,40).

Formaldehyde is a colorless, flammable gas with a strongly characteristic, pungent odor. It is marketed as formalin, an aqueous solution that is 37% to 50% formaldehyde by weight, with 10% to 50% methanol added to prevent spontaneous polymerization (3). Formalin is a disinfectant, antiseptic, and embalming fluid. Because it is highly reactive chemically, it is widely used in a variety of products, such as paints, adhesives, dyes, fuels, paper, and other chemicals. It can be a contaminant of air, originating from numerous sources including incinerators and engine exhausts. Atmospheric levels of 0.06 ppm have been reported near industrial sites or in areas of thick fog (40). Cigarette smoke contains high levels. Air concentration in some older mobile homes and other dwellings where urea formaldehyde foam insulation has been used may approach 1.9 ppm. The current NIOSH standard for formaldehyde in the occupational environment is 1 ppm for any 30-min sampling period (39). An individual who breathes contaminated air over many hours each day in enclosed quarters, such as in a mobile home, may be exposed to nearly twice the safe limit.

Mechanism of Toxicity

When formaldehyde is ingested in toxic amounts (60 to 90 mL is reported to be fatal), it produces a variety of effects. It quickly suppresses all cellular activity, leading to cell death. Tissue destruction (coagulative necrosis) is similar to that produced by mineral acids. Formaldehyde is oxidized to formic acid, and this accumulates quickly. Within minutes after ingestion, the victim may exhibit metabolic acidosis. All necrotic damage to gastrointestinal cells and other sites is secondary in importance to acidosis, which must be treated immediately.

Characteristics of Toxicity

Inhaled formaldehyde induces direct irritant action on the eyes and respiratory tract. Patients typically complain of tearing, rhinitis, itchy eyes, coughing, and dyspnea. Central nervous system effects include malaise, headache, insomnia, and anorexia. It has been suggested that inhalation of formaldehyde from urea formaldehyde foam insulation may be responsible for a significant number of cases of upper respiratory irritation.

Ingestion of formaldehyde causes immediate and intense GI tract irritation with severe abdominal cramping. This is quickly followed by metabolic acidosis, cardiovascular collapse, unconsciousness (due to CNS depression), and anuria (due to renal failure). Death usually occurs from circulatory collapse.

Management of Toxicity

Treatment is aimed at maintaining blood pressure and correcting the acid-base imbalance. Sympathomimetic amines may be necessary to achieve the former, and sodium bicarbonate is used for the acidosis. Since formaldehyde produces a corrosive action, dilution of gastric contents is the first-line treatment. Dialysis is effective in removing formic acid from the blood, and this removal will significantly aid treatment of acidosis.

ACETALDEHYDE

Acetaldehyde (ethanal, acetic aldehyde) is a colorless liquid or gas with a strongly penetrating, fruity odor. It is used in manufacturing dyes, plastics, flavors and perfumes, vinegar, and numerous other products.

Like formaldehyde, acetaldehyde is highly reactive. It is extremely irritating to all cells and can quickly inhibit cellular activity. Common routes of accidental exposure include inhalation of vapors and ingestion of solutions, although poisoning by the latter is rare.

One other source of acetaldehyde that may produce clinical symptoms is encountered by an individual taking disulfiram (Antabuse) who ingests ethanol. Typically, this person is a recovering alcoholic using disulfiram as a deterrent to drinking. Disulfiram inhibits aldehyde dehydrogenase. When ethanol is consumed, its metabolism is slowed at this step, and blood acetaldehyde concentrations may increase 10-fold (47). This, then, causes signs and symptoms reported by the individual as "unpleasant"—those that the person attempts to avoid by not consuming alcohol. Collectively, they are termed the *acetaldehyde syndrome* and include a hot and flushed feeling, throbbing pain in the head and neck, nausea and vomiting, dizziness, confusion, and hypotension.

Acetaldehyde intoxication by ingestion produces symptoms of narcosis. These are followed shortly by CNS depression, pulmonary edema, and albuminuria. Inhaled, it causes severe irritation of the eyes and respiratory system (7).

Treatment is symptomatic. There is no specific antidote.

ACETONE

Acetone (dimethylketone, propanone) is included in this chapter because of its relationship to isopropanol. Isopropanol is metabolized to acetone, and many symptoms of isopropanol toxicity are due to the metabolite.

Intoxication by acetone per se is a potential health hazard in industrial settings, where it is employed as a solvent. Most industrial poisonings occur by inhalation, with irritation of the eyes, nose, and throat produced at exposures of 500 to 1,000 ppm (11). The threshold limit value for acetone in an industrial setting for workers exposed 8 hr/day is 1,000 ppm (64). Higher concentrations cause CNS depression. Occasionally a case is reported where toxicity occurred after intentional inhalation of acetone vapors for recreational purposes.

In the home, acetone poisoning occurs infrequently. Acetone forms the basis for many commercial fingernail polish removers. Some products marketed for this use may also contain mineral seal oil, a hydrocarbon that is toxic in its own right (see chapter 7). The product's label should be carefully checked for contents in the event that the liquid is ingested. Acetone may be readily recognized on the breath by its characteristic fruity odor.

Ingestion of small quantities ranging from 10 to 20 mL does not normally produce symptoms. However, ingestion of 200 to 400 mL resulted in severe coma in adults, whereas in children 2 to 3 mL/kg is considered to be toxic (51,64).

Acetone is absorbed through the skin, but the quantity that reaches the blood from nail polish removers does not pose a threat. Acetone imparts an intense drying effect on the skin as it dissolves dermal lipids. Unless this occurs over a large area, it is not serious.

Symptoms following acute acetone ingestion include nausea, vomiting, gastric hemorrhage, sedation, respiratory depression, ataxia, and paresthesia. Depression resembles alcoholic stupor, but its onset is quicker than that with ethanol. Coughing and bronchial irritation may be the only clues to ingestion of quantities that are too small to produce sedation. Hyperglycemia and ketonemia with acidosis that resembles acute diabetic coma may be present. Treatment of acute acetone ingestion or inhalation of quantities sufficient to produce toxicity is symptomatic. Unless the patient is comatose, emesis or gastric lavage should be performed, followed by use of activated charcoal and catharsis. Diazepam will control seizures. Acidosis can be managed with sodium bicarbonate. The half-life of acetone in plasma is approximately 28 hr. Improvement in consciousness and other symptoms can, therefore, be expected to be a slow process (46).

SUMMARY

Numerous products around the home and workplace contain an alcohol or substance that reacts pharmacologically and toxicologically like alcohols. Aldehydes, glycols, and ketones are not as common as alcohol as causes of poisoning, but poisoning with these does occur. Immediate treatment with supportive therapy and more specific antidotes when appropriate are required for all alcohol/glycol/aldehyde/acetone intoxications.

Differential characteristics of alcohols and ethylene glycol are presented in Table 4.3.

Case Studies

CASE STUDY: ETHANOL INTOXICATION

History

A 23-year-old woman, weighing 45.8 kg, was involved in a hit-and-run automobile accident. She was arrested for suspicion of drunken driving. While in jail she became

TABLE 4.3. *Differential characteristics of alcohols and ethylene glycol*

Characteristic	Methanol	Ethanol	Isopropanol	Ethylene glycol
Toxic metabolites	Formaldehyde Formic acid	Acetaldehyde Acetic acid	Acetone	Glycoaldehyde Oxalate
Acidosis	Severe	Mild to moderate	Mild	Severe
Ketosis	Mild to none	Mild to moderate	Severe	None
Anion gap (>18 mEq/L)	+++	++	+	+++
Increased serum osmolality	Yes	Yes	Yes	Yes
CNS[a] depression	+	+++	++	+
Lethal dose	1–2 mL/kg	3–6 mL/kg	1–4 mL/kg	1–2 mL/kg

[a] CNS, central nervous system.

faint and passed out. After recovery, she related the following account of her activities.

On an empty stomach, the woman had consumed an entire fifth (26 ounces) of 100-proof bourbon over a 2-hr span. The accident occurred a few moments after she left the bar. She also later admitted that she had had a history of alcohol usage since she was 13 years old and had been discharged from an alcoholic rehabilitation center a week before this incident.

On arrival at an emergency facility, the patient was in stage 1 coma. Laboratory values were normal for pH, electrolytes, and glucose. Her blood alcohol concentration was 780 mg/dL; a toxicologic screen was negative for other drugs. Gastric lavage was performed, followed by administration of activated charcoal. Within 2 hr, her BAC was lowered to 730 mg/dL, and she began to respond to verbal commands. Three hours after activated charcoal administration, BAC was 420 mg/dL; at 11 hr, she was discharged with a BAC of 190 mg/dL. (See ref. 19.)

Discussion

1. Calculate the maximum BAC this individual should have attained after complete absorption of all she ingested. Does your value correspond to the BAC determined on admission to the ED? If it does not, suggest why the discrepancy exists.
2. How effective is forced diuresis in enhancing the elimination of ethanol?
3. Considering the ethanol blood concentrations, would hemodialysis have been useful in reducing the blood ethanol concentration? Did there seem to be an apparent need for dialysis?
4. Plot the blood ethanol concentrations (BAC) versus time. Comment on the rate of dissipation. Does it follow zero-order kinetics or first-order kinetics? Calculate the theoretical amount that should have dissipated over 11 hr, and relate this to the patient's BAC at 11 hr after admission.

CASE STUDY: INTOXICATION WITH MOUTHWASH

History

A 33-month-old, otherwise healthy girl was found by her parents in a stuporous condition. Beside her was a partially filled bottle of mouthwash. A paramedic team began intravenous therapy and then transported her to the emergency room.

On admission, the victim was comatose and nonresponsive to all stimuli except deep pain. Her pulse rate was 125 beats/min; respirations, 28/min; blood pressure, 88/50 mm Hg; and temperature, 35.4°C.

Laboratory data showed a blood alcohol concentration of 306 mg/dL (approximately 3.5 hr postingestion). Blood electrolyte measurement showed an anion gap of 28. It was estimated that the girl had ingested 11 ounces of 18.5% (v/v) ethanol (48.2 g absolute alcohol).

Treatment consisted of nasogastric lavage and intravenous fluids supplemented with bicarbonate. By 8 hr postingestion, blood alcohol concentration was reduced to 128 mg/dL. Eighteen hours after admission, all blood values had returned to normal, symptoms had disappeared, and the patient was discharged several hours later.

The ingestion of alcohol-containing products by children younger than 6 years of age is one of the most commonly reported poison exposures in the United States. The agents most commonly associated with ethanol ingestion in this group are perfumes, colognes,

TABLE 4.4. *Ethanol concentrations of leading mouthwashes*

Mouthwash	Ethanol (% v/v)	Approximate lethal dose (oz/12-kg child)
Cepacol	14.0	10.9
Listerine	26.9	5.7
Listermint	14.2	10.7
Scope	18.5	8.2
Signal	14.5	10.5

From ref. 62.

and aftershaves. The ingestion of mouthwash is also commonplace, probably because of its pleasing taste and odor. During an 18-month period, 422 cases in children under age 6 were reported by poison control centers. Ethanol content and the approximate lethal dose for five leading brands of mouthwash are listed in Table 4.4. (See ref. 62.)

Discussion

1. Assuming the child weighed 35 pounds and based on the history given, calculate the alcohol dissipation rate for this child. Is the calculated rate greater or less than the reported average dissipation rate? Why?
2. Does the clinical presentation of this child correlate well with the reported BAC?

CASE STUDY: POISONING BY WINE IN A CHILD

History

A previously healthy, 13-kg, 30-month-old boy was discovered unresponsive on the floor by his mother. The boy's 4-year-old brother told his mother that the younger brother had drank through a straw from a container that held Wild Irish Rose Wine (20% ethanol). Up to 16 ounces of the wine were believed to be missing. Paramedics were summoned and transported the child to the hospital.

Upon arrival at the ED, the child was comatose and unresponsive to deep pain but breathing spontaneously. Vital signs included temperature, 36.5°C rectally; blood pressure, 93/61 mm Hg; pulse, 88 beats/min; respirations, shallow, 24/min. Pupillary reflexes were sluggish. Deep tendon reflexes and gag reflex were intact. The rest of his physical examination was unremarkable.

A drug screen was negative except for ethanol which was determined to be 98.78 mmol/L (455 mg/dL, 0.46%). Treatment consisted of oxygen, 40% by face mask, and administration of 5% dextrose and normal saline.

Approximately 10 min after admission, the boy vomited spontaneously a large amount of rose-colored fluid smelling of ethanol. A nasogastric catheter was inserted and 200 mL fluid was aspirated. Gastric lavage with normal saline was continued until the returns were clear.

The patient remained unconscious and unresponsive to pain for slightly longer than 3 hr. By approximately 7 hr after admission, he was fully alert, behaving normally, and responding appropriately. He was discharged from the hospital 28 hr after admission.

An interesting observation about this case is shown by Fig. 4.8, which plots the semilogarithmic decline in blood ethanol concentration with time. The child appears to have metabolized ethanol by first-order elimination kinetics. (See ref. 32.)

Discussion

1. Comment on the extent of toxicity in this child based on his BAC of 455 mg/dL. Is this value higher or lower than expected? Were his symptoms characteristic of his BAC?
2. Calculate the actual amount of wine this child ingested.
3. Why is the discussion of elimination of ethanol in this patient of interest? (Hint: Over a 28-hr period, with BAC values as high as they were, what would have been

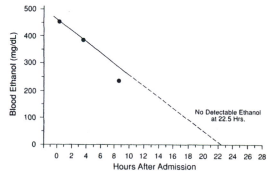

FIG. 4.8. Semilogarithmic decline in blood ethanol concentration with time. (From ref. 32.)

expected?) Can you explain the rate of elimination kinetics in this child?

CASE STUDIES: METHANOL INTOXICATION

History: Case 1

A well-nourished, otherwise healthy, female pathology resident complained of a "whiteness" in her vision, similar to "stepping out into a snow field." The previous evening she had consumed 2 to 3 ounces of 86-proof vodka and two glassfuls of wine. There had been nothing unusual about her activities the previous evening. She was admitted to the emergency room with irregular, rapid respirations (30/min); blood pressure, 170/105 mm Hg (previous history of labile hypertension); and pulse, 110 beats/min. Laboratory values are listed in Table 4.5.

Treatment consisted of ethanol, sodium bicarbonate, and hemodialysis for 6 hr. The patient did not complain of further disturbances during dialysis. Blood methanol levels were negative at the end of the dialysis procedure. Ophthalmologic examination revealed only slight pallor of the optic disc; otherwise, recovery was complete. (See ref. 5.)

History: Case 2

Seven days before admission to the hospital, this 8-month-old boy developed a cough accompanied by a low-grade fever. His parents treated the fever with aspirin.

The day before admission, the boy's respirations became progressively rapid and shallow. That afternoon the child seemed unusually drowsy and slept through his evening meal.

On the day of admission, the parents could not awaken the child, and he appeared to be severely dyspneic. On admission, he was in stage 3 coma. Pupils were dilated and unresponsive to light; he had slight papillary edema. Vital signs included blood pressure, 90/60 mm Hg; pulse, 132 beats/min; respirations, 25/min; and temperature, 37.8°C. Arterial pH was 6.50. Treatment consisted of antibiotics and sodium bicarbonate.

A toxicologic screen performed at the time of admission was negative. Due to the intense metabolic acidosis, another blood sample was taken for analysis. Methanol was confirmed, at a concentration of 40 mg/dL.

Specific treatment was started at once: ethanol, 0.33 g/kg intravenously initially, followed by 0.25 g/kg every 4 hr. Peritoneal dialysis was performed with dialyzing fluid containing sodium bicarbonate. In spite of treatment, the child's condition deteriorated rapidly. He experienced periods of hypothermia and episodes of bradycardia. Later that day, arterial blood pressure fell and the child died. A liver biopsy at the time of death revealed diffuse fatty degeneration. A lumbar puncture showed frank hemorrhage. A bacterial culture was negative.

Afterward, the parents were questioned about the child's exposure to methanol. They described an old family tradition used to "take off the cold" that consisted of applying warm compresses to the chest, which had been previously rubbed with olive oil. Compresses were soaked with alcohol and set on fire, then rapidly extinguished with a plate. The mother had had no alcohol on hand and unknowingly had purchased methanol, which she used to soak the compresses. Methanol-soaked pads had been applied to the child's chest throughout the night (approximately 12 hr) during the

TABLE 4.5. *Laboratory findings*

Na$^+$	= 135 mEq/L
K$^+$	= 4.7 mEq/L
Cl$^-$	= 107 mEq/L
HCO$_3^-$	= 6 mEq/L
Serum osmolality	= 325 mOsm/kg water
Blood methanol	= 140 mg/dL
pH	= 7.21
pCO$_2$	= 11 mm Hg
pO$_2$	= 123 mm Hg
BUN[a]	= 12 mg/dL
Creatinine	= 1 mg/dL

[a] BUN, blood urea nitrogen.

two nights before admission (total exposure, 24 hr). (See ref. 25.)

Discussion

1. What was the most likely source of methanol exposure in case 1?
2. Did this patient present in acidosis with a normal or elevated anion gap?
3. What is the significance in measuring the osmolality of serum? Can it be used to differentiate various alcohols from one another?
4. Why was gastric lavage not performed?
5. Give an explanation for the delayed onset of symptoms (i.e., visual disturbances) of methanol intoxication.
6. What is the most likely reason why the child in case 2 received peritoneal dialysis rather than hemodialysis?
7. Discuss a possible contributing role of aspirin in the child's death in case 2.
8. Was the child in case 2 poisoned by inhalation or percutaneous absorption of methanol?

CASE STUDIES: ETHYLENE GLYCOL POISONING

History: Case 1

A 51-year-old man was admitted to the emergency room 2.5 hr after ingesting 600 mL of an antifreeze solution containing 95% ethylene glycol. He was ataxic, dysarthric, and lethargic. Laboratory values are listed in Table 4.6.

Initial treatment consisted of gastric lavage and activated charcoal followed by sodium bicarbonate and ethanol infusion intravenously (5% ethanol, 0.98 g/kg). After 2 hr of treatment, the blood concentration of ethylene glycol decreased to 325 mg/dL. Hemodialysis was performed, and ethylene glycol concentrations decreased to 60 mg/dL after 6 hr of dialysis and were reduced to an undetectable quantity 80 hr after ingestion. Throughout the dialysis, etha-

nol concentrations were maintained between 100 and 140 mg/dL by hourly nasogastric doses of 20% ethanol. (See ref. 15.)

History: Case 2

This case involved an 18-year-old man who presented to the emergency department with symptoms of hysteria and hyperventilation. The patient gave a history that was essentially uneventful, and there was no indication of drug abuse. Laboratory tests for salicylates, methanol, and ethanol were negative, and urinalysis showed a large number of unidentifiable crystals.

Based upon the laboratory findings listed in Table 4.7, the patient was treated for acidosis. When bicarbonate therapy was unsuccessful, dialysis was initiated. Despite dialysis, the patient died less than 16 hr after he was admitted. (See ref. 15.)

History: Case 3

A 33-year-old woman with suicidal tendencies ingested 2 L of ethylene glycol. Upon admittance to the emergency room, she showed signs of mild intoxication. Laboratory values are presented in Table 4.4.

Gastric lavage recovered approximately 1 L of ethylene glycol. She was then given activated charcoal, castor oil, and an infusion of ethanol (absolute) at an initial volume of 600 mL, followed by 10 mL/hr for 25 hr. Serum ethylene glycol concentration dropped from 560 mg/dL to less than 100 mg/dL during the dialysis period. The patient recovered completely. (See ref. 55.)

Discussion

1. Compare case 3 to cases 1 and 2. The amount ingested in case 3 was greater than in the other two; why was there not a significant metabolic acidosis or elevated anion gap?
2. What are some probable reasons why the

TABLE 4.6. *Laboratory findings*

Measurement	Case 1	Case 2	Case 3
Quantity of ethylene glycol ingested	600 mL	Unknown	2 L
Arterial pH	7.18	7.03	7.31
pCO$_2$ (mm Hg)	14	13	39
pO$_2$ (mm Hg)	91	92	90
Anion gap (mEq/L)[a]	46	28.7	Normal
Osmolality (mOsm/kg)	422	331	383
Calculated osmolality (mOsm/kg)[b]	312	291	
Serum ethylene glycol (mg/dL)[c]	650	98	560

See the appendix for a table of normal laboratory values.

[a] Anion gap = $(N^+ + K^+) - (HCO_3^- + Cl^-)$

[b] $Osm = 2 (Na^+) + \dfrac{BUN}{2.8} + \dfrac{Glucose}{18}$

[c] Toxic concentration = 150 mg/dL.

patient in case 2 died, even though blood ethylene glycol concentration, when admitted to the emergency room, was less than that of the other two cases?

3. If patient 3 actually ingested 2 L, as reported, but half was still recovered, give the most probable explanation for why she survived.

4. Comment on the effectiveness of hemodialysis in each of the cases provided.

CASE STUDY: FORMALDEHYDE POISONING

History

A 41-year-old woman ingested 120 mL of a formaldehyde solution containing 37% (w/

TABLE 4.7. *Laboratory findings*

Blood	
Formaldehyde	= 0.48 mg/dL
Methanol	= 42.5 mg/dL
Formic acid	= 42 mg/dL
pH	= 6.87
HCO$_3^-$	= 10 mEq/L
Cl$^-$	= 60 mEq/L
Na$^+$	= 92 mEq/L
K$^+$	= 5.1 mEq/L
Serum creatinine	= 2.9 mg/dL
BUN	= 12.0 mg/L
pCO$_2$	= 35 mm Hg
pO$_2$	= 54 mm Hg
Liver enzymes	
LDH[a]	= 1,830 units/dL
SGOT[b]	= 1,520 units/dL

[a] IDH, lactate dehydrogenase.
[b] SGOT, serum glutamic-oxaloacetic transaminase.

v) formaldehyde and 12.5% (v/v) methanol. No formic acid was present in the solution. On admission to a hospital, the patient was cyanotic, apneic, and hypotensive.

Gastric lavage revealed a noticeable odor of formaldehyde. Fluid replacement included lactated Ringer's solution and 5% dextrose in water. Control of acidosis was attempted with sodium bicarbonate, 132 mEq/L. Her blood pressure was maintained with dopamine hydrochloride. Despite efforts to maintain her acid-base balance and blood pressure, the patient died 24 hr after admission. (See ref. 12.)

Discussion

1. If the patient ingested 120 mL of a formaldehyde solution containing methanol, why is the initial blood concentration for formaldehyde so low? What was the source of the high formic acid concentration?

2. Which laboratory values demonstrate that the patient presented with metabolic acidosis? Is the anion gap normal or elevated?

3. What was the probable cause of death (i.e., what did these poisons contain)?

4. Would hemodialysis have been of benefit? Was ethanol treatment indicated?

Review Questions

1. Which of the following is a product of isopropanol metabolism?

A. Acetic acid
B. Formaldehyde
C. Ethanol
D. Acetone

2. A victim of poisoning by Columbian spirits should receive treatment for which of the following substances?
   A. Ethanol
   B. Methanol
   C. Ethylene glycol
   D. Isopropanol

3. Which of the following symptoms appears at a blood ethanol concentration of 0.05%?
   A. Visual impairment
   B. Altered equilibrium
   C. Stupor
   D. Coma

4. The hallmark of isopropanol intoxication is:
   A. Severe metabolic acidosis
   B. Acetonemia
   C. Anemia
   D. CNS stimulation

5. Which of the following alcohols is the most commonly reported cause of poisoning in the general population?
   A. Ethanol
   B. Methanol
   C. Isopropanol
   D. Butanol

6. Oxalic acid is a metabolite of which of the following poisons?
   A. Methanol
   B. Ethylene glycol
   C. Acetaldehyde
   D. Isopropanol

7. The CNS symptoms associated with ethylene glycol toxicity may be attributed to accumulation of which of the following?
   A. Formic acid
   B. Calcium oxalate
   C. Glycoaldehyde
   D. NAD

8. A patient presenting with severe ketoacidosis with a high anion gap, hypoglycemia, and significant CNS impairment at blood levels >250 mg/dL would likely have ingested:

A. Methanol
B. Ethyl alcohol
C. Ethylene glycol
D. Formaldehyde

9. 4-Methylpyrazole has been used in the treatment of methanol and ethylene glycol poisonings. The beneficial actions are due to inhibition of:
   A. Alcohol dehydrogenase
   B. Aldehyde dehydrogenase
   C. Aldehyde transaminase
   D. Nicotinamide adenine dinucleotide

10. An ethylene glycol ingestion would be characterized by all of the following *except:*
    A. Anion gap metabolic acidosis
    B. Oxalate crystals in the urine
    C. Acute tubular necrosis
    D. Hepatic failure

11. Which of the following is related to ethanol metabolism?
    A. Disulfiram (Antabuse) increases the rate of ethanol metabolism.
    B. 4-Methylpyrazole increases the rate of ethanol metabolism.
    C. Diazepam inhibits the rate of ethanol metabolism.
    D. Alcohol dehydrogenase is the rate-limiting enzyme in ethanol metabolism.

12. Analeptic therapy is an important component of the treatment of ethanol intoxication.
    A. True
    B. False

13. In general, increasing the number of carbon atoms on a series of alcohols decreases the toxicity of the substance.
    A. True
    B. False

14. Pure "moonshine" liquor is a rich source of methanol.
    A. True
    B. False

15. Methanol is metabolized by the same enzymes that metabolize ethanol.
    A. True
    B. False

16. Which of the following is a symptom of

methanol toxicity: general CNS stimulation (I), metabolic alkalosis (II), or blurred vision (III)?

A. II only
B. III only
C. I and II only
D. II and III only
E. I, II, and III

17. Which of the following electrolyte abnormalities occurs often with an ethylene glycol poisoning?

A. Hypokalemia
B. Hypocalcemia
C. Hyperchloremia
D. Hyperphosphatemia
E. Hypercalcemia

18. Which of the following is a toxic metabolite of methanol metabolism: acetic acid (I), oxalic acid (II), or formaldehyde (III)?

A. II only
B. III only
C. I and II only
D. II and III only
E. I, II, and III

19. An ethylene glycol ingestion would be characterized by all of the following except:

A. Anion gap acidosis
B. Acute tubular necrosis
C. Hepatic failure
D. Oxalate crystals in the urine

20. The antidote for acute methanol intoxication is:

A. Atropine
B. BAL
C. Ethanol
D. Ethylene glycol

The next two questions refer to the following case history:

A 6-year-old boy attempting to mimic his father's nightly habit of drinking two martinis before bedtime mixes 3 ounces of rubbing alcohol (70% isopropyl alcohol) with some 7-Up and drinks the "cocktail" at about 7 p.m. The child awakens around midnight complaining of a burning stomachache, a bad headache, and dizziness. He vomits twice within a half-hour and finally admits to his mother what he had done earlier that evening.

21. All of the following are additional signs that might be expected to be observed in this case except:

A. Hypotension
B. Acetonemia
C. Acidosis
D. CNS depression
E. Optic nerve degeneration

22. A toxicologic analysis of the child's blood would likely reveal significant blood concentrations of:

A. n-Propanol
B. Acetaldehyde
C. Acetone
D. Oxalic acid
E. More than one of the above

23. Ethanol administration is often an important component of the acute treatment of methanol-intoxicated patients because:

A. Ethanol will enhance the oxidative detoxification of methanol
B. Ethanol will diminish the formation of toxic metabolites of methanol
C. Ethanol will inhibit metabolism of methanol by alcohol dehydrogenase
D. All of the above
E. Only two of the above

24. Ingestion of a mouthful of a "glycol" would most likely impart which of the following tastes?

A. Sweet
B. Sour
C. Salty
D. Bitter
E. Bland

25. Cite the reasons why ethanol is an antidote for methanol and ethylene glycol poisoning. What blood concentration of ethanol is recommended? How is it administered?

26. Discuss the relevance of using the anion gap value in assessing the probable cause of poisoning.

27. Discuss the information that the Widmark equation provides. Why is the formula different for men and women?

28. Describe the treatment protocol for methanol intoxication. What is the significance

of keeping a methanol-poisoned patient in a darkened room?

29. The term *glycol* was coined from the Greek stem that describes the taste of these substances. What is that taste?

References

1. Adinoff B, Bone GHA, Linnoila M. Acute ethanol poisoning and the ethanol withdrawal syndrome. *Med Toxicol* 1988;3:172–196.
2. Arulamantham K. Central nervous system toxicity associated with ingestion of propylene glycol. *J Pediatr* 1978;93:515–516.
3. Bardana EJ, Montanaro A. Formaldehyde: an analysis of its respiratory, cutaneous, and immunologic effects. *Ann Allergy* 1991;66:441–452.
4. Baud FJ, Bismuth C, Garrier R, et al. 4-Methylpyrazole may be an alternative to ethanol therapy for ethylene glycol intoxication in man. *J Toxicol Clin Toxicol* 1986–87;24:463–483.
5. Becker CE. Acute methanol poisoning—the blind drunk. *West J Med* 1981;135:122–128.
6. Berman L, Schreiner G, Feyes J. The nephrotoxic lesion of ethylene glycol. *Ann Intern Med* 1957;46:611–619.
7. Booze TF, Oehme FW. An investigation of metaldehyde and acetaldehyde toxicities in dogs. *Fundam Appl Toxicol* 1986;6:440–446.
8. Chow JY, Richardson KE. The effect of pyrazole in ethylene glycol toxicity and metabolism in the rat. *Toxicol Appl Pharmacol* 1978;43:33–44.
9. Clay KL, Murphy RC, Watkins WD. Experimental methanol toxicity in the primate: analysis of metabolic acidosis. *Toxicol Appl Pharmacol* 1975;34:49–61.
10. Day JH, Lees REM, Clark RH, Pattee PL. Respiratory response to formaldehyde, an off-gas of urea formaldehyde foam insulation. *Can Med J* 1984;131:1061–1065.
11. DiVincenzo GO, Yanno FJ, Astill BD. Exposure of man and dog to low concentrations of acetone vapor. *Am Ind Hyg Assoc J* 1973;34:329–330.
12. Eells JT, McMartin KE, Black K, et al. Formaldehyde poisoning—rapid metabolism to formic acid. *JAMA* 1981;246:1237–1238.
13. Freireich AW, Cinque TJ, Xanthary G, Lindau D. Hemodialysis for isopropanol poisoning. *N Engl J Med* 1967;277:699.
14. Geiling EMK, Cannon PR. Pathologic effects of elixir of sulfanilamide (diethylene glycol) poisoning. *JAMA* 1938;111:919–926.
15. Godolphin W, Meagher EP, Sanders HD, Frohlich J. Unusual calcium oxalate crystals in ethylene glycol poisoning. *Clin Toxicol* 1980;16:479–486.
16. Gonda A, Gault H, Churchill D, Hollomby D. Hemodialysis for methanol intoxication. *Am J Med* 1978;64:749–758.
17. Gosselin RE, Smith RP, Hodge HC. *Clinical toxicology of commercial products.* 5th ed. Baltimore: Williams and Wilkins; 1984.
18. Greear JN. The causes of blindness. In: Zahl PA, ed. *Blindness: modern approaches to the unseen environment.* Princeton: Princeton University Press; 1950:130.
19. Hammond KB, Rumack BH, Rodgerson DO. Blood ethanol—a report of unusually high levels in a living patient. *JAMA* 1973;226:63–64.
20. Harris JC, Rumack BH, Aldrich FD. Toxicology of urea formaldehyde and polyurethane foam insulation. *JAMA* 1981;245:243–246.
21. Holck HGO. Glycerin, ethylene glycol, propylene glycol and diethylene glycol. *JAMA* 1937;109:19.
22. Jacobsen D, McMartin KE. Methanol and ethylene glycol poisonings: mechanism of toxicity, clinical course, diagnosis and treatment. *Med Toxicol* 1986;1:309–334.
23. Jacobson D, Sebastian CS, Barron SK, Carriere EW, McMartin KE. Effects of 4-methylpyrazole, methanol/ethylene glycol antidote, in healthy humans. *J Emerg Med* 1990,8:455–461.
24. Jacobsen D, Webb R, Collins TD, McMartin KE. Methanol and formate kinetics in late diagnosed methanol intoxication. *Med Toxicol* 1988;3:418–423.
25. Kahn A, Blum D. Methyl alcohol poisoning in an 8-month-old boy: an unusual route of intoxication. *J Pediatr* 1979;94:841–843.
26. Kelner M, Bailey DN. Isopropanol ingestion: interpretation of blood concentrations and clinical findings. *J Toxicol Clin Toxicol* 1983;20:497–507.
27. Kini MM, Cooper JR. Biochemistry of methanol poisoning: 4. The effect of methanol and its metabolites on retinal metabolism. *Biochem J* 1962;82:164–172.
28. Kini MM, King DW, Cooper JR. Biochemistry of methanol poisoning: 5. Histological and biochemical correlates of effects of methanol and its metabolites on the rabbit retina. *J Neurochem* 1962;9:119–124.
29. Koivusalo M. Methanol. In: Tremolieres J, ed. *Alcohols and derivatives*, vol 2. London: Pergamon Press; 1970:465–505.
30. Lacouture PG, Wason S, Abrams A, Lovejoy FH. Acute isopropyl alcohol intoxication. *Am J Med* 1983;75:680–686.
31. Lewis BB, Chestner SB. Formaldehyde in dentistry: a review of mutagenic and carcinogenic potential. *J Am Dent Assoc* 1981;103:429–434.
32. Lopez GP, Yealy DM, Krenzelok EP. Survival of a child despite unusually high blood ethanol levels. *Am J Emerg Med* 1989;7:283–286.
33. Malmlund H, Berg A, Karlman G, Magnusson A, Ullman B. Considerations for the treatment of ethylene glycol poisoning based on analysis of two cases. *Clin Toxicol* 1991;29:231–240.
34. Martin G, Finberg L. Propylene glycol: a potentially toxic vehicle in liquid dosage forms. *J Pediatr* 1970;77:877.
35. McMartin KE, Ambre JJ, Tephley TR. Methanol poisoning in human subjects. *Am J Med* 1980;68:414.
36. McMartin KE, Hedstrom KG, Tolf BR, et al. Studies on the metabolic interactions between 4-methyl-pyrazole and methanol using the monkey as an animal model. *Arch Biochem Biophys* 1980;199:606–614.
37. Miller PD, Herring RE, Waterhouse C. Treatment of alcoholic acidosis. *Arch Intern Med* 1978;138:67–72.
38. NIH Report. Use of folate analogue in treatment of

methyl alcohol toxic reactions is studied. *JAMA* 1979;242:1961.

39. NIOSH Report. Criteria for a recommended standard: occupational exposure to formaldehyde. Rockville, MD: U.S. Government Publication; 1976: DHEW publication no. 77-126.

40. NIOSH Report. Formaldehyde: evidence of carcinogenicity. *Curr Intell Bull* 1981;34.

41. Palmer JP. Alcoholic ketoacidosis—clinical and laboratory presentation, pathophysiology and treatment. *Clin Endocrinol Metab* 1983;12:381–389.

42. Pappas AA, Ackerman BH, Olsen KM, Taylor EH. Isopropanol ingestion: a report of six episodes with isopropanol and acetone serum concentration time data. *Clin Toxicol* 1991;29:11–21.

43. Parry MF, Wallach R. Ethylene glycol poisoning. *Am J Med* 1974;57:143–150.

44. Peterson C. Oral ethanol doses in patients with methanol poisoning. *Am J Hosp Pharm* 1981;38:1024–1027.

45. Peterson CD, Collins AJ, Himes JM, et al. Ethylene glycol poisoning. *N Engl J Med* 1981;304:21–23.

46. Rall TW. Hypnotics and sedatives: ethanol. In: Gilman AG, Rall TW, Nies AS, Taylor P, eds. *The pharmacological basis of therapeutics*. 8th ed. New York: Pergamon Press; 1990:370–377.

47. Ramu A, Rosenbaum J, Blaschke TF. Disposition of acetone following acute acetone intoxication. *West J Med* 1978;129:429.

48. Roe O. Species differences in methanol poisonings. *Crit Rev Toxicol* 1982;10:275–286.

49. Rosansky SJ. Isopropyl alcohol poisoning treated with hemodialysis. *J Toxicol Clin Toxicol* 1982; 19:265.

50. Rothman A, Normann SA, Manoguerra AS, et al. Short-term hemodialysis in childhood ethylene glycol poisoning. *J Pediatr* 1986;108:153–155.

51. Rumack BH. *Poisondex*. Denver: Rocky Mountain Poison Center; 1983.

52. Ruprecht HA, Nelson IA. Preliminary toxicity reports on diethylene glycol and sulfanilamide: 5. Clinical and pathologic observations. *JAMA* 1937;109:1537–1540.

53. Scrimgeour EM. Outbreak of methanol and isopropanol poisoning in New Britain, Papua New Guinea. *Med J Aust* 1980;2:36–38.

54. Sporer KA, Ernst AA, Conte R, Nick TG. The incidence of ethanol-induced hypoglycemia. *Am J Emerg Med* 1992;10:403–405.

55. Stokes JB, Aueron F. Prevention of organ damage in massive ethylene glycol ingestion. *JAMA* 1980; 243:2065–2066.

56. Thompson CJ, Johnston DG, Baylis PH, Anderson J. Alcoholic ketoacidosis: an underdiagnosed condition? *Br Med J* 1986;292:463–465.

57. Turk J, Morrell L, Avioli LV. Ethylene glycol intoxication. *Arch Intern Med* 1986;146:1601–1603.

58. Vale J. Ethylene glycol poisoning. *Vet Hum Toxicol* 1979;21[Suppl]:118–120.

59. Vale J, Widdop B, Bluett N. Ethylene glycol poisoning. *Postgrad Med J* 1976;52:598–602.

60. Wagner JG, Wilkinson PK, Sedman AJ. Elimination of alcohol from human blood. *J Pharm Sci* 1976;60:152–154.

61. Walgreen H. Absorption, diffusion, distribution, and elimination of ethanol: effect on biological membranes. In: Tremolieres J, ed. *Alcohols and derivatives*, vol 1. London: Pergamon Press; 1970:161–188.

62. Weller-Fahy ER, Berger LR, Troutman WG. Mouthwash: a source of acute ethanol intoxication. *Pediatrics* 1980;66:302–304.

63. Wilkinson PK, Sedman AJ, Sakmar E. Pharmacokinetics of ethanol after oral administration in the fasting state. *J Pharmacokinet Biopharm* 1977;5:207–224.

64. Winchester JF. Methanol, isopropyl alcohol, higher alcohols, ethylene glycol, cellosolves, acetone, and oxalate. In: Haddad LM, Winchester JF, eds. *Clinical management of poisoning and drug overdose*. Philadelphia: WB Saunders; 1983:393–410.

5 || Nitrates and Nitrites

Nitrates are causing considerable concern among environmentalists and toxicologists (17,20,21). Nitrates, along with phosphates and several other ions, persist in the environment for long periods. Nitrates are being used with increasing frequency as synthetic nitrogen-gassed fertilizers become more popular. They are used in food production and processing to prevent food spoilage and are essential starting products and components or intermediate products formed during the manufacture of thousands of different chemicals and drugs. Animal waste products are also rich in nitrates.

The result of all of this activity is that high levels of nitrates have now contaminated soil and water supplies of many regions, especially from shallow wells in rural areas. Because of their high water solubility, nitrates eventually leach into soil and water supplies of adjacent areas. The time may be near when nitrate poisoning from drinking water will be a normal occurrence rather than an unusual one. A 1981 survey of more than 100 wells in a Midwestern community found that 27% of the wells had greater concentration of nitrate in the water than permitted by the Environmental Protection Agency (10 ppm) (15).

The use of amyl, butyl, and isobutyl nitrite as recreational drugs also has become a major problem. Each year approximately 250,000,000 doses are sold in the United States (16). These volatile nitrites are inhaled directly from their containers or are first allowed to volatilize in an enclosed area such as a plastic bag, from which they are then inhaled. They supposedly enhance the user's perception of certain social activities. While no fatalities have been reported, illicit use of these drug items can be considered to be potentially dangerous and should be curtailed (11). In one incident a 2-year-old girl was admitted with severe circulatory compromise and poor respiration after ingesting about 5 mL of an "aphrodisiac" product named Liquid Gold (8).

A special concern involves possible nitrosation of nitrites with amines (3). The resulting nitrosamines constitute one of the most potent classes of carcinogenic chemicals known. They have been shown to cause tumor growth in most animal models studied, including humans (24). A special problem is that nitrates readily undergo biologic conversion to nitrites, and nitrites may be subjected to nitrosamine formation *in vivo*. This has been demonstrated in animals, but whether such a reaction actually occurs *in vivo* in humans is questionable (7). The possibility that it does occur certainly must be taken seriously and cannot be brushed aside. This is why vitamin C, vitamin E, sulfamate, and antioxidants, such as butylated hydroxytoluene (BHT) and butylated hydroxyanisole (BHA), are frequently added to nitrite-treated foods and some drug products that have the potential for nitrosamine formation. These substances reduce the nitrosation process.

In the meantime, our consideration of nitrate/nitrite poisoning will not focus on suspected carcinogen formation. Rather, it will concentrate on acute poisoning from the nitrogenous substances that may be found around the home or workplace. It will also consider nitrate poisoning in infants from drinking contaminated water or ingesting foods that are rich in nitrate.

MECHANISMS OF NITRATE TOXICITY AND CHARACTERISTICS OF NITRATE POISONING

The two major toxicologic concerns resulting from nitrate poisoning are cardiovas-cular collapse and methemoglobinemia. Nitrates produce nonspecific relaxation of all smooth muscle, including the vasculature. Although this action is generalized throughout the body, the effect on postcapillary vessels is more prominent and results in venous pooling and, thus, a decrease in blood pressure. At therapeutic doses of nitrates, neither inotropy nor chronotropy is affected significantly, but at higher doses the myocardium is depressed.

As opposed to therapeutic actions, when nitrates are ingested in toxic quantities they produce intense vasodilation. This vasodilation can precipitate several outcomes, ranging from a throbbing headache and flushed face to rapid fall in blood pressure and cardiogenic shock. Normally, the heart would compensate for the effects of venous pooling and decreased blood pressure through baroreceptor stimulation and reflex sympathetic activation. Through these reflex mechanisms, sympathetic stimulation would result in increased heart rate and force of contraction in an attempt to elevate blood pressure to normal. However, when toxic blood concentrations of nitrates are present, the heart is unable to respond. The heart-related signs and symptoms of nitrate poisoning are listed in Table 5.1.

In addition to cardiovascular collapse, the other major toxic action of nitrates is methemoglobinemia. Methemoglobinemia is characterized by oxidation of ferrous ($HbFe^{2+}$) iron in hemoglobin to the ferric ($HbFe^{3+}$) state. Methemoglobin is unable to bind oxygen and, consequently, oxygen transport is in-

TABLE 5.1. *Signs and symptoms of nitrate poisoning*

Headache, pulsation feeling in head
Palpitations
Tachycardia
Hypotension, shock
Cardiovascular collapse
Dizziness, fainting
Weakness
Cyanosis
Shallow respirations
Methemoglobinemia

terrupted, resulting in cyanosis that is unresponsive to oxygen therapy.

As a result of this oxidation reaction, dried arterial blood will have a "chocolate-brown" appearance, which is pathognomonic (distinctively characteristic) for methemoglobinemia. Formation of methemoglobin also causes the oxygen dissociation curve to shift to the left, as will be discussed with cyanide and carbon monoxide in chapter 6. Although the mechanisms for various toxic substances are different, the end result, anoxia, is the same. Clinical characteristics of methemoglobinemia are listed in Table 5.2. All outcomes can be related to the inability of oxygen to be adequately transported to the body's tissues.

Any chemical that oxidizes ferrous iron to the ferric state can incite methemoglobin formation. This includes nitrates and nitrites, as well as other substances listed in Table 5.3. Nitrites are more potent than nitrates in producing methemoglobin. Heme oxidation also occurs spontaneously, probably because of environmental influences or from certain foods. At any time, approximately 1% to 2% of total hemoglobin exists in the oxidized (methemoglobin) form. This concentration is not pathologic.

Erythrocytes contain several enzyme systems that reduce methemoglobin back to hemoglobin (Fig. 5.1) (14). The most important is methemoglobin reductase (diaphorase I). A second methemoglobin reductase enzyme (diaphorase II) is dependent on concentrations of nicotinamide adenine dinucleotide phosphate (NADP, NADPH) for its action. This latter system is ordinarily of little importance, since the former normally maintains methemoglo-

TABLE 5.3. *Chemical agents reported to cause methemoglobinemia*

Acetophenetidin
Aminophenones
p-Aminosalicylic acid
Aniline
Antimalarials (i.e., chloroquine, primaquine)
Chlorates
Copper sulfate
Dapsone
Local anesthetics (i.e., benzocaine, lidocaine, prilocaine)
Methylene blue (high doses)
Naphthalene
Nitrates and nitrites
Amyl nitrite
Butyl/isobutyl nitrite
Nitroglycerin
Potassium nitrite
Sodium nitrite
Nitrate and nitrite meat preservatives
Vegetables (i.e., spinach and carrots in infants)
Nitrate and nitrite-contaminated well water
Nitrate and nitrite salts used in industry
Nitrobenzene
Nitrotoluene
Phenazopyridine
Resorcinol
Sulfonamides

From ref. 12.

bin levels below 1% to 2%. When methemoglobin concentrations increase, diaphorase II activity can increase 60-fold (1). Normal erythrocytic methemoglobin reductase can reduce methemoglobin to hemoglobin at a rate 250 times its rate of formation (19). As long as an individual can maintain an adequate level of these enzymes or does not ingest large quantities of oxidizing chemicals, the blood level of methemoglobin remains around 1% to 2%. It is only when the enzyme system becomes saturated, as occurs when large amounts of oxidizing substances are ingested, that methemoglobin accumulates in sufficient quantity to induce clinical signs and symptoms of poisoning.

There are several other ways, in addition to the oxidizing agents mentioned, in which the concentration of methemoglobin can be raised above normal. Toxic methemoglobin levels can result from a congenital disorder, hereditary methemoglobinemia. This condition is characterized by absence of NADH-depen-

TABLE 5.2. *Characteristics of methemoglobinemia*

Gray cyanosis, persistent even with oxygen therapy
Easy fatigability
Dyspnea; respiratory distress
Tachycardia
Dizziness with exertion
Arterial blood that is chocolate-brown
Oxygen-carrying capacity of arterial blood decreased; shift to the left of oxygen and dissociation curve

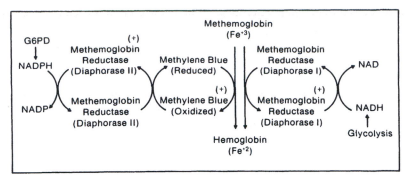

FIG. 5.1. Mechanisms of methemoglobin reduction.

dent methemoglobin reductase (18). The disorder is usually detected by the presence of cyanosis at birth.

The results of a study illustrate the effects of a challenge dose of sodium nitrite in an individual with hereditary methemoglobinemia versus a normal person (Fig. 5.2). Both individuals received a single 500-mg intravenous dose of sodium nitrite. From the figure, it may be seen that, by 6 hr after injection, the methemoglobin level had returned to near baseline in the normal person, but it was still abnormally elevated in the individual deficient in the enzyme. The total amount of methemoglobin formed in both subjects was essentially the same.

Nitrate-induced methemoglobinemia is of special concern in infants for several reasons

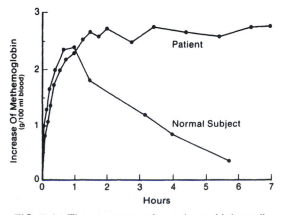

FIG. 5.2. The response of a patient with hereditary methemoglobinemia compared to the response of a normal person.

(5,15). First, the gastric pH of infants is characteristically less acidic than that of older children and adults. Normally, when gastric pH is low, growth of microorganisms, such as *Escherichia coli*, which convert nitrate to its more toxic form, nitrite, is retarded. When less acid is present, more bacteria proliferate (9). Therefore, when foods that are rich in nitrate, such as spinach or carrots, are given to these infants in excess or when baby formula is prepared from water containing high concentrations of nitrates, there is a possibility of nitrate poisoning and methemoglobinemia (5,9,22). It has been reported that water nitrate concentrations of 10 ppm are unsafe for infants. The same concentration typically causes no problems in older children or adults (1,20).

Second, fetal hemoglobin is more susceptible to oxidation to methemoglobin than is adult hemoglobin. This is because methemoglobin reductase is less active in infants under 3 months of age (20). Therefore, an excessive quantity of nitrates can easily cause methemoglobinemia. Infants may also consume more nitrate-contaminated well water per gram of hemoglobin than do adults (10).

The third reason why infants are more prone to methemoglobinemia is because they have an incompletely developed hepatic microsomal enzyme system. When ingested nitrates are converted to nitrites by intestinal bacteria, absorbed nitrite is not metabolized by the liver to its inactive form as rapidly as it is in older children and adults. Consequently, nitrite concentration in blood remains elevated longer, and the chance of oxidizing hemoglobin to methemoglobin is enhanced.

MANAGEMENT OF METHEMOGLOBINEMIA

Whenever cyanosis is present and persists after administration of oxygen, methemoglobinemia should be suspected. Diagnosis is aided when dried arterial blood appears chocolate-brown. This occurs when the methemoglobin concentration exceeds 15%. Definite confirmation can then be made by quantitative determination of methemoglobin in blood.

Cyanosis may be a manifestation of methemoglobin concentration as low as 10%. However, patients with levels less than 20% to 30% are usually asymptomatic and do not require immediate treatment (13,15). Even concentrations as high as 55% may be manifest by little more than shortness of breath in certain individuals (22). When blood methemoglobin concentrations reach 30% or more, signs and symptoms of methemoglobinemia are present and usually dictate that specific treatment should be initiated. Blood concentrations of 60% to 70% are considered lethal (6). Oxygen, alone or with methylene blue, is the treatment of choice. The offending agent should also be identified and removed.

Methylene blue (tetramethylthionine chloride) is a specific antidote for methemoglobinemia (2). It is a dye that serves as an intermediate in electron transfer between methemoglobin reductase (diaphorase II) and methemoglobin. The mechanism of action is outlined in Fig. 5.1 (13). A reversal of the toxic events of methemoglobinemia should be noted within an hour of initiation of methylene blue therapy. In patients with methemoglobin concentrations less than 30%, treatment consists of removing the offending agents and, if necessary, giving oxygen (100%). When methemoglobin concentrations exceed 30%, methylene blue (1% solution) is generally administered at 1 to 2 mg/kg intravenously. Special care is needed when using methylene blue, since larger doses may actually produce methemoglobinemia. A dose of 5 mg/kg has been reported to increase the methemoglobin level (23). Doses greater than 15 mg/kg are associated with hemolysis (14).

The suggestion is sometimes made that another reducing agent, such as ascorbic acid, will substitute for methylene blue in treatment of methemoglobinemia. Although ascorbic acid is occasionally used with some success, it normally is not suitable for serious cases because it does not reduce methemoglobin to hemoglobin quickly enough (13).

SUMMARY

Symptoms of nitrate/nitrite poisoning, for the most part, are similar regardless of the nature of the causative poison. Likewise, these poisons are treated in the same manner. It is important to understand what the symptoms of toxic nitrate and nitrite are and how they are treated.

Case Studies

CASE STUDY: METHEMOGLOBINEMIA FROM ETHYL NITRITE

History

After a suggestion from a relative, a parent of 4-month-old twin boys administered "sweet spirits of nitre" (4% ethyl nitrite in 70% ethanol) to the boys because they had an upper respiratory infection. The spirits of nitre would supposedly control their "fussiness." A "small amount" was added to each of the children's formula bottles.

After ingesting the entire contents of the formula bottle, one of the twins rapidly developed severe respiratory distress. He became cyanotic and unresponsive. On admission to an emergency facility, the baby was resuscitated. Arterial blood appeared chocolate-brown color when dried. Blood gases were: pO_2, 280 mm Hg; pCO_2, 176 mm Hg; and pH, 6.71. Total hemoglobin was 8.8 g/dL, of which methemoglobin composed 80%.

The mother reported giving the child 1 to 2 teaspoonfuls of ethyl nitrite. Ten milligrams of methylene blue were administered intravenously, and the methemoglobin concentration declined to 8.9% within a few hours. However, the baby continued to require ventilation assistance and died 12 hr later. An autopsy revealed acute hypoxemic changes in the tissues.

The other baby, who did not finish his bottle, was admitted at the same time because of respiratory distress, although less severe. His hemoglobin level was 9.8 g/dL, of which the methemoglobin concentration was 38%. He was also given 10 mg of methylene blue intravenously. The methemoglobin concentration was reduced to 0.4% within 4 hr, and he completely recovered. (See ref. 4.)

Discussion

1. Discuss the mechanism for inducing methemoglobinemia by ethyl nitrite.
2. What effect, if any, do you think the respiratory infection contributed to the outcome for the twin boys?

CASE STUDY: METHEMOGLOBINEMIA FROM AN INDUSTRIAL ACCIDENT

History

Two men were showered with molten chemicals in an industrial accident when a chamber, containing 50% sodium nitrate and 50% potassium nitrate heated to 246°C, exploded. Their clothing was immediately removed at the site, and they were rushed to a hospital.

On admission, patient 1, aged 23 years, had third-degree burns over 70% of his body. These were coated with a white, "salt-like" crust. The patient was alert and able to speak coherently. Vital signs included blood pressure, 90/60 mm Hg, and a weak pulse, 110 beats/min. Respirations were normal, although he admitted having trouble breathing. The patient had a generalized pallor. He complained of pain; opioids were not given because of his hypotension. The crust was washed away, but the damaged tissue was not debrided.

Within 10 to 15 min of arrival, the patient suddenly became cyanotic. He lapsed into unconsciousness and experienced a tonic seizure. He was intubated and given 100% oxygen but suffered cardiac arrest several minutes later and died. A postmortem blood sample showed a methemoglobin concentration of 65%.

The second patient, aged 49 years, was also alert and oriented when admitted. His burns were determined to be first and second degree, with 40% of his body affected. Burned areas were also coated with white crusts. Vital signs were all within normal limits except for a pulse of 100 beats/minute.

Attendants began to wash the white crust away. Approximately 20 min postadmission the patient experienced a generalized seizure. He then became intensely cyanotic.

He was intubated and administered 100% oxygen, but the cyanosis did not respond. A blood sample appeared chocolate-brown, so 100 mg methylene blue was administered intravenously. Despite this treatment, cyanosis continued.

The patient was transferred to an intensive care unit where he received an exchange transfusion with 30 units of whole blood. Before exchange, methemoglobin concentration was measured at 56%.

The patient tolerated the procedure well and, by 16 hr postadmission, he was awake, alert, and oriented. He received treatment for thermal burns and was eventually released without further complications.

Both of these victims illustrate that severe poisoning can occur after absorption of a toxic agent(s) through the skin. Absorption in these victims was no doubt enhanced by the hot temperature of the chemicals. (See ref. 13.)

Discussion

1. What is the mechanism for inducing methemoglobinemia by sodium and potassium nitrate?
2. What is considered to be a toxic concentration of methemoglobin?
3. Why was the arterial blood of these patients colored chocolate-brown? What does this mean?
4. Is it likely that the 10-mg dose of methylene blue given in case 1 was too high and actually caused the infant's death? Why, or why not, was it to blame?
5. The first victim probably died before attending physicians realized what was needed to save his life. Since his blood methemoglobin concentration was approximately equal to the level of the other victim, do you suppose the first patient would have survived his ordeal had he received methylene blue? Why or why not?

CASE STUDY: ENVIRONMENT-INDUCED METHEMOGLOBINEMIA IN AN INFANT

History

A 6-kg, 10-week-old girl was brought to the ED of a rural community hospital with severe cyanosis of sudden onset and irritability. An endotracheal tube was inserted, and she was given 100% oxygen. Laboratory results indicated metabolic acidosis with pH 7.31; paO_2, 231 mm Hg; $paCO_2$, 20 mm Hg; and bicarbonate, 10. Her blood was noted to be dark brown, and a methemoglobin concentration of 71.4% was detected.

Twelve milligrams of methylene blue was administered intravenously, resulting in a 98% reduction in the methemoglobin concentration within 8 hr. Sodium bicarbonate (6 mEq) corrected the acidosis. The infant was transferred to a children's hospital, where her methemoglobin concentration was measured as 1.3%. An erythrocyte reduction measurement determined this to be within normal limits, ruling out the possibility of congenital methemoglobinemia. There was no evidence of gastroenteritis and/or dehydration.

The child was extubated at 24 hr postadmission and resumed breast feeding. Her mother's methemoglobin concentration was less than 1%; that of the father and other siblings was negligible. She was discharged on day 3 of hospitalization with a methemoglobin concentration of 0.2%.

A family history later revealed a possible environmental cause of the infant's methemoglobinemia, creosote. Three days before the incident, the children's father had replaced a stove pipe leading from the wood-burning stove upward to the ceiling. Instead of replicating the existing angled construction, he had run a straight pipe from the stove to the chimney. The stove was the sole source of heat for the home, and green slab pine was continuously burned. The child's cradle was situated approximately 5 feet from the stove. It was hypothesized that, with a stove flue free of any angles, volatilized creosote dripped back into the stove, resulting in the emission of strong creosote fumes into the one-room home (6).

Discussion

1. Explain why only the child experienced severe symptoms. Why was her methemoglobin level so high, when concentrations in other family members were negligible to low?
2. The source of drinking water for this home was a well. Based on clues in this case study, what is the probability that the well water was contaminated and contributed to the child's poisoning?

Review Questions

1. Which of the following is a true statement?
   A. Methemoglobinemia exists when heme-

containing iron is in its oxidized state.

B. Methemoglobinemia is best treated with ascorbic acid.

C. Diaphorase I converts hemoglobin to methemoglobin.

D. A methemoglobin blood concentration of 30% is usually fatal.

2. Which of the following is a normal blood concentration of methemoglobin?
A. 0.5 to 1.0%
B. 1 to 2%
C. 3 to 5%
D. 7 to 10%

3. Nitrosamines are most often associated with which of the following disease states?
A. Gallbladder disorders
B. Renal tubular necrosis
C. Tumor growth
D. Gastric ulcers

4. Which of the following vitamins is sometimes advocated as an alternative treatment to methylene blue in methemoglobinemia?
A. Thiamine
B. Niacin
C. Ascorbic acid
D. Pantothenic acid

5. Nitrogen-containing poisons (e.g., aniline) most likely would cause which of the following toxic conditions if a toxic dose were ingested?
A. Methemoglobinemia
B. Cyanhemoglobin
C. Carboxyhemoglobin
D. Sulfmethemoglobin
E. None of the above

6. Which of the following clinical symptoms can be normally suspected in an individual with methemoglobinemia: tachycardia (I), lethargy (II), or dyspnea (III)?
A. II only
B. III only
C. I and II only
D. II and III only
E. I, II, and III

7. Nitrates are toxic because:
A. They oxidize iron in hemoglobin

B. They oxidize the iron in cytochrome oxidase

C. They reduce iron in hemoglobin

D. They reduce the iron in cytochrome oxidase

8. Indelible inks, shoe polish, and crayons are toxic, if ingested in sufficient amounts, because of the formation of:
A. Methemoglobinemia
B. Sulfmethemoglobin
C. Hypercalcemia
D. Nitrosamines
E. Electrophiles

9. Methylene blue, used as a specific antidote, is best termed a/an:
A. Chelating agent
B. Adsorbent
C. Sequestering agent
D. Oxidizing agent
E. Reducing agent

10. The "chocolate-brown" appearance of dried arterial blood of a person who has methemoglobinemia is caused by:
A. Oxidation of ferrous-iron in hemoglobin to the ferric valence.
B. Reduction of ferrous-iron in hemoglobin to the ferric valence.
C. Oxidation of ferric-iron in hemoglobin to the ferrous valence.
D. Reduction of ferric-iron in hemoglobin to the ferrous valence.

The next five questions pertain to the following case:

While his mother was in the basement doing the laundry, an experimenting 5-year-old attempted to help "season" the rather large pot of stew that was cooking on the stove.

He added the white crystalline contents of a bottle he acquired from his brother's chemistry kit. The chemical formula on the label was KNO_2, which seemed to this unknowing youngster to be the perfect flavoring ingredient for that night's supper. Later that evening, the entire family (father, 39 years; mother, 37 years; older son, 15 years; younger son, 5 years; and baby sister, 2 years) feasted on the "special formula" stew.

11. Which of the following symptoms would be expected to result from consuming a

significant portion of this adulterated stew?

A. Headache
B. Hypertension
C. Methemoglobinemia
D. All of the above
E. Only two of the above

12. The chemical name for KNO_2 is potassium:

A. nitrate
B. nitrite
C. nitride
D. nitrile
E. hyponitrite

13. The pharmacologic actions of KNO_2 include all of the following *except:*

A. Shift to the LEFT of the hemoglobin oxygen-dissociation curve
B. Reflex bradycardia
C. Oxidation of ferrous hemoglobin
D. Vasodilation
E. Vasoconstriction

14. The antidote that should be given to reverse significant methemoglobinemia is:

A. Oxygen
B. Phenacetin
C. Gentian violet
D. Phenolphthalein
E. Methylene blue

15. When an exogenous electron carrier, such as methylene blue, is used as an antidote to methemoglobinemia, all of the following are true *except:*

A. Glycolysis supplies the required reducing equivalents in the form of NADH.
B. Glucose 6-phosphate is oxidized.
C. The hexose monophosphate shunt provides the necessary cofactor NADPH.
D. Diaphorase II is activated.
E. High doses of the antidote may actually cause further methemoglobin production.

16. Cite the most probable cause of death in an individual poisoned with a massive overdose of a nitrate.

17. Infants have been reported to be more seriously affected by excessive nitrate ingestion than are adults. Discuss the factors that promote this action.

18. Discuss the consequence of administering nitrites to an individual with hereditary methemoglobinemia.

19. The dose of methylene blue must be closely monitored for what reason?

20. At what blood concentration of methemoglobin should treatment be initiated?

References

1. Angelakos ET. Coronary vasodilators. In: DiPalma JR, ed. *Drill's pharmacology in medicine.* 4th ed. New York: McGraw-Hill; 1975:809–823.
2. Berlin G, Brodin B, Hilden JO, et al. Acute dapsone intoxication: a case treated with continuous infusion of methylene blue, forced diuresis and plasma exchange. *Clin Toxicol* 1985;22:537–548.
3. Brunnemann KD, Hecht SS, Hoffman D. *N*-Nitrosamines: environmental occurrence, *in vivo* formation and metabolism. *J Toxicol Clin Toxicol* 1982–83;19:661–688.
4. Chilcote RC, Williams B, Wolff LJ, Baehner RR. Sudden death in an infant from methemoglobinemia after administration of "sweet spirits of nitre." *Pediatrics* 1977;59:280–282.
5. Comley HH. Cyanosis in infants caused by nitrates in well water. *JAMA* 1945;129:112–116.
6. Dean BS, Lopez G, Krenzelok EP. Environmentally-induced methemoglobinemia in an infant. *Clin Toxicol* 1992;30:127–133.
7. Doll R, Peto R. Avoidable risks of cancer in the U.S. *J Natl Cancer Inst* 1981;66:1196.
8. Forsyth RJ, Moulden A. Methaemoglobinaemia after ingestion of amyl nitrite. *Arch Dis Child* 1991;66:10.
9. Geffner ME, Powars DR, Choctaw WT. Acquired methemoglobinemia. *West J Med* 1981;134:7–10.
10. Gosselin RE, Smith RP, Hodge HC. Nitrite. In: *Clinical toxicology of commercial products.* 5th ed. Baltimore: Williams and Wilkins; 1984:III-314–319.
11. Haley TJ. Review of the physiological effects of amyl, butyl, and isobutyl nitrites. *Clin Toxicol* 1980;16:317–329.
12. Hall AA, Kulig KW, Rumack BH. Drug- and chemical-induced methaemoglobinaemia: clinical features and management. *Med Toxicol* 1986;1:253–260.
13. Harris JC, Rumack BH, Peterson RG, McGuire BM. Methemoglobinemia resulting from absorption of nitrates. *JAMA* 1979;242:2869–2871.
14. Jaffe ER. Methemoglobinemia and sulfhemoglobinemia. In: Wyngarden JB, Smith LH, eds. *Textbook of medicine.* 15th ed. Philadelphia: WB Saunders; 1979:1780–1782.
15. Johnson CJ, Bonrud PA, Dosch TL, Kilress AW, Senger KA, Busch DC, Meyer MR. Fatal outcome of methemoglobinemia in an infant. *JAMA* 1987;257:2796–2797.

16. Lowry TP. Amyl nitrite: an old high comes back to visit. *Behav Med* 1979;6:19–21.

17. Menzer RE, Nelson JO. Water and soil pollutants. In: Klaassen CD, Amdur MO, Doull J, eds. *Toxicology—the basic science of poisons.* 3rd ed. New York: Macmillan; 1986:825–853.

18. Scott EM. The relation of diaphorase on human erythrocytes to inheritance of methemoglobinemia. *J Clin Invest* 1960;39:1176–1186.

19. Scott EM. Congenital methemoglobinemia due to DPNH diaphorase deficiency. In: Bentler E, ed. *Hereditary disorders to erythrocyte metabolism.* New York: Grune and Stratton; 1968:102–113.

20. Shearer LA, Goldsmith JR, Young C, Kearns OA, Tamplin BR. Methemoglobin levels in infants in an area with high nitrate water supply. *Am J Public Health* 1972;9:1174–1180.

21. Smith RJ. Nitrites: FDA beats a surprising retreat. *Science* 1980;209:1100–1101.

22. Ten Brink WAG, Luijpen AFMG, Van Heijst ANP, Pikaar SA, Seldenrijk R. Nitrate poisoning caused by food contaminated with cooling fluid. *J Toxicol Clin Toxicol* 1982;19:139–147.

23. Whitwam JG, Taylor AR, White JM. Potential hazard of methylene blue. *Anesthesia* 1979;34:181–182.

24. Williams GM, Weisburger JH. Chemical carcinogens. In: Klaassen CD, Amdur MO, Doull J, eds. *Toxicology—the basic science of poisons.* 3rd ed. New York: Macmillan; 1986:99–173.

6 Carbon Monoxide, Cyanide, and Sulfide

Air may contain substances that, if inhaled, produce local toxic effects on the lungs and respiratory passageways and systemic effects throughout the body. These include particulate matter (such as dusts, fumes, and smokes) and gaseous products (including carbon monoxide, cyanide, sulfides, and other vapors and solvents).

Air quality in many areas is such that we continually breathe low levels of numerous solid and gaseous poisons without experiencing significant acute problems. Most airborne particles are either trapped by nasal hair or deposited on the moist walls within the respiratory system. They may be removed by coughing and sneezing or by the action of respiratory secretions aided by ciliary movement.

This chapter concentrates on three gases that exhibit significant toxicity: carbon monoxide, cyanide, and sulfide. Other gaseous or volatile substances that are associated with toxicity by inhalation are discussed in appropriate chapters (e.g., formaldehyde, gasoline, mercury vapor).

CARBON MONOXIDE

Acute carbon monoxide (CO) poisoning causes at least 10,000 persons each year in the United States to seek medical attention. About 1,500 die of accidental exposure, and another 3,500 commit suicide with CO each year (60). Chronic exposure to low concentrations of CO causes an array of complaints, including tiredness and lethargy, shortness of breath, irritability, and visual impairment. Chronic CO exposure also has been suggested to be a cause of heart disease and atherosclerosis, as well as numerous other abnormalities (2).

Toxic effects of CO are primarily due to its preferential affinity for hemoglobin and the production of carboxyhemoglobin (CoHb) (36). To appreciate the significance of this reaction, one must recall that a constant oxygen supply is essential for all bodily functions. Some tissues have greater oxygen requirements than others. The cells of the CNS and

myocardium, for example, become pathologically impaired when their oxygen requirement is compromised, even for short periods.

Atmospheric air contains approximately 21% oxygen. Oxygen is made accessible to body tissues by respiration. As oxygen diffuses across alveolar membranes, it combines with hemoglobin and is transported to various tissues.

Carbon monoxide is a ubiquitous product of incomplete combustion. Since it is odorless, colorless, tasteless, and nonirritating to the respiratory passages and readily mixes with air in all proportions, it is referred to as a *silent killer*. These features often prevent victims from recognizing the potential danger. A dangerous misconception is that, *as long as you can't smell smoke, there is no carbon monoxide*.

Carbon monoxide is normally present in the atmosphere at concentrations of less than 0.001% because most CO formed by incomplete combustion rises high into the atmosphere, where it is quickly oxidized to carbon dioxide. However, it is still the most abundant pollutant. Internal combustion automobile engine exhaust is the major source of CO (2,19). Natural gas (methane) does not contain CO, but its incomplete combustion, of course, will produce it. Charcoal fires produce CO, and this creates a potential hazard when hibachis and other charcoal grills are used in closed, poorly ventilated areas, such as camping trailers or apartments (see the case study at the end of this chapter). It is generally agreed that more people die in fire-related accidents from CO poisoning than by heat or burns.

Methylene chloride (CH_2Cl_2, dichloromethane), is another source of CO. It is a common industrial solvent used as a fumigant and in fire extinguishers and as a major component of many paint thinners and paint and varnish removers (11,39,65). Its use is increasing as a solvent in personal-care aerosol products. Unfortunately, methylene chloride is quickly absorbed and metabolized to CO, forming carboxyhemoglobin. Recall that one of the case studies at the end of chapter 1 described a fatal event in an unsuspecting victim by inhalation of methylene chloride.

Methylene chloride poisoning has become increasingly common since the early 1970s. At that time it was shown that, after methylene chloride inhalation, endogenous generation of carboxyhemoglobin follows. It is highly lipid soluble and deposited in a variety of body tissues, from which it is slowly released. In the liver, mixed-function oxidases convert methylene chloride to carbon dioxide and carbon monoxide. It is believed that over 70,000 workers are exposed to methylene chloride each year in the United States (52).

A significant source of inhaled CO is tobacco smoke. Cigarette smoke contains 3% to 6% CO, producing air concentrations that are up to 8 times greater than the level permitted in industry. Pipes and cigars normally burn at lower temperatures but may contain up to 15% CO. Smoking one or two packs of cigarettes per day produces CO blood concentrations of 1.9% or 3%, respectively (7). Firemen who do not smoke tobacco may have high CO blood concentrations due to excessive exposure to smoke from fires (8,53).

Blood normally contains low concentrations of CO, less than 1%. This is believed to occur through endogenous CO formation from metabolism of hemoglobin and other tetrapyrrols (16,23,56). These low concentrations are probably insignificant to an otherwise healthy individual.

Mechanism of Toxicity

The toxic effects of CO have been known for thousands of years. Political prisoners during Hippocrates' time were put to death with CO. Only since the last decade of the 19th century have its physiologic and biochemical effects been systematically studied.

The toxic effects of CO result from tissue hypoxia. This is achieved by (a) decreasing the amount of oxygen bound to erythrocytes, thus causing a reduction in tissue oxygenation, and (b) shifting the oxyhemoglobin dissociation curve to the left, thereby lowering the

partial pressure at which oxygen becomes available to tissues.

Carbon monoxide combines reversibly with hemoglobin to produce carboxyhemoglobin (36). This binding affinity is approximately 240 times greater than that of oxygen. Inhalation of relatively low concentrations of CO can, therefore, produce clinically significant decreases in the oxygen-carrying capacity of erythrocytes. In other words, a 50% COHb concentration can be achieved when the concentration of CO in ambient air is only $\frac{1}{240}$th that of oxygen, or about 0.08% (800 ppm). Breathing air that contains as little CO as 0.1% by volume can be lethal (41).

Binding of oxygen to hemoglobin displays a sigmoid relationship with respect to the partial pressure of oxygen. The binding of one oxygen molecule produces allosteric modification of the heme protein to enhance binding of the next three oxygen molecules.

Carbon monoxide also interferes with dissociation, or release of oxygen from hemoglobin; as stated above, CO shifts the oxyhemoglobin dissociation curve to the left. Graphically, this means that the normal oxygen association-dissociation curve now changes from a sigmoid to a hyperbolic relationship. The sigmoid curve indicates that oxygen can be readily released from hemoglobin when needed. Figure 6.1 shows that the slope of the S-curve is steep when pO_2 is low and levels off when pO_2 is high. When CO binds with hemoglobin and shifts the dissocia-

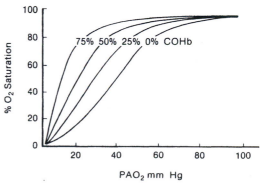

FIG. 6.1. Oxyhemoglobin dissociation curve in the presence of CO.

tion curve to the left, producing a hyperbolic curve, less oxygen is available to tissues or oxygen is only available to tissues at low pO_2.

Carbon monoxide also binds to myoglobin, a heme-containing protein that transports oxygen in skeletal and cardiac muscle, and to intracellular cytochrome oxidases (intracellular enzymes for respiration). This binding may also contribute to tissue and cellular hypoxia (67).

Absorption, Metabolism, and Excretion

The concentration of COHb in blood is a function of the CO concentration of inspired air, duration of exposure, and volume of pulmonary ventilation (tidal volume). Aqueous solubility of CO is low, but CO concentrations may be significantly high in the blood because of its binding affinity for hemoglobin. Table 6.1 correlates concentrations of CO in inspired air with the corresponding percentage of COHb saturation reached at equilibrium. From this table the COHb concentration, after exposure to a known concentration of CO, can be estimated for a particular time period and respiratory activity using the following equation:

Resting state: % COHb
$$= 6 \text{ L/min} \times \%CO \times \text{min exposure}$$

This relationship applies to an otherwise healthy individual, and several factors can influence the percentage of COHb saturation. Infants and others with hypermetabolic rates, patients with anemia (lower oxygen reserve)

TABLE 6.1. *Carboxyhemoglobin equilibrium at one atmosphere*

CO inhaled (ppm)	COHb (% saturation)
1	0.49
10	1.94
100	14.45
1,000	62.41
10,000	94.31
100,000	99.40
900,000	99.93

or chronic obstructive pulmonary disease (COPD), and those with arteriosclerotic cardiovascular heart disease will be much more susceptible to toxicity from CO. Of historical interest, canaries were once placed in mines to test the air quality. Birds are more susceptible to reduced oxygen concentrations. If the bird died, the oxygen concentration in the air was too low to sustain human life or perhaps a toxic gas (e.g., methane) was present, and the miners had to leave or protect themselves.

Carbon monoxide is eliminated from the lungs unchanged in an exponential manner. The rate of elimination can be increased by exercise or the administration of pure oxygen. Less than 1% is oxidized endogenously to carbon dioxide. The biologic half-life of CO in a healthy, sedentary adult at sea level is 4 to 5 hr. This half-life decreases to approximately 80 min with administration of 100% oxygen and to 23 min when hyperbaric oxygen is used (36).

Characteristics of Acute Poisoning

It was pointed out previously that the concentration of CO in ambient air does not need to be great for acute toxic exposure to occur. Table 6.2 correlates COHb concentrations and certain signs and symptoms. Toxic manifestations occur in organ systems with the greatest oxygen needs, the brain and heart. Not all manifestations will be observed.

Individuals with COHb concentrations of less than 10% are typically asymptomatic, and even COHb concentrations of 10% to 20% produce effects that are sometimes vague and nondescriptive. Effects become increasingly severe as COHb concentrations rise to the 30% to 50% range, with the victim showing irritability, headache, dizziness, confusion, disturbance of judgment, collapse, and fainting on exertion. Severe headache that often follows CO poisoning probably results from cerebral edema. Unconsciousness rarely occurs in individuals with COHb concentrations of less than 50%. If duration of exposure to CO is prolonged or acute exposure to high

TABLE 6.2. *Signs and symptoms at various concentrations of carboxyhemoglobin*

% COHb	Signs and symptoms
0–10	No symptoms; asymptomatic
10–20	Tightness across the forehead, possibly slight headache, dilation of the cutaneous blood vessels, exertional dyspnea
20–30	Headache and throbbing in the temples, easily fatigued, possible dizziness
30–40	Severe headache, weakness, dizziness, confusion, dimness of vision, nausea, vomiting, and collapse
40–50	Same as above, a greater possibility of collapse, syncope, and increased pulse and respiratory rate
50–60	Syncope, increased respiratory and pulse rate, coma, intermittent convulsions, and Cheyne-Stokes respiration
60–70	Coma, intermittent convulsions, depressed heart action and respiratory rate, and possibly death
70–80	Weak pulse, slow respirations, respiratory failure, and death within a few hours
80–90	Death in less than an hour
90+	Death within a few minutes

concentrations (0.5% to 1.0%) occurs and the resultant COHb concentration increases to 60% to 70%, then pulse rate, cardiac output, and respirations will be critically compromised. Death will follow soon.

It may be common knowledge that CO causes deleterious effects on the CNS, but its actions on the myocardium are not as well understood. Death often occurs from myocardial ischemia.

A study using monkeys placed in a chamber containing CO illustrated that the heart is markedly affected by CO concentrations. Twenty-five percent of the animals quickly developed ventricular arrhythmias and other ECG abnormalities (22). In another investigation, 40% of a group of individuals who had preexisting heart disease and were exposed to CO emissions on a freeway in a major metropolitan area experienced significant ECG abnormalities and increased anginal pain. Blood COHb concentrations in all affected individuals were below 5% (4). In another study, 7 of 21 persons (42 to 60 years old) who were exposed to CO resulting in blood concentrations of 5% to 9% COHb experienced ECG irregularities, with arrhythmias developing in 2 patients (37).

Individuals with coronary heart disease are at special risk from CO exposure because of their inability to compensate adequately for CO-induced increased myocardial oxygen demand (3,5,6). Various animal studies have demonstrated that focal areas of necrosis can be seen on the myocardium after prolonged CO exposure, but these necrotic areas are usually reversible. When COHb concentration is 5% or higher, people are 21 times more likely to develop atherosclerosis than when COHb is decreased to 3% (70).

Nonfatal exposure to CO usually results in complete recovery within 2 to 4 days. Survivors generally show little or no residual effects. It is only after the victim remains comatose for more than 24 hr that serious neurologic symptoms are likely to develop. Twitching, choreiform movements, and seizures may result from prolonged hypoxia. Delayed neuropathy, characterized by demyelination, may result as a late complication of CO poisoning. Patients may appear to be well immediately after recovery from the acute effects, only to show neurologic deficits later (21,74). Late sequelae in up to 45% of patients may develop gradually from 3 days to 3 weeks after initial exposure and therapy of acute poisoning (45). One study demonstrated that, in patients poisoned by CO who were evaluated 3 years after recovery, 13% displayed gross neuropsychiatric damage, 33% showed deterioration of personality, and 43% had some degree of memory impairment (42,50). Other complications of CO poisoning include visual and hearing impairment, neurologic and muscular deficiencies, blood and kidney damage, and skin lesions including erythema, blisters, and bullae.

The pathognomonic sign of CO poisoning is a pinkish to bright cherry-red discoloration of the skin. It begins around the mouth, when COHb concentrations exceed 25%, and spreads over the face and extremities as the percentage of saturation increases. In fatal CO poisonings, the bright discoloration persists and can be readily demonstrated on autopsy.

Management of Poisoning

Specific goals in management of acute CO poisoning are to (a) relieve cerebral and cardiac ischemia and (b) promote dissociation of COHb and increase the CO elimination rate. Each goal is best achieved by administering oxygen. The initial step, therefore, is to remove the victim from the CO source and administer pure oxygen. The victim should be kept quiet and resting. An increase in muscle movement may result in increased oxygen demand, leaving even less oxygen available to support CNS functions. Carbon monoxide poisoning is one of those rare situations where a direct antagonist, oxygen, is available. In general, the more oxygen administered, the better the outcome (41).

Carboxyhemoglobin concentrations can be easily determined in the laboratory. However, in most instances when the presence of signs and symptoms and positive conditions of CO exposure indicate that treatment is required, it should not be delayed until laboratory analysis is completed.

When COHb concentrations are less than 15%, fresh air and rest are all that are usually indicated. If COHb concentrations exceed 15%, 100% oxygen should be given, since dissociation of 50% of COHb will be achieved in 40 min in an oxygen atmosphere, as compared to 4.1 hr in ambient air (51).

The use of hyperbaric oxygen (oxygen at increased pressure) is recommended when the COHb concentration reaches 40% or greater (34). Oxygen at 2 atmospheres will reduce the half-life of CO to 20 min and causes almost instantaneous reversal of tissue hypoxia (33). This occurs because oxygen dissolved in plasma will oxygenate tissues directly. Also, hyperbaric oxygen accelerates the rate of dissociation of COHb and shifts the oxyhemoglobin dissociation curve back to the right (42). Other potential benefits include reduced cere-

bral edema and reduced cytochrome oxidase inhibition. Controversies to the selective use of hyperbaric oxygen exist, and a clinical judgment requires an evaluation of the potential risks and benefits (45). Some complications of hyperbaric oxygen therapy include decompression sickness, rupture of tympanic membranes, damaged sinuses, and oxygen toxicity.

As stated earlier, oxygen is transported through the body bound to hemoglobin and in lesser concentration dissolved in plasma. This concentration can be increased if the oxygen tension is increased. Breathing 100% oxygen can result in a dissolved oxygen concentration of 2.09 vol%. The body's normal arterial-to-venous oxygen difference is approximately 6%. Forcing oxygen at 100% concentration can supply up to one-third of the body's oxygen requirements (77). Giving oxygen at 2.5 atmospheres of pressure can result in a dissolved oxygen concentration of 5.62 vol% (18).

At high COHb concentrations, oxygen therapy at 100% concentration (10 L/min) may be administered over a prolonged period ranging up to 4 hr at normal atmospheric pressure and 1 hr at 2.5 atmospheres of pressure. A victim of hydrogen sulfide poisoning who is discussed in a case study at the end of this chapter received 100% oxygen for 10 hr. Although prolonged therapy with high concentrations of oxygen can be toxic, treatment of CO poisoning with high concentrations of oxygen for prolonged periods is not usually associated with seizures and other symptoms of oxygen poisoning (78).

From all indications, addition of 5% to 7% carbon dioxide to oxygen offers little advantage in treating CO poisoning. It is the opinion of some that carbon dioxide stimulates breathing. Others have shown that any possible advantage by carbon dioxide is overcome by the benefit that pure oxygen has on forcing the dissociation of COHb.

CYANIDE

Cyanide (hydrocyanic acid, prussic acid) is not a common poison, although today the pub-

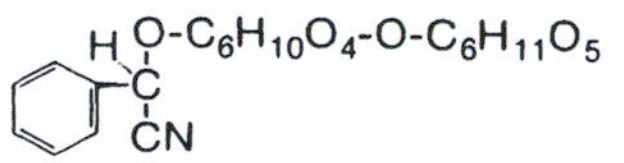

H—C—O-$C_6H_{10}O_4$-O-$C_6H_{11}O_5$
C
CN

FIG. 6.2. Structural formula for amygdalin.

lic is more aware of its occurrence than in the past. Most cyanide ingestions occur from accidental exposure or intentional ingestion of a cyanide-containing compound. There was an increased frequency in the number of case reports dealing with accidental cyanide poisonings a few years ago when use of laetrile was popularized. Occasionally, fruit seeds are ingested as part of a health food diet plan; some contain toxic levels of cyanide. Amygdalin (Fig. 6.2), one such cyanogenic glycoside, is present in apple, peach, plum, apricot, cherry, and almond seeds. As shown in Fig. 6.3, amygdalin is hydrolyzed to hydrogen cyanide (31,54). In addition, the public was grimly reminded of its rapidly induced toxicity when more than 900 suicide-murders occurred in Jonestown, Guyana, in 1978 as a result of drinking a cyanide-laced beverage.

The conventional means of cyanide exposure occur in industry. Hydrogen cyanide and its derivatives are used in electroplating, metallurgy, and extraction of gold and silver metals from ores; in production of synthetic fibers and plastics; and as fumigants and fertilizers. Table 6.3 lists many cyanide-containing compounds with their appropriate chemical formulas and names, as well as other relevant information.

A common error regarding cyanide poisoning is that it occurs only from ingestion, by swallowing a substance containing cyanide. Intoxication can occur also from inhalation or absorption through the skin (55). In the presence of cyanide gas, a gas mask alone

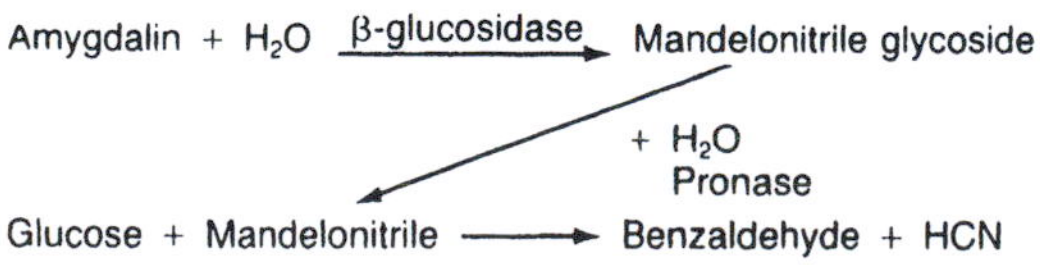

does not offer complete protection from intoxication.

The most rapidly acting cyanide compound, hydrocyanic acid, is readily volatilized to hydrogen cyanide, producing the characteristic odor of bitter almonds. Cyanide salts are the most frequently encountered of all cyanide-containing compounds. The LD_{50} for these salts is approximately 2 mg/kg, with ingestion of 50 to 75 mg of any one of them usually resulting in syncope and respiratory difficulty within a few minutes (29). Halogenated cyanides are irritating gases and produce pulmonary edema, tearing, and excessive salivation.

It is not uncommon on autopsy to find cyanide, as well as CO, in the blood of victims of smoke inhalation (9,43,64). Many plastics and polyacrylic fibers produce cyanide-containing gases when burned. Another source of cyanide toxicity is the administration of nitroprusside (50).

Mechanism of Toxicity

Cyanide produces histotoxic cellular hypoxia by binding to ferric (Fe^{3+}) iron. The body has over 40 enzyme systems that are reported to be inactivated by cyanide. The most significant of these is the cytochrome oxidase system, which consists of the cytochrome a-a_3 complex of the electron transport system (58). When cyanide binds to this enzyme complex, electron transport is inhibited—electron transfer from cytochrome a_3 to molecular oxygen is blocked. Consequently, no ATP can be generated because this is dependent on cytochrome oxidase at the last step in oxidative phosphorylation (71). This results in reduced cellular utilization of oxygen and increased venous pO_2. Cyanide intoxication has the same pathophysiologic effect as a complete lack of oxygen.

Since there are several metabolic pathways converging on the electron transport system, impairment of cellular oxygen utilization reduces aerobic respiration with a decrease in pyruvate conversion in the Krebs cycle. Therefore, lactate increases, producing metabolic acidosis.

Amygdalin + H_2O →(β-glucosidase) Mandelonitrile glycoside
+ H_2O
Pronase
Glucose + Mandelonitrile ← → Benzaldehyde + HCN

FIG. 6.3. Biochemical pathway for amygdalin metabolism.

TABLE 6.3. *Examples of cyanide-containing compounds*

Name	Commercial use	Fatal dose (TLV)[a]
Acetone cyanohydrin	—	15 mg/kg
Acetonitrile	Solvent	120 mg/kg
Acrylonitrile	Synthetic fibers & plastics	35–90 mg/kg (20 ppm)
Calcium cyanamide	Fertilizer	40–50 g
Calcium cyanide	Fumigant, pesticide	5 mg/kg
Cyanogen	Fumigant, blast furnace	13 ppm
Cyanogen bromide	Fumigant	13 ppm
Cyanogen chloride	Organic synthesis	13 ppm
Dimethyl cyanamide	Organic synthesis	75 mg/kg
Hydrocyanic acid	Fumigant	0.5 mg/kg (10 ppm)[a]
Nitroprusside	Antihypertensive, analytic reagent	10 mg/kg
Potassium cyanate	Herbicide, chemical reagent	1 g/kg
Potassium cyanide	Electroplating, organic synthesis	2 mg/kg
Potassium ferrocyanide	Metallurgy, graphic arts	1.6 mg/kg
Sodium cyanide	Electroplating, organic synthesis	2 mg/kg

From ref. 29.
[a] TLV, threshold limit value.

In cyanide toxicity, the quantity of oxygen that reaches tissues is not affected, but cells are unable to utilize the oxygen. Recall that this differs from CO poisoning, where tissue hypoxia is due to an insufficient amount of oxygen available for tissue utilization. In essence, a victim of cyanide poisoning suffocates from an inability to use oxygen. Since only the cellular utilization of oxygen is impaired, venous blood becomes almost as oxygenated as arterial blood. Consequently, cyanosis is not usually observed.

Characteristics of Poisoning

Cyanide is extremely rapid acting and capable of causing death within minutes. The classic odor of bitter almonds is not detected by everyone and seems to be genetically determined (10). Onset of symptoms of cyanide poisoning depends on the type of exposure. Hydrogen cyanide vapors are the most rapidly acting, with symptoms occurring within seconds and death within minutes. When cyanide salts are ingested, onset of toxicity is delayed somewhat due to slow absorption. The severity of acute poisoning is determined by the dose and exposure time.

Early symptoms of cyanide poisoning may include weakness, dizziness, headache, tachypnea, and tachycardia. This is followed by rapid progression to a stuporous, combative phase and, finally, by apnea, generalized convulsions, and death (62,69). A summary of signs and symptoms of cyanide poisoning is shown in Table 6.4.

Cyanide directly stimulates chemoreceptors of the carotid and aortic bodies, resulting in increased respiration. This produces increased tidal volume, minute volume, and frequency of breathing (71).

Nausea and vomiting associated with cyanide poisoning are probably due to local irritation to the gastric mucosa from cyanide salts. Tachycardia results from reflex actions after stimulation of chemoreceptors of the carotid and aortic bodies in response to cellular anoxia. Again, the patient usually does not appear cyanotic because of oxygenated venous blood.

As cyanide blood concentration increases, respiration rate slows and gasping occurs, but cyanosis is still usually absent. The presence of bradycardia and absence of cyanosis are strong evidence to support a suspected cyanide poisoning. As cyanide concentrations increase, sufficient CNS oxygen deprivation may cause hypoxic convulsions followed by death due to respiratory arrest. Also, lactic acidosis with a wide anion gap (see chapter

TABLE 6.4. *Correlation between blood cyanide concentrations and clinical manifestations of poisoning*

CN concentration (mg/L)	Degree of poisoning	Signs and symptoms
0.5–1.0	Mild	Conscious, flushed, rapid pulse, headache
1.0–2.5	Moderate	Stuporous but responsive to stimuli, tachycardia, tachypnea
2.5 and greater	Severe	Comatose, unresponsive, hypotension, respirations slow and gasping, mydriasis, cyanosis at high concentration, death unless treated immediately

4) should not be overlooked in these patients. Inhibition of aerobic respiration will shift glucose metabolism to anaerobic glycolysis, resulting in severe lactic acidosis (24).

Management of Poisoning

Treatment of acute cyanide poisoning is aimed at decreasing the amount of cyanide available for cellular binding. The primary objective is to maintain cellular utilization of oxygen by sequestering or interfering with cyanide to prevent its interaction with cytochrome oxidase. Treatment must be initiated immediately to be effective (55).

Unlike many other toxic exposures, cyanide poisoning is a good example of a situation where specific antidotes are available. The key to successful therapy is limited by how rapidly treatment can be initiated. It is rare for an intentional ingestion of cyanide to be discovered before death because cyanide acts so rapidly. In addition, many toxic exposures do not lend themselves to rapid, straightforward diagnosis of cyanide poisoning, and, therefore, specific treatment may be delayed.

At toxic concentrations, cyanide can dissociate from ferric iron binding sites and be converted to thiocyanate in the presence of sulfur transferase and an endogenous source of thiosulfate, as shown in Fig. 6.4. The thiocyanate is rapidly excreted by the kidney. When greater concentrations of cyanide are present,

this built-in detoxification system becomes saturated, and death results unless specific measures are taken.

Over the years, several antidotes have been suggested for treating cyanide poisoning. Pedigo (47) reported in 1888 that amyl nitrite was effective in treating cyanide-poisoned dogs. Methylene blue was later touted as effective (20). Methylene blue is an aniline dye that produces methemoglobinemia when taken in large doses (see chapter 5). Methemoglobin contains iron in its oxidized (Fe^{3+}) form and thus competes with cytochrome oxidase for binding to cyanide. It was subsequently shown that nitrites were successful antidotes (13–15) and was later confirmed that a combination of amyl nitrite and sodium nitrite was much more effective in producing methemoglobinemia (14). Also, a combination of nitrite and thiosulfate provided an effective treatment regimen (13).

This, then, formed the basis for the Cyanide Antidote Package (Fig. 6.5), which contains amyl nitrite inhalant, 3% sodium nitrite solution, and 25% sodium thiosulfate solution. First, amyl nitrite is administered by inhalation, followed by sodium nitrite intravenously. The purpose of these two agents is to oxidize ferrous iron of hemoglobin to its ferric form, producing methemoglobin, as shown in Fig. 6.6, Eq. A. Since amyl nitrite alone produces only about 5% methemoglobin, it must be combined with sodium nitrite to produce an

$$\text{CYANIDE + THIOSULFATE} \xrightarrow{\text{(sulfur transferase)}} \text{THIOCYANATE + SULFITE}$$

FIG. 6.4. Reaction of cyanide with thiosulfate in the presence of sulfur transferase.

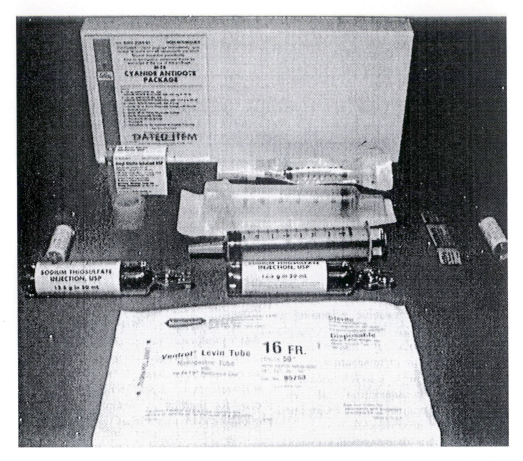

FIG. 6.5. Cyanide Antidote Package. (Photograph courtesy of Eli Lilly Company.)

adequate concentration of methemoglobin to bind with cyanide. In practice, a methemoglobin concentration close to 40% is desirable. Methemoglobin ($HbFe^{3+}$) can now compete with cytochrome oxidase for circulating cyanide.

Methemoglobin has greater affinity for cyanide than does cytochrome oxidase. Therefore, methemoglobin can bind to free cyanide (Fig. 6.6, Eq. B), as well as cause dissociation of the cyanide-cytochrome oxidase complex. This results in reactivation of cytochrome oxidase and permits it to resume its activity in the electron transport system. In addition, the released intracellular cyanide can now bind to methemoglobin to form cyanomethemoglobin, as shown in Fig. 6.6, Eq. C.

All of the discussed reactions that involve cyanide and its complexes are reversible and

may shift in either direction. Similarly, cyanomethemoglobin also has the potential to dissociate. This is partly the reason for instituting the second phase of the Cyanide Antidote Package. This involves the binding of cyanomethemoglobin with thiosulfate in the presence of sulfur transferase (rhodanese) to form a relatively nontoxic compound, thiocyanate, which is readily excreted by the kidney (Fig. 6.6, Eq. D).

Although the current treatment regimen just described for cyanide poisoning is effective, it does pose considerable potential toxicity. For example, when hemoglobin is converted to methemoglobin, it loses its ability to bind oxygen. This may cause the oxygen dissociation curve to shift to the left. As a result, the body can be placed in double jeopardy. Cellular oxygen utilization has first of all been di-

HEMOGLOBIN   AMYL NITRITE   METHEMOGLOBIN
(Fe^{+2})   +   or   →   (Fe^{+3})
SODIUM NITRITE

(Equation A)

CYANIDE + METHEMOGLOBIN ⇌ CYANOMETHEMOGLOBIN

(Equation B)

CYANIDE - CYTOCHROME   METHEMOGLOBIN ⇌ CYANOMETHEMOGLOBIN
OXIDASE COMPLEX   +   +
CYTOCHROME OXIDASE

(Equation C)

CYANOMETHEMOGLOBIN + THIOSULFATE ⇌ THIOCYANATE
+
SULFITE
+
METHEMOGLOBIN

(Equation D)

FIG. 6.6. Steps in treating cyanide intoxication.

minished by cyanide, and, with production of methemoglobin, the amount of oxygen available for tissues is potentially diminished. As can be expected, there is a fine line between reversing the toxicity of one agent and inadvertently initiating toxicity by another. It seems in practice that production of methemoglobin does not severely compromise the cyanide-poisoned patient unless the concentration reaches 40% to 50% or greater. However, this potential danger should not go unrecognized.

Another drawback is the possibility of critically lowering blood pressure with the use of nitrites. Nitrites induce vasodilation, which may result in cardiovascular collapse and render the treatment completely ineffective.

Oxygen is not a specific antidote for cyanide, but it has been advocated as a necessary adjunct in managing its toxicity (72,73). Oxygen therapy may be useful for two reasons: (a) it may displace cyanide from cytochrome oxidase and (b) increased intracellular oxygen tension may be sufficient to nonenzymatically

TABLE 6.5. *Effect of hyperbaric oxygen, sodium nitrite, and sodium thiosulfate on the LD_{50} of potassium cyanide in mice*

Experiment	Air	HBO^a	$NaNO_2$ (s.c.) (g/kg)	Na_2S_2O (i.p.) (g/kg)	LD_{50} values[b] (mg/kg)
1	+	0	0	0	11.8
2	0	+	0	0	11.2
3	+	0	0.1	0	21.2
4	0	+	0.1	0	21.3
5	+	0	0	1.0	34.8
6	+	0	0	1.0	39.0
7	0	+	0.1	1.0	51.7
8	0	+	0.1	1.0	73.0

From ref. 72.
s.c., subcutaneous; i.p., intraperitoneal.
[a] HBO, 100% oxygen at 4 atmospheres (hyperbaric oxygen).
[b] Each LD_{50} value was obtained from five graded doses of KCN administered to five or more groups of ten mice each; $p < 0.05$.

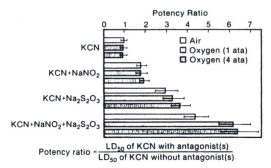

FIG. 6.7. Effect of hyperbaric oxygen (4 ata), oxygen, and air on the LD_{50} of KCN. (From ref. 72.)

convert reduced cytochrome to oxidized cytochrome, enabling the electron transport system to function again. Oxygen (100%) should be used routinely in patients with moderate to severe symptoms, even if pO_2 is normal.

Hyperbaric oxygen has been proposed as a treatment in cyanide toxicity, although evidence supporting its use is inconclusive (27,35,40). An animal study was conducted using mice given potassium cyanide followed by (a) nitrite and/or thiosulfate and (b) air and/or oxygen (72). Oxygen was given under atmospheric conditions and at hyperbaric pressures. Table 6.5 shows that oxygen at 4 atmospheric pressures reduces cyanide mortality in mice (not given along with nitrite and thiosulfate). When oxygen at 1 atmospheric pressure was compared with oxygen at 4 atmospheric pressures (Fig. 6.7), there was no significant difference between the two treatment groups. Hyperbaric oxygen does not seem to have additional benefits over 100% normobaric oxygen in cyanide poisonings. It may be considered, however, in patients who do not respond well to oxygen and the normal antidote (40).

Other antidotes used in Europe include aminophenols, cobalt salts, and hydroxocobalamin. Cobalt compounds such as Kelocyanor (dicobalt-EDTA) chelate cyanide but also can produce severe hypertension and cardiac arrhythmias (69). Hydroxocobalamin (vitamin B_{12a}) combines with cyanide to form cyanocobalamin (vitamin B_{12}) (57) and seems very promising as an antidote (9,38,69).

SULFIDES

Sulfide poisonings usually follow exposure to hydrogen sulfide (H_2S), carbon disulfide (CS_2), or one of the mercaptans. These compounds can produce systemic effects by inhalation or absorption through the skin.

Hydrogen sulfide is a colorless gas heavier than air (sp. gr. 1.192). For this reason, it accumulates in underground locations, such as sewers and wells. This gas has a characteristic odor of rotten eggs and is found wherever putrefaction occurs. It is generated in several industrial settings, including petroleum refineries, tanneries, and rubber and rayon factories (Table 6.6). Hydrogen sulfide has been the cause of intoxication from liquid manure tanks in agricultural settings and in rural latrines connected directly to septic tanks (17,44,46).

Hydrogen sulfide is classified as a primary irritant. When inhaled in high concentrations, it produces toxic effects almost as rapidly as does hydrocyanic acid (26,28). The threshold limit value (TLV) (i.e., the amount of substance a worker can be exposed to for 8 hr a day, 5 days a week) for hydrogen sulfide has been set at 10 ppm. Inhalation of 2,000 ppm can cause coma after a single breath and may be fatal (63). A victim typically loses consciousness without warning. The presence of apnea is a serious prognostic sign. Once respirations cease, spontaneous breathing does not resume. Apnea is quickly followed by hypoxic convulsions, cardiovascular collapse, and death (59). The rapidity of poisoning is illustrated by the case study entitled, ''Dung Lung

TABLE 6.6. *Sites of exposure of victims of hydrogen sulfide poisoning[a]*

Site	% (of all cases)
Gas plant	52
Pumping station	24
Oil rig	12
Sulfuric acid production	2
Oil refinery	1
Sewer	1
Other	8

From ref. 12.
[a] Total number of victims, 221.

Disease—Hydrogen Sulfide Poisoning,'' which is included at the end of this chapter.

Carbon disulfide is a colorless liquid that boils at 46°C but volatilizes at room temperature. In its pure state, it has a sweetish, aromatic odor, but most commercial grades smell like decaying cabbage or radishes. It is used as an insecticide, soil fumigant, and solvent for lipids, sulfur, rubber, phosphorus, waxes, and resins. Most exposures occur in industry, where it is used in production of viscose rayon fibers. The TLV for carbon disulfide has been set at 20 ppm to prevent serious systemic effects, especially damage to the central and peripheral nervous systems. This value may be lowered soon, perhaps to a low of 1 ppm. The World Health Organization has stated that over 20,000 workers are regularly exposed to carbon disulfide (68).

Inhalation is the major route of toxic exposure to carbon disulfide. Reports of skin contamination or ingestion are rare.

Both ethyl and methyl mercaptans are toxic flammable gases with a TLV of 0.5 ppm. They are used in production of jet fuels, plastics, and pesticides. They smell extremely foul and have been used in trace concentrations as *warning agents* for propane, butane, and natural gases. Mercaptan odors can be detected well below the concentrations necessary to produce toxicity.

Sulfides are not generally viewed by the public as being extremely toxic. This is probably the major reason that they are so hazardous. Also, the olfactory responses are quickly paralyzed when the gases are inhaled and the victim often fails to recognize the danger.

Mechanism of Toxicity

Hydrogen sulfide toxicity manifests similarly to hydrogen cyanide (i.e., inhibition of cytochrome oxidase) (58). Therefore, it also produces cellular hypoxia. *In vitro* experiments have shown that sulfide is a more potent enzyme inhibitor than cyanide (59). Also, the hydrosulfide anion (HS^-) forms a dissociable complex with ferric heme groups to produce

sulfmethemoglobin. Sulfmethemoglobin is relatively nontoxic and is reduced to hemoglobin by polysulfides, thiosulfate, or sulfate. In addition, hydrogen sulfide exerts a direct depressant effect on all parts of the CNS, including paralysis of the respiratory center. The heart continues to beat for several minutes, so artificial respiration with a mixture of oxygen and carbon dioxide may be beneficial, if given quickly.

Carbon disulfide has greater affinity for the CNS and the cardiovascular system than does hydrogen sulfide. Damage to the cranial nerves and peripheral neuropathies are prevalent in occupational exposures to carbon disulfide. Also, carbon disulfide poisoning may accelerate the atherosclerotic process and thus contribute to the onset of coronary heart disease. Recent epidemiologic studies of viscose rayon workers have shown a two- to fivefold increase in risk of coronary heart disease, as compared to workers not exposed to carbon disulfide (66).

Characteristics of Poisoning

In low concentrations, hydrogen sulfide is relatively harmless except for its unpleasant odor and irritation to the eyes, respiratory tract, and gastrointestinal system. It produces significant hyperpnea by direct chemostimulation of the carotid body (30).

Exposure to levels of 50 ppm for 1 hr or more can produce effects listed in Table 6.7.

TABLE 6.7. *Effects of hydrogen sulfide exposure*

Exposure to 50 ppm H_2S for 1 hr or more		Exposure to >700 ppm H_2S (high concentration)
Mucous membranes	Respiratory tract	
Conjunctivitis	Rhinitis	Respiratory collapse
Keratitis	Tracheitis	Sudden collapse
Photophobia	Bronchitis	Convulsions
	Pneumonia	Death
	Pulmonary edema	
	Greenish cyanosis	

TABLE 6.8. *Effects of carbon disulfide exposure*

Nervous system symptoms
  Paresthesias
  Unsteady gait
  Dysphagia
  Parkinson-like syndrome
Ocular changes
  Corneal anesthesia
  Decreased pupillary reflex
  Nystagmus
Gastrointestinal disturbances
  Chronic gastritis
  Achlorhydria
Renal impairment
  Albuminuria
  Elevated BUN[a]

[a] BUN, blood urea nitrogen.

These may include acute conjunctivitis with pain, lacrimation, and photophobia. Prolonged exposure can cause irritation and inflammation of the mucosal membranes of the respiratory tract, culminating in pulmonary edema and congestion. Inhalation of higher concentrations (greater than 700 ppm) results in instantaneous paralysis of the entire nervous system and can be rapidly fatal.

In deaths associated with hydrogen sulfide, the viscera and brain may have a greenish blue discoloration. This occurs as a result of tissue decomposition of sulfur and hemoglobin (1).

Carbon disulfide intoxication can involve all areas of the central and peripheral nervous systems. Centrally, it produces damage to the cranial nerves, caudate nucleus, and putamen. In the periphery, carbon disulfide causes axonal degeneration, which may be delayed in producing symptoms. The peripheral neuropathies can manifest as paresthesias, muscle weakness in the extremities, unsteady gait, or dysphagia. In extreme cases of intoxication, a Parkinson-like syndrome including tremors, loss of memory, mental depression, speech disturbances, and muscle twitches can occur. Table 6.8 lists some other reported effects of carbon disulfide exposure. Splashes of carbon disulfide in the eyes cause immediate and severe irritation and burns. Exposure of the skin can produce dermatitis and vesiculation. Carbon disulfide is reported to be one of the most potent known skin irritants, causing third degree burns within minutes (61).

Management of Poisoning

Since hydrogen sulfide produces toxic effects in a manner similar to that of hydrogen cyanide, the same treatment procedure has been proposed for hydrogen sulfide poisonings. This involves production of methemoglobin with nitrites (63). Sulfide ions combine with methemoglobin to form sulfmethemoglobin, instead of reacting with intracellular cytochrome oxidase. The sulfmethemoglobin is excreted through the kidney or gradually metabolized to nontoxic products. The sodium thiosulfate step is not required. Other treatment is symptomatic and supportive.

There is still significant doubt that nitrite therapy is beneficial. Animal studies have shown that LD_{50} doses of sulfide salts are increased when sodium nitrite is given immediately after exposure (25). However, once cytochrome oxidase has been bound, even for a short period, death is likely. To be effective, nitrite therapy would have to be instituted before or immediately after exposure. Also, induction of methemoglobin results in decreased oxygen-carrying capacity of blood and increases the chance for producing cellular hypoxia.

Oxygen is usually considered to be beneficial and, in some cases, is all that might be necessary (49). Oxygen decreases the severity of irritation to the eyes and lungs after hydrogen sulfide exposure.

For any sulfide, if exposure is not immediately fatal and adequate treatment is given, recovery is probable (1).

SUMMARY

One of the important points presented in this chapter is that poisoning by gases may occur indiscreetly, with symptoms appearing without prior warning. Risks should be avoided when working in any environment where these poisonous gases may be present.

Also, quick assessment and management is essential to prevent severe toxicity. This is one class of toxicants for which antidotes are available. However, they must be used under medical supervision and, except for oxygen, are not generally accessible at the site of exposure.

Case Studies

CASE STUDIES: CARBON MONOXIDE INHALATION

History: Case 1

On a cold night, a hibachi grill was used by a husband and wife camping team to cook their evening meal. After eating, the hibachi was taken inside to heat their camping trailer. The trailer was well insulated and closed, since it was rather cool that evening.

During the night, the wife was awakened with nausea and went to the bathroom to vomit. There, she collapsed. Later she awakened to find her husband in bed, dead. This was the first time they had used the hibachi inside the trailer to provide heat.

On autopsy, the husband's COHb concentration was 71%. Also, mitral valve damage from a previous episode of rheumatic heart disease was observed. (See ref. 76.)

History: Case 2

A family of five was spending a holiday in a permanently positioned camping trailer. After the evening meal they complained of nausea, vomiting, and abdominal cramping. A physician was summoned to the camper, who diagnosed the malady as gastroenteritis, apparently caused by something they ate. He prescribed prochlorperazine for all members. Approximately 30 hr later a neighboring camper became suspicious when he saw one of the curtains pulled from its mounting, after no notice of activity around the area for the past day. He looked inside the window and

saw the father slumped on the floor. He immediately called for help.

When investigators entered the camper, three of the family members were dead (Fig. 6.8). Only one small window at the end was slightly opened, near where the father lay. The deceased family members had bright pinkish skin. Survivors were unconscious and pale and were hyperventilating when removed from the camper to be taken to a hospital. Analysis of blood samples from the survivors taken 4 hr after removal revealed 30% COHb in the mother and 27% in the father. Blood, feces, and gastric contents from all family members and vomitus and food from the camper were analyzed and found to be free of possible causes of food poisoning.

Investigators learned that heating and cooking were done with propane gas burned in a gas stove. The flue had been altered so that ventilation was poor. When the family was found, the stove was not lit. Investigators lit it as a test and measured the CO output into the camper. The concentration quickly reached toxic levels. (See ref. 32.)

History: Case 3

A 13-year-old boy was found unconscious on the garage floor wedged between the car and garage door. The car's engine was not running, and there were no noticeable exhaust fumes. There did not seem to be open containers of gasoline, kerosene, or other volatile hydrocarbons sitting around. Previous to this incident, the boy had been in excellent health, and there were no reasons to suspect drug abuse. He often worked on his motorbike in the garage without experiencing difficulties.

He was admitted to the hospital in a coma. His breathing, which was rapid and labored, progressively worsened and required intubation. His pupils were equal and reactive, but a few retinal hemorrhages were present. There was no response to painful stimuli. Brief episodes of tonic contractions were periodically noted.

Laboratory data shown in Table 6.9 were

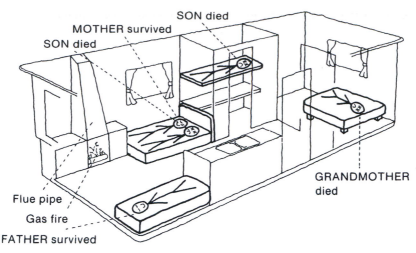

FIG. 6.8. Interior view of camping vehicle showing location of victims of carbon monoxide poisoning in relation to heating source. (From ref. 32.)

obtained on admission and 13 hr after discovery. The initial toxicology drug screen was negative for barbiturates and salicylates. The ECG showed sinus tachycardia, but computed tomographic scans and X-ray films were normal. Carbon monoxide poisoning was suspected. The patient's hospital stay was marked by anuria, pulmonary edema, ventricular tachycardia, hyperkalemia, and hypocalcemia.

Treatment included sodium polystyrene sulfonate, glucose, insulin, and calcium gluconate. Because of the elevated BUN (78 mg/dL) and serum creatinine (6.0 mg/dL) values on Day 6, peritoneal dialysis was started and maintained for 21 days. The boy remained intubated and dependent on a respirator for 11

days and was neurologically comatose for 12 days. The patient was then able to respond to vocal commands. He could feed himself by the 18th day, but it was not until the 21st day that he could speak and state that he remembered going into the garage to work on his bike. His memory improved over the next 5 weeks, and he was then able to move his lower extremities.

He was transferred to a rehabilitation facility, where he remained for the next 14 weeks. He made substantial progress and, at discharge, was speaking normally, although he had a poor ability to concentrate. He was able to walk with the aid of a walker and braces. (See ref. 79.)

TABLE 6.9. *Laboratory findings after poisoning by carbon monoxide*

Blood test	On admission	13 hr after discovery
Na^+ (mEq/L)	141	138
K^+ (mEq/L)	5.7	5.9
Cl^- (mEq/L)	90	100
HCO_3^- (mEq/L)	8	24
BUN (mg/dL)	28	42
Glucose (mg/dL)	155	183
Arterial pH	7.21	7.50
pO_2 (mm Hg)	97	88
pCO_2 (mm Hg)	16	25

Discussion

1. In all three case studies, the fact that carbon monoxide is a *silent killer* became evident. What precautions should have been taken to prevent exposure to CO?

2. In case 1, give a probable reason why the woman was not as acutely affected by the CO. Why did she not die? Why was she not treated at an emergency room?

3. Comment on the role of the husband's

heart disease (from case 1) as a probable factor in his susceptibility to CO poisoning.

4. Case 2 is a classic description of CO poisoning in several respects. First, all family members developed profound symptoms the evening before the incident. Neither they nor the attending physician recognized the symptoms as caused by CO. Second, the stove had a faulty flue and emitted a toxic concentration of CO into a small, poorly ventilated living area. Assuming that the camper was air-tight except for the one window that was opened slightly, how long do you think it would take to reach a potentially lethal CO concentration in the air?

5. Were the deceased family members in case 2 (two sons and a grandmother) those you would have expected to die? State your reasons for agreeing or disagreeing.

6. Describe the probable cause of the "pink coloration" of the skin of the three fatalities in case 2. Postulate whether the prochlorperazine had an effect on the outcome of this tragedy.

7. Comment on the possible use of hyperbaric oxygen in case 3.

8. The victim in case 3 showed periods of tonic contractions, even though he was comatose. Based on the information presented, what is the most likely cause of these events?

CASE STUDY: FATAL CARBON MONOXIDE POISONING IN A MOTEL

History

A 60-year-old man (patient 1) was discovered, dead, on the floor of his motel room. His wife (patient 2) was lying across the bed, comatose. She was transported to a local hospital.

Upon admission, serum bicarbonate was 16.0 mEq/L; arterial blood gases: oxygen, 59 mm Hg; carbon dioxide, 24 mm Hg. Serum pH was 7.31; oxygen saturation, 87.3%; and carboxyhemoglobin, 35.3%.

Upon autopsy, patient 1 displayed cherry-red livor mortis. Postmortem carboxyhemoglobin concentration was 90%.

In the motel room directly below the room occupied by patients 1 and 2 (Fig. 6.9), another couple (patients 3 and 4) slept through the day even though they had intended to check out earlier that morning. Patient 3 was a 65-year-old woman who later reported that she had awakened several times during the day but had been too weak to request assistance until late that day when she was finally able to telephone a relative for help. Twenty minutes later the relative and a security officer entered the room and removed the couple. Both patients survived.

Later that night (about 10.5 hr after the body of patient 1 had been discovered), a search of other guest rooms was undertaken. A fifth victim (patient 5), a 44-year-old man, was found comatose in a room adjacent to the room where patient 1 had died. At this point the motel was evacuated of all guests.

The three rooms occupied by the five victims were located close to a room containing a gas-fired water heater and purification system for the motel's swimming pool. The source of the carbon monoxide was the pool heaters, which were exhausted passively through vents on the roof. It was determined that, when the motel room doors were closed, there was a backdraft into the vents and that the room air-conditioning units pulled the gas into the three rooms through structural defects in the walls. In fact, patient 1 was a heavy smoker and his wife had set the room air conditioner to "high" to clear the air in the room. (See ref. 75.)

Discussion

1. Comment on why you think patient 1 died and his wife survived. Both breathed air containing the same concentration of carbon monoxide.

2. Patient 1 had a much higher blood carboxyhemoglobin concentration than his wife, even though both occupied the same room.

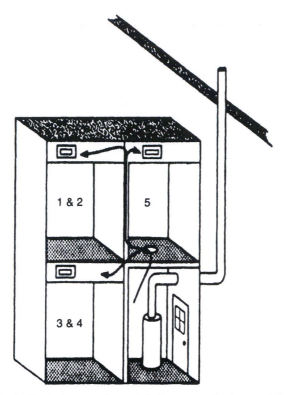

FIG. 6.9. Arrangement of affected rooms in motel. Room on the lower right contained the source of CO. (From ref. 75.)

What do you think contributed to this difference?

CASE STUDY: INTOXICATION FROM METHYLENE CHLORIDE

History

Four patients were transported to an emergency department (ED) at a local hospital after inhalation of methylene chloride for an unknown period. Patients 1 and 2 were working in an enclosed space where the substance was being used as a paint stripper. Patients 3 and 4 were rescuers.

Patient 1 was a 29-year-old man. Upon admission, he was in asystole without evidence of trauma. He was noted to have areas of purple discoloration or lividity on his forehead and left hand. There was no evidence of skin blistering. An endotracheal tube was placed and advanced life support started. The patient did not respond and was pronounced dead 15 min after admission. Arterial blood gases are shown in Table 6.10.

Patient 2 was a 32-year-old man who was found unconscious in the room with patient 1. Paramedics initially reported him in pulseless idioventricular rhythm (rate 40 beats/min). He failed to respond to prehospital cardiopulmonary resuscitation.

Upon admission, he was pulseless and apneic and had fine ventricular fibrillation. He was noted to have purple discoloration on the forehead and right arm, without other evidence of injury. Urine drug screen was positive for cocaine and ethanol.

Treatment consisted of cardiac defibrillation and routine pharmacologic agents including epinephrine. Cardiac rhythm changed from fine ventricular fibrillation to asystole to electrical-mechanical dissociation to idioven-

TABLE 6.10. *Arterial blood gases of patients poisoned by methylene chloride*

Patient	Time	FIO$_2$ (%)	pH	pCO$_2$ (mm Hg)	pO$_2$ (mm Hg)	HbCO (%)	HCO$_3$ (mm/L)
1	2200	100	6.48	129	16	8	9
2 2/2	2206	100	6.72	118	34	2	15
	2228	100	6.66	72	270	0	8
	2248	100	6.78	54	200	4	8
2/3	0008	100	7.09	42	349	4	12
	0054	50	7.11	46	166	4	14
	0132	50	7.14	49	105	2	16
	0230	40	7.16	47	91	2	16
	0408	40	7.17	50	71	4	18
	0517	40	7.26	50	76	6	22
	0627	40	7.30	43	55	6	21
	0705	50	7.31	42	74	8	21
	0900	50	7.35	35	66	7	19
	1445	50	7.31	33	61	6	16
	2200	50	7.24	37	55	2	15
3 2/2	2230	100	7.40	38	280	5	—
2/3	0055	100	7.38	39	193	3	22
4 2/2	2345	100	7.40	32	408	2	—
2/3	0200	100	—	—	—	2	—

From ref. 39.
FIO$_2$, fraction of inspired oxygen; HbCO, carboxyhemoglobin.

tricular rhythm with a rate of 80/min. Blood pressure was 90 mm Hg (palpable) systolic after 19 min in the ED. A total of 6 mg epinephrine and 2 mg atropine along with dopamine was administered during the resuscitation. Vital signs stabilized, and the patient was transferred to the intensive care unit. At no time did the patient awaken or breathe spontaneously.

In the intensive care unit, the patient remained unresponsive and required continued mechanical ventilation. Arterial blood gases (Table 6.10) showed gradual improvement of respiratory and metabolic acidosis with controlled respirations on the ventilator and the administration of sodium bicarbonate. Carboxyhemoglobin concentrations were low initially (0% to 2%) but increased to a maximum of 8% at 8 hr after administration.

The patient showed no evidence of electroencephalogram activity in the brainstem at 18 hr after admission. He required dopamine and mechanical ventilation to maintain the blood pressure and respiration status and showed no signs of neurologic recovery. His condition gradually deteriorated, and he died on the 4th hospital day.

Patient 3 was a 38-year-old male security guard who helped remove the two victims from the area of exposure. He performed mouth-to-mouth resuscitation on patient 1. He was given 100% oxygen at the scene. He complained of nausea and light-headedness and had three episodes of nonbloody emesis before arrival at the ED.

His physical examination was unremarkable. Arterial blood gases are shown in Table 6.10. He was discharged after 1.5 hr of observation. On follow-up examination 2 weeks later, he continued to complain of persistent headache and dizziness.

Patient 4 was a 24-year-old female security guard who helped remove patients 1 and 2 from the site. She subsequently spent 45 min in the hallway where the solvent odor was detectable.

She was asymptomatic for approximately 1 hr, when she developed slight dizziness, nausea, and belching, all of which resolved over 20 min. Physical examination was unremarkable. Arterial blood gases are listed in Table 6.10.

She was given 100% oxygen for 3 hr and then discharged to home. On follow-up examination 2 weeks later, she complained of intermittent headaches, nausea, and abdominal pain. (See ref. 39.)

Discussion

1. Carboxyhemoglobin concentrations in patient 2 increased over time, even though he was not continuously reexposed to methylene chloride at the time. What was the probable reason?
2. Patients 1 and 2 showed areas of purple discoloration on their body. Explain what these might have been.
3. Patients 3 and 4 continued to report symptoms at their 2-week follow-up examination. Would you expect this to occur as a typical outcome of exposure to methylene chloride?

CASE STUDIES: CYANIDE POISONING

History: Case 1

A 21-year-old man was admitted to an emergency facility unconscious, cyanotic, and with evidence of previous vomiting. Blood pressure was 168/112 mm Hg; pulse, 68 beats/min; and respirations (gasping), 24/min. A routine toxicology laboratory analysis on samples of blood and stomach contents was negative. Laboratory results are listed in Table 6.11. Pulmonary edema and lactic acidosis were characteristic throughout the clinical course.

The patient was ventilated and given 80% oxygen and intravenous fluids, including sodium bicarbonate and potassium chloride. Diuresis was initiated with furosemide. Nine hours postadmission, it was discovered that he had ingested potassium cyanide. Because at least 10 hr had elapsed since ingestion, treatment with sodium nitrite and sodium thiosulfate was not undertaken. Blood cyanide concentrations are listed in Table 6.11. In addition, the following ketoacids were elevated: beta-hydroxybutyrate, 1.2 mEq/L (normal, 0.6); acetoacetic acid, 1.6 mEq/L (normal,

TABLE 6.11. *Laboratory findings in two cases of cyanide poisoning*

Measurement	Case 1[a]	Case 2[b]
Amount of cyanide ingested	600 mg	Unknown
Respirations/min	24	20 (gasping)
Anion gap (mEq/L)	35	38
BUN (mg/dL)	21	9
Glucose (mg/dL)	245	313
pO_2 (mm Hg)	115	139
pCO_2 (mm Hg)	12	11
HCO_3^- (mEq/L)	5.6	—
pH	7.27	7.32
CN (μg/mL)	12 hr = 2.0	7.32
	22 hr = 1.6	
	84 hr = 1.2	

[a] From ref. 24.
[b] From ref. 69.

0.8); and lactic acid, 3.3 mEq/L (normal, 0.8). Also, note the high anion gap.

After recovery, the patient stated that he had ingested approximately 600 mg potassium cyanide. This means that he had been exposed to 3 to 6 times the lethal dose. Within 5 days, his chest X-ray findings were normal. He was discharged on the 9th day. (See ref. 24.)

History: Case 2

A 31-year-old male biochemist, with a previous history of alcohol abuse, was found comatose by his wife. She had last seen him awake about 1 hr earlier. He had been undergoing treatment for hypertension and an ulcer but otherwise was in good health. It was not revealed until 6 hr after admission that he had ingested an unknown quantity of potassium cyanide from his laboratory.

Laboratory values for this patient are also reported in Table 6.11. A routine toxicology drug screen was negative, although his blood alcohol concentration was 290 mg/dL.

The patient was given 0.4 mg naloxone (Narcan), but no improvement was shown. Gastric lavage was performed. Supportive treatment was continued, including 40% oxygen and forced diuresis with 5% dextrose in half-normal saline (D_5 NS). Three hours later, he was fully responsive, and 6 hr after admission he admitted ingesting a quantity of cyanide. The Cyanide Antidote Package was not used because of the long interval after ingestion, his continued stability, and the improvement of his clinical condition. The remainder of his clinical course was unremarkable. (See ref. 69).

Discussion

1. In case 1, gasping for air was noted. What is the pathophysiologic reason for this?
2. The patient in case 1 ingested more than the lethal dose of cyanide but survived. What is the most likely reason for his survival?
3. Neither patient was treated with nitrite and thiosulfate, even after the nature of their intoxication was determined. Why not?
4. What is the mechanism of cyanide-induced toxicity? Did either victim present with typical signs and symptoms associated with cyanide toxicity?
5. Explain the elevated anion gap in these patients.

CASE STUDY: HYDROGEN SULFIDE INTOXICATION

History

A 45-year-old man was overcome by fumes from a drain trap to which he was adding sulfuric acid (90%). The sink was located in a small basement cubicle of a hospital, which was used to prepare plaster casts. The drain had not been previously cleaned because of its high sludge content. Three other workers and a physician were less seriously affected when attempting to remove him from the area.

The man inhaled fumes for 2 or 3 min before being removed to fresh air. After exposure he was apneic, cyanotic, and comatose, and he displayed generalized tremors. Laboratory results listed in Table 6.12 were obtained. Poisoning by hydrogen sulfide was strongly suspected because of its strong odor.

Initial treatment consisted of sodium bicarbonate (44 mEq) and 100% oxygen. Five amyl

TABLE 6.12. *Laboratory findings after poisoning by hydrogen sulfide*

HCO_3^-	15 mEq/L		
K^+	3.4 mEq/L		
Na^+	152 mEq/L		
Cl^-	108 mEq/L		
Anion gap	29		
Sulfhemoglobin	7.9% (normal <0.5%)		
Blood gases (mm Hg)	pO_2	pCO_2	pH
Initial	127	26	7.27
After treatment with 100% O_2	270	32	7.30

From ref. 48.

nitrite ampules were broken over his airway during a 10- to 15-min period. He was given 300 mg of sodium nitrite and 12.5 g of sodium thiosulfate. He was also given dexamethasone (20 mg) and diazepam (15 mg), in divided doses. After 3 to 4 hr, the patient was able to breathe on his own, and after several more hours most symptoms disappeared except for headache and chest pains. (See ref. 48.)

Discussion

1. It was later discovered that sulfuric acid had been added to a drain blocked by calcium sulfide sludge, which had been produced by bacterial action on the plaster. The acid caused release of hydrogen sulfide gas. Discuss why the worker may not have smelled this gas, even though other persons who entered the room afterward were able to detect it. What is the characteristic odor?
2. How was acidosis produced from this toxic exposure?
3. What was the purpose of using amyl nitrite/sodium nitrite and sodium thiosulfate in treating this case?
4. Why did symptoms of headache and chest pains persist in this patient?

CASE STUDY: DUNG LUNG DISEASE—HYDROGEN SULFIDE POISONING

History

One day on a rural dairy farm, a cow kicked the lid to a large underground liquid manure tank into the tank. The farmer had gone into the tank before without incident, so he drained the manure to about a foot in depth and descended into the tank to retrieve the lid. Inside for only a few seconds, the farmer fell unconscious. His two sons sensed the emergency and entered to assist him. One immediately collapsed and fell face-up; the other escaped quickly to summon help. The county sheriff and village barber responded.

The barber entered the tank, lifted the still-gasping boy and then fell, unconscious. The sheriff entered to the rescue, but he, too, lost consciousness and fell.

The village ambulance arrived, and an emergency medical technician (EMT) entered the tank and quickly succumbed. Another technician (working swiftly and probably holding his breath!) entered the tank, tied a rope around the other technician's chest, and pulled him out. The first technician recovered rapidly and without further incident. Meanwhile, the barber was brought out of the tank by a fireman wearing a self-contained breathing apparatus. He was given cardiopulmonary resuscitation and survived. The barber did vomit a copious quantity of liquid manure. The farmer, his son, and the sheriff were soon removed by the protected fireman. Each was pronounced dead at the site.

The barber, age 41 years, was transported to a respiratory intensive care center. He was given 100% oxygen and required mechanical ventilation. On admission, his vital signs/symptoms were: blood pressure, 108/90 mm Hg (during dopamine administration); pulse, 155 beats/min; and rectal temperature, 38.5°C. He had intensive respiratory and cardiovascular distress. Blood pH was 7.31.

Treatment consisted of continuing oxygen for the next 10 hr. He received intravenous fluids, gentamicin, and clindamycin. Two days later, he did not have a fever or firm evidence of infection, and the antibiotics were discontinued. On the 4th hospital day, he developed a rectal temperature of 39.5°C. A gram stain of tracheal secretions disclosed multiple infectious pathogens, including *Klebsiella pneumoniae, Proteus mirabilis, Esche-*

richia coli, and *Pseudomonas aeruginosa.* Therapy was started with amikacin and ticarcillin.

By 2 weeks after the accident, chest X-ray films showed marked improvement with return of functions. By 6 weeks the barber returned to work and resumed jogging.

An autopsy was performed on the farmer, son, and sheriff. The farmer and sheriff suffered massive aspiration of liquid manure. The son did not. All three had significant blood sulfide concentrations: farmer, 5.0 mg/L; sheriff, 3.6 mg/L; and son, 0.8 mg/L. (Normal control concentrations are less than 0.05 mg/L). (See ref. 46.)

Discussion

1. Discuss the sequence of biochemical events that led to the deaths of these three victims.
2. Autopsy reports did not mention the pathognomonic sign that is characteristic for sulfide intoxication that usually involves the visceral and brain tissues. Assuming the victims did display this sign, how would these tissues have appeared?
3. Why was each person who went into the tank not able to smell hydrogen sulfide and thus avoid it?
4. Why did the son not experience aspiration pneumonia, while his father and the sheriff did?

Review Questions

1. Which of the following produces cyanomethemoglobin?
   A. Hydrogen sulfide
   B. Cyanide
   C. Methane
   D. Methylene chloride
2. Carbon monoxide exposure is more likely to produce toxicity in which of the following: athletes (I), geriatrics (II), infants (III)?
   A. I only
   B. II only

C. III only

D. II and III only

3. Which of the following is a specific antidote for CO poisoning: oxygen (I), sodium nitrite (II), sodium thiosulfate (III)?

A. I only

B. II only

C. III only

D. II and III only

4. Which of the following is a pathognomonic sign for CO poisoning?

A. Bitter almond odor

B. Cherry-red discoloration

C. Blue-green discoloration

D. Rotten egg odor

5. The binding affinity of hemoglobin with CO compared to its affinity with oxygen is:

A. One-fourth as great

B. Approximately the same

C. About 100 times greater

D. More than 200 times greater

6. All of the following cause the oxyhemoglobin dissociation curve to shift to the left *except:*

A. Carbon monoxide

B. Methemoglobin

C. Cyanide

D. Oxygen

7. Smoking two packs of cigarettes per day will produce CO blood concentrations that are closest to:

A. 1% to 2%

B. 3% to 4%

C. 7% to 8%

D. 10% to 12%

8. Although cyanide possesses affinity for binding to a number of different enzyme systems, it has strongest affinity for which of the following systems?

A. Sulfur transferase

B. Carboxyhemoglobin reductase

C. Cytochrome oxidase

D. Acetylcholine esterase

9. Which of the following is a true statement?

A. Hydrogen sulfide produces cellular hypoxia by reacting with sulfur transferase (rhodanese) enzyme.

B. Hydrosulfide ions readily combine with hemoglobin.

C. Carbon disulfide has a greater affinity for the CNS than does hydrogen sulfide.

D. After death by hydrogen sulfide poisoning, the brain will appear dark red in color.

10. Referring to Fig. 6.1 (the oxyhemoglobin dissociation curve), when CO binds to hemoglobin, which of the following is true?

A. The amount of oxygen available to tissues is reduced.

B. The oxyhemoglobin dissociation curve shifts to the right.

C. The percentage of oxygen saturation increases.

D. The oxyhemoglobin curve becomes sigmoid.

11. Cyanide is more tightly bound to iron in which of its valence states?

A. Fe^{2+}

B. Fe^{3+}

12. Hydrogen cyanide exerts its toxic effects via:

A. Direct inhibition of cellular utilization of oxygen

B. Prevention of adequate oxygenation alone

C. Combination with hemoglobin

D. Production of overt pulmonary edema

E. Medullary depression

13. Symptoms of cyanide toxicity include which of the following: headache (I), hyperpnea (II), or convulsions (III)?

A. II only

B. III only

C. I and II only

D. II and III only

E. I, II, and III

14. Which of the following is an antidote for carbon monoxide poisoning: sodium nitrite (I), sodium thiosulfate (II), or oxygen (III)?

A. II only

B. III only

C. I and II only

D. II and III only

E. I, II, and III

15. The proper sequence of therapy for treating cyanide is:
    A. Ventilate with oxygen; amyl nitrite; sodium nitrite; sodium thiosulfate
    B. Amyl nitrite; sodium nitrite; oxygen; sodium thiosulfate
    C. Sodium thiosulfate; oxygen; amyl nitrite; sodium nitrite
    D. Oxygen; sodium thiosulfate; amyl nitrite; sodium nitrite
    E. Sodium nitrite; amyl nitrite; oxygen; sodium thiosulfate

16. A farmer who has been seriously intoxicated by fumes from his liquid manure tank is most likely suffering from poisoning by:
    A. Methane gas
    B. Carbon monoxide
    C. Hydrogen cyanide
    D. Hydrogen sulfide

17. Upon metabolism, which of the following can produce significant concentrations of carboxyhemoglobin?
    A. Methylene chloride
    B. Amygdalin
    C. Laetrile
    D. All of the above
    E. Only two of the above

18. Which of the following best describes signs/symptoms of cyanide intoxication?
    A. Rapid fall of blood pressure with arterial blood that dries to a chocolate-brown color
    B. Severe diarrhea and abdominal pain and metabolic acidosis
    C. Depressed reflexes with flaccid paralysis and hyperthermia
    D. Increased respiratory rate, odor of rotten eggs on breath, and dyspnea
    E. None of the above

19. The half-life of carboxyhemoglobin in room air is 5 to 6 hr. If the patient receives 100% oxygen, the half-life will be:
    A. 9 to 10 hr
    B. 30 min
    C. 90 min
    D. Unchanged

20. To what substance does the term *silent killer* refer, and why is it used?

21. Discuss the physiologic barriers that normally prevent airborne particles from entering the lungs.

22. Infants are more susceptible than adults to the toxic effects of CO. Cite the reasons.

23. Carbon monoxide causes a characteristic discoloration of the skin. State the color and discuss why it appears.

24. What is meant by the term *hyperbaric oxygen?* At what carboxyhemoglobin blood concentration is hyperbaric oxygen recommended?

25. The blood normally has a low concentration of CO always present. What is this concentration, and what is its source?

26. Treatment of cyanide poisoning involves two primary steps. Name them, and specify the precise purpose of each step.

27. Oxygen is not a specific antidote for cyanide intoxication, although it may be administered. Cite the specific reasons why oxygen may be of benefit.

28. Prepare a chart listing methemoglobinemia (chapter 5), cyanide, and sulfide at the top and compare and contrast these with respect to the following:
    A. binding to heme (Fe^{2+})
    B. binding to cytochrome A_3 (Fe^{3+})
    C. arterial blood chocolate brown
    D. venous blood retains bright red color
    E. response to methylene blue
    F. response to oxygen
    G. response to cyanide antidote kit

References

1. Adelson L, Sunshine I. Fatal hydrogen sulfide intoxication. *Arch Pathol* 1966;81:375–380.
2. Amdur MO. Air pollutants. In: Klaassen CD, Amdur MO, Doull J, eds. *Toxicology—the basic science of poisons.* New York: Macmillan; 1980:801–824.
3. Atkins EH, Baker EL. Exacerbation of coronary artery disease by occupational carbon monoxide exposure: a report of two fatalities and a review of literature. *Am J Ind Med* 1985;7:73.
4. Ayres SM, Evans R, Light D. Health effects of exposure to high concentrations of automobile emissions. *Arch Environ Health* 1973;27:168–177.
5. Ayres SM, Giannelli S, Mueller H. Myocardial and systemic responses to carboxyhemoglobin. *Ann NY Acad Sci* 1970;174:268–293.
6. Ayres SM, Giannelli S, Mueller H, Criscitiello A.

Myocardial and systemic vascular responses to low concentrations of carboxyhemoglobin. *Ann Clin Lab Sci* 1973;3:440–447.

7. Ayers SM, Mueller HS, Gregory JJ, et al. Systemic and myocardial hemodynamic responses to relatively small concentrations of carboxyhemoglobin (COHb). *Arch Environ Health* 1969;18:699–709.

8. Barnard RJ, Weber JS. Carbon monoxide: a hazard to fire fighters. *Arch Environ Health* 1979;34:255–257.

9. Baud FJ, Barriot P, Toffis V, et al. Elevated blood cyanide concentrations in victims of smoke inhalation. *N Engl J Med* 1991;325:1761–1766.

10. Bonnichsen R, Maehly AC. Poisoning by volatile compounds. *J Forensic Sci* 1966;11:516–527.

11. Buie SE, Pratt DS, May JJ. Diffuse pulmonary injury following paint remover exposure. *Am J Med* 1986;81:702–704.

12. Burnett WW, King EG, Grace M, Hall WF. Hydrogen sulfide poisoning: review of 5 years' experience. *Can Med Assoc J* 1977;117:1277–1280.

13. Chen KK, Rose CL. Nitrite and thiosulfate therapy in cyanide poisoning. *JAMA* 1952;149:113–119.

14. Chen KK, Rose CL. Treatment of acute cyanide poisoning. *JAMA* 1956;162:1154–1155.

15. Chen KK, Rose CL, Clowes GH. Amyl nitrite and cyanide poisoning. *JAMA* 1933;11:1920–1922.

16. Coburn RF. Endogenous carbon monoxide production. *N Engl J Med* 1970;282:207–209.

17. Donham KJ, Knapp LW, Monson R, Gustafson K. Acute toxic exposure to gases from liquid manure. *J Occup Med* 1982;24:142–145.

18. End E, Long CW. Oxygen under pressure in carbon monoxide poisoning. *J Indust Hyg Toxicol* 1942;24:302.

19. Fawcett TA, Moon RE, Fracica PJ, et al. Warehouse workers' headache. *J Occup Med* 1992;92:12–15.

20. Geiger JC. Cyanide poisoning in San Francisco. *JAMA* 1932;99:1944–1945.

21. Ginsberg MD. Carbon monoxide intoxication: clinical features, neuropathology and mechanisms of injury. *Clin Toxicol* 1985;23(406):281–288.

22. Ginsberg MD, Myers RE. Experimental carbon monoxide encephalopathy in the primate: I. Physiologic and metabolic aspects. *Arch Neurol* 1974;30:202–208.

23. Goldsmith JR, Landaw SA. Carbon monoxide and human health. *Science* 1968;162:1352–1359.

24. Graham DL, Laman D, Theodore J, Robin ED. Acute cyanide poisoning complicated by lactic acidosis and pulmonary edema. *Arch Intern Med* 1977;137:1051–1055.

25. Gunter AP. The therapy of acute hydrogen sulfide poisoning. *Chem Abst* 1956;50:5916.

26. Haggard HW. Toxicology of hydrogen sulfide. *J Indust Hyg* 1925;7:113–121.

27. Hall AH, Rumack BH. Clinical toxicology of cyanide. *Ann Emerg Med* 1986;15:115–122.

28. Hamilton A, Hardy HL. *Industrial toxicology*. 2nd ed. New York: Paul B Hoeber; 1949.

29. Hanenson IB. *Quick reference to clinical toxicology*. Philadelphia: JB Lippincott; 1980.

30. Heymans C, Neil E. *Reflexogenic areas of the cardiovascular system*. Boston: Little, Brown; 1958.

31. Holzbecher MD, Moss MA, Ellenberger HA. The cyanide content of laetrile preparations, apricot, peach, and apple seeds. *J Toxicol Clin Toxicol* 1984;22:341.

32. Hopkinson JM, Pearce PJ, Oliver JS. Carbon monoxide poisoning mimicking gastroenteritis. *Br Med J* 1980;280:214–215.

33. Ilano AL, Raffini TA. Management of carbon monoxide poisoning. *Chest* 1990;97:165–169.

34. Kirkpatrick JN. Occult carbon monoxide poisoning. *West J Med* 1987;146:52–56.

35. Kizer KW. Hyperbaric oxygen and cyanide poisoning. *Am J Emerg Med* 1984;1:113.

36. Klaasen CD. Nonmetallic environmental toxicants: air pollutants, solvents and vapors, and pesticides. In: Gilman AG, Goodman LS, Rall TW, Murad F, eds. *The pharmacological basis of therapeutics*. 7th ed. New York: Macmillan; 1985:1628–1650.

37. Knelsen JH. United States air quality criteria and ambient standards for carbon monoxide. *UDI Berichte Nr* 1972;180:99–101.

38. Kulig K. Cyanide antidotes and fire toxicology. *N Engl J Med* 1991;325:1801–1802.

39. Leikin JB, Kaufman D, Lipscomb JW, et al. Methylene chloride: report of five exposures and two deaths. *Am J Emerg Med* 1990;8:534–537.

40. Litovitz TL, Larkin RF, Myers RAM. Cyanide poisoning treated with hyperbaric oxygen. *Am J Emerg Med* 1983;4:94–101.

41. Lowe-Ponsford FL, Henry JA. Clinical aspects of carbon monoxide poisoning. *Adverse Drug React Acute Poisoning Rev* 1989;8(4):217–240.

42. Mathieu D, Durocher A, Saulnier F, et al. Acute carbon monoxide poisoning—risk of late sequelae and treatment by hyperbaric oxygen. *Clin Toxicol* 1985;23(4–6):315–324.

43. Mohler SR. Air crash survival: injuries and evacuation toxic hazards. *Aviat Space Environ Med* 1975;46:86–88.

44. Morse DL, Woodbury MA, Rentmeester K, Farmer D. Death caused by fermenting manure. *JAMA* 1981;245:63–64.

45. Olson KR. Carbon monoxide poisoning: mechanisms, presentation, and controversies in management. *J Emerg Med* 1984;1:233–243.

46. Osbern LN, Crapo RO. Dung lung: a report of toxic exposure to liquid manure. *Ann Intern Med* 1981;95:312–314.

47. Pedigo L. Antagonism between amyl nitrite and prussic acid. *Med Soc Va* 1888;19:124–130.

48. Peters JW. Hydrogen sulfide poisoning in a hospital setting. *JAMA* 1981;246:1538–1539.

49. Ravizza AG, Carugo D, Cerchiari EL, et al. The treatment of hydrogen sulfide intoxication—oxygen versus nitrates. *Vet Hum Toxicol* 1982;24:241–242.

50. Rindone JP, Sloane EP. Cyanide toxicity from sodium nitroprusside—risks and management. *Ann Pharmacother* 1992;26:515–519.

51. Roughton FJW, Root WS. The fate of carbon monoxide in the body from mild carbon monoxide poisoning in man. *Am J Physiol* 1945;145:239–244.

52. Rudge FW. Treatment of methylene chloride induced carbon monoxide poisoning with hyperbaric oxygenation. *Milit Med* 1990;155:570–572.

53. Sammons JH, Coleman RL. Firefighters' occupa-

tional exposure to carbon monoxide. *J Occup Med* 1974;16:543–546.

54. Shrogg TA, Albertson TE, Fisher CJ. Cyanide poisoning after bitter almond ingestion. *West J Med* 1982;136:64–69.

55. Singh HB, Wasi N. Detection and determination of cyanide—a review. *Int J Environ Anal Chem* 1986;26:115–136.

56. Sjostrand T. Endogenous formation of carbon monoxide in man under normal and pathological conditions. *Scand J Clin Lab Invest* 1949;1:201–204.

57. Smith J, Brandon S. Morbidity from acute carbon monoxide poisoning at a three-year follow-up. *Br Med J* 1973;1:318–321.

58. Smith RP. Toxic responses of the blood. In: Klaassen CD, Amdur MO, Doull J, eds. *Toxicology—the basic science of poisons*. New York: Macmillan; 1986:223–244.

59. Smith RP, Gosselin RE. Hydrogen sulfide poisoning. *J Occup Med* 1979;21:93–97.

60. Spiller HA. Carbon monoxide exposure in the home: source and epidemiology. *Vet Hum Toxicol* 1987;29:383–386.

61. Spyker DA, Gallanosa AG, Suratt PM. Health effects of acute carbon disulfide exposure. *J Toxicol Clin Toxicol* 1982;19:87–93.

62. Stewart RD. Cyanide poisoning. *Clin Toxicol* 1974;5:561–564.

63. Stine RJ, Slosberg B, Beacham BE. Hydrogen sulfide intoxication: a case report and discussion of treatment. *Ann Intern Med* 1976;85:756–758.

64. Symington IS, Anderson RA, Oliver JS, et al. Cyanide exposure in fires. *Lancet* 1978;2:91–92.

65. Tariot PN. Delirium resulting from methylene chloride exposure: case report. *J Clin Psychiatry* 1981;44:340–342.

66. Tolonem M. Vascular effects of carbon disulfide: a review. *Scand J Work Environ Health* 1975;1:63–75.

67. Turino GM. Carbon monoxide toxicity: physiology and biochemistry. *Circulation* 1981;63:253A–259A.

68. United Nations Environment Programme, World Health Organization. *Environmental health criteria: 10. Carbon disulfide*. Geneva: World Health Organization; 1977.

69. Vogel SN, Sultan TR, TenEyck RP. Cyanide poisoning. *Clin Toxicol* 1981;18:367–383.

70. Wald M, Howard S, Smith PG, Kjedlsen K. Association between atherosclerotic diseases and carboxyhemoglobin levels in tobacco smokers. *Br Med J* 1973;1:761–765.

71. Way JL. Cyanide intoxication and its mechanism of antagonism. *Ann Rev Pharmacol Toxicol* 1984;24:451–481.

72. Way JL, End E, Sheehy MH, et al. Effects of oxygen on cyanide intoxication: IV. Hyperbaric oxygen. *Toxicol Appl Pharmacol* 1972;22:415–421.

73. Way JL, Gibbson SL, Sheehy M. Effect of oxygen on cyanide intoxication: I. Prophylactic protection. *J Pharmacol Exp Ther* 1966;153:381–385.

74. Werner B, Back W, Akerblom H, Barr PO. Two cases of acute carbon monoxide poisoning with delayed neurological sequelae. *Int Clin Toxicol* 1985;23(4–6):249–265.

75. Wharton B, Bistowish JM, Hutcheson RH, Schaffner W. Fatal carbon monoxide poisoning in a motel. *JAMA* 1989;261:1177–1178.

76. Wilson EF, Rich TH, Messman HC. Carbon monoxide poisoning following use of charcoal. *JAMA* 1972;221:405–406.

77. Winter PM, Miller JN. Carbon monoxide poisoning. *JAMA* 1976;236:1502–1504.

78. Winter PM, Smith G. The toxicity of oxygen. *Anesthesiology* 1972;37:210–241.

79. Zimmerman SS, Truxal B. Carbon monoxide poisoning. *Pediatrics* 1981;68:215–224.

7 ‖ Hydrocarbons

HYDROCARBON POISONING

Classification of Hydrocarbons

Hydrocarbons comprise a broad group of organic compounds that contain only hydrogen and carbon. They may be divided into two large categories: aliphatic (straight chain) or aromatic (benzene ring) compounds. Another group, which is of great toxicologic significance, consists of halogenated aliphatic and aromatic hydrocarbons. Some of these are discussed in this chapter; others, such as organochlorine insecticides, are described in other chapters. Hydrocarbons commonly encountered in acute poisonings consist of a mixture of saturated and unsaturated, aliphatic, alicyclic, or aromatic compounds and are usually distillates of crude oil, coal tar, and pine wood. Examples of each of these groups are presented in Table 7.1.

Characteristics of Hydrocarbons

Each hydrocarbon has unique characteristics, including molecular weight, volatility, surface tension, and viscosity. *Surface tension* refers to cohesiveness of molecules on a liquid's surface. *Volatility* is the tendency of a liquid to change into a gas or vapor. The most volatile hydrocarbons are low-molecular-weight (C_1 to C_5) gases and are asphyxiants. Aromatic hydrocarbons, such as benzene, toluene, and xylene, are also volatile and well absorbed from the GI tract. They can produce

TABLE 7.1. *Hydrocarbon classification*

Aliphatic
  Gases—methane, propane, butane
  Liquids—hexane, octane, etc.
  Waxes—paraffins
Aromatics
  Benzene, toluene, xylene, styrene, vinyl chloride
Halogenated
  Aliphatic—chloroform, carbon tetrachloride,
    methylene chloride
  Aromatic—DDT,[a] chlordane, lindane,
    p-dichlorobenzene, polychlorinated biphenyls
Petroleum distillates
  Petroleum ether (benzine), gasoline, naphtha
    kerosene, fuel oil, lubricating oil, paraffin,
    asphalt
Distillates of pine wood
  Turpentine
Distillates of coal tar
  Benzene, cumene, toluene, xylene

[a] DDT, dichlorodiphenyltrichloroethane.

significant systemic toxicity if absorbed. Some petroleum distillates, including naphtha, gasoline, and petroleum ether (benzine), are highly volatile but generally poorly absorbed after ingestion. Inhalation of their fumes may cause CNS depression.

Viscosity is defined as the resistance of a substance to flow over a surface and is measured in Saybolt seconds universal (SSU) units. Hydrocarbons with viscosity values below 45 SSU units have high aspiration risk, whereas those with a viscosity value greater than 100 SSU have a low aspiration potential (8).

Both volatility and viscosity are associated with hydrocarbon toxicity. Viscosity is the single most important index related to aspiration hazard (8).

Mechanism of Toxicity

The two most common routes of exposure for hydrocarbons are inhalation and ingestion. Ingestion is the more common route of exposure encountered in acute accidental hydrocarbon poisonings. When ingested, hydrocarbons produce toxic effects at several sites including the pulmonary, CNS, gastrointestinal, hepatic, and cardiovascular systems. Among these, the

most serious damage occurs to the pulmonary system. Aspiration pneumonitis is the greatest cause of morbidity and mortality with these compounds (6). Halogenated hydrocarbons, particularly those containing fluorine, sensitize the heart to catecholamines and induce arrhythmias in susceptible individuals (14).

PETROLEUM DISTILLATES AND TURPENTINE

Incidence of Poisoning

Although petroleum distillate ingestions involve a relatively small number of poisonings (reported to be approximately 7% of all cases), they do constitute a major cause of hospitalization of victims (21). Liquid products are more frequently encountered as causes of poisoning and include lubricants, mineral seal oil (in furniture polishes), fuels, cigarette and charcoal lighter fluids, solvents, paint and varnish thinners, and paint removers. Gasoline sniffing as a means of intentional abuse has been shown to cause toxicity (4,15,22).

Petroleum distillates are often stored in unmarked bottles or other common, unlabeled containers in the home or workplace. This puts them within easy reach of unsuspecting children who mistake them for something more palatable (13). Also, the ubiquitous nature of many household substances, such as lemon- or pine-scented furniture polish, room deodorants, and attractively colored and packaged cleaning aids, may invite more than a passing glance by a curious child. Table 7.2 lists some of the means by which children have been exposed to kerosene and illustrates the imaginative nature of children.

One of the major sources of petroleum distillate poisoning in adults is gasoline siphoning, resulting in pulmonary aspiration. During the world oil embargo of 1973 and other periods of gasoline shortages, reported instances of petroleum distillate poisonings increased.

Not all petroleum distillates are aspiration risks. Highly viscous substances (paint, glues,

TABLE 7.2. *Means by which children ingest kerosene*

Sniffed from a 30-gallon drum from which the top was missing.

Drank from a coffee can used to catch drippings from a leaky fuel line connected to an oil stove.

Drank from a can in the woodshed used for soaking paint brushes.

Drank from a cup left on the kitchen table by mother, who was treating the child for nits (lice eggs).

Sucked from an open vent pipe of an oil stove.

Drank from a soda bottle left on kitchen floor.

Dipped fingers into the fuel container of an oil stove and sucked them about 30 min.

Drank from a can of fluid used to start fires.

From ref. 7.

asphalt, rubber cement, etc.) pose little significant hazard of aspiration. Obstruction would be of greater concern after the ingestion of highly viscous products.

On the other hand, compounds with low viscosity and high volatility, such as gasoline, kerosene, and lighter fluid, can spread over mucosal surfaces easily and rapidly. Their risk for aspiration is great. Table 7.3 illustrates some common petroleum distillates listed by decreasing order of volatility and increasing order of viscosity.

Pathogenesis

The major target organs affected by petroleum distillates include the gastrointestinal, respiratory, and central nervous systems. Petroleum distillates produce gastrointestinal irritation and burning, often resulting in emesis and the risk of aspiration.

In the past, CNS depression was believed to be a serious complication of petroleum distillate ingestion. Therefore, the recommendation was to remove any ingested petroleum distillate quickly by emesis or gastric lavage. However, CNS depression occurs in fewer than 30% of patients who have ingested a petroleum distillate (18). In fact, it is not clear whether CNS involvement after hydrocarbon ingestion is due to a direct effect on the CNS or occurs secondary to hypoxic cerebral damage resulting from chemical-induced pneumonitis (13,30). Animal studies have demonstrated that kerosene is absorbed from the stomach only in small amounts (17,26,29).

Mann et al. (17) administered kerosene radiolabeled with ^{3}H-toluene or ^{14}C-hexadecane to primates to study gastrointestinal uptake and tissue distribution. Only small amounts were detected in tissues, including brain,

TABLE 7.3. *Petroleum distillates*

Hydrocarbon	Synonyms	Hydrocarbon composition
Low viscosity		
Benzin (benzine)	Petroleum ether	Low boiling point fractions (C_5–C_6)
Gasoline		Aliphatic (C_5–C_{12})
		Aromatic (xylenes)
Naphtha	Lighter fuel	Aliphatic (C_5–C_{13})
	Racing fuel	
VM&P naphthas	Mineral spirits	Aliphatic (C_7–C_{10})
Kerosene	Home heating oil #1	Aliphatic (C_{10}–C_{16})
	Kerosene	Aromatic (xylenes, naphthalenes)
Mineral seal oil	Signal oil	Aliphatic (over C_{20})
	Red furniture polish	
High viscosity		
Lubricating oil	Household oil	Aliphatic (over C_{16})
	Auto engine oil	Aromatic, polyaromatic
Diesel oil	Diesel fuel	Complex mixture, aromatic (over C_{11})
Fuel oil	Home heating oil #2	Complex mixture (over C_9)
	Gas oil	
Petrolatum	Petroleum jelly	Saturated, aliphatic (C_{14}–C_{18})
Paraffin	Wax	Saturated, aliphatic (C_{20}–C_{32})
Asphalt	Bitumen	Complex mixture of high-molecular-weight hydrocarbons,
	Mineral pitch	aromatic

heart, lung, liver, and kidney. They also showed that aromatic hydrocarbons are absorbed to greater degree than are aliphatic hydrocarbons. However, the amount absorbed is not sufficient to be directly responsible for CNS toxicity, except for the ingestion of large quantities (>15 mL/kg) of highly volatile aromatic hydrocarbons. They concluded that CNS manifestations associated with acute petroleum distillate ingestion result from hypoxia and acidosis, not systemic absorption (17,28).

From a chemical standpoint, such highly volatile hydrocarbons as gasoline, benzene, toluene, turpentine, and xylene are associated with greater risk of CNS toxicity because of their high lipid solubility. However, large amounts need to be swallowed and absorbed to produce significant CNS effects. These products have a disagreeable taste and, consequently, large volumes are rarely ingested. Although the precise amounts of petroleum distillate ingested are difficult to document, most children drink less than 30 mL (1,21).

The most serious and potentially lethal complication of petroleum distillate ingestion is the development of chemical pneumonitis (6,13). Pulmonary toxicity is primarily related to the aspiration of hydrocarbons during or after ingestion and vomiting (30).

Another controversy over the years has been whether hydrocarbons that are absorbed from the gastrointestinal tract reach the lung in sufficient concentration to produce direct toxicity. Several studies support the theory that pulmonary damage results from pulmonary aspiration of hydrocarbons and not from gastrointestinal absorption.

First, animal experimentation shows that, if a sublethal dose of kerosene is placed directly into the stomach, with the esophagus ligated to block the hydrocarbon mechanically from coming into contact with the trachea, little or no pulmonary damage occurs (11,17,26,29).

In a study by Dice et. al. (5), kerosene (20 mL/kg) was administered intragastrically in dogs that were protected from aspiration by esophageal transection and ligation. No clinical, radiographic, or histologic evidence of pulmonary abnormality was noted.

The second line of evidence is based on another series of animal studies by Gerarde (8). He showed that the LD_{50} ratio of oral-to-intratracheal instillation of kerosene is 140:1 and concluded that large quantities (amounts in excess of 100 mL) must be swallowed to allow the significant gastric absorption that would induce pulmonary damage. Most victims, especially children, whose volume of a swallow is estimated to be 4 to 5 mL, do not ingest such large quantities (1,12,21). Additionally, the time of onset of pathologic changes in the lung is too rapid and suggests that the pulmonary toxicity is caused by aspiration rather than absorption (8). Furthermore, studies have demonstrated that hydrocarbon-induced tissue damage was dependent on the site of administration. For example, if a hydrocarbon is injected into the portal vein, liver toxicity results; intratracheal administration causes significant pulmonary damage (2,28).

Overwhelming evidence supports the conclusion that lung damage after petroleum distillate ingestion does not result from gastrointestinal absorption, but is the result of pulmonary aspiration.

The physicochemical properties of hydrocarbons are also important factors responsible for the increased incidence of aspiration among certain hydrocarbons. From Gerarde's animal studies (8), the risk of aspiration and lung damage is directly proportional to volatility and indirectly related to surface tension and low viscosity. That is, hydrocarbons that are most likely to be aspirated are highly volatile and have low surface tension and viscosity. These properties permit the hydrocarbon to "creep" up the wall of the esophagus and enter the trachea. Hydrocarbons are also gastric irritants, and spontaneous vomiting sometimes occurs, during which there is greater chance for entry into the trachea (see chapter 3).

Characteristics of Poisoning

A variety of organ systems are affected by hydrocarbon toxicity. Symptoms are generally

TABLE 7.4. *Characteristics of hydrocarbon poisoning*

Petroleum distillates and turpentine
  Acute (inhalation, ingestion)
    GI—Nausea, vomiting, burning sensation
    Odor on breath
    Respiratory—Cough, shortness of breath, tachypnea, dyspnea, pulmonary edema, aspiration pneumonitis
    CNS—Dizziness, depressed reflexes, unconsciousness, convulsions
  Chronic (inhalation)
    Dizziness, anemia, weakness, weight loss, peripheral numbness, paresthesias
Aromatic hydrocarbons
  Acute (inhalation, ingestion)
    GI—Burning, vomiting, salivation
    Respiratory—Cough, aspiration pneumonitis
    CNS—Euphoria, dizziness, tremors, motor restlessness, hyperactive reflexes, violent excitement
  Chronic (inhalation, solvent sniffers)
    GI–Anorexia, vomiting
    CVS—Arrhythmias
    Blood—Anemia, bone marrow depression

GI, gastrointestinal; CNS, central nervous system; CVS, cardiovascular system.

similar regardless of the hydrocarbon ingested (24). Clinical manifestations of petroleum distillates, turpentine, and aromatic hydrocarbon poisoning are listed in Table 7.4. After acute ingestion, the most outstanding manifestations are CNS depression and chemical-induced pneumonitis.

Central nervous system symptoms may include lethargy, generalized weakness, dizziness, mental confusion, irritability, convulsions, and coma (30). Severe CNS involvement is not usually common. Although CNS symptoms were reported by Press (21) to occur in 91% of hydrocarbon poisonings, most patients experienced little more than lethargy. Another 5% were semicomatose, 3% were comatose, and 1% experienced seizures. Central nervous system symptoms are more likely to occur with highly volatile hydrocarbons (6).

Pulmonary toxicity is associated with aspiration and manifests as severe chemical pneumonitis. Initially, there is a burning sensation in the mouth and throat, which causes the victim to gag, choke, cough, and gasp for air. A persistent dry cough usually signals that the lungs have been severely damaged (24). Signs and symptoms of pulmonary toxicity after aspiration usually progress during the first 24 hr, reach a plateau, and then subside between the 2nd and 5th days (7). Chest roentgenograms show abnormalities within 30 min of aspiration, and almost all patients with lung involvement have positive signs of chemical pneumonitis within 12 hr. Furniture polish and lighter fluid caused more symptoms and positive roentgenographic evidence of pneumonitis in hospitalized children (7).

As the hydrocarbon enters the lung, it causes severe local irritation resulting in inflammation, edema, hemorrhagic bronchopneumonia, and atelectasis (6). Postmortem examination of the lung reveals interstitial inflammation, hyperemia, vascular thrombosis, intra-alveolar hemorrhage, bronchial and bronchiolar epithelial necrosis, and polymorphonuclear exudation (30).

A retrospective study of 950 children who ingested a petroleum distillate between 1969 and 1979 revealed the extent and outcome of the hydrocarbon ingestion problem (1). Eight hundred children were asymptomatic at the time of examination and remained so for a 6- to 8-hr observation period. None exhibited abnormal chest films, and all were treated as outpatients. The other 150 displayed symptoms of pneumonitis and were admitted for treatment.

The quantity of hydrocarbon ingested could be estimated in only 138 patients. In 67% of these, the quantity was believed to be less than 30 mL. Spontaneous vomiting occurred in 39% of the 150 patients who were hospitalized. Vomiting occurred more often when the ingested substance was furniture polish (mineral seal oil) rather than gasoline, paint thinner, kerosene, or lighter fluid. These differences were not significant. A definite correlation was shown between the presence of fever at or above 38°C and the observation of roentgenography-detected damage. There was no correlation between degree of fever and extent of pulmonary damage, however one hundred thirty-six (of the 150) children experienced no progressive pulmonary damage, and most were discharged within 72 hr of ingestion. Fourteen experienced progressive respiratory symptoms. Two died of respiratory failure, one developed secondary pneumonia due to *Staphylococcus aureus,* and four required ventilatory support.

MANAGEMENT OF HYDROCARBON POISONING

Numerous management protocols have been formulated for hydrocarbon poisonings. One of the early determinations that must be made is to identify the specific hydrocarbon ingested and determine its potential for aspiration and systemic toxicity.

Since morbidity and mortality from petroleum distillates and turpentine is related primarily to pulmonary damage after aspiration, preventing aspiration should have high priority in the management plan. Also, consideration must be given to the degree of respiratory distress, extent of CNS symptoms, and radiographic evidence of hydrocarbon-induced pneumonitis before specific treatment can be suggested.

An overriding question is whether the ingested hydrocarbon should be removed from the stomach. This question has been debated over the years and is still a controversial subject in clinical toxicology. Gastric decontamination is not recommended for most accidental petroleum distillate ingestions because of the risk of pulmonary aspiration. Some hydrocarbon ingestions, however, will require gastric emptying as outlined in Table 7.5.

When gastric decontamination is indicated, the preferred method is ipecac-induced emesis. In the past there was not a general consensus for either emesis or lavage. The dilemma was investigated by Ng et al. (19) in a retrospective study of 255 victims of petroleum distillate or turpentine poisoning. Twenty-nine percent of the victims received syrup of ipecac to induce vomiting, and 16% received gastric lavage. On careful follow-up of patients treated with ipecac, 19% were unchanged or worse than at the time of initial observation.

TABLE 7.5. *Hydrocarbon poisoning: indications for emesis*

Emesis not necessary for/with:
  High-viscosity, high-surface-tension compounds
    Grease, lubricating oils, petroleum jelly, paraffin wax, asphalt, rubber cement, fuel oil, diesel oil, mineral oil, baby oil
  Low-viscosity compounds
    Mineral seal oil, accidental ingestions of petroleum distillates or turpentine
Gastric evacuation by emesis recommended for:
  Large quantities of petroleum distillates, turpentine, aromatic hydrocarbons, halogenated hydrocarbons, and naphthalene
  Hydrocarbons containing camphor, insecticides, nitrobenzene, heavy metals

This contrasted with 39% of patients in the group that received gastric lavage. The conclusion was that pneumonitis was more significant after gastric lavage. Therefore, gastric lavage should be reserved for the drowsy or stuporous patient who recently ingested a large volume of a hydrocarbon or a hydrocarbon which was used as the vehicle for a more toxic substance. The airway must be protected when gastric lavage is indicated.

The following guidelines can be used to determine the necessity for ipecac-induced gastric emptying (9,23,30). Evacuation is indicated for hydrocarbon ingestion involving large quantities of petroleum distillates, turpentine, aromatic hydrocarbons, or halogenated hydrocarbons. For such hydrocarbons, gastric evacuation is recommended only when the amount ingested exceeds 1 mL/kg. Thus, an average 70-kg man would need to swallow more than 70 mL (2.3 ounces) before it should be removed. Emesis is indicated for ingestion of hydrocarbons containing heavy metals, camphor, or insecticides.

Accidental ingestion of low-viscosity hydrocarbons and accidental ingestions of petroleum distillates or turpentine seldom involves large quantities, and emesis would increase the risk of pulmonary aspiration. Therefore, gastric evacuation is not recommended. Also, gastric emptying is not warranted in individuals who have vomited spontaneously or ingested a nonvolatile, highly viscous hydrocarbon.

In the past, numerous attempts have been made to reduce absorption of ingested hydrocarbon by giving the patient doses of activated charcoal or various oily substances. Activated charcoal has not been shown to alter systemic absorption of hydrocarbons significantly. It may be given after emesis to adsorb any toxic additive that may be present. Various mineral or vegetable oils have been tried to increase the viscosity of ingested hydrocarbons in an effort to decrease absorption, as well as reduce the chance for aspiration. Oils also may produce demulcent and cathartic actions. However, most studies have not shown them to be significant in reducing hydrocarbon absorption, and they are not recommended. In fact, oils may actually enhance hydrocarbon absorption (Fig. 7.1). Gerarde (8) demonstrated that rats dosed with kerosene by intragastric intubation had higher blood concentrations when mineral oil was used. There is also the chance greater pulmonary damage (lipoid pneumonia) will occur should the added oil be aspirated during emesis.

Much of the management of hydrocarbon ingestion is symptomatic and largely supportive. This includes providing oxygen and fluids, and controlling fever with antipyretics.

Glucocorticoid and antibiotic usage has been advocated in past years, but neither is now considered beneficial. Antibiotics are indicated if infections occur but should be given only at that time. Most pulmonary complications are nonbacterial (3). Glucocorticoids may actually increase the patient's chance of developing pulmonary bacterial infections by lowering the immune system response (10,27). An intermittent positive pressure breathing (IPPB) device may be used, but, because of the extremely delicate nature of the distal alveoli and airways during hydrocarbon poisoning, this may worsen the condition (9,13).

SUMMARY

Numerous products in the home contain hydrocarbon substances. Many of these are obvious, such as gasoline and kerosene, and people take reasonable care to keep them out of the reach of children. Many others though, are not generally recognized as extremely potent poisons. Consequently, they are not stored or used properly. A good example is the red or lemon-scented furniture polish product that is carelessly left unattended.

Case Studies

CASE STUDIES: HYDROCARBON INTOXICATION

History: Case 1

A 19-month-old boy was admitted to an emergency facility 24 hr after the ingestion of an unknown quantity of kerosene. The baby was given castor oil at home before losing consciousness.

On admission, the child underwent gastric lavage. Respirations were rapid (rate not reported) but not grunting. His temperature was 101°F, and his pulse was 104 beats/min. He soon regained consciousness.

On roentgenographic examination, the medial aspect of both lower lung fields showed numerous coarse, mottled densities. The white blood cell (WBC) count was 11,500, and the

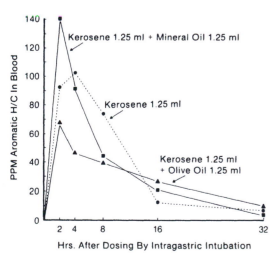

FIG. 7.1. Effect of olive oil and mineral oil on kerosene absorption. (From ref. 8.)

TABLE 7.6. *Clinical course of a charcoal lighter fluid-poisoned patient*

Hospital admission	24 hr later
Temperature: 38.1°C Blood pressure: 100/58 mm Hg Respiratory rate: 32/min Pulse rate: 100 beats/min Chest examination: tachypnea, bibasilar rales Chest roentgenogram: diffuse fluffy infiltrates	Temperature 38.1°C Respiration rate: 30–60/min Bloody sputum: gram stain, numerous polys Treatment: methylprednisolone

differential was normal. The child recovered in several days without additional treatment and with no apparent sequelae. (See ref. 16.)

History: Case 2

In a suicide attempt, a 40-year-old man injected himself intravenously with 3 mL of charcoal lighter fluid. He began complaining of burning chest pains and dyspnea about 2 to 3 hr later. He appeared at the emergency department on the following morning with severe pleuritic chest pain, epigastric discomfort, and shortness of breath. Table 7.6 depicts his clinical course.

Radiographic studies of the lungs made between the 4th and 12th days showed steady improvement in pulmonary abnormality. Repeated studies at 6, 12, and 18 months showed no residual abnormalities. (See ref. 25.)

Discussion

1. What is the significance of bloody pneumonitis? Would the same kind of pulmonary abnormality be observed if the hydrocarbon was ingested (assuming larger quantities were ingested, of course)?
2. Both cases involved the production of low-grade fever. Were antibiotics indicated? Why or why not?
3. In case 1, the baby was given castor oil at home. What do you think was the reason? What hazards are associated with the use of oils in hydrocarbon ingestions?
4. Where would the victim in case 2 have found naphtha (e.g., what types of products contain it)?

5. Why did the patient in case 2 display respiratory symptoms?

CASE STUDY: GASOLINE INGESTION

History

A 21-month-old boy was admitted to a hospital after consuming a large but unknown quantity of gasoline. Before admission he had been in good health, and he had no previous history of poison ingestion. On admission, a baby-sitter said that the boy had not vomited.

The youngster's breath smelled of gasoline, and he was in respiratory distress. A chest X-ray film revealed bilateral basilar infiltrates. He was given a slurry of activated charcoal and then transferred to a children's specialty hospital.

Upon reaching the emergency department of the second hospital, the child was lethargic and continued in respiratory distress. His systolic blood pressure was 110 mm Hg, and his pulse was 146 beats/min. Chest examination revealed suprasternal and intercostal retractions. Breath sounds were coarse. A second chest X-ray film identified bilateral alveolar infiltrates in the lower lobes and the right middle lobe. He also had traces of blood in the urine.

The child was given oxygen and a dose of magnesium citrate for catharsis while still in the emergency room. He was then admitted to the hospital in fair condition.

Over the next 24 hr, the patient's temperature rose to 39.8°C (rectally). He received acetaminophen. He remained tachypneic for 48 hr, with respiration rates as high as 60/min.

The patient progressively improved over a 48-hr period. No other medication was given. He was discharged on the 4th hospital day. All respiratory symptoms had disappeared, and the boy was playful. A final chest X-ray film revealed persistent pulmonary infiltrates without evidence of plural effusion. (See ref. 24.)

Discussion

1. Comment on the therapy this patient received in both hospitals (activated charcoal in one and magnesium citrate in the other). What do you think the rationale was and would you have treated him differently?
2. What was the purpose of acetaminophen given within the first 24 hr postingestion.
3. Describe the etiology of this child's tachypnea. Why did it persist so long?

CASE STUDY: FATAL LIPID PNEUMONIA AND LIQUID PARAFFIN

History

The patient was a 77-year-old man who was admitted for endoscopic prostatectomy. In addition to urinary symptoms, he also indicated that he was severely constipated, necessitating daily ingestion of liquid paraffin (the amount taken was not identified). He also smoked one pack of cigarettes each day.

A chest examination revealed normal breath sounds. There were no rhonchi or crepitations. Sounds suggestive of some degree of emphysema were heard. A preoperative X-ray film confirmed the presence of emphysema, but no active lung lesions were detected.

A prostatectomy was performed under epidural anesthesia. Twenty minutes postsurgery, the patient became confused and dizzy and developed numbness over his lower limbs and trunk. Blood pressure was 110/60 mm Hg. Pulse was 70 beats/min and regular. He suffered respiratory arrest and died despite attempts at resuscitation.

At autopsy, the stomach was found to contain mucoid exudates. There were scattered areas of gray consolidation in the lungs. There was no evidence of recent aspiration. Microscopic examination of the lungs revealed extensive lipid pneumonia. (See ref. 20.)

Discussion

1. Describe a sequence of events that contributed to this patient's death. How significant were the factors of smoking, emphysema, age, and epidural anesthesia on the patient's well-being.
2. What is the more common (i.e., household) name for liquid paraffin?
3. What are rhonchi and crepitations. When they are present on chest examination, what does this indicate?

Review Questions

1. Emesis is indicated in which of the following hydrocarbon poisonings?
   A. One swallow of lighter fluid
   B. One swallow of home heating oil or diesel fuel oil
   C. A large amount of gasoline in a suicide attempt
   D. One swallow of mineral seal oil furniture polish ingestion
2. Which of the following is the single most important predisposing factor in the occurrence of hydrocarbon-related pulmonary aspiration?
   A. Quantity ingested
   B. Viscosity of solution
   C. Age of victim
   D. Water solubility
3. Which of the following is a low-viscosity, highly volatile petroleum distillate?
   A. Turpentine
   B. Kerosene
   C. Mineral seal oil
   D. Benzene
4. Which of the following statements is true concerning acute hydrocarbon ingestion?

A. Hydrocarbons with a low viscosity are more likely to be aspirated.

B. Management of turpentine ingestion would be similar to management of naphtha ingestion.

C. Mineral seal oil ingestion produces minimal systemic toxicity.

D. All of the above are true.

E. Only A and B above are true.

5. Central nervous system depression is more significant in poisoning due to hydrocarbons with:

A. Aromatic rings

B. Low volatility

C. High surface tensions

D. High viscosity

6. The recommended management for the ingestion of a large volume of naphtha (>1 mL/kg) in a noncomatose patient may include:

A. Emesis with apomorphine

B. Dilution with milk and raw eggs

C. Emesis with syrup of ipecac

D. Lavage with peanut oil

7. Which of the following has proven to be effective in reducing the absorption of petroleum distillates?

A. Mineral oil

B. Activated charcoal

C. Milk and raw eggs

D. All of the above

E. None of the above

8. Petroleum distillates absorbed into the systemic circulation cause a high incidence of pulmonary pathology.

A. True

B. False

9. Many household cleaning products contain petroleum distillates. The treatment of the ingestion of approximately 1 teaspoonful of aliphatic hydrocarbon should involve:

A. Immediate induction of emesis using syrup of ipecac

B. Administration of mineral oil

C. Administration of activated charcoal

D. Dilution with vinegar

E. None of the above

10. The petroleum distillate with the least toxicity potential would have:

A. High surface tension and high volatility

B. Low surface tension and low volatility

C. High viscosity and low volatility

D. Low viscosity and low surface tension

E. High surface tension and high viscosity

11. A distinction must be made between incidence of poisoning by hydrocarbon substances and severity of intoxication. Discuss these points.

12. Describe the relationship between the surface tension of a given hydrocarbon and its potential for aspiration.

13. Discuss the feasibility of using intermittent positive pressure breathing devices in treating hydrocarbon poisoning.

14. Discuss reasons why the quantity of gasoline that actually enters the lungs during aspiration is probably small.

15. In cases of poisoning with insecticides that have a petroleum distillate base, which component is more toxic, the pesticide or hydrocarbon? What is the treatment priority in these cases?

16. Damage to the CNS by ingested hydrocarbons may be primary or secondary. What does this mean?

17. Antibiotics are sometimes indicated as part of the treatment protocol for hydrocarbon poisoning. What is the indication for anti-infective therapy?

References

1. Anas N, Namasonthi V, Ginsburg CM. Criteria for hospitalizing children who have ingested products containing hydrocarbons. *JAMA* 1981;246:840–843.

2. Bratton L, Waddow JE. Ingestion of charcoal lighter fluid. *J Pediatr* 1975;87:633–636.

3. Brown J, Burke B, Danani AS. Experimental kerosene pneumonia: evaluation of some therapeutic regimens. *J Pediatr* 1974;84:396–401.

4. Couleton JL, Hirsch W, Brillman J, et al. Gasoline sniffing and lead toxicity in Navajo adolescents. *Pediatrics* 1983;71:113–117.

5. Dice WH, Ward G, Kelley J, Kilpatrick WR. Pulmonary toxicity following gastrointestinal ingestion of kerosene. *Ann Emerg Med* 1982;11:138–142.

6. Eade NR, Taussig LM, Marks MI. Hydrocarbon pneumonitis. *Pediatrics* 1974;54:351–356.

7. Foley JC, Dreyer NB, Soule AB, Woll E. Kerosene poisoning in young children. *Radiology* 1954;62: 817–829.

8. Gerarde HW. Toxicological studies on hydrocarbons: V. Kerosene. *Toxicol Appl Pharmacol* 1959;1:462–474.

9. Goldfrank L, Kirstein R, Bresnitz E. Gasoline and other hydrocarbons. *Hosp Physician* 1979;9:32–79.

10. Hardman G, Tolson R, Haghdassarian O. Prednisone in the management of kerosene pneumonia. *Indian Practitioner* 1960;13:615.

11. Huxtable KA, Bolande RP, Klaus M. Experimental furniture polish pneumonia in rats. *Pediatrics* 1964;34:228–230.

12. Jones OV, Work CE. Volume of a swallow. *Am J Dis Child* 1961;102:427.

13. Karlson KH. Hydrocarbon poisoning in children. *South Med J* 1982;75:839–840.

14. Kaufman JD, Morgan MS, Marks ML, et al. A study of the cardiac effects of bromochlorodifluoromethane (halon 1211) exposure during exercise. *Am J Indust Med* 1992;21:223–233.

15. Kovanen J, Somer H, Schroeder P. Acute myopathy associated with gasoline sniffing. *Neurology* 1983; 33:629–631.

16. Lesser LI, Weens HS, McKey JD. Pulmonary manifestations following ingestion of kerosene. *J Pediatr* 1943;23:352–364.

17. Mann MD, Pirie DJ, Wolfsdorf J. Kerosene absorption in primates. *J Pediatr* 1977;91:495.

18. Moriarty RW. Petroleum distillate poisonings. *Drug Ther* 1979;9:135–139.

19. Ng RC, Darwish H, Stewart DA. Emergency treatment of petroleum distillate and turpentine ingestion. *Can Med Assoc J* 1974;111:537–538.

20. Paraskevaides EC. Fatal lipid pneumonia and liquid paraffin. *Br J Clin Pract* 1990;44:509–510.

21. Press E. Cooperative kerosene poisoning study: evaluation of gastric lavage and other factors in the treatment of accidental ingestion of petroleum distillate products. *Pediatrics* 1962;29:648–674.

22. Ross CA. Gasoline sniffing and lead encephalopathy. *Can Med Assoc J* 1982;127:195–197.

23. Rumack BH. Hydrocarbon ingestions in perspective. *J Am Coll Emerg Physicians* 1977;6:172–173.

24. Tinker TD. Hydrocarbon ingestion in children: its sequelae and management. *Okla State Med Assoc J* 1986;79:95–101.

25. Vaziri ND, Smith PJ, Wilson AF. Toxicity with intravenous injection of naphtha in man. *Clin Toxicol* 1980;16:335–343.

26. Wolfe BM, Brodeur AE, Shields JB. The role of gastrointestinal absorption of kerosene in producing pneumonitis in dogs. *J Pediatr* 1970;76:867.

27. Wolfe JE, Bone RC, Ruth WE. Effects of corticosteroids in the treatment of patients with gastric aspiration. *Am J Med* 1977;63:719–722.

28. Wolfsdorf J. Kerosene intoxication: an experimental approach to the etiology of the CNS manifestations in primates. *J Pediatr* 1976;88:1037–1040.

29. Wolfsdorf V, Kundig H. Kerosene poisoning in primates. *S Afr Med J* 1972;46:619.

30. Zieserl E. Hydrocarbon ingestion and poisoning. *Compr Ther* 1979;5:35–42.

8 ‖ Pesticides

Humans have long felt an obsession to rid their environment of pests. They are devastating to crops and food supplies, and life is basically more enjoyable without them. Indeed, the Old Testament makes several references to widespread destruction of crops in early Egypt by insects, especially locusts. Historical records confirm that insects have been a problem throughout the ages. Even with powerfully effective insecticides, locusts and other insects still damage food supplies in the Near East, Africa, and other parts of the world.

Pesticides are designed to kill various pests (both plants and animals) that interfere with our own comfort, health, or economic well-being. They are used in most countries around the world to protect agricultural and horticultural crops against damage. They are used at home and at work to assure a pest-free environment.

Overall, pesticides account for a small but significant number of human poisonings. Deaths reported from exposure are relatively rare. It is estimated that for each death there are another 100 nonfatal poisonings (27). In fact, a report representing 16 regional poison control centers in 1983 cited approximately 8,500 exposures to insecticides that resulted in no symptoms or minor effects (81).

Statistical surveys of morbidity and mortality have shown a reduction in the number of accidental deaths associated with pesticide use (29). This is probably due to increased awareness of pesticide toxicity through poison prevention programs. In occupational use, pesticide applicators are the high-risk group for both acute and chronic poisoning. Organophosphorus compounds are most commonly encountered. Morgan et al. (54), in 1980, noted that, among occupational users of pesticides, accidental trauma deaths were more common in pesticide applicators. Survivors showed an increased incidence of dermatitis and skin cancer.

Insecticides are the most commonly encountered pesticide in developing countries; *herbicides* are more commonly encountered in developed countries. The United States is the largest user of pesticides. A recent assessment of use, based on retail sales, confirmed the following data: United States, 45%; Western Europe, 25%; Japan, 12%; remaining countries combined, 18% (12). If all pesticide products in current use around the world were grouped together, their number would total in the tens of thousands. A few selected compounds have been purposefully chosen to exemplify those that are most generally encountered in poisoning cases.

Many of the poisons discussed elsewhere in this book can also be used to kill various pests. Arsenic and other heavy metals, such as mercury and copper, are effective and widely used herbicides. Hydrogen cyanide is a fumigant that controls insects and certain rodents. Creosote (a petroleum product) protects wood against insect damage. Lime (an alkali) protects against fungus.

Most poisoning by pesticides occurs as a result of misuse or accidental exposure. At home, poisoning usually occurs by oral ingestion; occupational users most frequently encounter dermal exposure or inhalation (73,87).

INSECTICIDES

Organophosphorus Compounds

More than 50,000 organophosphorus compounds have been synthesized and tested for insecticidal activity. The number actually used for this purpose today probably does not exceed three dozen. In addition to use as insecticides, organophosphorus compounds also have several medical applications. Physostigmine (eserine), edrophonium, and neostigmine are used for their cholinomimetic (cholinergic) activity. They are used in diagnosis or treatment of several neuromuscular disorders, including myasthenia gravis. Physostigmine is also an important antidote for treating toxic ingestion of anticholinergic substances, including tricyclic antidepressants, atropine, and jimsonweed. Its role as an antidote is discussed in subsequent chapters. Physostigmine, echothiophate iodide, and other organophosphorus drugs may be used in treatment of glaucoma to reduce intraocular pressure.

TABLE 8.1. *Toxicity of selected organophosphorus insecticides*

Insecticide	LD$_{50}$ (mg/kg)	
	Oral	Dermal
Highly toxic		
TEPP (tetraethyl pyrophosphate)	1.1	2.4
Mevinphos (Phosdrin)	3.7	
Chlorpyrifos (Lorsban, Dursban)	8	
Ethyl parathion (Parathion)	13	21
Methyl parathion (Dalf, Penncap-M)	14	67
Fenthion (Baytex, Lysoff)	15	
Moderately toxic		
Leptophos (Phosvel, Abar)	53	
Dichlorvos, DDVP (Vapona, No Pest Strip)	80	107
Trichlorfon (Dylox, Dipterex)	630	>2,000
Ronnel (Korlan, Trolene, Viozene)	1,250	>4,000
Malathion (Cythion, Karbofos, Malamar)	1,375	>4,444
Temophos (Abate, Abathion)	2,000	>4,000

From refs. 15 and 21.

Organophosphorus insecticides are among the most toxic of all substances that cause human poisoning and are the most frequently encountered insecticide poisons (26). Ingestion of as little as 2 mg in children may be lethal (15).

LD$_{50}$ data are useful to predict the potential hazard of a substance to humans. Table 8.1 lists organophosphorus insecticides in order of decreasing toxicity based on oral LD$_{50}$ values. Highly toxic ones generally have oral LD$_{50}$ values of less than 50 mg/kg and are restricted largely to agricultural use. Those with oral LD$_{50}$ values greater than 50 mg/kg are considered moderately toxic and diluted for household use. Differences between oral and dermal LD$_{50}$ values provide an additional safety feature during application of the product (15,21).

Discovery of Organophosphorus Compounds

Organophosphorus compounds were first synthesized in Germany during World War II. Their use as nerve gases in chemical warfare was quickly recognized. In fact, much of our understanding of clinical manifestations of organophosphorus insecticide poisoning was derived from the development of nerve gases, such as tabun, sarin, and soman (69). Early syntheses included compounds such as tetraethyl pyrophosphate (TEPP), parathion, and schradan, which were not only extremely effective insecticides, but also quite toxic to mammals. Research continued toward development of additional compounds, such as malathion, that maintained insecticide potency with less risk of toxicity to humans. The chemical structures of a few are shown in Fig. 8.1.

Mechanism of Toxicity

Understanding the mechanism of toxicity requires prior knowledge of actions of the cholinergic neurotransmitter, acetylcholine (ACh). Muscarinic and nicotinic ACh receptors exist in both the central and peripheral nervous systems (Fig. 8.2). In the peripheral system, ACh is released in autonomic ganglia at (i) sympathetic and parasympathetic preganglionic synapses, (ii) parasympathetic postganglionic synapses, and (iii) neuromuscular junctions of skeletal muscle (Fig. 8.2). In the central nervous system, most ACh receptors of greatest importance to organophos-

$$(C_2H_5O)_2\text{-}\overset{\overset{O}{\|}}{P}\text{-O-}\overset{\overset{O}{\|}}{P}\text{-}(OC_2H_5)_2$$

TEPP

$$(C_2H_5O)_2\text{-}\overset{\overset{S}{\|}}{P}\text{-O-}\langle\ \rangle\text{-}NO_2$$

PARATHION

$$(CH_3O)_2\text{-}\overset{\overset{S}{\|}}{P}\text{-S-CHCOOC}_2H_5$$
$$\qquad\qquad\quad |$$
$$\qquad\qquad CH_2COOC_2H_5$$

MALATHION

FIG. 8.1. Structural formulae for representative organophosphorus insecticides.

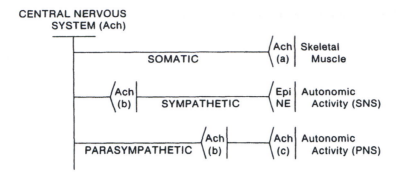

FIG. 8.2. Distribution of acetylcholine (*Ach*) throughout the body. Location includes the CNS, neuromuscular junctions (**a**), autonomic ganglia (**b**), and muscarinic sites (**c**).

phorus insecticide toxicity are located within the medulla at the respiratory and vasomotor centers.

When ACh is released, it acts as an excitatory neurotransmitter to propagate nerve conduction in the peripheral and central nervous systems or to initiate muscle contraction. The actions of ACh are terminated by hydrolysis in the presence of the enzyme acetylcholinesterase (AChE). There are two forms of AChE. *True cholinesterase,* or acetylcholinesterase, is located in erythrocytes, neurons, neuromuscular junctions, lungs, spleen, and gray matter of the brain. *Pseudocholinesterase,* or serum cholinesterase, is located primarily in serum and plasma but is also in the liver, pancreas, heart, and white matter of the brain.

Acetylcholinesterase has two points of attachment, and ACh binds to it in a sequential manner. First, ACh binds to an anionic site on the enzyme, and then the acetyl moiety binds at an esteratic site (enzyme-substrate complex). Choline is cleaved, leaving an acetylated enzyme (Fig. 8.3A). The acetyl portion is rapidly hydrolyzed to acetic acid and the regenerated active enzyme.

Organophosphorus insecticides and carbamates inhibit AChE by phosphorylating the esteratic site of the enzyme (Fig. 8.3B). The phosphate moiety is bound so tightly that it is considered irreversible. Acetylcholinesterase activity remains inhibited until new enzyme is generated or cholinesterase reactivator (i.e., pralidoxime) is administered. Depression of RBC acetylcholinesterase is considered a spe-

cific response to organophosphorus poisoning and reflects the degree of inhibition of neuronal synaptic cholinesterase (57). However, both erythrocytic (true) cholinesterase and pseudocholinesterase activities can be increased. Which enzyme is measured must be specified in the clinical assessment of potential organophosphorus (OP) poisoning.

As a result of AChE inhibition by organophosphorus insecticides, ACh accumulates and binds to muscarinic and nicotinic receptors throughout the nervous system. Consequently, OP poisoning may produce a variety of clinical manifestations. Low-dose exposure to the compounds generally produces signs and symptoms attributed to stimulation of pe-

A. ACh + AChE $\rightleftharpoons$ ACh-AChE $\rightleftharpoons$ Choline + Acetyl-AChE
 (Enzyme-substrate
 complex)

Acetyl-AChE + H$_2$O $\rightleftharpoons$ Acetic acid + AChE
 (Reactivated
 enzyme)

B. OP + AChE $\rightleftharpoons$ Phosphorylated-AChE

Phosphorylated-AChE + H$_2$O $\longrightarrow$ No reaction*

Phosphorylated-AChE + ACh $\longrightarrow$ No reaction

FIG. 8.3. Scheme showing deactivation of acetylcholine by acetylcholinesterase (**A**) and events that occur when an organophosphorus compound (e.g., insecticide) is present (**B**). *ACh,* acetylcholine; *AChE,* acetylcholinesterase; *OP,* organophosphorus compound; *, very slow hydrolysis may occur with some organophosphorus compounds or carbamates.

ripheral muscarinic receptors. Larger doses also bind with nicotinic receptors and central muscarinic receptors. Two to 4 weeks are required for plasma pseudocholinesterase, and 4 weeks to several months are required for erythrocytic and synaptic cholinesterase activity to return to normal (3).

Characteristics of Poisoning

As shown in Table 8.2, organophosphorus insecticide poisoning may produce a variety of toxic actions. Signs and symptoms are attributed to persistent acetylcholine hyperstimulation at muscarinic and nicotinic receptor sites.

Early signs and symptoms of low doses of organophosphorus insecticides are due to excess cholinergic stimulation at muscarinic re-

TABLE 8.2. *Characteristics of organophosphorus poisoning*

Muscarinic
  SLUD: Salivation, lacrimation, urination, diarrhea
    (or defecation)
  Abdominal cramping
  Nausea and vomiting
  Bradycardia and heart block
  Bronchoconstriction; wheezing
  Increased bronchial secretions
  Miosis
  Sweating
Nicotinic
  Muscle fatigue; weakness
  Twitching and fasciculations; tremor
  Paralysis
  Dyspnea
  Pallor
  Tachycardia (from ganglionic stimulation);
    hypertension
Central nervous system
  Anxiety, restlessness, insomnia, nightmares,
    confusion, neurosis
  Headache
  Ataxia
  Confusion
  Emotional instability
  Giddiness
  Slurred speech
  Generalized weakness
  Convulsions
  Depressed respiration and cardiovascular
    functions
  Cheyne-Stokes respiration
  Coma

ceptors. With moderate to larger doses, nicotinic and central stimulation predominate over most muscarinic effects. Clinical manifestations can be grouped into three categories: muscarinic, nicotinic, and central nervous system effects. The muscarinic effects are the result of ACh accumulation at autonomic effector cells and usually appear early, within minutes after ingestion. Symptoms include nausea, sweating, miosis (pinpoint pupils), blurred vision, and a syndrome identified by the acronym *SLUD* (salivation, lacrimation, urination, and diarrhea). Respiratory effects include bronchoconstriction with wheezing and increased bronchial secretions.

Nicotinic effects (autonomic ganglia and skeletal muscles) of organophosphorus insecticide poisoning usually appear after the muscarinic effects have been noted. The nicotinic effects include muscle twitches, weakness, fatigue, and fasciculations as a result of excess ACh at neuromuscular junctions causing persistent depolarization followed by paralysis of skeletal muscles. The most profound effect of paralysis is on the respiratory muscles. In severe organophosphorus insecticide poisoning, transient hyperglycemia due to stimulation of sympathetic ganglia and adrenal glands may be observed.

The central nervous system manifestations of organophosphorus insecticide poisoning include an initial stimulation followed by depression of the respiratory and cardiovascular centers in the medulla. Other CNS effects include anxiety, restlessness, confusion, headaches, slurred speech, convulsions, and coma. Even a single episode of significant organophosphorus poisoning may result in a persistent decline in neuropsychologic function tests (67).

Death associated with organophosphorus insecticide poisoning is the result of respiratory muscle paralysis, depression of the central respiratory center, bronchoconstriction, and accumulation of bronchial secretions.

Organophosphorus insecticides may be absorbed by various routes of exposure, which influences the onset of clinical manifestations. After inhalation of vapors, for example, symptoms may appear within minutes. Oral ingestion or dermal exposure generally requires a longer period to exhibit signs and symptoms of toxicity. Limited exposures may cause only localized effects. For example, percutaneous absorption of an organophosphorus compound over a confined area of skin may cause intense sweating and twitching of the muscles in the affected area only. Eye exposure to vapors may result in only miosis or blurred vision. Inhalation of a small concentration may cause only wheezing and coughing.

Complications of poisoning are usually related to prolonged neurotoxicity (38,42,49) and organophosphorus-induced delayed neuropathy (OPIDN) (36,46). The onset of symptoms may be delayed for days to weeks (1). Symptoms typically begin in the distal portion of the lower limbs and progress to generalized muscular weakness and flaccidity of the entire limb. In some instances, there is complete loss of control of arms and legs. In OPIDN, symptoms usually peak in a few weeks and then subside gradually. Complete recovery is not always apparent. The delayed neuropathy is not related to continued inhibition of acetylcholinesterase, and it is not reversible with atropine or pralidoxime.

The mechanism of toxicity of OPIDN is related to neuronal degeneration rather than demyelination. Animal models have shown the mechanism to involve phosphorylation and inhibition of a neurotoxic esterase. A marker for these neurologic changes seems to be 1′,3′-cyclic nucleotide 3′-phosphohydrolase, which eventually may be of clinical significance.

Management of Organophosphorus Poisoning

Treatment of organophosphorus insecticide poisoning should begin immediately after a probable diagnosis is made. Hesitation for just a few minutes following severe exposure will greatly decrease the victim's chance for surviving a potentially lethal dose.

A presumptive diagnosis can be made based on the patient's exposure history and characteristic cholinergic signs and symptoms and response to antidotes (57). A confirming diagnosis, measuring inhibition of erythrocytic acetylcholinesterase activity, may be useful. However, treatment should not be withheld until laboratory results are known. In severe intoxication or when chronic exposure to organophosphorus poisoning is suspected, cholinesterase activity should be measured.

Clinical manifestations of acute poisoning generally occur when more than 50% of cholinesterase is inhibited, and severity of signs and symptoms often parallels the degree of inhibition. For example, in mild poisoning 20% to 50% of normal enzyme activity remains; moderate, 10% to 20%; and severe intoxication, less than 10% (57).

Initial management of acute toxicity must include establishing an adequate airway and maintaining respiration. Suction may be required to remove bronchial secretions. If exposure involved ingestion, removal by ipecac-induced emesis or gastric lavage, with protection of the airway, is indicated. Since organophosphorus insecticides are rapidly absorbed from the gastrointestinal tract, gastric decontamination is most effective within 30 min postingestion.

Most organophosphorus insecticides are mixed with petroleum distillate solvents. Caution must be exercised to protect against the risk of pulmonary aspiration. If gastric decontamination was not undertaken within several hours after ingestion, activated charcoal may be considered to decrease absorption.

The antidotes for organophosphorus insecticide are atropine and pralidoxime (2-PAM, Protopam). Atropine should be given immediately if severe poisoning is suspected. Atropine antagonizes peripheral muscarinic effects and many of the central cholinergic effects. It will not reverse neuromuscular paralysis associated with nicotinic stimulation or respiratory failure in severe poisoning.

A test dose of atropine (adults, 1 mg; children, 0.015 mg/kg) may be used in mild to moderate organophosphorus insecticide poisoning to confirm diagnosis. Pupil size is helpful in assessing the effects of atropine. After the initial test dose, atropine is administered at doses of 2 to 4 mg intravenously (children, 0.015 to 0.05 mg/kg) and repeated every 10 to 15 min as needed until cholinergic effects (such as bradycardia, salivation, and increased bronchial secretions) diminish and signs of atropine action (such as mydriasis, tachycardia, and dry mouth) appear (44). The organophosphorus insecticide-poisoned patient is usually resistant to atropine, and high doses given for long periods may be necessary to control cholinergic signs effectively (42,49,53). Management of poisoning using 50 mg of atropine over a 24-hr period or 7 g over a week has been reported (57,85). A case study at the end of this chapter documents the large amount of atropine needed in one patient. Normal therapeutic doses of atropine that achieve an antimuscarinic action in nonintoxicated patients are as low as 0.4 mg every 4 hr.

Pralidoxime is a specific antidote for organophosphorus insecticide poisoning. It is commercially available as the chloride salt, packaged in 1-g ampules (Fig. 8.4). Its action is to reactivate acetylcholinesterase and promote hydrolysis of accumulated acetylcholine. It combines directly with the organophosphorus insecticide portion of the phosphorylated enzyme complex and breaks the covalent bond between AChE and insecticide. Removal of the phosphate completely restores enzyme activity (28).

Pralidoxime is a quaternary amine and does not penetrate the CNS readily. It is, therefore, without significant effect on brain acetylcho-

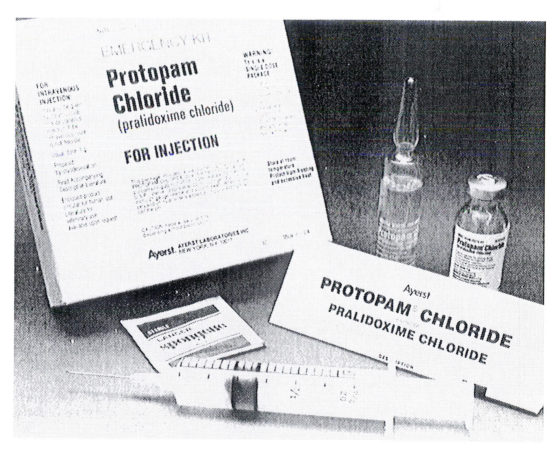

FIG. 8.4. Pralidoxime chloride (*2-PAM*) antidote for organophosphorus poisoning. (Photograph courtesy of Wyeth-Ayerst Laboratories, Inc.)

linesterase enzyme inhibition. It also has minimal effect on autonomic muscarinic receptors. Its greatest affinity is for phosphorylated acetylcholinesterase at the neuromuscular junction. Therefore, most of its beneficial actions are directed toward reestablishing skeletal muscle activity. Skeletal muscle normally begins to respond within several minutes. Because of these limitations, atropine must be continued if the patient is to be managed successfully (44).

The data presented in Table 8.3 show that pralidoxime alone provides limited protection to mice treated with an organophosphorus insecticide. Atropine alone gives about twofold protection. The synergistic protective action of pralidoxime and atropine is approximately 100-fold (62).

Pralidoxime should be administered as soon as the patient has been given atropine. If oxime treatment is delayed more than 24 hr after poisoning, its effectiveness is questionable. This may be due to aging of AChE.

In enzyme aging, once phosphorylation occurs, additional chemical changes, such as loss of an alkyl or alkoxy group, also occur to strengthen the phosphorylated complex even more. Aging occurs more readily with organophosphorus insecticides that contain tertiary alkoxy groups. The process may begin within minutes to hours after the complex forms. Once it occurs, the enzyme complex is then resistant to reactivation by pralidoxime (36,46,69).

Pralidoxime is normally administered in a 1- to 2-g dose for adults (25 to 50 mg/kg in children) over 5 to 10 min. If muscular weakness is not reversed, the dose may be repeated in 1 to 2 hr. Treatment is usually continued for no longer than 24 hr, except in cases of severe exposure or exposure to highly lipid-soluble compounds (18). Side effects of pralidoxime are minimal in organophosphorus insecticide-poisoned patients.

Dermal exposure may be managed by removing and discarding contaminated clothing and then washing contaminated skin with water followed by a mild soap (e.g., tincture of green soap). Rubber gloves should be worn by emergency personnel to avoid exposure. Ocular exposure is treated by rinsing the eyes with tap water for at least 15 to 20 min.

Some drugs are contraindicated in the treatment of organophosphorus insecticide poisoning. Parasympathomimetic agents, such as physostigmine and succinylcholine, should be avoided because they potentiate anticholinesterase activity. Also, potentiation of organophosphorus insecticide toxicity may occur with phenothiazines and H_1 antagonists that possess anticholinesterase activity. Morphine and other CNS depressants may compromise the respiratory status of the patient and should be avoided, also.

TABLE 8.3. *Reduction of sarin toxicity in mice by atropine and pralidoxime*[a]

Treatment	LD_{50} (μg/kg)	Protective ratio
None	14.5	—
Atropine	38.0	2.63
Pralidoxime	18.4	1.27
Atropine (5 mg/kg) and pralidoxime	365	25.17
Atropine (10 mg/kg) and pralidoxime	1,321	91.10

From ref. 62.

[a] Neither atropine nor pralidoxime alone significantly reduced toxicity of this organophosphorus compound. However, when the two antidotes were combined, the LD_{50} dose of sarin was greatly increased, showing a protective action of these antidotes.

Carbamates

Carbamate insecticides are reversible cholinesterase inhibitors that have a shorter duration of action and are generally less toxic than are organophosphorus compounds. Carbamates are frequently used as agricultural and household insecticides. A list of commonly used carbamates is given in Table 8.4.

The mechanism of carbamate toxicity is via carbamoylation of AChE. Unlike organophosphorus insecticide binding to AChE, carbamates dissociate easily from the enzyme.

Clinical manifestations of carbamate poisoning are similar to those of organophospho-

TABLE 8.4. *Toxicity of selected carbamate insecticides*

Compound	LD$_{50}$ (mg/kg)
Highly toxic	
Aldicarb (Temik)	0.9
Carbofuran (Furadan)	5
Oxamyl (Vydate)	5
Methiocarb (Mesurol)	15
Methomyl (Lannate, Nudrin)	17
Aminocarb (Matacil)	21
Dimetilin	50
Moderately toxic	
Carbaryl (Sevin)	89
Propoxur (Baygon)	95
Isocarb	128
Bendiocarb (Ficam)	143
Bufencarb (Bux)	170
Terbucarb (Azak)	34,000

From refs. 15 and 21.

rus insecticides (see Table 8.2). Generally, CNS effects are minimal and most manifestations are due to accumulation of ACh at muscarinic and nicotinic sites. Treatment of symptomatic carbamate exposure is managed as described for organophosphorus insecticides. Some animal studies have shown that oxime reactivators, such as pralidoxime, increase carbamate toxicity (58). Therefore, they are not recommended in carbamate poisoning (28,53,57).

Organochlorine Insecticides

Organochlorine insecticides represent a group of fat-soluble, low-molecular-weight, stable compounds. Representative examples are listed, in decreasing order of toxicity, in Table 8.5. This class of insecticides also has low water solubility. The compounds are not very biodegradable and may persist in the environment. For example, the half-life of chlorophenothane (DDT) and its metabolites is approximately 10 years (53).

As a result of their lipid solubility, organochlorine insecticides are stored in adipose tissue. The rate of elimination of stored DDT from the body is only 1% per day. Although these insecticides persist in body stores and

the environment, they are relatively safe compared to organophosphorus insecticides. Acute poisoning and death due to organochlorine exposure are rare. This relative safety may be due in part to their lipid solubility and storage in adipose tissue. The fact that these compounds are highly lipid soluble also accounts for selective toxicity to insects. They can easily penetrate the exoskeleton of insects, but percutaneous absorption in mammals is relatively poor. To illustrate, the oral LD$_{50}$ for DDT in rats is approximately 113 mg/kg, whereas the dermal LD$_{50}$ is 2,510 mg/kg.

Mechanism of Toxicity

Organochlorine insecticides are neurotoxins that stimulate sensory and motor nerve fibers and the motor cortex. These compounds alter the movement of sodium and potassium across neuronal membranes and affect membrane-related enzymatic reactions adversely (47, 60,75). Thus, acute toxicity results in abnormal electrical activity. The severity of signs denoting toxicity is correlated to CNS concentrations of these insecticides (13).

Liver necrosis and sensitization of the myocardium to catecholamines are distinct features of this class of insecticides. These effects, however, may be more significant in animals than humans.

Characteristics of Organochlorine Poisoning

Signs and symptoms associated with organochlorine insecticide poisoning are attrib-

TABLE 8.5. *Toxicity of selected organochlorine insecticides*

Compound	LD$_{50}$ (mg/kg)
Endrin	18
Aldrin	39
Dieldrin	48
Lindane	88
DDT[a]	113
Heptachlor	100
Chlordane	335
Mirex	740
Methoxychlor	5,000–7,000

From refs. 15 and 21.
[a] DDT, dichlorodiphenyltrichloroethane.

TABLE 8.6. *Clinical characteristics of organochlorine insecticides*

Nausea, vomiting
Paresthesia of tongue, lips, and face
Restlessness
Apprehension, irritability
Tremor
Convulsions
Hypersusceptibility to stimuli
Coma
Respiratory failure
Death

uted mostly to CNS stimulation resulting in behavioral changes, sensory and equilibrium disturbance, involuntary muscle activity, and depression of vital centers (Table 8.6) (8). Sensitization of the myocardium to catecholamines may lead to life-threatening ventricular arrhythmias. Neurotoxicity is generally associated with misuse of commercial products in children, but neurotoxicity in adults has also been shown to occur with proper use (76).

Management of Organochlorine Poisoning

Treatment of acute poisoning by organochlorine insecticides is largely supportive and symptomatic. For ingestion, gastric decontamination with ipecac-induced emesis, gastric lavage, or activated charcoal and saline cathartics may be indicated. Central nervous system depressants and anticonvulsants are necessary to control tremors and convulsions. Diazepam has largely replaced phenobarbital for treating tremors and convulsions because of its lower incidence and severity of respiratory depressant action. Epinephrine and other sympathomimetics must be avoided. There is no specific antidote for organochlorine poisoning.

Insecticides from Botanical Origin

Pyrethrum (Pyrethrins)

Pyrethrum is obtained from the yellow flower *Chrysanthemum cinerariaefolium*. Its active principles include pyrethrin I and II and cinerin I and II. The pyrethrins are esters formed from two acids, chrysanthemic acid and pyrethric acid, and three alcohols, jasmolone, cinerolone, and pyrethrolone. Pyrethrins are incorporated into a large variety of household insecticidal products because of their rapid knockdown action and mammalian safety (56).

Severe poisoning with pyrethrum is rare, although injecting or inhaling a pyrethrum insecticide can cause nausea, vomiting, muscular paralysis, and death. Massive doses may induce CNS stimulation symptoms including excitation and convulsions that terminate in paralysis. Death occurs from respiratory failure (27).

Contact dermatitis is the most frequent adverse effect to pyrethrum and, in allergic individuals, asthma and rhinitis may occur. Pyrethrum is poorly absorbed across intact mammalian skin and, once absorbed, is rapidly metabolized. The human fatal dose is reported to be 50 g for a 70-kg man (27). Most reports show toxicity to pyrethrum-containing products is due to other ingredients in the preparation, usually a petroleum distillate solvent (4).

Commercially marketed pediculicide products combine pyrethrum, 0.17% to 0.33%, with piperonyl butoxide, 2% to 4%. Piperonyl butoxide is a pharmacologic synergist to the pyrethrins. It interferes with insect's ability to destroy pyrethrum by oxidative degradation (10,83). Piperonyl butoxide is poorly absorbed after cutaneous application to mammals and is relatively nontoxic. The fatal human dose is reported to be 11.5 g/kg (15).

Generally, no treatment is required for acute ingestion of pyrethrum insecticides. Management is symptomatic. Poisoning by products containing petroleum distillate solvent must be managed accordingly to prevent aspiration and pulmonary toxicity (see chapter 7). Individuals with hypersensitivity reactions to pyrethrum may require treatment with epinephrine.

Rotenone

An insecticide of botanical origin, rotenone has long been used to control a large variety of insect pests. For many centuries, plants containing rotenoids have been used as fish poisons. The poisonous substituents dissolved in water were absorbed through the gills. Because much of the early investigations of rotenone, one of the rotenoid poisons, used the substance obtained from plants of the genus *Derris,* the term *derris* persists as a synonym for rotenone. Rotenone is a widely used insecticide that has a low order of toxicity to humans. The oral LD_{50} is reported to be 132 mg/kg (15).

Signs and symptoms of acute rotenone poisoning include gastrointestinal irritation associated with nausea and vomiting. Liver and kidney damage may be detected after chronic exposure. Death from massive exposure occurs from respiratory paralysis.

Rotenone exposure by inhalation is considered to be of greater toxicologic concern. In the lungs, rotenone can cause intense respiratory stimulation followed by depression and convulsions. In the stomach, however, a significant amount of an ingested dose is frequently expelled because of its irritant gastrointestinal action. Thus, the toxic potential of ingested rotenoids is less significant.

Management of rotenone poisoning is largely supportive. There is no specific antidote.

Nicotine

Nicotine is extracted from tobacco and is a potent contact insecticide against a large variety of insects. It stimulates autonomic sympathetic and parasympathetic ganglia, neuromuscular junctions, and certain neuronal pathways in the CNS. Its initial effects (Table 8.7) are stimulatory, mimicking excessive acetylcholine at nicotinic receptors. Dizziness, miosis, vomiting, and the SLUD syndrome are encountered shortly after poisoning (41). These effects progress rapidly to persistent muscular weakness and tremors, followed by convulsions, and eventually to respiratory paralysis and CNS depression. Death occurs from respiratory failure due to paralysis of respiratory muscles and blockade of central respiratory mechanisms.

TABLE 8.7. *Progression of signs and symptoms in acute nicotine poisoning*

Nausea, vomiting, diarrhea
Salivation
Abdominal cramps
Cold sweat
Dizziness
Bradycardia
Hypotension
Dyspnea
Cardiovascular collapse
Convulsions
Death

Overall, clinical characterization of nicotine poisoning is complex, and presenting symptoms after exposure may vary widely among different people. The ultimate response represents a summation of several opposing forces.

For example, nicotine may cause tachycardia by stimulating ganglia or blocking parasympathetic ganglia. It may induce bradycardia by blocking sympathetic ganglia or by stimulating the parasympathetic ganglia. It is difficult to predict, *a priori,* just how an individual will respond.

Nicotine acts quickly, with death often occurring within minutes to a few hours. It readily penetrates the skin and is absorbed by inhalation of its vapors, whereas absorption from the GI tract is low because of reduced gastric emptying (74).

Nicotine-containing insecticide products should be quickly washed off the skin, and all contaminated clothing removed. Ingested nicotine usually involves spontaneous emesis. Any remaining nicotine may be removed by gastric lavage and activated charcoal along with a cathartic. Other treatment is purely symptomatic (41). Atropine sulfate is effective in reversing early cholinergic signs. An alpha-adrenergic blocking agent, such as phentolamine, may reverse severe hypertension when refractive to fluid replacement and sympathetic stimulation. Seizures can be managed with diazepam or barbiturates.

INSECT REPELLENTS

Diethyltoluamide (DEET) was synthesized in 1954 and marketed in 1957. Today, this

TABLE 8.8. *Characteristics of diethyltoluamide (DEET) poisoning*

CVS[a]
Decreased blood pressure
Decreased heart rate
CNS[b]
Ataxia
Confusion
Slurred speech
Muscle cramping
Insomnia
Tremor; clonic jerking
Psychosis
Seizures
Coma
Skin
Erythema
Contact urticaria
Anaphylaxis

[a] CVS, cardiovascular system.
[b] CNS, central nervous system.

compound is widely used and generally considered to be safe. The major adverse reactions associated with it involve the CNS, although dermatologic and allergic reactions are also reported (Table 8.8). The mechanism of toxicity is not entirely understood (16).

Commercial insect repellents contain 15% to 95% DEET. The rate and amount absorbed through the skin is variable and dependent largely on the quantity used, concentration, and location of application. Topically applied insect repellents are effective for 1 to several hours.

Toxic exposure to DEET in children, both dermal and oral, has been reported (65,72). Most exposures showed characteristic CNS effects. The case described at the end of the chapter, however, illustrates primarily the cardiovascular effects of DEET in an adult.

HERBICIDES

Chlorophenoxy Compounds

Two substances, *2,4-dichlorophenoxyacetic acid* (2,4-D) and *2,4,5-trichlorophenoxyacetic acid* (2,4,5-T), and their esters and salts are among the most widely used herbicides to control many broadleaf woody plants. They are also the subject of extensive contemporary public interest. A contaminant of 2,4,5-T called 2,3,4,8-tetrachlorodibenzo-*p*-dioxin (TCDD or dioxin) is a potent teratogen and possible carcinogen and mutagen (2,52,56).

Dioxin is reported to be one of the most toxic synthetic chemicals known, with toxic doses for most animals in the microgram range. Because of the widespread and sometimes careless use of 2,4,5-T, it is believed that many have been exposed to dioxin. The controversy over dioxin will undoubtedly continue for the next several decades. At present, the concentration of dioxin in 2,4,5-T is closely regulated at 0.1 ppm or less.

The LD_{50} value for these compounds ranges from 300 to 700 mg/kg (12). The acute human toxic dose of chlorophenoxy herbicides is approximately 3 to 4 g. One victim of poisoning did not survive a dose of 2,4,5-T that was at least 6.5 g (59).

Although these compounds act as growth hormones in plants, they do not possess hormonal action in humans. Their mechanism of toxicity is unknown. Nonspecific liver and kidney changes can be seen after exposure (27). The substances do not accumulate in the body, and the plasma half-life in animals is about 24 hr (23).

Signs and symptoms of acute chlorophenoxy herbicide poisoning are listed in Table 8.9. The principal findings of 2,4-D poisoning in animals and humans include muscular weakness and hypotension. Death after massive ingestion is believed to be caused by ventricular fibrillation (32,56). A commonly reported form of severe dermatitis, *chloracne*, may be due to dioxin.

Management of acute oral 2,4-D poisoning involves its removal from the GI tract by emesis or gastric lavage followed by activated charcoal and a saline cathartic. Dermal exposure should be managed by thorough scrubbing with soap and water after removal of contaminated

TABLE 8.9. *Toxicity characteristics of acute chlorophenoxy herbicide poisoning*

Burning pain in the nose, eyes, throat, and bronchi
Vomiting, diarrhea
Abdominal pain
Lethargy
Weakness
Muscle twitching

clothing. Specific symptoms are treated as needed (e.g., lidocaine for ventricular fibrillation and diazepam for convulsions). Since the pKa for 2,4-D is 2.6, alkaline diuresis will enhance excretion (19). In one case, the half-life of 2,4-D decreased from an initial 39.5 hr to 2.7 hr when alkaline diuresis was used to produce a urinary pH of 7.5 to 8.5 (20).

Bipyridyl Compounds

Paraquat and *diquat* are nonselective herbicides that destroy plant tissue on contact. These compounds are rapidly inactivated on contact with soil (68). This unique property facilitates spraying to control broadleaf weeds and reseeding the next day.

These compounds produce herbicidal action by competing with nicotinamide adenine dinucleotide phosphate (NADP) and interfering with intracellular electron transport systems during photosynthesis. This reaction involves the production of methyl viologen, which reacts with molecular oxygen to generate toxic products, such as superoxide anion (24).

Hundreds of cases of paraquat toxicity due to inhalation of sprays, dermal exposure, intravenous injection, and oral ingestion have been reported (7,25,26,51). Paraquat was at one time the subject of considerable public interest and concern (79). It was used to control illicit production of marijuana growing in selected areas in the southern states and in Mexico. Consequently, high concentrations of paraquat were reported in some marijuana cigarettes. It is suggested that "scarring" of lung tissue could occur from smoking these cigarettes or ingesting baked goods made with the plant. There is little evidence to document this claim (34). However, common sense dictates that such "tainted" marijuana products should be avoided.

Mechanism of Toxicity

The fatal dose of paraquat for humans may be as low as 4 mg/kg. The reported LD$_{50}$ values for paraquat and diquat are 120 mg/kg and 200 to 300 mg/kg, respectively (15).

Several mechanisms have been proposed for paraquat toxicity (51,70,71). Much of the recent evidence has pointed to the inhibition of superoxide dismutase in lung, generation of free radicals, and lipid peroxidation. A proposed mechanism is outlined in Fig. 8.5. Paraquat undergoes single electron reduction, forming a superoxide anion that is responsible for inhibition of quinolate phosphoribosyl transferase. This enzyme is essential in the biosynthesis of NAD. Since NAD is the main electron acceptor of cellular respiration, blockade results in decreased oxygen utilization. In addition, the superoxide anion can be nonenzymatically dismutated to singlet oxygen, which reacts with unsaturated lipids of cell membranes to form lipid hydroperoxides. Lipid hydroperoxides are unstable in the presence of trace metal ions and spontaneously decompose to lipid-free radicals, ultimately resulting in membrane destruction and lipid peroxidation (9,70).

Paraquat also produces a corrosive action when in contact with eyes, skin, and mucous membranes of the GI tract, producing pain, ulcerations, inflammation, and tissue damage (51). Paraquat accumulates in lung tissue in a concentration- and time-dependent manner (61,66). There is no preferential subcellular localization (35). Pulmonary pathologic response has been divided into two phases (71). The early, destructive phase is marked by damage to pneumonocytes with intra-alveolar hemorrhage and inflammatory cell infiltration. The later, proliferative phase involves alveolar and interstitial fibrosis.

Although paraquat is associated with pulmonary toxicity, which accounts for its high mortality rate, the target organ for diquat seems to be the kidney. Diquat exposure results in acute renal failure.

Characteristics of Paraquat and Diquat Poisoning

Dermal and eye exposure may result in severe irritation, but systemic absorption is unlikely. Inhalation of sprays produces local irritation, but significant systemic toxicity is not expected. In-

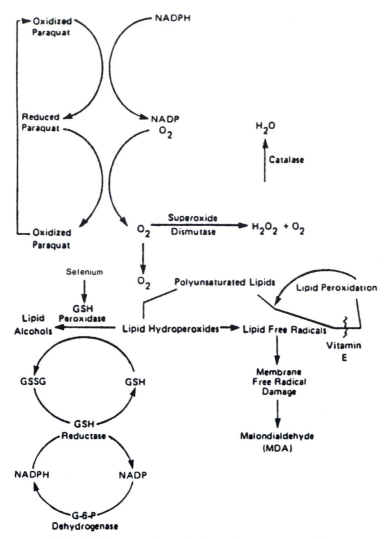

FIG. 8.5. Proposed mechanism of paraquat toxicity.

gestion of paraquat produces severe gastrointestinal irritation followed by toxic damage to the liver, kidney, and heart. The toxicity profile culminates with severe pulmonary fibrosis and hemorrhagic pulmonary edema. Signs and symptoms associated with acute ingestion of paraquat are listed in Table 8.10.

Initial symptoms of poisoning, such as gastrointestinal irritation, may occur within 1 hr, but the onset of respiratory problems and death may occur several days later. For example, a victim who ingested a small quantity (probably no more than several milliliters) of paraquat did not develop respiratory distress until 2 weeks later (28). Massive doses may be fatal within 24 hr (33).

Management of Paraquat and Diquat Poisoning

Management of acute poisoning by paraquat or diquat includes gastrointestinal decontamination, increase of elimination, and reduction of pulmonary damage (77). Once lung damage presents, chances for survival are limited (51,53).

TABLE 8.10. *Clinical manifestations of paraquat poisoning*

Stage I	1–5 days	Local corrosive action
		Hemoptysis
		Ulcerations of mucous membranes
		Nausea, diarrhea
		Oliguria
Stage II	2–8 days	Signs of liver, kidney, cardiac damage
		Jaundice
		Fever
		Tachycardia, myocarditis
		Respiratory distress, cyanosis
		Elevated BUN, serum alkaline phosphatase, serum bilirubin, serum transaminases
Stage III	3–14 days	Pulmonary fibrosis
		Cough, dyspnea, tachypnea
		Edema, pleural effusions
		Atelectasis
		Low arterial oxygen tension
		Increased alveolar oxygen tension gradient
		Respiratory failure

From refs. 24 and 25.

Initial management is directed at removing unabsorbed paraquat as quickly as possible. Several methods have been proposed. Paraquat and diquat are cationic compounds that are not absorbed quickly. Therefore, gastric lavage is recommended. The lavage solution may consist of a 30% suspension of Fuller's earth, a 6% to 7.5% suspension of bentonite, or a slurry of activated charcoal (1 g/kg) (24,53). Activated charcoal should be repeated every 2 to 4 hr and followed by a cathartic, such as sorbitol. Whole gut lavage, using a nasogastric tube and a polyethylene glycol-electrolyte solution, has been used with some success to decrease paraquat absorption (61,66).

Efforts to increase elimination of these herbicides have included forced diuresis, peritoneal or hemodialysis, and hemoperfusion (35,61,77,78). Each method has met with limited success because paraquat has a large volume of distribution. Forced diuresis is effective only within the first 24 hr. The most satisfactory results have been obtained with long-term, continuous hemoperfusion or hemodialysis in renally compromised patients (6,61,78). If plasma paraquat concentrations are kept below 0.1 μg/mL, survival is enhanced (15).

Reducing pulmonary damage has been attempted by using glucocorticoids and vitamins C and E, as well as D-propranolol and superoxide dismutase (5). Animal experiments have shown promising results, but therapeutic efficacy has yet to be established (6). Oxygen seems to accelerate pulmonary toxicity, and hypoxic concentrations of 15% to 16% oxygen should be given to reduce pulmonary fibrosis (64).

RODENTICIDES

Rodenticides are substances that kill rodents, especially mice, rats, and squirrels. They have different mechanisms of action, as well as potential for human toxicity. The Federal Insecticide, Fungicide, and Rodenticide Act (FIFRA) classified these products according to their potential for toxicity, as estimated by LD_{50} determinations. Examples are given in Table 8.11. Some of these compounds, such as strychnine and arsenic, are covered in other chapters.

Highly Toxic Rodenticides

Thallium

Thallium has been used as a rodenticide and insecticide for many years. At the turn of the century it was used therapeutically for syphi-

TABLE 8.11. *Toxicity of rodenticides*

Highly toxic (LD_{50} < 50 mg/kg)
   Thallium
   Sodium fluoroacetate (Compound 1080)
   Strychnine
   Elemental phosphorus—yellow phosphorus
   Arsenic
   Zinc phosphate
Moderately toxic (LD_{50} 50–500 mg/kg)
   α-Naphthyl thiourea (ANTU)
Low toxicity (LD_{50} 500–5,000 mg/kg)
   Hydroxy coumarins
   Red squill
   Warfarin
   Norbromide

lis, tuberculosis, dysentery, and ringworm. It was used topically as a depilatory agent until the early 1950s. At present, its use as a depilatory agent or as a pesticide in the United States is prohibited. The incidence of poisoning has declined in recent years; however, thallium is still the cause of an occasional report of toxicity (14,22,31,82).

Thallium is extremely toxic, with doses of approximately 1 g being lethal (15). It is odorless and tasteless, which adds to its potential for accidental ingestion. Toxicity occurs from a variety of potential mechanisms. Thallium inhibits sulfhydryl-containing enzymes and interferes with oxidative phosphorylation (30).

Signs and symptoms of acute thallium poisoning are listed in Table 8.12. Gastrointestinal manifestations begin within hours after acute ingestion and persist for several days. Painful paresthesia occurs within days of ingestion, followed by motor neuropathy, generalized weakness, and the Guillain-Barré syndrome. Mental capacity decreases over time. Severe cases terminate in coma with death from respiratory depression, pneumonia, or cardiac failure. Alopecia is often regarded as a pathognomonic sign and begins within 1 to 3 weeks. Alopecia occurs because thallium prevents incorporation of cysteine into protein and keratin. Unlike other metals, including arsenic, which deposit in hair, thallium is not incorporated into the hair matrix.

Various chelators (see chapter 9) have been used in an attempt to reduce thallium blood concentrations. Although thallium forms chelates with calcium ethylenediaminetetraacetic acid (Ca-EDTA), dimercaprol, and other substances, renal and pancreatic toxicity is reported. Thus, no clear-cut benefit can be derived from their use.

There is no known effective antidote for thallium. Management of acute thallium poisoning involves gastric evacuation with ipecac-induced emesis or lavage, followed by activated charcoal and a cathartic.

Since thallium and potassium have similar chemical properties, potassium chloride has been recommended to hasten thallium excretion (50,55). Potassium chloride apparently competes with thallium for reabsorption in the renal tubules. The half-life of thallium with potassium chloride therapy is lowered from 30 days to 3 to 10 days (55). However, potassium therapy is hazardous for two reasons. First, it causes temporarily increased plasma thallium concentrations. Second, potassium itself may be toxic, especially if renal function is impaired.

Prussian blue (potassium ferricyanoferrate

TABLE 8.12. *Characteristics of thallium poisoning*

Location	Signs and symptoms
Gastrointestinal	Nausea, vomiting, diarrhea
Neurologic	Agitation, confusion, paresthesias, intense pain, neuropathy, motor weakness, Guillain-Barré syndrome, convulsions, memory loss (short term), poor concentration, vision changes (blurred, distorted, "spots," loss)
Cardiovascular and respiratory	Respiratory depression, pneumonia, orthostatic hypotension, cardiac failure
Other	Alopecia,[a] renal and hepatic damage, smooth and cardiac muscle necrosis

[a] Diagnosis is often difficult because signs and symptoms are nonspecific. However, the appearance of alopecia, along with the other manifestations, asserts a positive diagnosis for thallium poisoning.

II) adsorbs thallium and may be used to prevent gastrointestinal absorption. In the alkaline pH of the intestine, thallium is substituted for potassium and prevented from being absorbed.

Phosphorus

Elemental yellow (or white) phosphorus is an extremely lethal protoplasmic poison that disturbs carbohydrate, fat, and protein metabolism. It impairs the circulation and, with chronic exposure, interferes with bone growth, leading to necrosis, especially in the mandible. This is the source of the so-called "phossy jaw." Red phosphorus, on the other hand, is not absorbed and, consequently, is not toxic. Match heads contain about 50% red phosphorus.

Yellow phosphorus has been accidentally encountered in a number of industrial settings, although most cases of human toxicity involve use as a rodenticide. It is incorporated into a paste in concentrations up to 5%, and this paste is spread on bread, cheese, or other food to attract rodents. Unfortunately, it can also be ingested by children.

Phosphorus intoxication occurs in three stages. Initially (stage I), intense gastrointestinal irritation with nausea, vomiting, diarrhea, abdominal pain, and mucosal burning is present. A characteristic garlic odor on the breath is detected. The vomitus and stool may be phosphorescent. Phosphorus poisoning has been described as the "smoking stool syndrome." Stage II may last several hours to a few days and is characterized by apparent recovery. Stage III (systemic toxicity) follows, with convulsions, jaundice and hepatomegaly, coma, and death, usually due to irreversible shock or cardiovascular failure.

The phosphorus-poisoned patient may not show signs of toxicity until stage III. Many patients quickly pass through stage I or do not interpret the period as a toxic reaction because of its lack of severity. Not all patients will have a garlic odor on their breath or phosphorescent vomitus or feces. Too frequently, the severity of intoxication may be underestimated because the victim does not have the classic symptoms (48).

Chronic exposure to low concentrations frequently causes tooth pain or sore jaws as the earliest symptom. Necrosis of the mandible, loss of appetite, weight loss, and anemia are signs of possible phosphorus exposure.

The mortality rate for acute phosphorus poisoning is approximately 25% for victims who had early symptoms of nausea and vomiting, nearly 50% when both gastrointestinal and CNS symptoms were present, and almost 75% when the first manifestation of poisoning was restlessness, irritability, drowsiness, stupor, or coma (48). This difference in survival rates most likely reflects the interval between time of ingestion and treatment. The toxic dose is 15 mg, and as little as 50 mg may be lethal (27).

Management of acute phosphorus ingestion is directed at preventing absorption from the gastrointestinal tract, removing unabsorbed phosphorus, and providing good supportive care, since there is no specific antidote. Gastric lavage with potassium permanganate solution (1:5,000) is recommended to oxidize phosphorus to harmless phosphates (48).

Low-Toxicity Rodenticides

Warfarin

Warfarin is almost universally accepted as the most effective means to control rodents. It is effective in killing rodents but is generally safe for humans, if used properly. It is commercially available at concentrations ranging from 0.025% to 0.5%. It is used in baits or added to drinking water placed where rodents congregate. Serious toxicity occurs when these preparations are repeatedly ingested by humans.

Warfarin inhibits synthesis of the vitamin K-dependent clotting factors in the liver, specifically factors II (prothrombin), VII, IX, and X (Fig. 8.6). Prothrombin synthesis is, therefore, reduced. This promotes hemorrhage

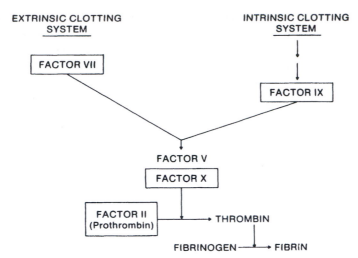

FIG. 8.6. Sites of action of warfarin on the blood clotting system. Factors II, VII, IX, and X are inhibited.

throughout the body, which is the cause of death. Warfarin is reported to have a direct pathologic action on capillary walls (27), but this response is secondary to action on prothrombin synthesis. The reason for this is that the half-lives of the four clotting factors are long (i.e., VII, IX, X, and II; 6, 24, 40, and 60 hr, respectively). Warfarin does not affect clotting factors already formed, just those that have not yet formed. Therefore, 1 to 3 days of warfarin administration are required before a hypoprothrombinemic effect will be seen.

It is estimated that a single dose of 15 g of warfarin would be required to cause death. As little as 1 to 2 mg/kg for 6 days caused severe illness in a patient attempting suicide (37). A family of 14 persons accidentally consumed cornmeal containing warfarin for 15 days. Their intake of poison was estimated at 102 mg/kg/day (40). All but two of the family survived, although all family members experienced severe hemorrhage.

Severe toxicity or death is rare after single or a few repeated doses. Major characteristics of poisoning are related to hemorrhage. These include bleeding from the nose (epistaxis) and gums, easy bruising of the skin, and, ultimately, hemorrhagic shock and death. Pain in the joints, abdomen, and back probably re-flects hemorrhage into those areas. Weakness results from anemia.

During the past several years, several hydroxycoumarin anticoagulants have been synthesized to deal with the growing problem of warfarin resistance in rodents. Resistance develops rapidly because it is genetically transmitted as a dominant trait (37,43). One derivative, brodifacoum (Talon) is highly effective against warfarin-resistant rodents. Its anticoagulant action in humans is similar to that in rodents (63). Studies in dogs show that its half-life is approximately 120 days (43). Successful treatment for poisoning requires weeks to months of active therapy with vitamin K_1 to reverse severe, prolonged coagulopathy (84,86).

Warfarin ingestion should be treated by ipecac-induced emesis or gastric lavage if a dose known to induce symptoms was ingested within the preceding 2 to 3 hr. This may be followed by activated charcoal. In smaller ingestions, emesis or adsorbents are not necessary. The victim should be monitored for development of symptoms.

Management of overdose or of undetermined doses when symptoms are present includes the use of the specific antidote, vitamin K_1 (phytonadione). Prothrombin should return to normal within 24 hr. Vitamins K_3 (menadione) and K_4 (menadiol) are not effective. Fresh blood or plasma transfusions or plasma concentrates of the vitamin K-dependent clotting factors are indicated if hemorrhage is severe.

Prognosis is good when vitamin K_1 is given. However, because death may occur 1 to 2 weeks after poisoning, the victim must be observed carefully.

Red Squill

Red squill bulbs contain at least two glycosides, scillaren A and scillaren B, which possess potent cardiotoxic actions similar to those of digitalis. Signs and symptoms of toxicity are treated similarly to digitalis poisoning. Those that indicate probable red squill poisoning include blurred vision, cardiac arrhythmias, and convulsions.

Red squill has been used as a rodenticide for many years. It is considered to be of low toxicity in humans because it possesses a powerful emetic action, and little is absorbed. Rodents do not have a vomiting reflex and, consequently, cannot vomit. Interestingly, rodents die of chronic convulsions with respiratory failure rather than from the cardiac effects (27).

SUMMARY

Pesticides, unlike some other substances found in the home, are often considered by most people to be extremely toxic. Instead of being handled with the caution they deserve, however, pesticidal products are used carelessly and often in great excess of amounts actually required to control the pests for which they are intended. This then leads to human poisoning and needless suffering.

Case Studies

CASE STUDY: MYSTERIOUS POISONING IN A CHILD

History

Eleven hours before admission to an emergency facility, a 3-year-old boy began to

vomit. His mother gave him children's aspirin and lemon juice. Two hours later he began to experience tremors and complained of abdominal pain and headache. He gradually became tremulous and limp. These symptoms continued to worsen, so he was brought to a hospital.

At the hospital, the boy was awake but lethargic. Eventually, he became flaccid and comatose. Pupils were miotic (1 mm). At no time were seizures noted. He did have prominent fasciculations on one thigh.

There was no evidence suggesting ingestion of any toxic substance or prior trauma. Other family members remained well.

Physical examination revealed that his blood pressure was 130/60 mm Hg; pulse, 130 beats/min; and respirations, 30/min.

Laboratory findings are shown in Table 8.13. A toxicology screen was negative for sedative-hypnotic drugs, alcohol, heavy metals, salicylates, phenothiazines, and opioids.

Several different diagnostic avenues were pursued to determine the reason for these symptoms. First, a 0.2-mg dose of naloxone was given intravenously. Neither respirations nor pupil size changed. Other treatment consisted of 20% mannitol, 20% dexamethasone, 20% ampicillin, and 40% oxygen.

Eight hours after admission, the boy was given 0.15 mg atropine intravenously, but no response was seen until 500 mg pralidoxime was given. An increase in electroencephalogram (EEG) activity was noted within 2 min, and eventually consciousness was restored.

A ketchup bottle found at the child's home contained a white, milky liquid that was identified as a 20% solution of parathion. The mother had brought the liquid back from El

TABLE 8.13. *Laboratory findings*

Na^+	=133 mEq/L
CO_2	=18 mEq/L
BUN[a]	=18 mg/dL
Serum creatinine	=0.7 mg/dL
Hematocrit	=35
pH	=7.27
pCO_2	=43 mm Hg
pO_2	=150 mm Hg

[a] BUN, blood urea nitrogen.

Salvador for treatment of lice. The substance had been placed on the child's head for 20 min the evening before admission. (See ref. 45.)

Discussion

1. Given the information in this case study and in this chapter, can you predict in what class the pesticide in this case study belongs?
2. Is the delayed onset of symptoms consistent for this group of pesticides?
3. When the test dose of naloxone was given and neither respirations nor pupil size changed, what type of possible poison was ruled out?
4. Explain the origin of fasciculations noted in this child.
5. Is pralidoxime expected to relieve CNS manifestations of insecticide poisonings? How does it convey pharmacologic activity overall?

CASE STUDY: ORGANOPHOSPHORUS POISONING

History

A 68-year-old man with a history of depression attempted suicide by consuming 3 ounces of concentrated Cygon 2-E (23.4% dimethoate), an organophosphorus insecticide. (If the concentrated solution had been diluted as directed, it would have yielded 15 gallons of insecticidal mixture.) The man was brought to a hospital within 20 min. Thirty milliliters of syrup of ipecac and 60 g of activated charcoal were given immediately to decontaminate the GI tract.

Physical examination revealed normal cardiovascular, pulmonary, and neurologic functions. Pupils were dilated but reactive to light. The abdomen was soft and not tender. The patient became progressively more lethargic over the next hour and soon lost consciousness, responding only to deep pain. Blood pressure at this time was 46/0 mm Hg, and

pulse was 116 beats/min. He was intubated and given pralidoxime, 1 g. He was kept in the intensive care unit (ICU) until 24 hr after exposure and then transferred to a general care ward after his condition stabilized.

Within 8 hr the patient relapsed and was sent to the coronary care unit (CCU). There he was started on atropine, 5 mg every 10 min, which was continued for 24 hr. He was given a 4-g dose of pralidoxime and then was transferred to an atropine drip delivered at the rate of 0.5 to 2.4 mg/kg/hr. This was maintained for the next 5 weeks.

He continued to experience episodes of respiratory and cardiac difficulty which progressed to asystole. He showed typical symptoms of hypercholinergic activity: miosis, hyperactive bowel sounds, salivation, and fasciculations. He also developed generalized seizures, which were controlled with intravenous phenytoin, diazepam, and phenobarbital.

Overall, this patient required a total dose of 30 g atropine, and this is reported to be the largest therapeutic dose of that drug ever given to a human, with survival. Control of hypersecretions was the criterion followed for monitoring this patient.

All the while, the patient required full supportive measures, including total parenteral nutrition and bronchopulmonary hygiene. By 5 weeks he was markedly improved, and atropine was withdrawn.

The patient was discharged on the 42nd hospital day. He was in good health except for a noticeable hearing deficit and a slight, nonspecific personality change. (See ref. 42.)

Discussion

1. List as many factors as you can to explain reasons for the severity of this exposure.
2. Comment on the benefit that syrup of ipecac and activated charcoal may have had on the outcome of this patient. Would other methods of gastrointestinal decontamination have been useful?
3. The initial 1-g dose of pralidoxime was standard, according to the package label.

Based on the therapeutic response, should a larger dose have been used?

4. What was the most compelling reason for switching this patient to a continuous atropine drip after about 24 hr of intermittent bolus dosing?

CASE STUDY: PROLONGED TOXICITY TO ORGANOPHOSPHORUS POISONING

History

A 39-year-old woman was admitted to an emergency facility. She had a history of chronic depression and had attempted suicide 6 hr earlier by taking, among other items, about 2 ounces of fenthion. This is a long-acting organophosphorus insecticide that has a high lipid solubility. It also contains a sulfate group in its chemical structure that makes it highly resistant to hydrolysis. It is sold commercially for agricultural use.

On admission the patient was treated with naloxone, 4 mg; activated charcoal; magnesium citrate; and pralidoxime, 1 g. Her hospital course of therapy and enzyme activity are summarized in Fig. 8.7.

On transfer to the ICU, she was lethargic but oriented. She responded to verbal stimuli, and physical examination was otherwise normal. A blood sample was taken to determine erythrocyte acetylcholinesterase and serum pseudocholinesterase activity. All routine laboratory tests were in the normal range.

Over the next 24 hr, the patient appeared to be anxious. She experienced occasional diarrhea. She was transferred to a medical-psychiatric ward the next day.

On her 5th hospital day, she experienced cardiac and respiratory arrest. She was successfully resuscitated and returned to the ICU. At that time, a blood sample showed that pseudocholinesterase activity was significantly depressed (<1% of normal). By 5 hr after readmission to the ICU, the patient became hypotensive and developed sialorrhea and generalized muscle fasciculations. Another 1-g dose of pralidoxime caused cholinergic symptoms to resolve. She was slowly weaned off artificial ventilation and was extubated on day 12.

She again developed respiratory problems and was reintubated on the evening of the 13th day. At this time, muscular spasms, bronchospasm, profuse sialorrhea, lacrimation, and tachycardia (150 beats/min) were noted. She received atropine and pralidoxime (1 g/12 hr). Symptoms resolved, except for occasional periods of delusions. Atropine and pralidoxime were withdrawn on day 18. By day 22 she appeared to

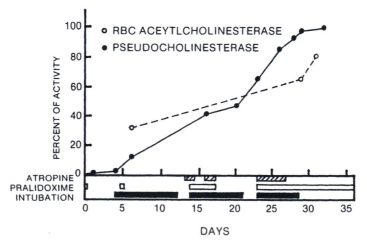

FIG. 8.7. Graphic summary of hospital course of a patient poisoned with an organophosphorus insecticide. (From ref. 49.)

be doing well and was extubated; supplemental oxygen was continued. A sample of fat tissue was obtained for insecticide analysis.

On the morning of day 24, the patient was weak and tremulous. Mild fasciculations of muscles around her eyes and in her legs were noted. Shortly, she had a major motor seizure, followed by a second one. She was intubated and again given atropine and pralidoxime (1 g/12 hr). All cholinergic symptoms and seizure activity resolved. She continued to experience persistent delusions. She was extubated on day 27.

By day 30 the patient's mental status improved markedly. Atropine was withdrawn, with no reappearance of cholinergic symptoms. Pralidoxime was continued until analysis of tissue samples on day 37 revealed that all traces of insecticide had disappeared. The patient was discharged on the 38th day of hospitalization. (See ref. 49.)

Discussion

1. Discuss the pharmacologic implication of the lipid solubility and resistance to hydrolysis of fenthion, as they relate to the toxicologic outcome of poisoning.
2. Why did this patient receive naloxone on admission? Why were activated charcoal and magnesium citrate given?
3. Symptoms of delusion were constant and sometimes the singular symptom for 18 days (days 13 to 30). What caused the problem? Atropine? Support your answer with the facts of this case study.
4. Would this patient have responded better overall if pralidoxime had been started on admission and continued without interruption? Support your answer.
5. The patient experienced tachycardia on day 13 and had fasciculations on day 24. What caused them?

CASE STUDY: LINDANE INTOXICATION

History

An 18-month-old boy had been treated prophylactically with lindane since his older sister had been diagnosed as having scabies. He was healthy, without any other apparent medical problems. The instructions were to apply a lindane lotion product for two consecutive nights, from neck to toes, after a hot bath and to wash it off the following morning. (This is a standard protocol for scabies).

The morning after the second treatment, the infant's mother forgot to wash off the lindane. Approximately 12 hr after the second treatment, the infant experienced a generalized convulsive seizure that lasted about 30 min. Shortly thereafter, he had another seizure. He was then taken to a hospital.

When he arrived, he was experiencing tonic-clonic movement. He was restless, lethargic, and disoriented. He was given diazepam intravenously to control seizure activity and improved. There were no signs of head trauma or systemic illness to account for the clinical findings.

A toxicology screen of blood and urine for drugs was negative, but a qualitative test for lindane was positive. He received a thorough washing. Later, blood samples showed lindane concentrations of 0.450 ppm at 12 hr, 0.080 ppm at 24 hr, and 0.029 ppm at 96 hr after the second application.

Electroencephalograms obtained within the first 48 hr and liver function tests were both normal. The infant was discharged. Complete recovery was evident during a checkup 3 weeks later. (See ref. 75.)

Discussion

1. Would the toxic effects of lindane be more or less prominent if the solution were ingested, as opposed to percutaneous absorption? Why or why not?
2. Why was the onset of seizures delayed for at least 12 hr?
3. Lindane lotion was applied after a hot bath. Did this possibly make a difference in the amount of poison absorbed versus application to cold skin?
4. Is lindane effectively removed by (a) hemodialysis, (b) charcoal hemoperfusion, or (c) peritoneal dialysis?

5. To what general class of insecticide poisons does lindane belong?

CASE STUDY: FATAL NICOTINE INGESTION

History

A 17-year-old boy who had been under "house arrest" at his parents' home for drug-related offenses was threatened with being taken to the juvenile detention center because of a domestic dispute with his family. He told his family that "they'll never take me alive" and promptly swallowed a brownish liquid from an unlabeled test tube. He had obtained this solution from a fellow Satanic cult member, expressly to take his own life in such a circumstance.

Approximately 1 to 2 min later, the patient vomited and collapsed, pulseless, to the ground. Responding medics performed immediate cardiopulmonary resuscitation (CPR) and advanced cardiac life support in less than 7 min. His initial rhythm of asystole converted to ventricular fibrillation with 1 mg of intravenous epinephrine 1:10,000. He was defibrillated, placed on lidocaine for premature ventricular contractions, given 50 % dextrose in water ($D_{50}W$), 2 mg naloxone, and transported to a hospital.

On arrival, the patient was in coma (scale 3). His pulse was 100 beats/min; blood pressure was 70 mm Hg systolic. Vomitus was present at the nares. Breath sounds were remarkable for the presence of extensive rhonchi. Bowel sounds were absent. Extremities were flaccid, with response to deep pain. No corneal or deep tendon reflexes were present. A urine toxicology screen was positive for nicotine; a serum toxicologic screen was negative.

Mechanical ventilation was maintained. The patient received gastric lavage with 2 L normal saline followed by instillation of 50 g activated charcoal.

With the preliminary diagnoses of overdose of an unknown agent, cardiopulmonary arrest, and probable aspiration pneumonitis, the patient was managed supportively and admitted to the intensive care unit. Some time later, detectives arrived with an old bottle of pesticide labeled *nicotine alkaloid,* which they had obtained from a friend of the patient. The solution contained 870 mg of nicotine per mL. The patient's serum nicotine concentration, subsequently, was shown to be 13,600 ng/mL.

Over the next couple of hours, the patient had multiple seizures, which were controlled with diazepam, phenytoin (Dilantin), mannitol, and dexamethasone (Decadron). A CT scan showed cerebral edema, and EEG and evoked potential testing showed no cortical function. The patient was assumed to have suffered anoxic brain death. Intractable hypotension occurred on the 2nd hospital day, and the patient died 64 hr postingestion. (See ref. 41.)

Discussion

1. What was the purpose of giving naloxone and $D_{50}W$ before transporting this patient to the hospital?
2. The patient had a urine toxicologic screen that was positive for nicotine but a negative serum toxicologic screen. What is the significance of this finding?
3. What was the cause of this patient's "anoxic brain death"?
4. What effect did the fact that this patient was a smoker have on the outcome of his poisoning with an overdose of nicotine?

CASE STUDY: INSECT REPELLENT TOXICITY

History

A 61-year-old woman in otherwise good health was admitted to the hospital. After covering herself with sunscreen and a DEET-containing insect repellent, she had begun working in her yard. Shortly, she had developed lightheadedness and returned to the house to sit down and drink a cup of coffee. Symptoms resolved at that time.

She returned to the yard then developed presyncope and fell to the ground but did not lose consciousness. She reported that she was unable to speak at that time. She also developed nausea, vomiting, and explosive diarrhea. She was able to crawl inside to telephone her husband. Her husband, an internist, found her systolic blood pressure to be 80 mm Hg and immediately took her to the emergency department. On arrival, blood pressure varied from a palpable systolic of 70 to 100/60 mm Hg. She had orthostatic hypotension.

Treatment consisted of intravenous sodium chloride, which resulted in improvement in blood pressure. She was then admitted to the hospital for observation because of her orthostatic hypotension, nausea, vomiting, and diarrhea.

The patient was in obvious distress and had her eyes closed. She was having noticeable "chills." She denied chest pain or palpitations. She also denied any recent upper respiratory infection, abdominal pain, melena, or hematemesis.

Examination was significant for relative hypotension and orthostatic change in blood pressure. Temperature was 36.6°C; heart rate, 70 beats/min; respirations, 18/min. Her skin felt warm to the touch.

Electrocardiogram recording showed marked sinus bradycardia (heart rate, 44 beats/min) but was otherwise normal. A repeat recording 1 hr later revealed sinus rhythm at a rate of 64 beats/min and no abnormalities.

The patient became completely asymptomatic and had a stable blood pressure several hours after admission. No rechallenge with DEET was attempted. She was dismissed in her usual state of health the following day with a presumptive diagnosis of DEET toxicity. (See ref. 11.)

Discussion

1. The patient wore only shorts and a halter top when doing her yard work on the eventful morning. She reported it as a "hot summer day." Also, she applied a sunscreen product along with the DEET. Postulate how the factors described here may have increased absorption of repellent.
2. What was the source of orthostatic hypotension for which this patient was hospitalized?

CASE STUDY: PARAQUAT POISONING

History

A 17-year-old boy accidentally ingested a mouthful of paraquat. An unprovoked vomiting episode occurred about 10 min later. He was brought to a local hospital 5 days after ingestion complaining of nausea, vomiting, and burning pain in the mouth and throat. He remained at this hospital for 4 days, during which time he developed a low-grade fever and was lethargic and confused. He had elevated SGOT levels and increased serum creatinine.

The patient was then transferred to a large medical center. His admitting examination revealed a lethargic individual with respirations, 32/min; blood pressure, 112/82 mm Hg; temperature, 99.5°F; and pulse, 84 beats/min. Laboratory values are shown in Table 8.14.

Initial treatment consisted of 7 g methylprednisolone intravenously per day, along with hemodialysis. The patient remained on

TABLE 8.14. *Laboratory findings*

Hematocrit	=45%
WBC	=21,000/mm
BUN	=100 mg/dL
Serum creatinine	=9 mg/dL
pH	=7.42
pO_2	=58 mm Hg
pCO_2	=33 mm Hg
CPK	=6,996 mU/mL
LDH	=493 mU/mL
SGOT	=128 mU/mL
Alkaline phosphatase	=122 mU/mL

WBC, white blood cells; CPK, creatinine phosphokinase; LDH, lactate dehydrogenase; SGOT, serum glutamate oxaloacetate transaminase.

dialysis for 7 days, at which time his renal function recovered and an adequate urine output was maintained.

Despite this apparent recovery, the patient had a steady decline in respiratory function and increased oxygen requirement as a result of irreversible lung damage. He died approximately 3 weeks after ingestion. (See ref. 17.)

Discussion

1. Do the symptoms and laboratory values presented in this case study correlate with the expected toxic effects of paraquat?
2. Would gastric lavage with fuller's earth have been of any benefit when he was admitted? (Read the case study that follows.) What about activated charcoal?
3. Is it a consistent finding in paraquat intoxication that lung damage is delayed?

CASE STUDY: THE CASE OF THE "DEADLY" ANTIDOTE

History

A 39-year-old man attempted suicide by ingesting 100 mL of 20% paraquat solution. He was admitted to an emergency facility, decontaminated by gastric lavage, and then given 30% Fuller's earth suspension (in isotonic saline) at a rate of 250 mL every 4 hr. On the 3rd day peristalsis disappeared, and an abdominal X-ray film showed distension of the small and large bowel, with the appearance of enormous fecaliths. All the while the patient also continued to receive enemas and purgatives (not identified by the case study).

On the 3rd day, serum calcium concentrations were noted to be increased, as shown in Table 8.15. The patient did not receive calcium salts or vitamin D, and thus neither could be considered as a cause of the hypercalcemia.

This case study concluded with: "The patient died six days after intake as a result of paraquat-induced lung edema." (See ref. 80.)

TABLE 8.15. *Laboratory findings*

Day	Serum calcium (mg/dL)
1	9.3
2	9.2
3	11.9
4	13.0
5	10.9
6	10.8

Discussion

1. Can you suggest what might have actually caused this patient's death? (Hint: Fuller's earth contains 4.2 g CaO per 100 g.) Do you believe that the amount of paraquat solution he drank would have been sufficient to cause his death? If you choose this latter cause, then does paraquat per se cause hypercalcemia?
2. What are fecaliths? How did they form in this patient?

CASE STUDY: POISONING BY 2,4-D

History

A 26-year-old male mental patient intentionally ingested 75 mL of a herbicide product containing 2,4-dichlorophenoxyacetic acid and 4-chloro-2-methylphenoxypropionic acid. He was brought to an emergency facility 10 hr after ingestion.

On admission, he was in grade 4 coma but did not require mechanical respiratory assistance. Gastric lavage was performed. Physical examination revealed dilated pupils, but reflexes were normal and there was no indication of muscle damage. The chest and abdomen were normal. There were no corrosive burns in the mouth, but a phenolic smell was detected on his breath.

Laboratory findings revealed slight hypoxia, metabolic acidosis, and slight liver damage. Even though urinary output and adequate hydration were maintained, his blood urea nitrogen (BUN) increased to 159 mmol/L and serum creatinine to 165 μmol/L. On admission, serum 2,4-D concentration was 79.6 mg/L.

Forty-eight hours after admission, the patient responded to sounds and apparently did well from that point forward. (See ref. 87.)

Discussion

1. Would herbicides such as 2,4-D adsorb onto activated charcoal?
2. Would forced alkaline diuresis help promote the excretion of 2,4-D? If so, why was it not used?
3. Overall, this case was unremarkable. Compared to 2,4,5-T, the herbicide 2,4-D is much less toxic. Had this patient been seriously intoxicated, what organ would have been affected?

CASE STUDY: PHOSPHORUS INTOXICATION

History

A 24-year-old woman ingested 45 mL of Stearn's Electric Brand Paste (containing approximately 2.5% phosphorus) along with a quantity of ethanol. Forty-five minutes later, she began to vomit and experience abdominal cramping. This continued off and on for about 4 days. Afterward, she sought medical attention at a hospital.

On admission, she was alert and cooperative but still complained of abdominal pain, jaundice, and decreased urine output. Physical examination revealed blood pressure, 80/68 mm Hg; pulse, 108 beats/min; respirations, 28/min; and temperature, 98.2°F. Her sclera were yellowed, and she had shallow burns on the lips and diffuse abdominal tenderness. Arterial blood gases showed pH, 7.51; pO_2, 94 mm Hg; and pCO_2, 27 mm Hg.

Other laboratory findings are shown in Table 8.16. She was stable throughout her 16-day hospital stay.

The patient was treated with calcium chloride, vitamin K, and fluids. Urine output was severely depressed, and her BUN increased

TABLE 8.16. *Laboratory findings*

BUN	=133 mg/dL
Na^+	=129 mEq/L
K^+	=6.3 mEq/L
Cl^-	=74 mEq/L
HCO_3^-	=22 mEq/L
Ca^{2+}	=6.4 mg/dL
SGOT	=2,574 U
SGPT	=371 U
Amylase	=1,826 U
PT	=40% of normal
PTT	=86.1 sec (control, 275 sec)
Creatinine	=7.6 mg/dL
Total bilirubin	=4.4 mg/dL

SGPT, serum glutamate pyruvic transaminase; PT, prothrombin time; PTT, partial thromboplastin time.

to 108 mg/dL, creatinine to 9.5 mg/dL, and amylase to 2.083 U/L.

At this point, she received 50 passes of peritoneal dialysis. It was not until the 8th day postadmission that liver function tests improved, and 10 days after admission diuresis began. She left the hospital against medical advice on the 16th day and appeared well. She was reexamined in the medical clinic for the next 2 months and continued to make steady improvement. (See ref. 48.)

Discussion

1. Why did the phosphorus product cause burning in the oral cavity?
2. Was the patient's serum calcium concentration normal? If not, with what symptoms does it correlate?
3. Are the liver function tests normal or elevated? What does this suggest?
4. Can you give an explanation for the hypotension observed?
5. What is the significance of the patient's prothrombin time (PT) and partial thromboplastin time (PTT) values?
6. What does the elevated BUN, serum creatinine, and total bilirubin suggest?

CASE STUDIES: THALLIUM POISONING

History: Case 1

About 3 weeks before hospital admission, a 35-year-old female schoolteacher began to notice numbness in her extremities. She was always tired, often vomited, and no longer had an appetite. She also noticed some hair loss. Eventually, her vision deteriorated and became "fuzzy," and she experienced episodes of visual hallucinations. She had trouble judging distances, and concentration became progressively more difficult.

Two weeks before the hospital admission mentioned above, she was observed at a local hospital. Physical examination revealed blood pressure of 150/100 mm Hg with marked orthostatic changes and pulse of 100 to 120 beats/min. Neurologic examination showed decreased sensation in the hands and feet with decreased muscle strength, especially in the legs. Stretch reflexes were normal. Serum potassium concentration were 3.5 mEq/L. She was discharged pending urinary heavy metal analysis.

She was later admitted to a medical center hospital where she presented with severe pain in the lower extremities and marked alopecia. Her supine blood pressure was 160/110 mm Hg and, while sitting erect, 140/100 mm Hg. A neurologic examination did not show major pathologic disturbance. There were some problems with attention span and with making calculations.

Serum electrolytes were decreased, but hematologic values were within normal limits. Suspected thallium intoxication was confirmed when urinary thallium concentrations were shown to be 3,100 μg/dL.

The patient was treated with 15 mg of 10% KCl every 8 hr. No other indication of additional therapy was stated, and the source of intoxication was not determined. (See ref. 22.)

History: Case 2

A 52-year-old man deliberately ingested 20 g thallium iodide (12 g thallium), which he calculated from a chemical reference book to be 20 times the fatal dose. He was brought to the emergency facility while complaining of intense abdominal cramping and nausea.

Treatment consisted of administering 1 g of activated charcoal 4 times a day for 5 days; a cathartic, 40 mEq of KCl, 4 times a day for 6 days; and peritoneal dialysis.

The progression of signs and symptoms is presented as given below:

Week 1: Abdominal colic, constipation, severe pain. Motor weakness of the lower extremities.
Week 2: Severe postural hypotension. Agitation, confusion, short-term memory loss.
Week 3: Alopecia.

Improvement of motor weakness and postural hypotension was noted within 1 month. The patient was discharged to a nursing home to regain muscle strength and returned home a year later with some persistent neurologic problems, particularly muscular weakness and difficulty walking. (See ref. 39.)

Discussion

1. In both cases, marked orthostatic hypotension was noted. Why did this occur?
2. How does thallium manifest its toxicity?
3. What was the purpose for giving 1 g activated charcoal every 4 hr for 5 days in case 2? Was it of any value?
4. In both cases, potassium therapy was given. Why?
5. Alopecia was present in both patients. What caused it?

CASE STUDY: PROLONGED POISONING BY A COUMARIN DERIVATIVE

History

A 17-year-old boy attempted suicide by consuming approximately 7.5 mg (0.12 mg/kg) brodifacoum (a long-acting hydroxycoumarin derivative) contained in a commercially available rodenticide. He was admitted to a regional hospital with flank pain and gross hematuria, and subsequently he developed bleeding gums and epistaxis. He had a prolonged prothrombin time and activated partial

TABLE 8.17. *Treatment regimens for brodifacoum poisoning in a 17-year-old boy*

Product	Day postingestion
Vitamin K_3, 10 mg i.v./day	24–34
Vitamin K_3, 10 mg orally/day	38–44
Vitamin K_1, 5 mg s.c. twice/day	45–48
Vitamin K_3, 10 mg s.c. twice/day	49–56
Prothrombin complex, 1,700 units i.v.	25
Stored plasma, 2 units i.v.	37
Fresh-frozen plasma, 2 units i.v.	40 and 49
Phenobarbital, 50 mg orally, twice/day	52–56

From ref. 37.
i.v., intravenous; s.c., subcutaneous.

thromboplastin time (aPTT), both exceeding 120 sec. He was given large doses of vitamin K and plasma-product infusions. Despite treatment, PT and aPTT values remained prolonged. The patient was transferred to another hospital 23 days later for further evaluation.

On admission, vital signs were normal. He had a large, painful hematoma on his left thigh. His PT was 25.2 sec (reference range, 11.5 to 12.5) and aPTT was 54.5 sec (reference range, 20 to 29). Hemoglobin was 8.5 g/L, and platelet count was 487×10^9/L. A fecal occult blood test was positive. Vitamin K-dependent coagulation factors were reduced.

Because of concern about potential intracranial bleeding, a single dose of prothrombin complex was given. He continued to receive vitamin K, plasma, and iron supplements. Near the end of his hospital stay, he was prescribed phenobarbital. This therapy is summarized in Table 8.17.

By day 51 postingestion, PT and aPTT had returned to normal values. Therapy was continued to day 55 and then was discontinued. (See ref. 37.)

Discussion

1. Name the vitamin K-dependent coagulation factors. What are their normal half-lives?
2. Discuss the meanings of the terms *hematoma, epistaxis,* and *flank pain.*
3. Why was phenobarbital added to this pa-

tient's regimen beginning on day 52? Should it have been added earlier, or was it inappropriate to give it at all?
4. The text states that vitamin K_3 is not effective in treating warfarin overdosage. Why then was this form of vitamin K given to this patient on days 38 to 44?

Review Questions

1. After ingestion of an organophosphorus insecticide, which of the following effects can be expected to occur?
   A. Massive nicotinic response
   B. Massive muscarinic response
   C. Both of the above
   D. Neither of the above
2. Which of the following is a characteristic symptom of thallium intoxication?
   A. Arrhythmia
   B. Hypercalcemia
   C. Hemorrhage
   D. Alopecia
3. Which of the following is a true statement?
   A. Carbamate insecticides are generally more toxic than organophosphorus compounds.
   B. After phosphorylation of plasma cholinesterase, several days are needed for activity to return to normal.
   C. Organophosphorus insecticides cause miosis and tachycardia.
   D. Erythrocytic anticholinesterase levels

correlate with levels of enzyme in the brain.

4. Appearance of a SLUD syndrome characterizes poisoning by which of the following?
   A. Phosphorus
   B. Organophosphorus compounds
   C. Warfarin
   D. Paraquat

5. Which of the following is true about organochlorine insecticides?
   A. They are water soluble and, hence, biodegradable.
   B. Their toxic effects are treated with 2-PAM.
   C. They are less toxic, on a milligram-to-milligram basis, than organophosphorus compounds.
   D. Percutaneous absorption in humans is rapid and complete.

6. The major site of toxicity of organochlorine insecticides is the:
   A. Liver
   B. Brain
   C. Kidney
   D. Heart

7. Which of the following produces symptoms of poisoning largely identical to those of DDT: lindane (I), methoxychlor (II), or TEPP (III)?
   A. I only
   B. II only
   C. I and II only
   D. II and III only

8. A victim of "derris" intoxication should receive treatment for poisoning by:
   A. 2,4-D
   B. Diquat
   C. Rotenone
   D. Pyrethrins

9. The major site of toxicity to paraquat is the:
   A. Lung
   B. Liver
   C. Brain
   D. Kidney

10. Polychlorinated biphenyls are chlorinated hydrocarbon insecticides.
    A. True
    B. False

11. Which of the following pesticides inhibits synthesis of vitamin K-dependent clotting factors?
    A. Thallium
    B. Lindane
    C. Warfarin
    D. Phosphorus

12. Symptoms of diquat poisoning are identical to those caused by paraquat.
    A. True
    B. False

13. A victim of paraquat ingestion will expect the most significant toxic symptoms in which of the following systems?
    A. Brain
    B. Kidney
    C. Lung
    D. Heart
    E. Liver

14. All of the following are true statements about pralidoxime *except:*
    A. Another name for pralidoxime is 2-PAM.
    B. It has the same mechanism of action as atropine.
    C. It is not useful in poisoning by carbamates.
    D. It should be used cautiously in persons with myasthenia gravis.

15. Which of the following is true concerning insecticide toxicity?
    I. Enzyme aging to organophosphorus poisoning implies that the enzyme that metabolizes these poisons is no longer active.
    II. A benzodiazepine derivative is the antidote of first choice for DDT- or lindane-induced convulsions.
    III. The major symptoms of pyrethrin intoxication would be the result of inhibition of AChE.
    A. I only
    B. II only
    C. III only
    D. I and II only
    E. II and III only

16. A victim of poisoning presented with the following symptoms and signs:

CNS: apprehensive, irritable, hypersusceptible to stimuli

Cardiovascular system (CVS): within normal limits

Eyes: normal

GI tract: nausea, vomiting, normal activity otherwise

Lungs: no perceived abnormality

Kidneys: no perceived abnormality

Hepatic functions: no perceived abnormality

Which of the following poisons did this individual most likely encounter?

A. Parathion

B. Paraquat

C. 2,4,5-T

D. Ethylene glycol

E. Kwell

17. Which of the following is true about organochlorine insecticides?

A. They are water soluble and, hence, biodegradable.

B. Their use as ectoparasiticides is contraindicated.

C. They are less toxic, on a milligram-to-milligram basis, than organophosphorus compounds.

D. Percutaneous absorption in humans is rapid and complete.

E. The SLUD syndrome is characteristic of ingestion by humans.

18. Excretion of 2,4-D can be hastened by altering the pH of urine. This may be accomplished best by:

A. Increasing urinary pH with sodium bicarbonate

B. Increasing urinary pH with ammonium chloride

C. Decreasing urinary pH with sodium bicarbonate

D. Decreasing urinary pH with ammonium chloride

19. The *delayed neurotoxic effect* after ingestion of pesticides is rare, but is closely related to which of the following?

A. Pyrethrins

B. Organochlorine compounds

C. Organophosphorus insecticides

D. Paraquat

E. Coumarin derivatives

20. The defoliant *Agent Orange,* which was used extensively in the Vietnam War, consisted of:

A. Lindane and DDT

B. Paraquat and diquat

C. Thallium and phosphorus

D. Pyrethrum and piperonyl butoxide

E. 2,4-D and 2,4,5-T

21. Explain the probable cause of the "delayed neurotoxic effects" sometimes seen with organophosphorus insecticides.

22. In treating severe organophosphorus toxicity, why is it essential that both atropine and 2-PAM be given to assure maximum patient benefit?

23. What is the specific rationale for performing gastric lavage with solutions of copper sulfate in victims of phosphorus ingestion?

24. Discuss the major symptoms associated with each stage of phosphorus poisoning.

25. Describe the mechanism of toxic action of warfarin. What are the biochemical events that lead to the appearance of symptoms of toxicity?

26. Labels of products containing pyrethrum warn persons with hay fever or severe allergies to avoid inhaling the solutions. What is the specific reason for this precaution?

27. An acute poisoning with nicotine causes initial muscle stimulation followed by muscular weakness. How does nicotine cause this cyclic effect?

28. Discuss the toxic potential of dioxin. What is its source(s), and how can accidental exposure to it best be avoided?

29. A victim of insecticide ingestion was admitted to the hospital for observation. The symptoms that developed did not correlate to those expected from the specific insecticide contained in the bottle. List all of the various factors that could cause the appearance of these unexpected symptoms.

References

1. Aldridge WN, Johnson MK. Side effects of organophosphorus compounds: delayed neurotoxicity. *Bull World Health Organ* 1971;44:259–263.

2. [Anonymous]. EPA halts most use of herbicide 2,4,5-T. *Science* 1979;203:1090–1091

3. [Anonymous]. Organophosphate insecticide poisoning. *Clin Toxicol* 1979;15:189–191.

4. Arena JM. *Poisoning: toxicology, symptoms, treatment.* 4th ed. Springfield, IL: Charles C Thomas; 1979.

5. Autor AP. Reduction of paraquat toxicity by superoxide dismutase. *Life Sci* 1974;14:1309–1319.

6. Bismuth C, Garnier R, Baud FJ, et al. Paraquat poisoning—an overview of the current status. *Drug Safety* 1990;5:243–251.

7. Bismuth C, Scherrman JM, et al. Elimination of paraquat. *Hum Toxicol* 1987;6:63–68.

8. Blain PG. Aspects of pesticide toxicology. *Adverse Drug React Acute Poisoning Rev* 1990;9:37–68.

9. Bus JS, Aust SD, Gibson JE. Paraquat toxicity—proposed mechanism of action involving lipid peroxidation. *Environ Health Perspect* 1976;16:139–146.

10. Casida JE. Mixed-function oxidase involvement in the biochemistry of insecticide synergists. *J Agric Food Chem* 1970;18:753.

11. Clem JR, Havemann DF, Raebel MA. Insect repellent (*N,N*-diethyl-*m*-toluamide) cardiovascular toxicity in an adult. *Ann Pharmacother* 1993;27:289–293.

12. Cremlyn R. *Pesticides—preparation and mode of action.* New York: John Wiley; 1978.

13. Dale WE, Gaines TB, Hayes WJ, Pearce GW. Poisoning by DDT: relation between clinical signs and concentration in rat brain. *Science* 1963;142:1474–1476.

14. DeGroot G, vanLeusen R, vanHeipt ANP. Thallium concentrations in body fluids and tissues in a fatal case of thallium poisoning. *Vet Hum Toxicol* 1985;27:115–119.

15. Dreisbach RH, Robertson WO. *Handbook of poisoning.* 12th ed. Los Altos, CA: Appleton and Lange Publications; 1982.

16. Edwards DI, Johnson CE. Insect repellent-induced toxic encephalopathy in a child. *Clin Pharm* 1987;6:490–498.

17. Fairshter RD, Rosen SM, Smith WR, et al. Paraquat poisoning: new aspects of therapy. *Q J Med* 1976;180:551–565.

18. Farrar HC, Wells TG, Kearns GL. Use of continuous infusion of pralidoxime for treatment of organophosphate poisoning in children. *J Pediatr* 1990;116:658–661.

19. Flanagan RJ, Merideth TJ, Ruprah M, et al. Alkaline diuresis for acute poisoning with chlorophenoxy herbicides and ioxynil. *Lancet* 1990;335:454–458.

20. Friesen EG, Jones GR, Vaughan D. Clinical presentation and management of acute 2,4-D oral ingestion. *Drug Safety* 1990;5:155–159.

21. Gaines TB. Acute toxicity of pesticides. *Toxicol Appl Pharmacol* 1969;14:515–534.

22. Gastel B. Thallium poisoning. *Johns Hopkins Med J* 1978;142:27–31.

23. Gehring PJ, Krames CG, Schultz BA, et al. The fate of 2,4,5-trichlorophenoxyacetic acid (2,4,5-T) following oral administration to man. *Toxicol Appl Pharmacol* 1973;26:352–361.

24. Gosselin RE, Smith RP, Hodge HC, eds. *Clinical toxicology of commercial products.* 5th ed. Baltimore: Williams and Wilkins; 1984:III-328–336.

25. Haley TJ. Review of the toxicology of paraquat. *Clin Toxicol* 1979;14:1–46.

26. Harley JB, Grinspan S, Root RK. Paraquat suicide in a young woman—results of therapy directed against the superoxide radical. *Yale J Biol Med* 1977;50:481–488.

27. Hayes WJ. *Clinical handbook on economic poisons.* Washington: US Government Printing Office; 1963; Public Health Service publication no 476.

28. Hayes WJ. Epidemiology and general management of poisoning by pesticides. *Pediatr Clin North Am* 1970;17:629–644.

29. Hayes WJ, Vaughn WK. Mortality from pesticides in the United States in 1973 and 1974. *Toxicol Appl Pharmacol* 1977;42:235–252.

30. Herman MM, Bensch KG. Light and electron microscopic studies of acute and chronic thallium intoxication in rats. *Toxicol Appl Pharmacol* 1967;10:199–222.

31. Heyl T, Barlow RJ. Thallium poisoning: a dermatological perspective. *Br J Dermatol* 1989;121:789–792.

32. Hill EE, Carlisle H. Toxicity of 2,4-dichlorophenoxyacetic acid for experimental animals. *J Ind Hyg Toxicol* 1947;29:85–89.

33. Hoffman S, Jedeikin R, Korzets Z, et al. Successful management of severe paraquat poisoning. *Chest* 1983;84:107–109.

34. Howard JK. The myth of paraquat inhalation as a route for human poisoning. *J Toxicol Clin Toxicol* 1983;20:191–193.

35. Ilett KF, Stripp B, Menard RH, et al. Studies on the mechanism of the lung toxicity of paraquat. *Toxicol Appl Pharmacol* 1974;28:216–226.

36. Johnson MK. The target for initiation of delayed neurotoxicity by organophosphorus esters: biochemical studies and toxicological applications. *Rev Biochem Toxicol* 1982;4:141–212.

37. Jones EC, Grove GH, Naiman SC. Prolonged anticoagulation in rat poisoning. *JAMA* 1984;252:3005–3007.

38. Karczmar AG. Acute and lasting central actions of organophosphorus agents. *Fundam Appl Toxicol* 1984;4:S1–S17.

39. Koshy KM, Lovejoy FH. Thallium ingestion with survival: ineffectiveness of peritoneal dialysis and potassium chloride diuresis. *Clin Toxicol* 1981;18:521–525.

40. Lange PF, Terveer J. Warfarin poisoning: report of fourteen cases. *US Armed Forces Med J* 1954;5:872–877.

41. Lavoir FW, Harris TM. Fatal nicotine ingestion. *J Emerg Med* 1991;9:133–136.

42. LeBlanc FN, Benson BE, Gilg AD. A severe organophosphate poisoning requiring the use of an atropine drip. *J Toxicol Clin Toxicol* 1986;24:64–76.

43. Lipton RA, Klass EM. Human ingestion of a super-warfarin rodenticide resulting in a prolonged anticoagulant effect. *JAMA* 1984;252:3004–3005.

44. Lotti M. Treatment of acute organophosphate poisoning. *Med J Aust* 1991;154:51–55.

45. Lotti M, Becker CE. Treatment of acute organophosphate poisoning: evidence of a direct effect on central nervous system by 2-PAM (pyridine-2-aldoxime methyl chloride). *J Toxicol Clin Toxicol* 1982;19:121–127.

46. Marquis JK. Central neurotoxicity of organophosphate insecticides. *Concepts Toxicol* 1986;2:53–61.
47. Matsumura F, Ghiasuddin SM. DDT-sensitive Ca-ATPase in the axonic membrane. In: Narahashi T, ed. *Neurotoxicology of insecticides and pheromones.* New York: Plenum Press; 1979:245–257.
48. McCarron MM, Gaddis GP, Trotter AT. Acute yellow phosphorus poisoning from pesticide pastes. *Clin Toxicol* 1981;18:693–711.
49. Merrill DG, Mihm FG. Prolonged toxicity of organophosphate poisoning. *Crit Care Med* 1982;10:550–551.
50. Moeschlin SN. Thallium poisoning. *J Toxicol Clin Toxicol* 1980;17:133–146.
51. Mofenson HC, Greensher J, Caraccia TR, D'Agostino RD. Paraquat intoxication—report of a fatal case: discussing pathophysiology and rationale of treatment. *J Toxicol Clin Toxicol* 1981–83;19:821–824.
52. Moore JA, Courtney KD. Teratology studies with the trichlorophenoxyacid herbicides, 2,4,5-T and Silvex. *Teratology* 1971;4:236–240.
53. Morgan DP. *Recognition and management of pesticide poisoning.* 3rd ed. Washington: US Environmental Protection Agency; 1982.
54. Morgan DP, Lin LI, Saikaly HH. Morbidity and mortality in workers occupationally exposed to pesticides. *Arch Environ Contam Toxicol* 1980;9:349–382.
55. Moses HH, Innis R. Thallium poisoning. *Johns Hopkins Med J* 1978;142:27–31.
56. Murphy SD. Pesticides. In: Klaassen CD, Amdur MO, Doull J, eds. *Toxicology—the basic science of poisons.* 3rd ed. New York: Macmillan; 1986:519–581.
57. Namba T, Nolte CT, Jackrel J, Grob D. Poisoning due to organophosphate insecticides. *Am J Med* 1971;50:475–492.
58. Natoff II, Reiff B. Effect of oximes on the acute toxicity of anticholinesterase carbamates. *Toxicol Appl Pharmacol* 1973;25:569–575.
59. Nielsen K, Koempe B, Jensen-Holm J. Fatal poisoning in man by 2,4-dichlorophenoxyacetic acid (2,4-D)—determination of the agent in forensic materials. *Acta Pharmacol Toxicol* 1965;22:224–234.
60. Norahashi T. Nerve membrane ionic channels as the target site of insecticides. In: Narahashi T, ed. *Neurotoxicology of insecticides and pheromones.* New York: Plenum Press; 1979:211–243.
61. Okonek S, Hofmann A, Henningsen B. Efficacy of gut lavage, hemodialysis, and hemoperfusion in the therapy of paraquat or diquat intoxication. *Arch Toxicol* 1976;36:43–51.
62. O'Leary JF, Kunkel AM, Jones AH. Efficacy and limitations of oxime-atropine treatment of organophosphorus anticholinesterase poisoning. *J Pharmacol Exp Ther* 1961;132:50–55.
63. Park BK, Leck JB. A comparison of vitamin K antagonism by warfarin, difenacoum and brodifacoum in the rabbit. *Biochem Pharmacol* 1982;31:3635–3639.
64. Rhodes M, Zavala D, Brown D. Hypoxic protection in paraquat poisoning. *Lab Invest* 1976;35:496–500.
65. Roland EG, Jan JE, Rig JM. Toxic encephalopathy in a child after brief exposure in insect repellents. *Can Med Assoc J* 1985;132:155–156.
66. Rose MS, Smith LL, Wyatt I. Evidence for the energy-dependent accumulation of paraquat into the lung. *Nature* 1974;252:314–315.
67. Rosenstock L, Keifer M, Daniell WE, et al. Chronic central nervous system effects of acute organophosphate insecticide intoxication. *Lancet* 1991;338:223–237.
68. Sager GR. Uses and usefulness of paraquat. *Hum Toxicol* 1987;6:7–11.
69. Sidell FR, Borak J. Chemical warfare agents: II. Nerve agents. *Ann Emerg Med* 1992;21:865–871.
70. Smith L. Mechanism of paraquat toxicity in lung and its relevance to treatment. *Hum Toxicol* 1987;6:31–36.
71. Smith PH, Heath D. Paraquat. *Crit Rev Toxicol* 1976;4:411–445.
72. Snyder JW, Poe RD, Stubbins JF, Garrettson LK. Acute manic psychosis following the dermal application of N,N-diethyl-m-toluamide (DEET) in an adult. *J Toxicol Clin Toxicol* 1986;24:429–439.
73. Spigiel RW, Gourley DR, Holcslaw TL, et al. Organophosphate pesticide exposure in farmers and commercial applicators. *Clin Toxicol Consul* 1981;3:45–50.
74. Taylor P. Anticholinesterase agents. In: Gilman AG, Goodman LS, Rall TW, Murad F, eds. *The pharmacological basis of therapeutics.* 7th ed. New York: Macmillan; 1980:110–129.
75. Telch J, Jarvis DA. Acute intoxication with lindane (gamma benzene hexachloride). *Can Med Assoc J* 1982;126:662–663.
76. Tenebein M. Seizures after lindane therapy. *J Am Geriatr Soc* 1991;39:394–395.
77. Vale JA, Crome P, Volans GN, et al. The treatment of paraquat poisoning using oral sorbents and charcoal haemoperfusion. *Acta Pharmacol Toxicol* 1977;41:109–117.
78. Vandenbogaerde J, Colardyn F. Untractable fecalith's and hypercalcemia, both associated with fuller's earth therapy in a fatal case of paraquat poisoning. *J Toxicol Clin Toxicol* 1983;19:1011–1012.
79. VandeVyver FL, Giuliano RA, Paulus GJ, et al. Hemoperfusion—hemodialysis inefficient for paraquat removal in life-threatening poisoning? *J Toxicol Clin Toxicol* 1985;23:117–131.
80. Vandijk A, Maes RAA, Prost RH, Daize JMC. Paraquat poisoning in man. *Arch Toxicol* 1975;34:129–136.
81. Veltri JC, Litovitz TL. 1983 annual report of the American Association of Poison Control Centers national data collection system. *Am J Emerg Med* 1984;2:420–443.
82. Villanueva E, Hernandez-Cueto C, Emilia L, et al. Poisoning by thallium: a study of five cases. *Drug Safety* 1990;5:384–389.
83. Wachs H. Synergistic insecticides. *Science* 1947;105:530.
84. Wallace S, Worsnop C, Paull P, Mashford ML. Covert self poisoning with brodifacoum, a "superwarfarin." *Aust NZ J Med* 1990;20:713–715.
85. Warriner RA, Niles AS, Hayes WJ. Severe organophosphate poisoning complicated by alcohol and turpentine ingestion. *Arch Environ Health* 1977;32:203–205.
86. Watts RG, Castleberry RP, Sadowski JA. Accidental poisoning with a superwarfarin compound (brodifacoum) in a child. *Pediatrics* 1990;86:883–887.
87. Wolfe HR, Durham WF, Armstrong JF. Exposure of workers to pesticides. *Arch Environ Health* 1967;14:622–633.

9 ‖ Metals

Over 40 substances are classed as metals. Although many have the potential to cause toxicity, most do not produce significant human poisoning. This chapter will focus on five metallic poisons: arsenic, cadmium, iron, lead, and mercury. Three additional metals are also discussed to a lesser extent. These are either reported less commonly than the other five as causes of toxicity (copper) or are contemporary sources for potential poisoning because of their use as part of fad diets or "nutritional" dietary programs (e.g., selenium and zinc).

Metals have been carelessly used in the past and casually discarded into the air, water, or food supply. They have been used as medicinals (e.g., sugar of lead, calomel) for centuries or as legitimate insecticides or pesticides. Fossil fuels rich in metal content have been freely burned with the metal spewed into the air.

As new technologies develop, additional uses will undoubtedly unfold for metals. As a result, poisoning by the classic ones, such as lead, mercury, and arsenic, may continue to decrease in incidence, only to be replaced by nickel, selenium, and others.

Toxicity from metals may occur by any route of exposure—inhalation, ingestion, or percutaneous absorption. In industry, inhalation of metallic fumes is the most significant route. Around the home, ingestion is more frequently encountered. On occasion, a metallic salt will be absorbed across inflamed or abraded skin to cause systemic effects. Rarely, someone will inject a metal salt or metallic mercury, usually with suicidal intentions.

CHELATION TREATMENT OF METAL POISONING

Using chemical antidotes to specifically treat metal toxicity is a relatively new concept. Several substances (Fig. 9.1) are called *chelators* (Gr. *chela* = claw) because they bind directly with metal ions to form stable complexes that remove the metal from competition with the body's cells (90). Because a *chelated* metal is water soluble, it can be excreted readily by the kidney. By definition, then, a *chelate* is a cyclic complex formed between a metal and a compound that contains two or more ligands (binding sites). The most sta-

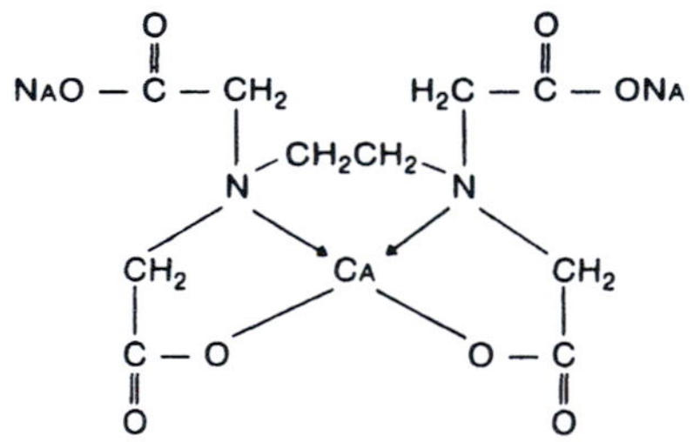

CALCIUM DISODIUM EDETATE

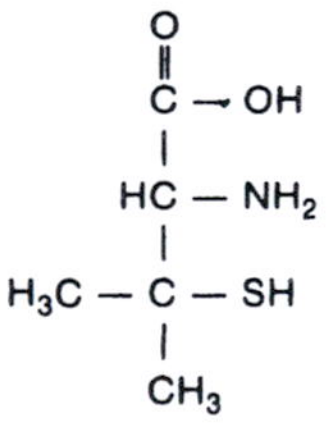

PENICILLAMINE

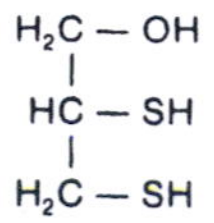

DIMERCAPROL

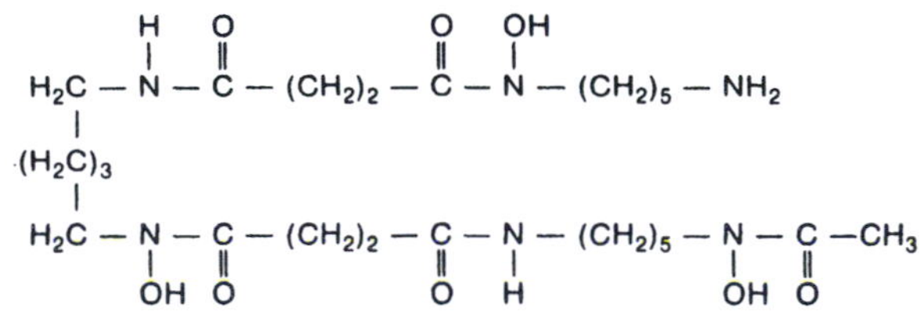

DEFEROXAMINE

FIG. 9.1. Chelators used as antidotes for metal poisoning.

TABLE 9.1. *Properties of an ideal chelating agent*

Have greater affinity for metals than ligands of tissue
Possess high water solubility
Be able to penetrate into tissue sites of metal storage
Be resistant to metabolism or degradation
Form tight bonds with metals that are stable and nontoxic at physiologic pH values
Be readily excreted as a chelate with little or no dissociation
Have a low affinity for calcium
Possess minimal inherent toxicity
Be absorbed via oral administration

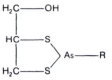

FIG. 9.2. Chelate formed when dimercaprol binds with arsenic.

ble chelates are those with a five- or six-membered ring.

Although chelators are generally perceived as having specific affinity for a particular metal, this is not always the case. Sometimes there is nonspecific binding as well. To illustrate, ethylenediaminetetraacetic acid (EDTA) can be used to treat lead ingestion. It will also form tight complexes with several other metals including calcium. The possibility exists, therefore, for producing hypocalcemic tetany with EDTA.

Another problem is that chelators are less stable at lower pH values. They may partially dissociate in an acidic urine, releasing free metals into the urine. These may be reabsorbed into the body or may cause local kidney damage because of their high concentration in the urine.

The properties of an ideal chelator are listed in Table 9.1. Unfortunately, there is no such item available for clinical use.

METAL CHELATORS

The pharmacologic adage that *no drug has a single effect* (*drugs are two-edged swords*) also applies to chemical chelators. Each chelator has its own array of side effects, and special precautions must be closely observed when they are used. The physician is often confronted with the difficult task of deciding whether to start or withhold chelation therapy.

Dimercaprol

Dimercaprol (British antilewisite) was designed specifically to bind with the arsenical gas, lewisite (Fig. 9.2) (80). Subsequent investigation showed that it would also chelate other metals (Table 9.2).

The dosage of BAL is designed to assure the formation of a 2:1 complex (i.e., 2 molecules of dimercaprol and 1 molecule of metal). These complexes are both more stable and more soluble in water than a 1:1 complex. This assures that BAL will chelate strongly with the metal and, at the same time, that the complex will be readily excreted from the body. British antilewisite blood concentrations are best achieved and maintained by giving repeated doses within the first 4 hr after

TABLE 9.2. *Clinical usefulness of chelating agents*

Chelating agent	Metals reported to be chelated
Calcium disodium EDTA	Beryllium
	Cadmium
	Cobalt
	Copper
	Iron
	Lead
	Manganese
	Nickel
	Zinc
Deferoxamine	Iron
Dimercaprol (BAL)	Arsenic
	Lead
	Mercury
Penicillamine	Copper
	Lead
	Mercury
	Zinc
Succimer	Lead

EDTA, ethylenediaminetetraacetic acid; BAL, British antilewisite.

TABLE 9.3. *Toxicity reported for dimercaprol*

Increased systolic and diastolic pressures
Tachycardia
Nausea and vomiting; abdominal cramps
Headache; sweating forehead
Painful or burning sensation in mouth, lips, throat,
   and penis
Conjunctivitis, rhinorrhea, lacrimation, salivation
Constriction in throat and chest
Paresthesia
Painful (sterile) abscesses at injection site
Anxiety and unrest
Fever in children

poisoning. It must be given parenterally. Excessive single doses should be avoided because of possible side effects. The antidote causes a variety of toxic actions (Table 9.3), which are reported to occur in up to 50% of those who receive it.

British antilewisite is clinically useful for treating acute and chronic poisoning by organic or inorganic arsenicals and for protecting against mercury-induced renal damage. It is generally not effective in treating mercury-induced neurologic conditions or symptoms of brain damage (33). Although theoretically active as a chelator for cadmium, the chelate may partially dissociate in urine and enhance renal damage. British antilewisite should be avoided in cadmium poisoning (27,31). This is also true for iron and selenium.

Calcium Disodium Edetate

Calcium disodium edetate ($CaNa_2$-EDTA) will chelate any metal that has a higher binding affinity than Ca^{2+} (e.g., lead, iron, zinc, manganese, beryllium, and copper). Providing EDTA as the calcium disodium salt ($CaNa_2$-EDTA) largely prevents it from binding with calcium to cause hypocalcemic tetany.

The chelator does not enter host cells but relies on excretion of lead into blood from bone (its major storage site) (38,39). Lead chelates with $CaNa_2$-EDTA to form a complex that is 10^7 times greater than that of the calcium complex (35). Lead that remains in

blood and soft tissues redistributes into bone, where it can later be removed through chelation.

Toxicity to $CaNa_2$-EDTA partly restricts its usage. After intravenous administration, severe proximal nephron degeneration may occur. Other symptoms including fever, nasal congestion, and dermatitis are occasionally seen but are secondary to the renal effects.

Penicillamine

Penicillamine is formed from hydrolysis of penicillin. It forms tight chelates with copper, lead, mercury, and zinc. It is not universally recognized as the first-choice antidote for lead or mercury. An advantage of this chelator is that it is well absorbed from the GI tract after oral administration. Consequently, penicillamine is often given for long-term treatment of chronic metal poisoning, after the patient has been removed from immediate danger, using a parenterally administered chelator (i.e., $CaNa_2$-EDTA for lead; BAL for mercury). An added advantage is that penicillamine, unlike BAL, facilitates removal of methyl mercury (5) and enhances urinary mercury excretion after inhalation of mercury vapor (78). Penicillamine may cause acute allergy-like reactions that are thought to be due to histamine release. In large doses, symptoms appear identical to those of pyridoxine deficiency. In both animal and human studies, these symptoms were reversed when the vitamin was given.

Allergy to penicillin must be carefully considered before penicillamine is given. Patients who are allergic to the antibiotic may also be sensitive to the chelator.

Deferoxamine

Deferoxamine possesses high affinity for both ferrous and ferric iron. It readily binds with iron of hemosiderin and ferritin, sparing iron contained in transferrin, the cytochrome enzymes, and hemoglobin, which bind iron more tightly. It is given parenterally, since less than 15% is absorbed from the GI tract.

Toxicity includes sequelae related to histamine release. These are urticaria, generalized erythema, and pain at the site of injection. Anaphylactic reactions, hypotension, tachycardia, and fever have also been reported.

Succimer

In 1991, succimer was approved as an effective oral chelating agent indicated when blood lead concentrations are greater than 45 μg/dL (55). Succimer is chemically similar to dimercaprol (BAL) but is more water soluble, has a high therapeutic index, and is absorbed well from the gastrointestinal tract. It produces a lead diuresis comparable to that of CaNa$_2$-EDTA and reverses the biochemical toxicity of lead, as indicated by normalization of circulating delta-aminolevulinic acid (ALA) dehydratase (3,14,36). The primary indicators of efficacy are lowered blood lead concentrations and increased urinary lead excretion. Secondary indicators include restoration of red blood cell aminolevulinic acid dehydratase (ALA-D) activity, an enzyme necessary for heme synthesis, and a reduction in urinary aminolevulinic acid and coproporphyrin (36,55). The most common adverse effects include nausea, vomiting, diarrhea, and anorexia (55).

The recommended initial dose in children is 10 mg/kg or 350 mg/m^2 every 8 hr for 5 days, followed by 10 mg/kg or 350 mg/m^2 every 12 hr for 14 days (55). Outpatient administration of 700 mg/m^2/day was shown to delay the typical rebound blood lead concentration without significant adverse effects (37).

TOXIC ACTIONS OF METALS

Metals are toxic because they bind with ligands of biologic structures. Major sites are various enzyme systems of the body. Binding causes inactivation of the enzyme system with resultant diminution of function.

It is difficult to isolate a single target tissue or enzyme system that is acted upon by each metal. The affinity of metals for many enzymes is strong. However, for each metal there is usually a *most sensitive* target. Inhibiting it produces most of the signs and symptoms of toxicity associated with that particular metal. The specified site is based on the tissue that is most sensitive at the lowest dose that will cause toxicity. When larger doses are encountered, additional sites (enzymes) may also be affected. The dose of the metal, therefore, is an important factor in determining the toxicologic outcome.

ARSENIC

Arsenic is a legend in folklore history. It was used as a therapeutic agent more than 2,000 years ago and as a poison for as many years.

Metallic arsenic is a gray, brittle metal that is nontoxic. The most common commercial form is arsenic trioxide (As$_2$O$_3$), an inorganic salt of the trivalent form of arsenic acid (H$_3$AsO$_4$). Arsenic also exists in the pentavalent state (As$_2$O$_5$). Arsenates (e.g., lead arsenate: PbHAsO$_4$) are salts of arsenic acid and are the most abundant forms in nature. They are less toxic than trivalent arsenic. Organic arsenicals also exist and, in this form, arsenic is covalently bonded to an aliphatic carbon chain or ring, with arsenic existing in either the trivalent or the pentavalent state. Organic arsenicals are less toxic than are trivalent inorganic salts.

Arsine gas (AsH$_3$) is the most toxic form of arsenic. It is generated when acids combine with arsenic-containing metals. Poisoning by arsine gas is relatively rare.

Acute arsenic poisonings commonly result from suicidal or accidental ingestion. Some references also list homicide as still being a common cause of arsenic poisoning (60). Arsenic trioxide is odorless and tasteless; thus, it can be added to most liquids without notice. Chronic arsenic poisonings usually occur from environmental or industrial exposures.

Table 9.4 lists a variety of sources of arsenic exposure. It is a common industrial nuisance around factories where ores, such as gold and

TABLE 9.4. *Sources of arsenic exposure*

Environmental
　　Water, soil, air
　　Fish, shellfish
Industrial
　　Metallurgy
　　Manufacturing of glass
　　Pigment production
　　Manufacturing of arsenical
　　　chemicals
Household
　　Weed killers
　　Ant and roach control products
　　Arsenic-containing
　　　pharmaceuticals

copper, are smelted. It is used in manufacturing of certain kinds of glass, in pigment production, and in hardening of copper and lead alloys. It may be a contaminant of water supplies and soil samples. It is also an excellent insecticide and herbicide that continues to be a source of poisoning in children and a significant public health issue (63). Medicinal uses of arsenic are now limited to treatment of a few tropical diseases.

Daily arsenic exposure in humans reaches 900 μg (53). About four-fifths of absorbed arsenic is stored in the body, especially the liver, kidney, walls of the GI tract, spleen, and lung. Arsenicals are deposited in fine hair and nail beds and can be detected in these tissues several years after chronic exposure. The body burden is approximately 21 mg. Normal, unexposed blood concentrations are in the range of 2.0 to 7.0 μg/dL. Arsenic has a short half-life. Arsenic concentrations in blood are only

useful if determined within a few days after acute exposure and are not reliable in assessing chronic toxicity. The best biologic indicator of recent exposure is the concentration in urine, which is usually greater than 100 μg/L (8).

Mechanism of Toxicity

Arsenic is a general protoplasmic poison. Toxicity results when it combines with sulfhydryl (-SH) groups, particularly those contained within enzymes. One sensitive enzyme system is the pyruvate dehydrogenase complex, necessary for oxidative decarboxylation of pyruvate to acetyl CoA and CO_2 before it enters into the TCA cycle. This system comprises several enzymes and cofactors, as shown in Fig. 9.3.

One reaction in this system involves a transacetylase enzyme that combines with coenzyme A (CoA-SH) to form acetyl CoA and a dihydrolipoyl-enzyme complex that contains two sulfhydryl groups. These sulfhydryl groups are extremely vulnerable to chelation by trivalent arsenic. The dihydrolipoyl-arsenite chelate prevents reoxidation of the dihydrolipoyl group necessary for continued enzymatic activity. As a result of binding with arsenic, pyruvic acid accumulates in the blood (see *far left side* of Fig. 9.3).

Arsenic also uncouples oxidative phosphorylation in the second stage of glycolysis by competing with phosphate in the glyceraldehyde dehydrogenase reaction. As shown in

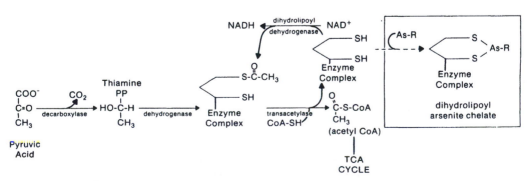

FIG. 9.3. The effect of arsenic on sulfhydryl-related enzyme systems.

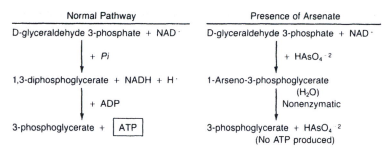

FIG. 9.4. Binding of arsenic to glyceraldehyde-3-phosphate resulting in inhibition of ATP production.

Fig. 9.4, the binding of arsenic to glyceraldehyde-3-phosphate and its subsequent nonenzymatic hydrolysis to 3-phosphoglycerate does not produce ATP, in contrast to the normal glycolytic pathway. Since arsenic has strong affinity for -SH groups and there are several SH-containing enzymes, it is reasonable to expect high concentrations of arsenic to be found in the liver.

Characteristics of Poisoning

Acute

If the amount of arsenic ingested is small, signs and symptoms discussed below may not be seen and a positive diagnosis may be difficult. On the other hand, ingestion of large doses may result in rapid death. A garlic-like odor on the breath or in perspiration should suggest arsenic poisoning. Death is due to circulatory collapse, preceded by intense gastroenteritis. The acute toxic dose ranges from 5 to 50 mg, whereas lethal doses of arsenic trioxide range from 70 to 120 mg. Acute arsenic ingestion usually has a delayed onset of toxic action, up to 30 to 60 min.

The clinical characteristics of acute arsenic poisoning are listed in Table 9.5. The most dramatic effects after acute exposure are on the GI tract. The corrosive action of arsenic produces extreme gastroenteritis, beginning with burning esophageal pain, difficulty in swallowing, and unbearable stomach pain. Nausea, projectile vomiting, and explosive diarrhea ensue. The irritant action of arsenic causes bleeding and capillary transudation into the gastrointestinal mucosa, with vesicle formation. Eventually, these vesicles rupture into the GI tract and the tissue sloughs off, producing *rice-water* (*ricey*) stools, bloody diarrhea, and vomitus. Excessive bleeding compromises the circulatory system, and blood pressure progressively decreases. If the patient survives an acute exposure, ECG abnormalities may still be seen months later.

Renal damage results from glomerular de-

TABLE 9.5. *Characteristics of arsenic poisoning*

Acute arsenic toxicity
  Severe nausea
  Profuse diarrhea; rice-water stools
  Projectile vomiting
  Abdominal pain
  Skin eruptions
  Severe irritation of the nose, throat, conjunctiva
  Loss of fluid
  Uremia
  Cardiac arrhythmias
  ST-segment and T-wave abnormalities
  Hypoxic convulsions
Chronic arsenic toxicity
  Weight loss
  Anorexia
  General malaise
  Garlic odor on breath
  Hyperpigmentation—mottled brown spots
  Hyperkeratosis—palmar and plantar surfaces
  Mee's lines—white lines on the lunulae of the nails
  Peripheral neuritis
  Tremors
  Ulceration of gastrointestinal tract
  Chronic hepatitis
  Liver cirrhosis
  Pancytopenia
  Anemia

struction and dilation of renal capillaries and tubules. Urine outflow is decreased, and the condition may progress to uremia.

Delayed actions of acute arsenic poisoning include alopecia and peripheral neuropathy characterized by paresthesia of the lower extremities, foot-drop, wrist-drop, abnormal gait, and slow reflexes. The liver shows fatty infiltration with central necrosis and cirrhosis.

Chronic

At one time, arsenic (as Fowler's solution) was a popular treatment for certain skin diseases. Low doses caused a *milk and roses* appearance due to vasodilation of facial capillaries. Prolonged usage also produced hyperkeratosis, keratosis of the palms and soles, and dermatitis, especially in areas where there was a high concentration of sweat glands. Dermatitis was due to the primary irritation and sensitization action of arsenic.

Chronic arsenic poisoning usually begins insidiously, with the victim complaining of weakness, tiredness, lack of appetite, weight loss, and irritability. It is obvious that these nonspecific indicators could result from a number of different toxic exposures. More specific characteristics of chronic poisoning are related to effects of arsenic on the integumentary system, causing dark brown pigmentation and a thickening of the keratin layer. Nails thicken and characteristic white bands (referred to as Mee's lines) develop above the lunulae.

Peripheral neuropathies sometimes develop in the latter stages. The legs are affected more than the arms, resulting in paralysis of both motor and sensory pathways. Gastrointestinal effects result in ulcerations in the GI tract. Hepatic injury is evidenced by hepatitis and cirrhosis.

Laboratory examination of peripheral blood shows pancytopenia, especially neutropenia. Prominent features of chronic poisoning include decreased erythrocyte production and basophilic stippling. Occasionally, hypochromic normoblasts and megaloblastic anemia associated with folic acid deficiency is observed.

Management of Poisoning

For *acute* arsenic poisoning, management consists of supportive and symptomatic treatment. Gastric decontamination with ipecac-induced emesis or gastric lavage should be performed for ingestion. Chelation therapy should be started as soon as possible. British antilewisite is the specific chelator used most often in all serious acute arsenic exposures except arsine gas.

Treatment for *chronic* arsenic poisoning should begin with removal of the source of poisoning. Chelation therapy with BAL or penicillamine may be indicated.

CADMIUM

Although sporadic cases of toxicity to cadmium have been reported since the mid-1850s, it was not until nearly a century later that its toxic potential was realized. Cadmium now ranks as one of the heavy metals of greatest toxicologic concern (25).

Cadmium and its salts are widely used in numerous industrial processes, and it is a component of many commercial products. Electroplating is the major use of the pure metal.

Cadmium is found in nature in close association with lead and zinc (90). During mining of these metals, they may be released into the environment.

Cadmium is only poorly absorbed from the GI tract, with as little as 5% entering the blood (71). Most of this burden accumulates from contaminated food and water and inhalation of airborne cadmium, including cigarette smoking.

There is no known biologic need for cadmium. It is the heavy metal most prone to accumulate in the body. Its level increases throughout life as its biologic half-life is 10 to 30 years (48). The average 50-year-old American has about 30 mg in his or her body (28).

Mechanism of Toxicity

Cadmium inhibits enzymes that contain sulfhydryl groups. It also binds to other ligands, including carboxyl, cysteinyl, histidyl, hydroxyl, and phosphatyl groups of protein and purines. Its major toxic effects probably result from enzyme inhibition. One of the plasma enzymes that is inhibited by cadmium is (alpha)$_1$-antitrypsin (15). This may be one of the mechanisms that is at least partially responsible for cadmium-induced pulmonary symptoms. Cadmium has also been reported to compete with cellular uptake of various other metals in the body, such as copper and zinc.

Characteristics of Poisoning

Inhalation of cadmium produces the greatest toxic hazard. Within several hours, the victim complains of intense irritation to the respiratory passages, nausea and vomiting, dizziness, and chest pains (85). Death is usually attributed to severe pulmonary edema (81). If the patient survives, life-long complications of emphysema and other respiratory abnormalities will be encountered. Cadmium also produces nephrotoxicity. Proteinuria, glycosuria, and aminoaciduria are noted, and the glomerular filtration rate is decreased. Important clinical manifestations of toxicity are summarized in Table 9.6.

Of major research interest in recent years has been the effects of chronic exposure on the cardiovascular system. Several studies have suggested that cadmium causes hypertension (75,84,87). However, hypertension is not a consistent finding in chronic industrial poisonings.

Cadmium is reported to cause osteomalacia, perhaps by interfering with calcium and phosphate balance in the kidney. Residents of Toyama, Japan, were shown several years ago to suffer severe cadmium poisoning, with symptoms largely referable to bone and muscle pain. Their disease was termed *I'tai-I'tai Byo* (the *ouch-ouch* disease) and resulted from contamination of rice fields by cadmium released from a metal-processing plant upstream. Osteomalacia was a prominent feature of these victims (86).

Acute and chronic exposures of animals have demonstrated that cadmium causes growth retardation and testicular damage and is carcinogenic. The clinical significance of these effects is not completely known.

Management of Poisoning

Management of acute cadmium poisoning is not as standardized as with some other metals. Treatment should consist of supportive care for pulmonary edema. Vitamin D has been recommended for bone pain. Effectiveness of chelators is questionable. Although chelators increase cadmium excretion after acute exposure, they may increase renal toxicity (27,31). This occurs because the chelated complexes readily dissociate in the kidney, as explained above. Chelators are usually ineffective in chronic cadmium poisoning.

IRON

Accidental ingestion of iron-containing preparations is relatively common among children; intentional overdoses with iron are seen occasionally in adults (7). Between 2,000 and 5,000 cases of toxicity are reported in the United States each year (22,43). The reason for the high incidence of accidental iron poisoning among children is easily understood if

TABLE 9.6. *Characteristics of cadmium toxicity*

Oral
  Severe nausea, vomiting, diarrhea
  Muscular cramps
  Salivation
  Dizziness
  Proteinuria
  Glycosuria
  Osteomalasia
Inhalation
  Rhinorrhea
  Dyspnea
  Chest pain
  Pulmonary edema
  Progressive emphysema
  Azotemia
  Proteinuria

we examine the types of dosage forms available for iron-containing preparations. Comparing iron tablets with pieces of candy (refer back to chapter 1, Fig. 1.5) reminds us of their similarity in appearance, shape, and color. At one time the death rate in children from iron poisoning exceeded the rate for aspirin (77).

Iron is commonly available in many pharmaceutical preparations, including iron supplement tablets, multiple vitamin-mineral products, and prenatal vitamin-mineral preparations. It may be found in oral products as the sulfate, gluconate, and fumarate salts. It is important to remember that all discussion about iron toxicity is related to the amount of elemental iron that is actually absorbed. Therefore, for salt forms, the actual iron content (Table 9.7) must be calculated (77).

Iron is absorbed from the small intestine in its divalent (ferrous) form and converted to the trivalent (ferric) form, which combines with apoferritin to form ferritin. Ferrous iron is absorbed more easily than the ferric form in the intestinal mucosal cell. Ferritin-iron complex passes into the blood and then is attached to transferrin. In the blood, iron remains in the trivalent state or is stored either as ferritin or hemosiderin. Toxicity occurs whenever serum iron concentrations exceed the iron-binding capacity of transferrin.

The daily diet of an average man contains about 15 to 40 mg of elemental iron, only a small portion of which is actually absorbed. The normal iron intake for children is about 10 to 20 mg/kg. The body burden of iron is near 4 g. Ingestion of <20 mg/kg of elemental iron is considered nontoxic. Mild to moderate toxicity occurs with 20 to 60 mg/kg. Ingestion of greater than 60 mg/kg is potentially serious. The minimum lethal dose (MLD) for iron is about 200 to 300 mg/kg body weight (51).

TABLE 9.7. *Iron salts and content*

Salt	Elemental iron (%)
Ferrous sulfate	20
Ferrous sulfate, exsiccated	30
Ferrous gluconate	11.6
Ferrous fumarate	33

Serious acute poisoning in children can occur after ingestion of as little as 1 g, although most ingestions involve larger quantities (24). Most deaths occur in children 12 to 24 months old (23).

Mechanism of Toxicity

Iron toxicity occurs when serum iron concentrations exceed the total iron-binding capacity (TIBC) of transferrin. Circulating free iron is responsible for injury to the GI tract, heart, and liver, producing metabolic alterations.

Iron produces corrosive action on gastrointestinal mucosal cells, leading to stomach and intestinal ulceration, hemorrhage, and coagulative necrosis. The severity of the corrosive action depends on the quantity of ingested elemental iron, duration of local exposure, and contents of the stomach. Hematemesis and bloody stools are common features of acute iron poisoning. Also, severe gastritis may lead to scarring and obstruction of the GI tract.

Cardiovascular effects include decreased cardiac output and shock. Free circulating iron causes damage to blood vessels, producing massive postarteriolar dilation and, consequently, venous pooling. The vascular effects are thought to be due to the direct effect of free iron, ferritin release, or histamine and serotonin release from damaged blood vessels. Free circulating iron also increases capillary permeability, leading to plasma loss and decreases in blood volume, tissue perfusion, and venous pressure (43,73).

Hepatic damage resulting from circulating free iron begins when iron accumulates in Kupffer cells, moves into hepatocytes, and becomes localized in mitochondria. Mitochondrial dysfunction may result from free radical formation and lipid peroxidation. Iron catalyzes lipid peroxidation, leading to altered membrane permeability. Altered membrane permeability results in loss of aerobic respiration. In addition, iron may act as an electron sink, shunting electrons away from the electron transport system, thereby reducing ATP production. Consequently, iron-induced mitochondrial damage results in cellular dysfunction, metabolic acidosis, and, ultimately, cell death (70,73).

Histologic changes in the liver have ranged from no alterations to cloudy swelling, fatty degeneration, and massive hemorrhagic periportal necrosis (32,92). Liver damage may lead to hepatic failure with hypothrombinemia, hypoglycemia, and hepatic encephalopathy. Circulating free iron also inhibits the thrombin-induced conversion of fibrinogen to fibrin. The resultant coagulopathy may aggravate early gastrointestinal blood loss.

Characteristics of Poisoning

There are five critical stages associated with iron poisoning. These are listed in Table 9.8.

The first phase lasts 30 min to 2 hr after ingestion, is characterized by gastrointestinal irritation, and includes abdominal pain, bloody diarrhea, and emesis. Cardiovascular alterations lead to severe hypotension and compensatory tachycardia. Lethargy, irritability, and restlessness may be apparent during this phase, also. Victims seldom die during phase 1, but shock or coma during this early phase is considered to be a poor prognostic sign.

Assessment of poisoning may be difficult during phase 1. Iron is rapidly cleared from plasma and deposited in the liver (73). Thus, by the time the patient is observed, iron blood concentrations may be normal or nearly normal. However, even in the absence of elevated blood concentrations, iron toxicity is progressing.

The second phase is one of quiescence. Recovery is suspected, but the patient still continues to progress into the third phase, which occurs 12 to 48 hr after phase 1. Phase 3 is characterized by persistent gastrointestinal hemorrhage, abrupt onset of shock, and metabolic acidosis, resulting in hyperventilation, hypoglycemia, cyanosis, severe lethargy, or coma.

The fourth phase occurs 2 to 4 days postingestion and is characterized primarily by hepatic injury. It is thought that necrosis is due to a direct toxic action of iron on hepatic mitochondria or possibly depletion of sulfhydryl enzymes. Hepatic necrosis may be evidenced by elevated serum bilirubin, transaminases, and alkaline phosphatase concentrations, as well as jaundice, hypoglycemia, and coagulation defects. Oliguria and renal failure, due to volume depletion, may occur during this phase.

The final phase of iron toxicity begins ap-

TABLE 9.8. *Characteristics of acute iron poisoning*

Phase	Time	Signs and symptoms
Phase 1	30 min–2 hr	Irritability
		Seizures
		Restlessness
		Abdominal pain
		Vomiting
		Bloody diarrhea
		Tachypnea
		Tachycardia
Phase 2	Immediately follows phase 1	"Period of apparent recovery"
Phase 3	12–48 hr after phase 1	Shock
		Refractive acidosis
		Cyanosis
		Fever
Phase 4	2–4 days postingestion	Hepatic necrosis
		Elevated SGOT, SGPT
Phase 5	2–4 weeks postingestion	Gastrointestinal obstruction

SGOT, serum glutamate oxaloacetate transaminase; SGPT, serum glutamate pyruvic transaminase.

proximately 2 to 4 weeks after ingestion. It is generally characterized by gastrointestinal obstruction, including pyloric stenosis and gastric fibrosis. Perfusion and stricture are common. If the victim survives the initial poisoning episode, life-long gastrointestinal problems necessitating abdominal surgery may ensue.

Management of Poisoning

The most important consideration in treating acute iron poisoning is to prevent continued absorption. Ipecac-induced emesis is indicated in the alert patient when large amounts of iron have been ingested. The minimum toxic dose of iron is not well established. Doses of elemental iron of 20 to 60 mg/kg are not likely to cause serious toxicity and probably can be managed at home with ipecac-induced emesis (49).

Gastric lavage is an alternative method of gastric decontamination if the patient is obtunded or lacks a gag reflex. However, there is much controversy surrounding the use of intragastric complexation agents in acute iron poisoning. Complexation agents, such as phosphates, deferoxamine, or bicarbonate, have been suggested.

Sodium dihydrogen phosphate (Fleet Phospho-Soda enema) converts ferrous phosphate to less soluble ferric phosphate and was previously recommended. It is no longer recommended because of the possibility of causing life-threatening hyperphosphatemia and hypocalcemia (4,29).

The use of oral deferoxamine has been suggested to reduce absorption of iron, but its efficacy has not been clearly established. There is evidence that the iron-deferoxamine complex is absorbed and may be toxic itself (91). Another consideration includes the fact that deferoxamine is effective in chelating only ferric iron and medicinal preparations contain ferrous salts (70). Also, large volumes would be required. At this time, intragastric deferoxamine seems to be of little value.

Sodium bicarbonate also complexes with iron to form insoluble ferrous and ferric carbonate and is usually the recommended complexation agent because of its relative safety. However, animal studies have questioned the efficacy of this regimen, and the safety of large volumes of sodium bicarbonate has not been established (18,70).

Whole gut irrigation, with a polyethylene glycol-electrolyte solution, has been suggested in cases of slow-release iron formulations or if an abdominal radiograph after gastric lavage shows persistence of tablets in the stomach or small intestine (10,70,83).

Iron tablets may form concretions in the stomach and small intestine. Adherence to the mucosal lining and continued iron release have resulted in severe hemorrhagic infarction, with subsequent perforation peritonitis and scarring (30,42). In situations where conventional methods of gastric decontamination were ineffective in removing the concretion or if the concretion failed to move through the gastrointestinal tract, a gastrotomy has been performed to reduce the corrosive effects of iron and prevent perforations (52,67).

Deferoxamine (Desferal) is a selective chelator of ferric ions, with little affinity for calcium, copper, magnesium, or zinc. Deferoxamine combines with iron to form an iron-deferoxamine complex (brownish-red), which is water soluble and readily excreted by the kidneys. Deferoxamine (100 mg) will bind approximately 9 mg of free circulating iron but does not chelate iron bound to transferrin or iron in cytochrome and hemoglobin (54,73). Its volume of distribution is about 60% of body weight. Its plasma half-life is 10 to 30 min. Toxicity of deferoxamine is minimal. Adverse effects, however, may include gastrointestinal distress and hypotension.

Use of deferoxamine in iron poisonings is based on severity of symptoms and serum iron concentrations. Any patient with serum iron concentrations greater than 350 μg/dL who is symptomatic or who exhibits serious systemic toxicity with unknown serum iron concentrations is a candidate for chelation therapy (70). Chelation therapy is not necessary if (a) the patient is asymptomatic, (b) the total iron-binding capacity is greater than the serum iron concentration, or (c) the patient ingested 150 to 300 mg of elemental iron per kg. Peak serum iron concentrations greater than 500 μg/dL should be treated promptly with deferoxamine.

Chelation therapy with deferoxamine is recommended when serum iron concentration exceeds 300 μg/dL, even if clinical signs of poisoning are not evident (70). This therapy should be given quickly after acute iron ingestion, since efficacy decreases with time (65). Deferoxamine complexes preferentially but not exclusively with ferric ions. It can be given orally to bind with iron in the gut and reduce its absorption. Deferoxamine is typically administered intravenously. It should be administered cautiously to minimize drug-induced hypotension. If poisoning is mild, it can be administered intramuscularly. Urine should be monitored for the characteristic reddish orange (*vin rosé*) color, which indicates excretion of the chelated complex. Chelation therapy should be continued until urine returns to normal color, indicating termination of iron complexation.

LEAD

Lead toxicity has probably plagued humans since earliest civilization. It was found in almost all early utensils, storage containers, and vessels used for cooking. Besides metallic lead, it can exist in both inorganic and organic forms. For all practical purposes, inorganic lead salts have the same action on the body. Organic lead compounds, primarily the tetraethyl and tetramethyl forms (TEL, TML), act similarly to each other but differently from inorganic salts.

Sources of exposure to lead are listed in Table 9.9. Lead is a cumulative poison that causes both acute and chronic intoxication. Acute poisoning with lead is rare; chronic poisoning is more common and serious.

Lead toxicity is of special concern to workers, such as miners and smelters, automobile finishers, foundry and storage battery workers,

TABLE 9.9. *Sources of lead exposure*

Environmental
  Water
  Air
  Soil
  Food
Household
  Crayons and toys
  Paper and clothes
  Dirt and sand
  Paint flakes
  Furniture
  Wallpaper
  Lead-glazed dishes, cups, glasses, etc.
Persons at high industrial risk
  Miners
  Smelters
  Automobile finishers
  Storage battery workers
  Sheet metal workers
  Spray painters

typesetters, sheet metal workers, and spray painters. Lead (as well as potentially toxic levels of copper and zinc) may also be a contaminant in *moonshine* whiskey. Sometimes old automobile radiators are used as condensers, and the beverage becomes contaminated with lead from solder used in the original construction of the radiator (34). Before World War II, paints containing lead concentrations up to 40% dry weight were used for both exterior and interior surfaces.

The Lead Poisoning Prevention Act, passed by Congress in 1971, limited the acceptable lead concentration to 1%. In 1977, this legislation was amended to reduce the acceptable level to 0.06%. Although the use of paint with a high concentration of lead has been largely discontinued, there still exists a potential hazard for children obsessed with pulling paint chips from walls and woodwork of older homes and buildings. A tiny paint chip from one of these old buildings may contain as much as 100 mg lead. If a child ingested a few chips, this would exceed the daily permissible intake by a factor of at least 30.

Some children possess abnormal craving for placing unnatural, non-nutritional substances in their mouths. Such substances include paint chips, plaster, pencils, and paper. This habit is referred to as *pica*. Although the term is often used to describe a craving for paint or plaster chips alone, pica is, in reality, a generic term that describes a craving for placing anything abnormal in the mouth. Most lead poisoning in children occurs between ages 1 and 5 years. There is a higher incidence of child-related lead poisoning during the warmer months.

There are a number of sources of lead exposure (11). It has been estimated that the average body burden among children and adults in the United States is 100 times greater than the so-called *natural* burden.

Organic lead intoxication occurs less frequently than inorganic lead poisoning. Organic lead compounds have been used in gasoline as *antiknock* additives. With the nation converted to *nonleaded* gasoline, the risk of organic lead poisoning may decline even more.

Pharmacokinetics of Lead

Adults absorb approximately 10% of ingested lead per day; in some children the amount of dietary lead absorbed is much greater. Inorganic lead salts do not penetrate through skin very well. However, alkyl derivatives (tetraethyllead) are capable of penetrating intact skin. Inhalation of lead vapor results in rapid alveolar absorption.

Inorganic lead salts are distributed first from blood to such soft tissues as the kidney, lung, liver, and spleen and later are redistributed and deposited in teeth, hair, and bone as insoluble lead triphosphate. Bone is the major storage depot of lead, comprising nearly 90% of the total body lead burden. In the absence of toxic blood lead concentrations and with good renal function, the kidney accounts for 75% of the daily lead loss.

Mechanism of Toxicity

Lead manifests toxicity primarily by binding to sulfhydryl groups of protein molecules, which inactivates several vital enzyme systems. Lead produces many structural and functional changes within the mitochondria of cells. The resultant inhibition of cellular respiration produces a variety of deleterious effects on cell function, particularly the gastrointestinal system, hematopoietic system, and central nervous system.

The earliest effect of lead poisoning is inhibition of heme formation. Lead interferes with heme synthesis by preventing conversion of delta-aminolevulinic acid (delta-ALA) to porphobilinogen and incorporation of iron into protoporphyrin IX to form heme in bone marrow normoblasts (erythrocyte precursors) by inhibiting delta-aminolevulinic acid dehydratase (ALA-D) and ferrochelatase, respectively (Fig. 9.5). This causes increased urinary coporphyrin and delta-ALA excretion and decreased heme synthesis.

To compensate for decreased heme synthesis, bone marrow erythrocyte production is increased. These cells are released as immature reticulocytes and stippled cells. Basophilic stippling occurs as part of the metabolic disturbance of heme synthesis, which occurs with

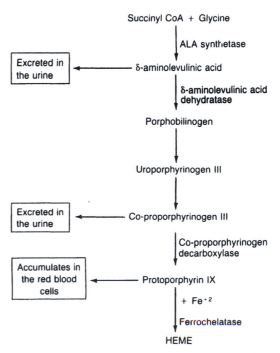

FIG. 9.5. The inhibition of heme production by lead.

lead poisoning. Erythrocytes fail to mature completely and retain some of the cellular organelles that usually disappear during cell maturation. When peripheral blood smears are stained, the irregular polyribosomes and associated RNA aggregate and produce the characteristic stippled cell.

Basophilic stippling is not pathognomonic of lead poisoning. The ultimate effect of lead on the hematopoietic system is microcytic hypochromic anemia, which is usually not severe, even in children. Anemia results from a decrease in the life-span of erythrocytes, as well as interference with hemoglobin synthesis.

In vitro experiments suggest that accumulation of delta-ALA and protoporphyrin may produce a toxic effect on some tissues. For example, animal studies have shown that quantities of delta-ALA have been found in the hypothalamus and that protoporphyrin accumulates in the dorsal root ganglion. This may be responsible for lead encephalopathy. Peripheral neuropathies associated with lead poisoning seem to be related to demyelination and degeneration of peripheral nerves.

Lead circulates bound to erythrocytes. It is initially distributed to soft tissues, such as the kidney and liver, but it eventually incorporates into bone, hair, and teeth for storage (11). Up to 90% will be stored as tertiary lead phosphate in bones (40).

Any factor that affects calcium absorption or desorption can modulate the stability of stored lead. A diet low in phosphate, for example, favors release of lead into blood, whereas a high phosphate intake promotes storage. Vitamin D promotes lead deposition if phosphate concentration is sufficient, and parathyroid hormone causes its removal.

Characteristics of Poisoning

Acute lead poisoning is rarely observed. Most acute poisoning results from accidental ingestion of large quantities of one of the acid-soluble salts. Characteristics of lead poisoning are listed in Table 9.10. Presenting signs and

TABLE 9.10. *Characteristics of lead poisoning*

Acute lead poisoning (rare)
  Sweet metallic taste
  Salivation
  Vomiting
  Intestinal colic
Chronic lead poisoning (plumbism)
  Hematologic
    Basophilic stippling
    Hypochromic microcytic anemia
  Neurologic (lead encephalopathy)
    Ataxia, nausea, vomiting
    Restlessness
    Irritability
    Convulsions
    Coma
  Gastrointestinal (lead colic)
    Anorexia
    Constipation
    Metallic taste
  Neuromuscular (lead palsy)
    Wrist-drop, foot-drop
    Fatigue
    Muscular weakness
  Renal
    Fanconi-like syndrome (reversible)
    Chronic nephritis (irreversible)

symptoms of acute lead poisoning are nonspecific and related to gastrointestinal inflammation. Stools may be black from formation of lead sulfide. Urinary output decreases because of renal damage. Massive ingestion may cause death as a result of cardiovascular collapse. If the patient survives the initial toxic effects of acute poisoning, symptoms of chronic toxicity are commonly seen.

Chronic lead poisoning (plumbism) results in a variety of signs and symptoms that primarily involve the hematopoietic system, GI tract, and nervous, renal, and neuromuscular systems. In early stages of plumbism, anemia causes tiredness and weakness. Hematologic changes result from a decreased life-span of erythrocytes due to interference in the synthesis of the heme portion of hemoglobin. As a result, hypochromic, microcytic anemia and reticulocytosis are evident. Hypochromic cells are due to reduction in heme synthesis. Increased reticulocyte count is a compensatory process responding to the decreased number of erythrocytes. The effects of lead on the hematopoietic system are seldom life threatening.

Lead stimulates the smooth muscle of the GI tract; abdominal pain is a striking feature of plumbism. It may become so severe as to suggest possible bowel obstruction on preliminary diagnosis. Early symptoms are mild and nondescript. However, as lead intoxication progresses, anorexia and constipation (adults) or diarrhea (children) appear, and intestinal spasms increase in frequency and intensity to produce even more severe abdominal cramping, commonly referred to as *lead colic*. There are complaints of persistent metallic taste in the mouth.

Lead is toxic to the kidney. Damage to proximal tubules results in impaired tubular reabsorption of glucose, phosphate, amino acids, bicarbonate, and uric acid. Lead also causes irreversible nephritis characterized by progressive interstitial fibrosis, sclerosis of renal blood vessels, and glomerular atrophy. This irreversible damage is usually observed in individuals who have been exposed to high concentrations for prolonged periods.

Lead palsy is another characteristic of chronic lead poisoning, resulting from action of lead on the neuromuscular system. Lead causes demyelination of the median nerve, which innervates extensor muscles of the hand to produce a *wrist-drop* phenomenon. A similar effect is seen on the foot, but with less frequency and severity.

The most serious manifestation of lead poisoning is encephalopathy, which occurs more often in children than adults. Local edema, hemorrhage, and necrosis of brain tissue are seen. The first indications of lead encephalopathy include clumsiness, lethargy, insomnia, restlessness, and irritability. Symptoms may eventually progress to delirium, convulsions, and coma. Projectile vomiting and visual disturbance are common. One-fourth of all victims with lead encephalopathy will not survive. Up to 40% of survivors experience severe neurologic dysfunction (74,79). Low-level lead exposure has led to deficits in gross- and fine-motor development, as well as intel-lectual and academic deficits up to 10 years later (9,19).

Lead sulfide may deposit as a thin line along the gingival margin. This line appears blue to black and is called a *Burtonian* line. It is characteristic of chronic lead poisoning. A similar discoloration of the gums along a line just above the teeth may also be caused by chronic accumulation of other metals, such as silver, iron, or mercury.

Management of Poisoning

The Centers for Disease Control established guidelines for the standardization of lead intoxication (12). These guidelines are presented in Table 9.11.

New data indicate significant adverse effects of lead exposure in children at blood lead concentrations previously believed to be safe. Some adverse health effects have been shown to occur at 10 μg of lead per dL of blood. For 1985, the intervention blood lead concentration of concern was reduced to 25 μg/dL. In years to come, this intervention value will likely be lowered to 10 μg/dL. Blood lead concentrations of less than 10 μg/dL are not considered to be indicative of poisoning, whereas concentrations between 20 and 69 μg/dL require a complete medical evaluation. Blood lead concentrations greater than 45 μg/dL probably will require chelation therapy. See Table 9.11 for a description of the appropriate action required for children.

The erythrocyte protoporphyrin (EP) test measures the amount of erythrocyte protoporphyrin in whole blood; results greater than 35 μg/dL are considered abnormal. Lead inhibits ferrochelatase in the final step of heme synthesis and prevents the insertion of iron into protoporphyrin IX (Fig. 9.5). Inhibition of these steps results in the accumulation of free erythrocyte protoporphyrin (FEP) in red blood cells, with zinc generally occupying the position normally taken by iron. The resulting complex is referred to as zinc protoporphyrin (ZnPP). Analytical methods are available to measure zinc protoporphyrin by direct fluo-

TABLE 9.11. *Children grouped by class and recommended action according to blood lead measurement*

Class	Blood lead concentration (μg/dL)	Action
I	<9	Low risk for high-dose exposure; a child in Class I is not considered to be lead poisoned.
IIA	10–14	High risk for high-dose exposure; rescreen. If many children in the community have blood lead concentrations of 10 or higher, community interventions (primary prevention activities) should be considered by appropriate agencies.
IIB	15–19	Take a history to assess possible high-dose sources of lead. Educate parents about diet, cleaning, etc. Test for iron deficiency. Consider environmental investigation and lead hazard abatement if levels persist.
III	20–44[a]	Conduct a complete medical evaluation. Identify and eliminate environmental lead sources. Such a child may need pharmacologic treatment.
IV	45–69[a]	Begin medical treatment including chelation therapy, and environmental assessment and remediation within 48 hr.
V	70+[a]	Begin medical treatment and environmental assessment and remediation IMMEDIATELY. A child with Class V is a medical emergency.

[a] Based on confirmatory blood lead concentration.

rescence or free erythrocyte protoporphyrin extracted from RBCs by fluorometry. Results are reported in EP equivalents.

An elevated EP can be caused by lead absorption or iron deficiency. The EP test is a more sensitive indicator of iron status than of elevated blood lead. The combination of a blood lead test and an EP test is required in screening children for potential toxic lead exposure (66,94).

For blood lead concentrations of 25 to 44 μg/dL, a CaNa$_2$-EDTA mobilization test can be performed to assess lead stores and the necessity for subsequent treatment (58,69). An abnormal or increased blood lead concentration in urine after administration of CaNa$_2$-EDTA is a very good predictor of a significant risk of lead toxicity.

A variety of chelators are used in treatment of lead poisoning. These drugs are capable of chelating lead from blood, soft tissues and bone, reducing its acute toxicity (69).

Chelation therapy is advised for patients in groups III and IV (see Table 9.11) according to the CDC guidelines, including asymptomatic children. Symptomatic plumbism (colic, seizures, acute encephalopathy) is usually associated with blood lead concentrations greater than 70 μg/dL, and chelation therapy should be administered promptly.

Calcium disodium EDTA is the drug of choice for acute and chronic lead poisoning and lead encephalopathy. Calcium disodium EDTA increases urinary lead excretion by 20- to 50-fold. Calcium disodium EDTA removes lead from the extracellular compartment of soft tissue only (62). Use of CaNa$_2$-EDTA should continue no more than 5 days and be followed by a rest period of at least 5 days to allow recovery of zinc depletion. It should be used in conjunction with dimercaprol (BAL) when blood lead concentrations are greater than 70 μg/dL, since use of CaNa$_2$-EDTA alone may aggravate symptoms in patients with very high blood lead concentrations (69).

Dimercaprol chelates lead intracellularly and extracellularly. Two molecules of dimercaprol combine with one atom of lead to form a stable complex that is excreted in urine.

Until the recent approval of succimer, D-penicillamine was the only commercially available oral chelating agent. The FDA has approved its use for treatment of Wilson's disease, cystinuria, and severe, active rheumatoid

TABLE 9.12. *Chelation therapy in lead poisoning*

Type	Blood lead concentration ($\mu g/dL$)	Action
Asymptomatic lead poisoning	70+	BAL and CaNa$_2$-EDTA
	45–69	CaNa$_2$-EDTA for 3–5 days
	25–44	CaNa$_2$-EDTA mobilization test
	20–24	No chelation
Symptomatic lead poisoning	70+	BAL and CaNa$_2$-EDTA
	45–69	CaNa$_2$-EDTA and penicillamine succimer

arthritis. It is used by some for the treatment of lead poisoning. Although D-penicillamine is not as effective as CaNa$_2$-EDTA in enhancing urinary lead excretion, it has been used with blood lead concentrations less than 45 $\mu g/dL$. One advantage is that it can be given over a long period (weeks to months). Adverse effects to D-penicillamine occur at a rate of 33% (76). The use of chelation therapy in lead poisoning is summarized in Table 9.12.

MERCURY

Mercury compounds are divided into three chemical classes: elemental mercury (quicksilver, mercury vapor, Hg^0), inorganic mercury salts, and organic mercury salts. Inorganic mercury salts exist either in the mercurous (Hg^{1+}) or mercuric (Hg^{2+}) state. Mercuric salts are more toxic. Aryl, alkyl, and alkoxyalkyl mercury compounds represent the organic mercury compounds that are of greatest toxicologic significance.

Through the years mercury has been used in medicine, agriculture, and industry. Medicinal uses to treat syphilis originated as early as 1500 A.D. Calomel (mercurous chloride) was used as a cathartic until a few decades ago. Organic mercury compounds, used for a number of years as diuretics, have been replaced by safer, more effective nonmercurial diuretics. An amalgam of mercury is used in dentistry.

Mercury is popular in agriculture because of its ability to counteract fungi and mold growth. It, therefore, has been widely used to prevent grain spoilage. A serious outbreak of mercury poisoning occurred in the early 1970s when grain treated with methyl mercury was inadvertently mixed with flour and consumed. Over 500 people died in Iraq (6).

Elemental mercury vapor is the most volatile of all mercury compounds. Intoxication of mercury vapor is mainly an occupational problem, usually from chronic exposure. Elemental mercury has a high vapor pressure. At a saturated atmosphere at 20°C, approximately 15 mg mercury vapor is present per m^3; at 24°C, 18 mg/m^3, and at 40°C, 80 mg/m^3 is present. Exposure to an atmosphere of 0.7 mg/m^3 for 5 hr/day is associated with symptoms of mercury poisoning (40,61). One of the case studies at the end of this chapter illustrates this principle very well.

Suicide attempts by injecting elemental mercury have been documented (1,41). Elemental mercury is nontoxic when ingested due to lack of absorption but can be toxic when introduced subcutaneously (82). Toxic mercury salts may form and enter the blood to cause dangerously high concentrations.

Inorganic mercury salts exist in two oxidation states. Mercurous salts include mercurous chloride (Hg$_2$Cl$_2$) and mercuric chloride (HgCl$_2$, corrosive sublimate), formerly used as an antiseptic. Mercuric chloride is still widely used in industry. Mercuric nitrate was commonly used in the felt hat industry, and occupational exposure has been associated with neurologic changes. In fact, the phrase *mad as a hatter* describes symptoms characteristic of chronic exposure to mercury. One wonders if Lewis Carroll knew a real-life hatter after whom he patterned the character in *Alice's Adventures in Wonderland*.

Differences in toxicity among organic mercurials are due to ease of dissociation between the organic moiety and the anion attached. Alkyl mercury salts are of greatest toxicologic importance because they are incorporated into the food chain. The most toxic of all alkyl mercurials is methyl mercury. Characteristic and usually irreversible CNS damage has been associated with methyl mercury exposure (61,68).

Mechanism of Toxicity

Mercury ions produce toxic effects by protein precipitation, enzyme inhibition, and generalized corrosive action. Mercury binds to sulfhydryl groups, as well as to phosphoryl, carboxyl, amide, and amine functional groups. Mercury also reacts with several enzymes and other proteins that contain these functional groups. Thus, mercury interferes with cellular enzyme reactions.

The toxic effects produced by various compounds of mercury are functions of their chemical form, route of administration, and duration of exposure. For example, it was mentioned previously that mercuric salts are more toxic than mercurous salts. This is partly because divalent inorganic mercury compounds (e.g., $HgCl_2$) are more soluble than are monovalent mercury compounds (e.g., Hg_2Cl_2). Therefore, when ingested, $HgCl_2$ will be more rapidly absorbed and thus produce greater toxicity.

On the other hand, at least 90% of a methyl mercury ingestion is absorbed from the GI tract, compared to about 10% with the soluble inorganic salts. Organic mercurials are less corrosive to intestinal mucosa than are inorganic compounds such as mercuric chloride. The organic mercurials also cross the blood-brain barrier and placenta and cause neurologic and teratogenic disorders more readily than do inorganic salts (59).

Elemental mercury vapor presents unique toxicologic problems. There are two important properties of elemental mercury that make it a potential health hazard. First, it crosses cell membranes with little difficulty because of its high lipid solubility. Second, elemental mercury is easily oxidized to the mercuric form. Chronic exposure to mercury produces significant toxic effects to two separate organ systems (16).

To illustrate, in mercurialism due to chronic inhalation of mercury vapor, mercury preferentially attacks the CNS (45). Chronic exposure to inorganic mercury compounds leads to renal complications. Again, this difference can be explained on the basis of high lipid solubility. After elemental mercury has rapidly accumulated in the brain, it oxidizes to the mercuric form, and the expected reactions occur.

Independent of the chemical form of mercury, two major target organs affected are the CNS and kidney. Central nervous system specificity is characteristic of elemental mercury vapor and short-chain alkyl mercury compounds. When they enter the CNS, degenerative changes occur from the action of mercury on structural proteins and enzyme systems. Synaptic and neuromuscular transmission is blocked.

Although the kidney is the principal target organ for inorganic mercurials, all mercury compounds concentrate in the kidney to some extent. Inorganic compounds, however, produce the majority of toxic renal effects.

Characteristics of Poisoning

Signs and symptoms are qualitatively and quantitatively dependent on the chemical structure of the compound, amount and duration of exposure, and individual sensitivity to the particular compound. Table 9.13 lists clinical manifestations according to the chemical form encountered.

Prolonged exposure to mercury vapor at concentrations greater than 100 mg/m^3 results in insidious onset of symptoms. Anorexia, weight loss, fatigue, and muscular weakness are some nonspecific clinical manifestations of chronic exposure. Chronic mercury toxicity is evidenced by a variety of neurologic and behavioral problems due to accumulation of mercury in the cerebral and cerebellar cortex (17).

TABLE 9.13. *Characteristics of mercury poisoning*

Characteristic	Elemental	Inorganic	Organomercurial
Primary route of exposure	Inhalation	Oral	Oral, food chain
Target organ	CNS, kidney	Kidney	CNS, liver
Clinical manifestations			
Local			
Lungs	Bronchial irritation	—	—
	Pneumonitis		—
GI tract	Metallic taste	Metallic taste	—
	Stomatitis	Stomatitis	—
	Gingivitis	Gastroenteritis	—
	Excessive salivation	—	—
Skin	—	Urticaria	—
	—	Vesication	—
Systemic			
CNS	Erethism	—	Ataxia, chorea, athetosis, tremor
	Tremors	—	Convulsions, paresthesia, erethism
Kidney	Tubular necrosis	Tubular necrosis	—
Treatment	BAL	BAL	Chelators are not effective
	CaNa$_2$-EDTA		
	Penicillamine		
Biologic half-life	10−15 days	65−70 days	70−90 days

GI, gastrointestinal; CNS, central nervous system.

Fine muscle tremors are among the early signs of mercurialism. Tremor usually begins in the eyes, tongue, or fingers, with progression to an entire limb. Handwriting suffers severely and can be used as a qualitative measurement of the success of treatment. The magnitude of tremors may also affect the facial muscles, resulting in slurred speech. In extreme cases, there can be generalized tremor involving the entire body.

The emotional state of the individual who has been repeatedly exposed to mercury is also altered. Sudden attacks of anger, increasing irritability, loss of memory, and drowsiness occur. The person loses interest in life and withdraws from society. The syndrome is referred to as *erethism,* with the origin of the word based on the blushing and sweating that also occurs.

At one time, mercuric chloride was available as a blue coffin-shaped tablet with the skull and crossbones depicted on one side and the inscription POISON on the other (Fig. 9.6). Despite obvious warnings, the tablets were commonly ingested, usually accidentally. A 0.5-g tablet dissolved in water and swallowed will produce immediate corrosive injury to the mucosa of the mouth, throat, esophagus, and stomach. As a result the mouth, pharynx, and gastric mucosa appear ashen and are severely painful. If a large quantity of an inorganic salt is ingested, intense epigastric pain, profuse vomiting of mucoid material, bloody diarrhea, circulatory collapse, shock, and sudden death may occur. A metallic taste is usually present.

Organomercuric compounds are classed into two separate groups, based on chemical structure and relative toxicity. These groups are the long-chained aryl mercury compounds and short-chained alkyl mercury compounds. The group that poses the greater hazard to humans is the short-chained alkyl compounds such as methyl mercury. These are more hazardous because they possess greater inherent toxicity and because they are a major threat to the environment (21).

The alkyl mercury compounds are almost completely absorbed from the GI tract; distributed to the brain, liver, and kidney; and excreted primarily in the feces. The aryl mercury compounds are excreted as mercuric ions.

Differences between acute and chronic toxicity are minimal. A characteristic feature is that symptoms may occur weeks to months after an acute exposure. Neurologic manifestations of organic mercury poisoning are due to toxic effects on the cerebellum and can lead

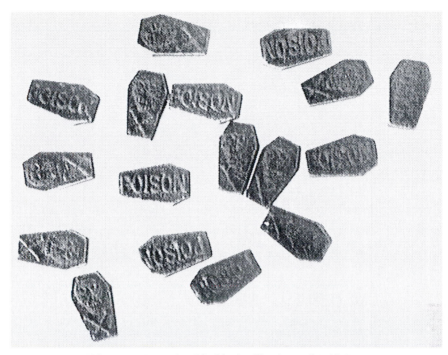

FIG. 9.6. Mercuric chloride (coffin-shaped) tablets.

to ataxia, tremors, unsteady gait, and difficulty in maintaining equilibrium. Simple tasks, such as buttoning a shirt, become difficult to perform. Illegible handwriting and slurred speech are noted also. Sensory involvement includes paresthesia of the lips, hands, and feet, as well as visual and hearing impairment. Emotional disturbances and erethism are also manifestations of organic mercury poisoning. If poisoning is severe, symptoms may not be reversible.

Organic aryl mercury poisonings are rare. When they occur, poisonings show signs of gastrointestinal and renal toxicity because these compounds are metabolized to mercuric ions.

The biologic half-life of methyl mercury is approximately 70 to 90 days. Elimination is slow and irregular, and accumulation can easily produce toxicity. Mercury concentrations in the blood at about 10 to 20 μg/dL are usually not associated with toxic symptoms, but blood concentrations around 50 to 100 μg/dL are considered toxic.

Management of Poisoning

Choice of treatment depends on the form of mercury involved. Mild exposure to mercury vapor may require only that the victim be removed from the source of the vapor. In the case of acute oral inorganic mercury poisoning, the initial concern is removal of mercury from the GI tract. A considerable amount of mercuric chloride can be removed by spontaneous or ipecac-induced emesis or gastric lavage. This can be followed with a generous slurry of activated charcoal and a cathartic. Shock, due to peripheral vascular collapse, can be treated with fluid replacement.

The most effective means to eliminate inorganic mercury for both chronic and acute poisoning is with chelators. A chelator is indicated in all mercury poisonings except alkyl mercuric compounds. The choices include dimercaprol, penicillamine, and its *N*-acetyl derivative, *N*-acetylpenicillamine (78). Calcium disodium EDTA should not be used because it binds poorly to mercury and is potentially nephrotoxic.

Dimercaprol is indicated as the chelator of choice in severe inorganic mercuric salt poisonings, in which the critical target organ is the kidney, but its effectiveness in elemental and organic mercury poisoning is doubtful.

It is much less effective in chronic mercury poisoning, also. Dimercaprol is maximally effective when given early. It enhances the renal excretion of mercury, which may aggravate mercury-induced renal damage, and should be used with caution in patients with acute renal insufficiency.

OTHER METALS

In addition to the metals already discussed, several others occasionally cause toxic reactions. They are discussed in this chapter. An additional metal, thallium, was discussed in chapter 8.

Copper

Copper occurs throughout nature in a variety of salt forms and as the pure metal. It is widely used in industry and at home as metallic copper in electrical wiring and components. Copper sulfate is added to farm ponds and swimming pools as an algicide. It is also occasionally recommended for use as an emetic, although this use is outmoded and dangerous. Death has resulted from the ingestion of 10 g.

Poisoning usually results from acute oral ingestion of a copper salt, such as copper sulfate. It has also resulted from repeated washing of burned skin with copper sulfate (44).

Although not a form of poisoning in the true sense, patients with Wilson's disease have abnormally high blood copper concentrations. An inborn error of metabolism, Wilson's disease is a hereditary disorder in which ceruloplasmin is decreased. Ceruloplasmin is one of the plasma alpha-globulins that normally transports copper through the body. Wilson's disease is an uncommon disorder resulting in accumulation of copper in the CNS, which destroys nerve cells in the putamen, caudate nucleus, and cerebral cortex. The neurologic syndrome consists of tremors of the extremities, muscle rigidity, choreoathetoid movements, and personality changes progressing to dementia. Centrilobular hepatic necrosis de-

velops, producing cirrhosis with ascites, edema, and progressive hepatic failure. Also, a golden-brown ring of accumulated copper is deposited on the cornea and is known as Kayser-Fleischer rings. They are present in 50% of patients with Wilson's disease. Although Wilson's disease is incurable, therapy with chelating agents can control copper concentrations so that the patient can lead a nearly normal life.

Characteristics of Poisoning

After ingestion of an excessive dose of copper, victims experience severe nausea with vomiting, bloody vomitus and stool, diarrhea, hypotension, and jaundice (Table 9.14). Repeated exposures have been associated with hemolytic anemia (57). Death usually occurs within 24 hr, preceded by coma. If there are hepatic or renal complications, death may be hastened.

Management of Poisoning

The most effective medical means to manage copper poisoning is with penicillamine. This chelator is also widely used in treating patients with Wilson's disease and certain other diseases such as rheumatoid arthritis.

TABLE 9.14. *Characteristics of copper toxicity*

Acute exposure
  Nausea, vomiting
  Bloody diarrhea
  Hypotension
  Hemolytic anemia
  Uremia
  Cardiovascular collapse
Chronic exposure
  Sporadic fever
  Vomiting
  Epigastric pain
  Diarrhea
  Jaundice
Inhalation
  Ulceration and perforation of nasal septum
  Necrotic hepatitis

Selenium

Selenium is produced mainly as a by-product of copper refining. Although technically not a metal from a purist's standpoint, it possesses metallic characteristics. It has a variety of industrial applications, including use in the electronics, glass, and paint industries. Selenium is a vulcanizing agent for rubber. Selenious acid is a gun bluing agent. Selenium is used as a drench for sheep and cattle, and selenium sulfide is employed as a shampoo for dandruff control. Aside from causing irritation to the eyes or mucous membranes, this latter form of selenium is nontoxic. More recently, selenium has been widely promoted as a nutritional element and food additive. It is because of these uses that contemporary interest in potential selenium toxicity has emerged.

Mechanism of Toxicity

The precise mechanism of toxicity is not understood. Selenium has a high affinity for thiol groups (20). It may thus inhibit certain sulfhydryl-containing enzymes.

Characteristics of Poisoning

Acute poisoning causes a variety of gastrointestinal and CNS effects (Table 9.15). Nervousness, drowsiness, and convulsions are common. The bizarre behavior experienced when horses grazed on *loco weed* in western movies of the 1930s and 1940s may be attributed to selenium at 15,000 ppm or more (89). This plant concentrates selenium. A fatal case of poisoning from ingestion of gun bluing showed widespread focal hemorrhages and edema. Death is usually due to depression of the respiratory or cardiovascular centers.

Chronic poisoning may induce pallor, a *garlic* breath, metallic taste, liver and spleen damage, and anemia, in addition to gastrointestinal and CNS effects. Fatty necrosis of the liver is a frequent finding. Selenium is believed to be teratogenic in humans (72), and it may be carcinogenic.

Management of Poisoning

Treatment of poisoning by ingestion or inhalation includes symptomatic and supportive care. Influenza-like symptoms may be controlled with salicylates. The individual must be immediately removed from inhalation exposure. Contaminated skin and eyes should be thoroughly rinsed.

Zinc

Zinc is widely used in industry in the galvanizing processes, in paints, and as $ZnCl_2$ for preserving wood. Zinc is an essential trace element, necessary for enzyme reactions, protein synthesis, and carbohydrate metabolism. It is a component of numerous enzymes, including alcohol dehydrogenase, carbonic anhydrase, carboxypeptidase, and lactic dehydrogenase.

Over the years, various zinc salts have been used in medicinal preparations as a topical astringent, antiseptic, and antifungal agent.

Characteristics of Poisoning

Poisoning occurs most commonly by inhalation of zinc oxide fumes or ingestion of one

TABLE 9.15. *Characteristics of selenium toxicity (selenosis)*

Acute exposure
  Nervousness
  Drowsiness
  Fever
  Vomiting
  Decreased blood pressure
  Convulsions
  Death due to respiratory or cardiovascular failure
Chronic exposure
  Depression
  Garlic-like odor on breath
  Pallor
  Loss of nails and hair
  Hemolytic anemia
  Liver and spleen damage
  May be teratogenic and carcinogenic
Inhalation
  Chemical pneumonitis

TABLE 9.16. *Characteristics of zinc toxicity*

Oral
 Lassitude
 Enteritis
 Diarrhea (bloody, watery)
 Intense abdominal pain
 CNS depression
 Tremors
Inhalation
 "Fume fever"—sudden onset of thirst,
  fever, chills, myalgias, and headaches

of the salts. A syndrome known as *metal fume fever* results from inhalation of fumes of zinc oxide produced when zinc is heated to high temperatures, such as during welding, metal cutting, or smelting zinc alloys. Victims complain of nausea and vomiting, chills and fever, muscular aches and pains, and weakness (Table 9.16). Zinc chloride fumes have caused fatalities, with death from pulmonary edema. Although metal fume fever may occur from heating other metals, it is most common with zinc.

Management of Poisoning

Treatment of poisoning includes immediate removal of the victim from the source of poisoning. The victim is treated symptomatically. Salicylates help control influenza-like symptoms. Corticosteroids are useful in management of pulmonary edema.

SUMMARY

The clinical characteristics of poisoning with individual metals are classic and often predictable. Management is directed at minimizing gastrointestinal absorption, providing symptomatic and supportive care, and applying specific chelating antidotes.

Case Studies

CASE STUDY: ACUTE ARSENIC EXPOSURE

History

When found in her backyard, a 16-month-old, 10-kg girl was holding a wafer from a package of Grant's Ant Control. Her face had traces of a gel-like substance around the mouth. Her parents washed her hands and face. Approximately 30 min later, the child began to vomit and experienced a watery bowel movement.

She was rushed to a local emergency facility and given 15 mL of syrup of ipecac, which provoked further vomiting. After a bout of copious emesis, she was given 20 g of activated charcoal and 2.5 g of sodium sulfate. A short while later, the child became lethargic and had three rice-water stools. At this point she was transported to a larger medical facility for further care.

It was later estimated that she ingested 2 to 3 g of ant killer, resulting in consumption of 9 to 14 mg of arsenic trioxide. Because of the severity of symptoms, it was assumed she had swallowed a toxic dose.

While she was being transported, she was given 25 mg BAL intramuscularly. She presented with a pulse that varied between 130 and 156 beats/min. Blood pressure was 110/55 mm Hg; respirations, 36/min; and rectal temperature, 36.7°C. Arterial blood gases, electrolytes, and renal and liver function tests were all within normal limits. A total of 185 mg of BAL was administered over 18 hr. This was followed by 250 mg of penicillamine every 6 hr for 5 days.

A charcoal stool was passed about 22 hr postingestion. During her hospital stay, there were no seizures, arrhythmias, vomiting, watery diarrhea, or changes in laboratory values. .

The patient was released from the hospital on her 3rd day. Penicillamine treatment was continued by her private physician for 5 days. Her arsenic blood concentration on admission was in excess of 7 μg/dL and on the 2nd day had decreased to approximately 2 μg/dL. (See ref. 88.)

Discussion

1. With the exception of some early gastrointestinal symptoms, this young patient did not experience many of the symptoms

listed in Table 9.5. What are some possible reasons for this omission?

2. Why was penicillamine initiated and BAL discontinued?
3. Was the initial blood arsenic concentration suggestive of a mild, moderate, or severe toxic exposure?
4. Compare the toxic effects produced by arsenic trioxide with arsenic pentaoxide.
5. What is the significance of knowing that a charcoal stool was passed?

CASE STUDY: CADMIUM FUME POISONING

History

A 25-year-old male sailor was cleaning the sanitary tank (approximately 428 ft³) of a submarine. The job required heating a pipe joint that had been brazed previously with a cadmium-containing grade of silver braze alloy. After heating the joint he began coughing. He discontinued his work and left the area. He had worked about 8 min in the confined area.

The coughing ceased upon exposure to fresh air, but he experienced a mild sore throat and dyspnea, which rapidly improved. Dyspnea and cough reappeared 4 hr later, and his cough worsened, forcing him to report to the sick bay the following morning.

The patient presented with moderate respiratory distress. Auscultation of the chest revealed bilateral rales over the posterior aspect of the thorax. Vital signs were blood pressure, 130/80 mm Hg; pulse, 120/min; and respirations (shallow), 40/min. A chest X-ray film revealed a diffuse, bilateral infiltrate in the lungs, indicating pulmonary edema.

Treatment consisted of furosemide and dexamethasone. The patient recovered completely within 2 days. No arrhythmias were noted. He was discharged 2 days later and returned to full duty. (See ref. 85.)

Discussion

1. In this case study, there was an asymptomatic period after initial pulmonary irrita-tion. Is this typical of cadmium intoxication?
2. Is chelation therapy indicated for most acute cadmium exposures?
3. Would the clinical manifestations presented by this patient have been different if the route of exposure was by ingestion?
4. Explain why furosemide and dexamethasone were given.

CASE STUDIES: IRON POISONING

History: Case 1

A 19-year-old woman ingested 50 to 60 ferrous sulfate tablets, representing 9.8 to 11.7 g elemental iron. Within 1 hr she developed abdominal cramping and vomited a dark brown liquid. She later indicated that there were no tablet fragments in the vomitus. Over the next several hours, she vomited bright red blood. She was admitted to a hospital approximately 8 hr postingestion.

On admission she appeared slightly intoxicated but was not in acute distress. Vitals included blood pressure, 110/80 mm Hg; pulse, 80 beats/min; respirations, 16/min; and oral temperature, 37°C. Neurologic examination was normal. Physical examination revealed slight epigastric tenderness. There were no masses or organomegaly. Bowel sounds were normal. Laboratory values are shown in Table 9.17.

The patient underwent gastric lavage with 5% sodium bicarbonate and normal saline for approximately 1 hr. The return was blood tinged; no tablet fragments were recovered.

TABLE 9.17. *Laboratory values*

Na⁺	=142 mEq/L
K⁺	=3.4 mEq/L
Cl⁻	=116 mEq/L
pH	=7.34
Hematocrit	=34.2%
Hemoglobin	=11.3 g/dL
Prothrombin time	=normal
Partial thromboplastin time	=normal
Blood glucose	=223 mg/dL
Blood ethanol	=225 mg/dL
Serum iron	=915 μg/dL

Deferoxamine therapy (15 mg/kg/hr intravenously) was initiated approximately 1 hr after admission and was continued for 4 hr. A red-tinged urine was noted within 2 hr of initiating the chelator. After checking the literature to assure that continued therapy with deferoxamine was safe, therapy was reinstituted and continued for a total period of 52 hr.

Over this period the patient experienced a low-grade fever. She had no change in vital signs or renal function and displayed no other difficulties. She was discharged after 5 days of hospitalization with no sequelae. She did not return for follow-up. (See ref. 65.)

History: Case 2

In a suicide attempt, a 17-year-old pregnant girl ingested 90 ferrous sulfate capsules (325 mg each). On admission to an emergency department 30 min later, physical examination revealed no strikingly abnormal values, and vital signs were all within normal limits.

Vomiting was induced with 30 mL of syrup of ipecac. The vomitus contained many partially digested iron capsules. An unprovoked emesis resulted about 4 hr later. This was followed by diarrhea. Both were positive for blood. Physical examination was still unremarkable, except for hypoactive bowel sounds. About 12 hr after admission, the patient began vomiting bloody material.

Laboratory results revealed hypoglycemia, metabolic acidosis, bleeding tendencies, and renal dysfunction. She had tachycardia and eventually developed renal impairment.

Treatment consisted of fluids, dextrose, sodium bicarbonate, and diuretics. Deferoxamine was not given because the patient was pregnant and had renal failure. Instead, she underwent an exchange transfusion 30 min after admission, after which she spontaneously aborted a 16-week fetus.

Her condition became progressively worse. In addition to hypotension, hypoglycemia, and clotting deficiency, she became febrile (105°F), tachypneic, and cyanotic. She contin-

ued vomiting dark brown material and experienced a seizure 74 hr after admission. She was intubated and given a pressor agent because of progressively decreasing blood pressure, but she died 80 hr after admission.

It was later reported that the victim did not mean to commit suicide. She intended only to draw attention to herself. (See ref. 56.)

Discussion

1. Identify which lab results for patient 1 (Table 9.17) are not within the normal ranges and cite reasons for each of these discrepencies.
2. A red-colored urine was noted within 2 hr of the initiation of deferoxamine treatment in patient 1. What does this color indicate and how long will the color of the urine remain affected?
3. Based on your knowledge of the organ specific toxicity of ferrous sulfate, what pathologic findings would you expect from an autopsy of patient 2?
4. Comment on the production of hypoglycemia with iron poisoning. Is it a common characteristic of iron toxicity? Why do you think it occurred in patient 2?
5. What led to the death of patient 2? What caused the fetus to abort?
6. Did patients 1 and 2 exhibit all five clinical phases of toxicity?

CASE STUDIES: INTOXICATION WITH LEAD

History: Case 1

A 3-year-old girl was brought to the emergency facility by her parents after they tried unsuccessfully to awaken her. Her father had noticed over the past 2 days that she was lethargic, easily fatigued, and sleepy. Her personality had changed, and she complained of abdominal pains and headaches.

She had been given acetaminophen 3 times daily for aches and pains. The previous day she had vomited 3 times. Her dietary intake had been restricted to orange juice, which was one of her favorite beverages. The family suspected that the little girl had picked up some kind of a virus while vacationing, causing flu-like symptoms.

When responding to a physician's questioning to obtain a complete history, the father remembered that his daughter had taken a special interest in a pink funny-faced Indian mug. Whenever she drank liquids she used this particular mug. She drank at least five to six mugfuls of orange juice per day.

The girl was admitted with a pulse of 80 beats/min; temperature, 101°F; and blood pressure, 130/90 mm Hg. She was in lighter stages of coma and able to awaken on verbal commands. Physical examination revealed questionable blurring of the optic disc and hyperactive reflexes.

Laboratory values showed a hemoglobin content of 12 g/dL, hematocrit of 38%, and mean corpuscular volume of 78. Her WBC count was 8,000 cells/mm^3; the differential count showed 60% leukocytes, 35% polys, 3% eosinophils, and 2% mononucleocytes. The free erythrocytic protoporphyrin concentration was 300 μg/dL. Lead poisoning was the diagnosis at this point.

The patient received treatment with CaNa$_2$-EDTA and improved with time. She was discharged without apparent sequelae. (See ref. 64.)

History: Case 2

A 59-year-old woman was admitted to the hospital with diffuse pains and anemia. About

1 year previously, she had injured her back. She had been treated with acupuncture by an herbalist-chiropractor on two separate occasions. She was given two herbal products to be ingested daily.

A few months after initiating therapy, she had begun to complain of pain in her knees, hips, and abdomen. Also, she became unusually irritable and could not sleep well. It was difficult for her to hold objects in her hands, and she often felt constipated.

On admission, the laboratory results shown in Table 9.18 were obtained. Symptoms and laboratory values suggested lead poisoning. Her husband's blood and urine showed lead levels within normal limits. The herbal pills were therefore suspected to be a possible source. They were analyzed and found to contain 0.5 mg of lead. She had ingested 30 pills per day for 2 to 3 months. Therefore, she had a daily lead intake of 15 mg.

The patient was started on CaNa$_2$-EDTA at 2 g/24 hr intravenously, along with intravenous fluids. Marked reduction in symptoms occurred within 24 hr. She was also given antibiotics, chlordiazepoxide for anxiety, and vitamins. Her improvement was remarkable and quick. After the 1st day of treatment, blood lead concentration decreased to 70 μg/dL. She was released after 10 days. (See ref. 47.)

History: Case 3

A 23-year-old male amateur painter was admitted to the hospital after experiencing violent

TABLE 9.18. *Signs and symptoms in a patient poisoned with lead*

	Results	Normal[c]
Hematocrit	27%	36–42%
Reticulocyte count	5.6%	0.5–2.0%
Blood iron	98 μg%	80–160 μg%
Total iron-binding capacity	260 μg%	250–350 μg%
RBC[a] (protoporphyrin)	403 μg%	40–100 μg%
Urine delta-ALA[b] (24 hr)	51.9 mg	1.5–7.5 mg
Urine lead (24 hr)	0.281 mg	<0.100 mg
Blood lead	90 μg%	<60 μg%
Peripheral blood smears showed marked basophilic stippling		

From ref. 47.
[a] RBC, red blood cells.
[b] ALA, aminolevulinic acid.
[c] Reflects 1977 standards.

abdominal cramps. The only physical findings were facial pallor and mild icterus. Laboratory findings shown in Table 9.19 were obtained.

At the time of admission, the source of his intoxication was not established, and the patient denied exposure to lead. Treatment was initiated with $CaNa_2$-EDTA and continued over the next 50 days. Chelation therapy caused reversal of his abdominal colic and hyperbilirubinemia within 2 weeks. Thirty days after the final $CaNa_2$-EDTA treatment, laboratory values were again obtained.

The patient finally identified the source of lead exposure. He had ingested about 15 g of lead white (basic lead carbonate) within a month. His intent was to produce hallucinations so that he could be more artistically creative. (See ref. 13.)

History: Case 4

The patient was a 63-year-old timber cutter living in a rural environment, who had been admitted to the hospital because of recurrent painful abdominal colic of 4 months' duration. Although the laboratory tests on admission suggested lead poisoning (basophilic stippling of some erythrocytes), at that time this diagnosis had been rejected as being incompatible with the man's work. Because of the onset of

TABLE 9.19. *Signs and symptoms in a patient poisoned with lead*

On admission	
Hematocrit	25.5%
Hemoglobin	8.9 g%
RBC count	288×10^4 cells/mm³
Total bilirubin	4.3 mg%
Indirect bilirubin	2.7 mg%
Serum iron	205 µg%
Total iron-binding capacity	86%
Urine delta-ALA	144 mg/day
Urine coproporphyrin	1,800 µg%
Serum lead	112 µg%
30 days after final $CaNa_2$-EDTA treatment	
Urine delta-ALA	1.9–3.9 mg/day
Urine coproporphyrin	60–140 µg/day
Serum lead	47 µg%
Serum iron	67 µg%

From ref. 13.

severe weakness in the upper and lower limbs on both sides, he was referred to the neurology department.

Neurologic examination disclosed marked weakness, mainly affecting the limb girdle, extensors of the hands and fingers, and extensors of the feet and toes. Deep tendon reflexes were absent. Clinical examination revealed no sensory impairment. Neurophysiologic studies demonstrated severe axonal damage in the sensory and motor fibers of the median, radial, common peroneal, and sural nerves and severe denervation of the deltoid, biceps, abductor pollicis brevis, and tibialis anterior muscles. Laboratory investigations revealed the following: moderate normochromic, normocytic anemia (hemoglobin, 10.7 g/dL; mean corpuscular volume, 90 fL) with basophilic stippling of some erythrocytes, increased reticulocytes (180,000/mm³), indirect hyperbilirubinemia, negative direct and indirect Coombs' test results, and erythroblastic hyperplasia on bone marrow examination; altered porphyrin metabolism and abnormal lead concentrations in urine and blood, with or without chelating agents (Table 9.20); normal cerebrospinal fluid levels of proteins, glucose, immunoglobulins, and cellularity. Nerve biopsy showed axonal degeneration with segmental demyelination secondary to axonal damage.

The patient underwent a chelating course with slight improvement in the laboratory data. Nevertheless, his clinical picture worsened and was complicated by respiratory failure. Despite respiratory assistance, the patient died 14 days later.

The blood lead content of persons living in the same building was within the normal range, and no water pollution was detected. These results suggested a poisoning source within the household environment, to which only the woodcutter was exposed. Tests revealed lead contamination in a batch of home-produced wine. The source of pollution was finally identified as the container used for storing the wine, which was lined with lead-glaze ceramic tiles. (See ref. 2)

TABLE 9.20. *Lead and porphyrin concentrations in a woodcutter with wine lead poisoning*

Measurement	On admission	After 1 week of therapy
In blood		
Lead (μg/dL)	130	—
Zinc protoporphyrin (μg/dL)	335	—
Total porphyrins (μg/24 hr)	1,554	125
In urine		
Lead (μg/dL)	67	4,700
Coproporphyrins (μg/24 hr)	543	78
Uroporphyrins (μg/24 hr)	1,011	47
Porphobilinogen (mg/dL)	0.40	0.04
Urinary aminolevulinic acid (mg/dL)	10	0.7
In wine	61	
Lead in red wine (ppm)	20	
Lead in white wine (ppm)		

From ref. 2.

Discussion

1. The preceding case studies deal with a variety of sources of lead exposure. What clinical findings are common to all three cases?
2. In case 1, what role do you think the orange juice that the little girl drank, played in the lead exposure?
3. In case 3, which laboratory tests were indicative of jaundice? Is lead poisoning usually associated with hepatotoxicity?
4. Is CaNa$_2$-EDTA the only chelator used for lead toxicity? If not, what others could be used? Note the blood lead concentration in these cases. How do they compare to the new guidelines for chelator therapy in lead poisoning?

CASE STUDY: MERCURY POISONING

History

A 49-year-old, somnolent woman ingested 125 g of a fungicide containing 3.5% methoxyethylmercury chloride in a suicide attempt. She vomited a blue liquid. She presented with no outstanding physical signs or symptoms related to the corrosive nature of mercury poisoning.

Two hours after ingestion she was admitted to an emergency facility where she was intubated and gastric lavage was performed. Forced diuresis was initiated. Two hours after ingestion, charcoal hemoperfusion was given for 4 hr. This was repeated 15 hr after ingestion. The chelators used included penicillamine and BAL.

All laboratory results were within normal limits except for a slight increase in SGOT. The patient continued under examination for the next 3 months without experiencing further problems. Blood concentrations of mercury remained high throughout the period. (See ref. 50.)

Discussion

1. What organ systems are affected by this type of mercury poisoning?
2. Three months after ingestion, the patient had no toxic symptoms but had high blood concentrations of mercury. Why?
3. Do you believe chelators were effective in this case? What is the role of chelators in this type of mercury poisoning?

CASE STUDIES: METALLIC MERCURY POISONING

History: Case 1

A 53-year-old man had been working on an amateur ore distillation experiment. He had heated mercury on his kitchen stove on two separate occasions within a 2-week period.

After the first exposure he presented to the emergency room, cyanotic, with chills, fever, dyspnea, and severe abdominal cramping. He often saw red spots in front of his eyes and became partially blinded. Symptoms gradually disappeared over 2 days from the first exposure to mercury vapor.

On the second occasion, he noted the room becoming dark, and the red spots reappeared. He was again admitted to the hospital with acute respiratory distress and severe abdominal cramping. He was given a tracheostomy and mechanical assistance for breathing. Urinary mercury concentration at this time was 5 mg/dL (normal, 0 to 2.0 μg/dL). He was transferred to another facility so that charcoal hemoperfusion could be initiated.

Physical examination showed that the blood pressure was 130/100 mm Hg; respirations, 18/min; and pulse, 76 beats/min. A chest X-ray film depicted extensive bilateral pulmonary infiltrates, but no signs of cardiomegaly. Laboratory findings are shown in Table 9.21.

The patient was given 500 mL 5% dextrose over 4 hr. He also received a course of BAL. Urinary mercury concentrations were 0.06 mg/dL by the 7th day, and renal function improved. He temporarily recovered but later developed a nosocomial pneumonia, which proved to be fatal. He died during his 3rd week of hospitalization. (See ref. 46.)

History: Case 2

The patient was a 17-year-old male storekeeper who ingested the metallic mercury

TABLE 9.21. *Laboratory findings*

Na$^+$	=131 mEq/L
Cl$^-$	=94 mEq/L
Glucose	=172 mg/dL
BUN	=45 mg/dL
Uric acid	=9.6 mg/dL
LDH[a]	=2,400 U
Urinary Hg	=0.37 mg/dL
Serum creatinine	=1.5 mg/dL

From ref. 46.
[a] LDH, lactate dehydrogenase.

content of a clock pendulum (i.e., approximately 204 g or 15 mL). (For comparison, a clinical fever thermometer contains approximately 1 g mercury.) He arrived at the hospital asymptomatic 2 hr after ingestion. Blood urea, electrolyte, and hematologic findings were normal.

Treatment consisted of a mild laxative and bed rest. X-ray films of the abdomen were used to follow passage of the mercury through the GI tract, and by 3 weeks all mercury had been excreted in the feces. Daily urine mercury excretions were all less than 15 μg. There were no gastrointestinal symptoms, and apparently the mercury was not absorbed. He was discharged without further problems. (See ref. 93.)

History: Case 3

A 14-year-old boy took apart two thermostats 4 months before coming to medical attention. He poured the mercury (estimated volume, 5 mL) into a test tube and toyed with it repeatedly. Three weeks later, he spilled the mercury on the carpet and managed to pick up about half. He vacuumed the remainder repeatedly. The vacuum cleaner did not have a disposable bag, but instead a filter over the motor, with dust gathering in the canister. During the next 3 months, the vacuum was used exclusively by the patient once every 2 to 3 weeks. The canister had not been emptied up to the time when health inspectors surveyed the home 4 months later.

Two months before admission, the patient had a brief "flu-like" illness and then gradually developed progressive weakness until he was barely able to hold a cup, button his buttons, or climb stairs. Over 6 weeks, he slept and ate poorly and lost 4 kg.

On admission, 4 months after the mercury spill, he was cachectic and depressed but alert and oriented. He showed moderate proximal and distal weakness with diffuse muscle wasting. He walked with bilateral foot-drop and rose from the floor with a partial Gower's sign. His hand grip was very weak with striking wasting of the small muscles of the hands. Deep tendon reflexes were present but reduced without sensory loss. Tandem gait was poorly performed. There was no tremor. Cranial nerves and skin examination were normal with no signs of acrodynia. (See ref. 95)

Discussion

1. Is the delayed onset of respiratory distress with mercury vapor exposure typical? What are some of the signs and symptoms related to this type of exposure?
2. In case 2, do you think chelation therapy was indicated for metallic mercury ingestion?
3. If anuria or renal shutdown had occurred with either of these patients, describe the procedure that could be used to decrease the concentration of mercury.
4. Patient 2 ingested a much greater amount of mercury than did patient 1. However, patient 1 was more seriously intoxicated. Discuss the reasons why this occurred.

CASE STUDY: ZINC ABUSE

History

The patient, a 34-year-old man, presented with a 10-day history of feeling tired and "run-down." He noted, in addition, heart palpitations and shortness of breath with minimal activity. His history was notable for the treatment of schizophrenia, for which he was taking chlorpromazine, thiothixene, and benztropine mesylate. He denied any incidences of melena, hematuria, or a change in urine color. Three years before admission he had stopped using street drugs and alcohol.

On physical examination, he was pale and obese but apparently in no acute distress. His blood pressure was 130/74 mm Hg, and his pulse rate was 112 beats/min and regular. He had no lymphadenopathy, petechiae, hepatosplenomegaly, or cardiopulmonary abnormalities.

Pertinent normal laboratory values included

the platelet count, the mean corpuscular volume, serum B_{12}, and folic acid, liver function studies [except for a serum albumin concentration of 29 g/L (normal, 35 to 50)], and renal function studies. Serum iron concentrations, total iron-binding capacity, and iron saturation were normal. Ferritin concentration was elevated at 485 μg/L (normal, 125 to 350). A serum zinc concentration determined on the 2nd hospital day was elevated at 23.4 μmol/L (normal, 11.5 to 18.5). A serum copper concentration measured at the same time was 0.16 μmol/L (normal, 11.0 to 22.0).

The patient received 2 units of erythrocytes during the first 2 days, with a rise in his hematocrit from 0.10 to 0.15. At this time the results of the bone marrow aspiration done on admission indicated myeloid hyperplasia with vacuolation of both the erythroid and myeloid precursors. Minimal megaloblastic changes were seen in the erythroid series. Iron stores were greatly increased, with 15% of the erythroblasts showing ring forms. A pronounced increase in reticuloendothelial cell iron stores was noted (4+/5). No other abnormal forms were seen in the bone marrow. The peripheral blood smear did not show any abnormalities.

At this point, copper replacement therapy was begun. An intravenous solution of copper, 2 mg in 1 L of 5% dextrose in saline solution, was infused over 12 hr daily. This regimen was continued until discharge on day 15. No side effects were noted. By day 7 of therapy, his reticulocyte count reached a maximum of 176×10^{-3}. He was discharged on a regimen of copper sulfate, 2.0 mg/day by mouth. After 10 weeks of oral therapy, his blood counts had become normal, and the copper therapy was discontinued. No further problems were noted. During outpatient follow-up, he confided that he had abused vitamins A, C, and D in the past. (See ref. 26.)

Discussion

1. The patient admitted to consuming large amounts of vitamin and mineral products. In addition, it was later shown that he took

1 to 2 g elemental zinc each day over several months. This case study illustrates what can happen when people abuse such products without knowing what can happen.

Review Questions

1. Chronic exposure to which of the following metals is referred to as *ouch-ouch* disease?
   A. Cadmium
   B. Lead
   C. Mercury
   D. Selenium
2. Which of the following is characteristic of BAL toxicity: bradycardia (I), sedation (II), or paresthesia (III)?
   A. I only
   B. III only
   C. I and II only
   D. II and III only
3. Which of the following is the antidote of first choice for treating iron poisoning?
   A. CaNa$_2$-EDTA
   B. Deferoxamine
   C. Dimercaprol
   D. Penicillamine
4. Which of the following mercury salts is extremely toxic, and which one has limited toxic potential?
   A. HgCl$_2$
   B. Hg$_2$Cl$_2$
5. Which of the following is the principal site of toxicity of inorganic mercury compounds?
   A. Kidney
   B. Brain
   C. Heart
   D. Bone
6. Which of the following forms of organomercuric compounds is more toxic?
   A. Long-chain aryl compounds
   B. Short-chain alkyl compounds
7. Which of the following is a true statement?
   A. *Pica* refers solely to ingestion of lead-based substances.

B. Each of the inorganic forms of lead produces symptoms of poisoning that are specific for that form.
   C. Acute poisoning from lead is rare; chronic intoxication is a serious problem.
   D. Inorganic lead poisoning is more rare than organic lead poisoning.
8. A request to supply BAL refers to which of the following?
   A. CaNa$_2$-EDTA
   B. Deferoxamine
   C. Dimercaprol
   D. Penicillamine
9. Which of the following is a true statement about deferoxamine?
   A. It imparts a greenish blue color to urine.
   B. It complexes more tightly with ferric iron.
   C. Rapid injection is associated with hypertensive crisis.
   D. Therapy is indicated when the serum iron concentration exceeds 100 mg/dL.
10. Which of the following forms of mercury has the most potential for CNS toxicity?
    A. Hg^0
    B. Hg^{1+}
    C. Hg^{2+}
11. The term *plumbism* refers to toxic symptoms produced by chronic ingestion of which of the following metals?
    A. Zinc
    B. Lead
    C. Iron
    D. Arsenic
12. Which of the following is the chelator of first choice for treating a toxic ingestion of arsenic?
    A. CaNa$_2$-EDTA
    B. Deferoxamine
    C. BAL
    D. Penicillamine
13. A victim of heavy metal poisoning has an odor of garlic on his breath. Of the following, which is the most probable cause of poisoning?
    A. Mercury

B. Lead

C. Zinc

D. Arsenic

14. The chelator of first choice for treating a toxic ingestion of copper is:

A. $CaNa_2$-EDTA

B. Deferoxamine

C. BAL

D. Penicillamine

15. Arsine gas is produced when acid reacts with arsenic-containing metals.

A. True

B. False

16. The toxic action of lead on erythrocytes is usually life-threatening.

A. True

B. False

17. Gastric lavage with a bicarbonate solution is recommended as a means of gastric decontamination after acute ingestion of which of the following metals?

A. Iron

B. Zinc

C. Arsenic

D. Cadmium

18. Which of the following metal poisonings is associated with erethism?

A. Mercuric chloride

B. Arsenic trioxide

C. Elemental mercury

D. Lead acetate

19. Which of the following will *least* benefit a victim who has ingested a toxic dose of iron?

A. Syrup of ipecac

B. Gastric lavage with $NaHCO_3$

C. Gastric lavage with sodium phosphate

D. Deferoxamine i.m. or i.v.

E. Prussian blue p.o.

20. Which of the following mercury exposures is *least* likely to produce mercury toxicity?

A. $HgCl_2$ p.o.

B. Elemental mercury p.o.

C. Inhalation of elemental mercury vapor

D. Methyl mercury p.o.

E. Elemental mercury s.c.

21. Which of the following is a true statement about deferoxamine?

I. It readily competes for the iron of ferritin and hemosiderin.

II. It does not remove iron from cytochromes and hemoglobin.

III. Administration sometimes causes hypertensive episodes.

A. II only

B. III only

C. I and II only

D. II and III only

E. I, II, and III

22. Which of the following is an expected toxic symptom of dimercaprol administration?

I. Paresthesias

II. Hypotension

III. Headache

A. II only

B. III only

C. I and II only

D. I and III only

E. II and III only

F. I, II and III

23. Which of the following target organs is associated with Ca-EDTA toxicity?

A. Heart

B. Brain

C. Liver

D. Kidney

E. Lung

24. Which of the following is seen with elemental mercury poisoning?

A. Pneumonitis

B. Erethism

C. Stomatitis

D. All of the above

E. A and B only

25. Which of the following is a true statement?

A. Pica refers solely to ingestion of lead-based paints.

B. Each of the inorganic forms of lead produces symptoms of poisoning that are specific for that form.

C. Acute poisoning from lead is rare; chronic intoxication is a serious problem.

D. Lead is best chelated with dimercaprol.

26. Which of the following chelators is effective if administered orally?
    A. Succimer (Chemet)
    B. CaNa$_2$-EDTA (Calcium Disodium Versenate
    C. Dimercaprol (BAL)
    D. Deferoxamine

27. Succimer (2,3-dimercaptosuccinic acid; Chemet) is a heavy metal chelating agent indicated for increasing the urinary elimination of which of the following?
    A. Mercury
    B. Arsenic
    C. Cadmium
    D. Lead
    E. Iron

28. Lead poisoning can be positively identified by determining the urinary concentrations for precursors to heme synthesis. A positive indication for lead intoxication would be:
    A. Increased delta-ALA; increased coproporphyrins
    B. Increased delta-ALA; decreased coproporphyrins
    C. Decreased delta-ALA; decreased coproporphyrins
    D. Decreased delta-ALA; increased coproporphyrins

29. Throughout the chapter, reference is made to the *body burden* of various metals. What does this term mean?

30. What characteristic odor may be detected on the breath after selenium ingestion?

31. A young girl has been brought to an emergency facility. A fever thermometer had been broken within her rectum. Discuss the problem.

32. What is lead colic? What are the major symptoms?

33. Describe major symptoms associated with various stages of iron poisoning. What are the inherent dangers of stage 2?

34. A delayed symptom of arsenic poisoning is the presence of Mee's lines. What are they?

35. Discuss the pros and cons of using a chemical chelator to treat heavy metal intoxication. Why might a physician decide against using a chelator, even if the victim has seriously high blood levels of metal?

References

1. Annest JS, Pirkle JL, Makug D, et al. Chronological trend in blood levels between 1976 and 1980. *N Engl J Med* 1983;308:1373–1377.
2. Antonini G. Wine poisoning as a source of lead intoxication. *Am J Med* 1989;87:238–239.
3. Aposhian HV, Aposhian MM. Meso-2,3-dimercaptosuccinic acid: chemical, pharmacological, and toxicological properties of an orally effective metal chelating agent. *Ann Rev Pharmacol Toxicol* 1990;30:279–306.
4. Bachrach L, Correa A, Levin R, Grossman M. Iron poisoning: complications of hypertonic phosphate lavage therapy. *J Pediatr* 1979;94:147–149.
5. Bakir F, Damluji SF, Amin-Zaki L, et al. Methyl mercury poisoning in Iraq: an interuniversity report. *Science* 1973;181:230–241.
6. Bakir F, Al-Khalidi A, Clarkson TW, Greenwook R. Clinical observations on treatment of alkylmercury poisoning in hospital patients. *Bull World Health Organ* 1976;53:87–92.
7. Banner W, Czajka PA. Iron poisoning. *Am J Dis Child* 1981;135:484–485.
8. Baselt RC, Cravey RH. A compendium of therapeutic and toxic concentrations of toxicologically significant drugs in human biofluids. *J Anal Toxicol* 1977;1:81–103.
9. Bellinger DC, Stiles KM, Needleman HL. Low-level lead exposure, intelligence and academic achievement—a long-term follow-up study. *Pediatrics* 1992;90:855–861.
10. Bock GW, Tenenbein M. Whole bowel irrigation for iron overdose. *Ann Emerg Med* 1987;16:184–184.
11. Bushnell PJ, Jaeger RJ. Hazards to health from environmental lead exposure: a review of recent literature. *Vet Hum Toxicol* 1986;28:255–261.
12. Centers for Disease Control. *Preventing lead poisoning in young children.* Atlanta: US Department of Health and Human Services, Public Health Service; 1990.
13. Chiba M, Toyoda T, Inaba Y, et al. Acute lead poisoning in an adult from ingestion of paint. *N Engl J Med* 1980;303:459.
14. Chisolm JJ Jr. Evaluation of the potential role of chelating therapy in the treatment of low to moderate lead exposures. *Environ Health Perspect* 1990;89:67–74.
15. Chowdhury P, Louria DB. Influence of cadmium and other trace metals on human alpha-antitrypsin: an *in vitro* study. *Science* 1976;191:480–481.
16. Clarkson TW. The pharmacology of mercury compounds. *Ann Rev Pharmacol* 1972;12:375–406.
17. Curtis HA, Ferguson SD, Kell RL, Samuel AH. Mercury as a health hazard. *Arch Dis Child* 1987;62:293–295.
18. Dean BS, Krenzelok EP. *In vivo* effectiveness of oral complexation agents in the management of iron poisoning. *Clin Toxicol* 1987;25:221–230.

19. Dietrich KN, Berger OG, Sucoop PA. Lead exposure and motor developmental status of urban six-year-old children in the Cincinnati prospective study. *Pediatrics* 1993;91:301–307.

20. Diplock AT. Metabolic aspects of selenium action and toxicity. *Crit Rev Toxicol* 1976;4:271–329.

21. Elhassani SB. The many faces of methyl mercury poisoning. *J Toxicol Clin Toxicol* 1982–83;19:875–906.

22. Engle JP, Polin KS, Stile IL. Acute iron intoxication: treatment controversies. *Drug Intell Clin Pharm* 1987;21:153–159.

23. Fairbanks VF, Fahey JL, Beutler E. *Clinical disorders of iron metabolism.* 2nd ed. New York: Grune & Stratton; 1971.

24. Finch CA. Drugs effective in iron-deficiency and other hypochromic anemias. In: Gilman AG, Goodman LS, Gilman A, eds. *The pharmacological basis of therapeutics.* 6th ed. New York: Macmillan; 1980:1315–1330.

25. Flick DF, Kraybill HF, Dimetroff JM. Toxic effects of cadmium: a review. *Environ Res* 1975;4:71–85.

26. Forman WB. Zinc abuse—an unsuspected cause of sideroblastic anemia. *West J Med* 1990;152:190–192.

27. Friberg L. Edathamil calcium-disodium in cadmium poisoning. *Arch Ind Health* 1956;13:13–23.

28. Friberg L, Piscator M, Norberg G, Kjellstrom T. *Cadmium in the environment.* 2nd ed. Cleveland: CRC Press; 1974.

29. Geffner ME, Oas, LM. Phosphate poisoning complicating treatment of iron ingestion. *Am J Dis Child* 1980;134:509–510.

30. Gezernik W, Schmaman A, Chappell J. Corrosive gastritis as a result of ferrous sulfate ingestion. *S Afr Med J* 1980;57:151–153.

31. Gilman A, Philips FS, Allen RP, Koelle E. The treatment of acute cadmium intoxication in rabbits with 2,3-dimercaptopropanol (BAL) and other mercaptans. *J Pharmacol Exp Ther* 1946;87:85–101.

32. Gleason WA, deMello DE, deCastro FI, et al. Acute hepatic failure in severe iron poisoning. *J Pediatr* 1979;95:138–140.

33. Glommer J, Gustavson KH. Treatment of experimental acute mercury poisoning by chelating agents BAL and EDTA. *Acta Med Scand* 1959;164:175–182.

34. Goldman RH, Baker EL, Hannan M, et al. Lead poisoning in automobile radiator mechanics. *N Engl J Med* 1987;317:214–218.

35. Goldstein A, Aronow L, Kalman SM. *Principles of drug action: the basis of pharmacology.* 2nd ed. New York: John Wiley; 1974.

36. Graziano JH, LoIacono NJ, Meyer P. Dose-response study of oral 2,3-dimercapatosuccinic acid in children with elevated blood lead concentrations. *J Pediatr* 1988;113:751–757.

37. Graziano JH, LoIacono NJ, Moulton T, et al. Controlled study of meso-2,3-dimercaptosuccinic acid for the management of childhood lead intoxication. *J Pediatr* 1992;120:133–139.

38. Hammond PB. The effect of chelating agents on the tissue distribution and excretion of lead. *Toxicol Appl Pharmacol* 1971;18:296–310.

39. Hammond PB, Aronson AL, Olson WC. The mechanism of mobilization of lead by ethylenediaminetetraacetate. *J Pharmacol Exp Ther* 1967;157:196–206.

40. Hammond PB, Bilikes RP. Metals. In: Doull J, Klaassen CD, Amdur MO, eds. *Toxicology—the basic science of poisons.* 2nd ed. New York: Macmillan; 1980:409–467.

41. Hannigan BG. Self-administration of metallic mercury by intravenous injection. *Br Med J* 1978;2:933.

42. Henretig FM, Karl SR, Weintraub WH. Severe iron poisoning treated with enteral and parenteral deferoxamine. *Ann Emerg Med* 1983;12:306–309.

43. Henretig FM, Temple AR. Acute iron poisoning in children. *Emerg Med Clin North Am* 1984;2:121–132.

44. Holtzman NA, Elliott DA, Miller RH. Copper intoxication: report of a case with observations on ceruloplasmin. *N Engl J Med* 1966;275:347–352.

45. Hryhorczuk DO, Meyers L, Chen G. Treatment of mercury intoxication in a dentist with *N*-acetyl-D,L-penicillamine. *J Toxicol Clin Toxicol* 1982;19:401–408.

46. Jung RC, Aaronson J. Death following inhalation of mercury vapor at home. *West J Med* 1980;132:539–543.

47. Kalman SM. The pathophysiology of lead poisoning: a review and a case report. *J Anal Toxicol* 1977;2:277–281.

48. Klaassen CD. Heavy metals and heavy-metal antagonists. In: Gilman AG, Goodman LS, Rall TW, Murad F, eds. *The pharmacological basis of therapeutics.* 7th ed. New York: Macmillan; 1985:1605–1627.

49. Klein-Schwartz W, Oderda GM, Gorman RL, et al. Assessment of management guidelines—acute iron ingestion. *Clin Pediatr* 1990;29:316–321.

50. Koppel C, Baudisch J, Keller F. Methoxymethylmercury chloride poisoning: clinical findings on *in vitro* experiments. *J Toxicol Clin Toxicol* 1982;19:391–400.

51. Lacouture PG, Lovejoy FH. In: Haddad LM, Winchester JF, eds. *Clinical management of poisoning and drug overdose.* Philadelphia: WB Saunders; 1983;644–648.

52. Landsman I, Bricker TJ, Reid BS, Bloss RS. Emergency gastrotomy: treatment of choice for iron bezoar. *J Pediatr Surg* 1987;22:184–185.

53. Lisella FS, Long KR, Scott HG. Health aspects of arsenicals in the environment. *J Environ Health* 1972;34:511–518.

54. Lovejoy FH. Chelation therapy in iron poisoning. *J Toxicol Clin Toxicol* 1982–83;19:871–874.

55. Mann KV, Travers JD. Succimer, an oral lead chelator. *Clin Pharm* 1991;10:914–922.

56. Manoguerra AS. Iron poisoning: report of a fatal case in an adult. *Am J Hosp Pharm* 1976;33:1088–1090.

57. Manzler AD, Schreiner AW. Copper-induced acute hemolytic anemia: a new complication of hemodialysis. *Ann Intern Med* 1970;73:409–412.

58. Markowitz ME, Rosen JF. Need for lead mobilization test in children with lead poisoning. *J Pediatr* 1991;119:305–310.

59. Marsh DO, Myers GJ, Clarkson TW, et al. Dose-response relationship for human fetal exposure to methyl mercury. *Clin Toxicol* 1981;18:1311–1318.

60. Massey EW, Wold D, Heyman A. Arsenic: homicidal intoxication. *South Med J* 1984;77:848–850.

61. McIntyre AR. The toxicities of mercury and its compounds. *J Clin Pharmacol* 1971;11:397–401.
62. Osterlok J, Becker CE. Pharmacokinetics of Ca-Na₂EDTA and chelation of lead in renal failure. *Clin Pharm Ther* 1986;40:686–693.
63. Park MJ, Currier M. Arsenic exposures in Mississippi—a review of cases. *South Med J* 1991;84:461–464.
64. Pearce J, Burg FD. Lead poisoning in children. *Drug Ther* 1982;5:May 87–102.
65. Peck MG, Rogers JF, Rivenbark JF. Use of high doses of deferoxamine (Desferal) in an adult patient with acute iron overdosage. *J Toxicol Clin Toxicol* 1982–83;19:865–869.
66. Peter F, Bourdean J. Screening for undue lead absorption: correlation between lead and erythrocyte protoporphyrin. *Can J Public Health* 1983;74:356–359.
67. Peterson CD, Fifield GI. Emergency gastrotomy for acute iron poisoning. *Ann Emerg Med* 1980;9:262–264.
68. Pierce PE, Thompson JF, Likosky WH, et al. Alkyl mercury poisoning in humans—report of an outbreak. *JAMA* 1972;220:1439–1442.
69. Piomelli S, Rosen JF, Chisolm JJ Jr, Graef JW. Management of childhood lead poisoning. *J Pediatr* 1984;105:523–532.
70. Proudfoot AT, Simpson D, Dyson EH. Management of acute iron poisoning. *Med Toxicol* 1986;1:83–100.
71. Rahola T, Aaran RK, Mietinen JK. Half-time studies of mercury and cadmium by whole body counting. In: *Assessment of radioactive contamination in man.* Vienna: International Atomic Energy Agency; 1972:1–25.
72. Robertson DSE. Selenium—a possible teratogen. *Lancet* 1970;1:518–519.
73. Robotham JL, Lietman PS. Acute iron poisoning. *Am J Dis Child* 1980;134:875–879.
74. Sanford HN. Lead poisoning in young children. *Postgrad Med* 1955;17:162–169.
75. Schroeder HA. Cadmium as a factor in hypertension. *J Chronic Dis* 1965;18:217–228.
76. Shannon M, Graef J, Lovejoy FH Jr. Efficacy and toxicity of D-penicillamine in low-level lead poisoning. *J Pediatr* 1988;112:799–804.
77. Sisson TRC. Acute iron poisoning in children. *Q Rev Pediatr* 1960;15:47–49.
78. Smith ADM, Miller JW. Treatment of inorganic mercury poisoning with *N*-acetyl-D,L-penicillamine. *Lancet* 1961;1:640.
79. Smith HD, Boehner RL, Carney T, Majors WJ. The sequelae of pica with and without lead poisoning. *Am J Dis Child* 1963;105:609–616.
80. Stocken LA, Thompson RHS. Reactions of British antilewisite with arsenic and other metals in living systems. *Physiol Rev* 1949;29:168–194.
81. Taylor A, Jackson MA, Patil D, et al. Poisoning with cadmium fumes after smelting lead. *Br Med J* 1984;288:1270–1271.
82. Teitelbaum DT, Ott JE. Elemental mercury self-poisoning. *Clin Toxicol* 1969;2:243–248.
83. Tenenbein M. Whole bowel irrigation in iron poisoning. *J Pediatr* 1987;111:142–145.
84. Thind GS, Fischer G. Plasma cadmium and zinc in human hypertension. *Clin Sci Mol Med* 1976;51:483–486.
85. Tibbits PA, Milroy WC. Pulmonary edema induced by exposure to cadmium oxide fume: case report. *Milit Med* 1980;145:435–437.
86. Tsuchiya K. Causation of ouch-ouch disease, an introductory review. *Keio J Med* 1969;18:181–194.
87. Voors AW, Shuman MS. Liver cadmium levels in North Carolina residents who died of heart disease. *Bull Environ Contam Toxicol* 1977;17:692–696.
88. Watson WA, Veltui JC, Metcalf TS. Acute arsenic exposure treated with oral D-penicillamine. *Vet Hum Toxicol* 1981;23:164–165.
89. Wilber CG. Toxicology of selenium: a review. *Clin Toxicol* 1980;17:171–230.
90. Williams DR, Halsted BW. Chelating agents in medicine. *J Toxicol Clin Toxicol* 1982–83;19:1081–1115.
91. Witten CF, Gibson GW, Good MH. Studies in iron poisoning I. Deferoxamine in the treatment of acute iron poisoning: clinical observations, experimental studies, and theoretical considerations. *Pediatrics* 1965;36:322–335.
92. Witzelben CL, Chaffey NJ. Acute ferrous sulfate poisoning: a histochemical study of its effect on the liver. *Arch Pathol* 1966;82:454–460.
93. Wright N, Yeoman WG, Carter GF. Massive oral ingestion of elemental mercury without poisoning. *Lancet* 1980;1:206.
94. Yip R, Schwartz S, Deinard AS. Screening for iron deficiency with the erythrocyte protoporphyrin test. *Pediatrics* 1983;72:214–219.
95. Zelman M, Camfield P, Moss M, et al. Toxicity from vacuumed mercury: a household hazard. *Clin Pediatr* 1991;30:121–123.

10 Corrosives

The category of corrosive substances is broad in nature. It includes *acids* such as hydrochloric, sulfuric, oxalic, and phenol; and *alkali*, including potassium hydroxide, sodium hydroxide, sodium phosphate, and potassium permanganate *per se*, and a larger variety of miscellaneous products found around the home and workplace (e.g., creosote, electric dishwasher detergents, hydrogen fluoride, drain cleaners, toilet bowl cleaners). Their chemical and physical properties vary widely, although expected outcomes after a toxic exposure are similar. All corrosives produce extensive tissue damage, but the site at which damage occurs and the specific form of damage depends on the type of corrosive involved. Table 10.1 lists common acidic and alkaline corrosive products.

Most households contain a wide variety of corrosive substances that invite curious children to explore, or adults to use inappropriately. The toxic potential of many of these substances is obvious to adults, and generally, they avoid them. All of these substances are extremely irritating to mucous membranes. Thus, massive intentional ingestions are rare.

TABLE 10.1. *Examples of common acids and alkali*

Acid
  Hydrochloric acid
    Metal cleaners
    Muriatic acid
    Swimming pool cleaners
    Toilet bowl cleaners
  Sulfuric acid
    Battery acid
    Toilet bowl and drain cleaners
Alkali
  Sodium or potassium hydroxide
    Clinitest tablets
    Detergents
    Drano crystals
    Drain pipe and toilet bowl cleaners
    Lye
    Paint removers
    Washing powders
Others
  Ammonia (NH_4OH) solutions (hair products, jewelry cleaners, household cleaners)
  Electric dishwashing granules
  Potassium permanganate
  Sodium carbonate (nonphosphate) detergents
  Sodium hypochlorite (bleach)

Even small quantities (in the range of 1 mL of liquid or a single granule of crystalline solid) can produce severe irritation or burning to a child within a short period of time. Children have been known to suffer serious injury from corrosive ingestions that required many years of reconstructive surgery to correct. These injuries have occurred, for example, when they drank the remaining few drops of a liquid corrosive from an apparently empty container that had been carelessly discarded in a wastebasket (17,46).

Some corrosive substances are not generally recognized as being dangerous. Special precautions are, therefore, seldom taken to keep them away from an inquisitive child's reach, or to make sure that adults use them properly. Rust remover products (oxalic acid), electric dishwasher detergents, and citrus-scented bowl cleaners are in this category. Tissue damage from corrosives is listed among the more common type of poisoning emergencies that occur around the home.

It has been reported that 1.7% to 9.6% of all accidental ingestions by children involve alkali or acids (54). The major reason for this high incidence among children is that too many of these toxic substances are stored in old, unmarked beverage containers (68). Among adults, poisonings with corrosives are often related to suicide attempts (10).

Traditionally the term *corrosive* denotes an acidic substance capable of inflicting tissue injury. *Caustic* describes an alkaline substance having similar properties. The Federal Hazardous Substance Act of 1967 specifically defines as corrosive any substance that, in contact with living tissue, will cause destruction by chemical action (42). This definition does not differentiate acids from alkali. Throughout this chapter and book, the term corrosive is used to encompass both extremes of pH, except where specifically indicated.

ACIDS

Strong acids are substances with a pH below 2. Some substances, such as lemon juice and carbonated beverages, can have a strongly acidic pH, but not be corrosive. Acidic compounds include a wide variety of inorganic (e.g., sulfuric, hydrochloric/muriatic, nitric, phosphoric) and organic (e.g., oxalic, tartaric, acetic, etc.) acids. Even though all acids can produce similar tissue damage, they differ in intensity of damage. Not all acids are common causes of poisoning. Nitric and phosphoric acids, for examples, are less commonly encountered. Also, not all acids are sufficiently corrosive to be of major toxicologic concern. Acetic and tartaric acids exemplify these.

Mechanism of Toxicity

Corrosive damage is caused by direct chemical action on the involved tissue. Acids denature tissue proteins. The resulting lesion causes cell death that is represented as coagulative necrosis. Consequently, both structural and enzymatic proteins are denatured but cellular morphology is not grossly interrupted. In addition, a tough, leathery scab (eschar) forms, which delays further corrosive damage and helps reduce systemic absorption. Thus, damage, especially with small quantities of acid, is often limited to local sites of injury to the skin or gastrointestinal tract.

Characteristics of Poisoning

After an acid ingestion, intense corrosive damage to the oral mucosa and esophagus may occur, but most significant damage occurs in the lower two-thirds of the stomach (Table 10.2). The involved areas frequently

TABLE 10.2. *Sites and types of damage after ingestion of a corrosive[a]*

Corrosive	Site of injury	Type of injury
Acid	Stomach	Coagulative necrosis
Alkali	Esophagus	Liquefactive necrosis

[a] Tissue damage by corrosives is a function of numerous factors (see text). The information presented in this table represents the classic situation; the actual damage may vary depending on these factors.

appear brown or black (except when damaged by picric and nitric acids, which stain tissue yellow). Precipitated blood may be found in the stomach, and is described as having a *coffee grounds* consistency. Damaged gastric glands are usually not regenerated, but are replaced by a thin epithelial layer. Gastric motility is disrupted also (50).

Ingested acid normally passes through the esophagus quickly and causes little damage to this area. Studies have shown that esophageal damage occurs in as few as 6% to 20% of all acid ingestions (10,24). This is not to imply that significant damage could not result if acid were left in contact with esophageal tissue. For example, 30 seconds contact with 9% sulfuric acid solution causes coagulative necrosis *in vitro* (2). The extent of esophageal damage is a function of the volume of acid ingested, its strength, and length of contact. This is why emetics are contraindicated in acid ingestion because they increase the contact time between acid and esophageal mucosa.

Strong acids, such as sulfuric, are more likely to cause gastric necrosis and perforation than weaker ones, such as hydrochloric. However, chronic gastric problems have been reported more frequently after hydrochloric acid ingestion, rather than sulfuric acid. This may be due to the severity of damage that occurs from sulfuric acid ingestion. Poisoning victims are more likely to die shortly after ingestion of the latter.

The premorbid condition of the stomach is a fairly good predictor of the site of toxic gastric injury. In patients with a full stomach before acid ingestion, damage is confined mainly to pyloric and lesser curvature regions. For those victims with a fluid-filled stomach, damage is proximal and generalized. For fasting persons, acid ingestion causes antral damage, as well as a wide variety of other toxic involvement (50).

Damage to the small intestine as a result of acid ingestion is rare. This most likely relates to pylorospasm induced by the acid, which limits its entry into the duodenum.

Table 10.3 lists major clinical manifestations that have been reported for acid and

TABLE 10.3. *Clinical manifestations of corrosive toxicity in acute poisoning*

Route of exposure	Signs and symptoms
Ingestion	Severe burning pain in mouth, throat, and abdomen
	Vomiting, possibly blood-tinged
	Diarrhea—bloody, mucoid
	Stains around mouth
	Dysphagia
	Drooling
	Hypotension
Inhalation	Bronchial irritation
	Pulmonary edema
	Frothy sputum
	Moist rales
	Hypotension
	Hemoptysis
	Dyspnea
Dermal	Staining of skin
	Burning pain
Ocular	Conjunctivitis
	Corneal destruction
	Pain, lacrimation
	Photophobia

alkali poisonings, according to the route of exposure. An excellent review of the pathogenesis of acid toxicity is provided by Penner (50).

Management of Poisoning

Poisoning by acid, whether localized or systemic, is a medical emergency and treatment must be initiated at once. Unfortunately, though reports of acid ingestion and resultant toxicity continue to appear in the literature, there is an insufficient number of controlled clinical studies that identify the best therapeutic management. The rules of treatment that follow are based on clinical experience, and do not always receive universal acceptance.

Skin or Eye Contact

Contamination of the skin or eye with acid must be given immediate attention. The area should be washed thoroughly with large quantities of room-temperature water. A 15- to 20-min wash is usually necessary to completely

neutralize and remove all residual traces of contaminant. Contaminated clothing and jewelry should be removed. Contact lenses, if present, should be removed to avoid prolonged contact of acid with ocular tissues.

A mild soap solution may be used to wash the skin and aid in neutralizing the acid, but soap should not be placed in the eye. After washing, no cream, ointment, or dressing of any kind should be applied to the affected area. These may cause further tissue injury to an already damaged area, and make it difficult for emergency personnel to remove them without inflicting additional irritation, trauma, and intense pain.

Ingested Acid

Management of a corrosive acid ingestion is outlined in a decision flow chart, Fig. 10.1. The immediate concern for acid solutions that are not mineral acids or in high concentrations is to dilute them with copious amounts of water or milk. Antacids may be given as a demulcent. Under no circumstance should carbonated beverages or sodium bicarbonate be used because carbon dioxide gas is released, which quickly distends the stomach wall. Distention imposes a greater chance for perforation of already weakened tissues and may hasten the time for gastric emptying. If the ingested acid was concentrated (mineral or organic) it is unlikely that the patient will be able to swallow, and dilution becomes a mute point.

Emesis must be avoided to prevent recurrent damage to the esophagus. Spontaneous emesis is common enough with corrosive ingestion. If emesis is prolonged, antiemetics may be necessary to control vomiting. The use of opioids for pain management and fluid replacement to correct circulatory shock may be necessary.

If a large quantity of acid has been swallowed, gastric lavage may be considered (50). It is best performed as soon as diagnosis of acid ingestion has been confirmed and the extent of mucosal damage evaluated by esophagoscopy and gastroscopy. First, acid is suc-

Corrosive (Caustic, Acid) Ingestion

possible ingestion

IMMEDIATELY: *Dilute* ingested material. *Irrigate* exposed surfaces.
REVIEW HISTORY: Clarify *ingredients* of product. Determine *concentration*.
Determine if *exposure* was real.
DETERMINE PATIENT SYMPTOMS: Any pain, irritation, dysphagia, excess drooling, obvious burns.

product concentration sufficient to produce corrosive effect
and exposure potentially toxic or unknown
or   patient is symptomatic

product too dilute to be corrosive
or exposure clearly non-toxic and
patient asymptomatic

ESTABLISH AIRWAY CONTROL AND IV/CP SUPPORTIVE
MEASURES AS NECESSARY. EXAMINE ESOPHARYNX

OBSERVE FOR SYMPTOMS

product is caustic (alkaline)   product is acid

REFER FOR ESOPHAGOSCOPY

esophagoscopy cannot be   esophagoscopy can be
performed within 24 hours   performed within 24 hours

INITIATE CORTICOSTEROID THERAPY→PERFORM ESOPHAGOSCOPY   PERFORM
PENDING ESOPHAGOSCOPY   ·ESOPHAGOSCOPY
                                                         AND ENDOSCOPY
burns present   no burns

INITIATE CORTICOSTEROID THERAPY

PROVIDE SUPPORTIVE CARE AND FOLLOW UP AS INDICATED

FIG. 10.1. Flow chart illustrating the steps involved in assessment and management of a victim of corrosive ingestion. (Reproduced with permission of the Soap and Detergent Association.)

tioned out of the stomach as completely as possible to reduce the risk of heat formation when the lavage fluid is added. Then, cold water or milk can be used as the lavage fluid, followed by antacid washes. The tube should be repositioned frequently to assure that all traces of acid have been removed.

Surgical resection of damaged tissue is sometimes advised. It is not always possible to easily identify the damaged area and after resection, leaking may occur at anastomoses. When tissue has been damaged beyond repair, it is usually removed surgically (17).

The remaining treatment is largely supportive. Antibiotics should be used only if infection occurs. The value of corticosteroids after acid ingestion is questionable because esophageal stricture is less common than alkali (50). Acids, unlike alkali, do not produce their entire range of toxic damage immediately. In fact, injury may continue to develop over 90 min or longer (52). The patient must be closely monitored during this period and treatment continued, even in the absence of perceptible or worsening symptoms.

Controversy of Dilution

Frequently, while managing a victim of acid ingestion, the corrosive agent is treated by dilution but damage due to exothermic heat production is ignored. This results in the following dilemma: To dilute (neutralize) or not to dilute—that is the question! Considerable heat is released when strong acids come in contact with water or antacids. For example, 55 mL of sulfuric acid, 91.6% by weight, mixed with 54 mL of water results in an almost instantaneous solution temperature of 79°C (50). When water is added to sulfuric acid (as opposed to mixing in the reverse order), it results in an explosive release of steam and heat. The resulting diluted solution, however, is still strongly acidic and highly corrosive (41).

Moreover, heat is released when acids react with antacids. The heat of neutralization of 1 mole of sulfuric acid with magnesium hydroxide suspension (80 mg/mL) is about 40 kcal. Approximately 730 mL of antacid would be required to neutralize the acid, resulting in a final mixture temperature of about 62°C (50).

SPECIFIC ACID CORROSIVES

Fluorides

Hydrogen fluoride (hydrofluoric acid, HF) induces damage that differs from other corrosives, and it is described separately. Hydrofluoric acid is a widely used industrial compound that exists as an extremely corrosive, colorless volatile liquid. Its commercial uses include glass and computer chip etching, and cleaning metal, and production of various synthetic chemicals. Some rust remover agents contain hydrofluoric acid (32). Industrial smoke often contains high levels of HF because it is evolved from burning coal. The exposure limit for HF is 3 ppm.

Sodium fluoride is a soluble salt that is used as a rodenticide, insecticide, and anthelmintic for swine. As expected, fluoride salts are more commonly encountered around the home than HF, and it is this group of products that is responsible for most acute fluoride poisonings (47).

Fluorides are rapidly absorbed after inhalation, ingestion, dermal, or even rectal exposures (7,18,59). Systemic absorption results in acute fluoride poisoning. The amount absorbed is dependent principally on the solubility of the fluoride, and the duration of exposure. Sodium fluoride, which is very soluble, is readily absorbed 75% to 90% (43).

Knowledge of the relative solubility of various fluoride salts is beneficial in understanding one of the mechanisms for treating fluoride toxicity. Administration of calcium gluconate (oral or dermal) is used to convert soluble fluorides to insoluble calcium fluoride (43). As a result, absorption is limited.

Mechanism of Fluoride Toxicity

Hydrogen fluoride causes deep corrosive lesions on tissues. It has a high affinity for water and rapidly hydrolyzes to hydrofluoric acid. All fluorides are protoplasmic poisons. Fluorides bind many cations, most notably calcium. The binding of calcium results in the arrest of many cellular enzymatic processes and decreases the coagulation process. Although many believe that the cardiovascular collapse associated with fluoride toxicity is due to the precipitous fall in serum calcium concentrations, others support a theory involving fluoride-induced potassium efflux from cardiac cells (43). The neurologic effects of fluoride toxicity are related also to the calcium-binding effect of fluorides.

Toxic symptoms from sodium fluoride may appear after ingestion of as little as 200 mg. The lethal dose may be closer to 4 g (11). Death usually results from cardiac or respiratory failure, preceded by intense gastrointestinal symptoms (Table 10.4), hypotension, and convulsions. If death does not occur immediately, jaundice and oliguria may onset later. Chronic exposure has produced skeletal fluorosis (i.e., osteosclerosis, periosteal apposition of bone, and calcification of ligaments and joints) (5).

Management of Toxicity

Quick treatment is necessary if the fluoride-intoxicated patient is to survive. Fluoride is

TABLE 10.4. *Characteristics of fluoride poisoning*

Location	Signs and symptoms
Gastrointestinal	Abdominal pain, nausea, vomiting, diarrhea, salivation
Neurologic	Paresthesia, hyperactive reflexes, clonic-tonic convulsions, positive Chvostek's sign, muscular pain and weakness
Blood	Hypocalcemia, hypoglycemia
Cardiovascular/ respiratory	Hypotension, respiratory stimulation followed by depression

best inactivated by converting it to an insoluble form, e.g., calcium fluoride. Treatment of HF burns of the skin consists, first of all, of decontamination with copious amounts of water (7). Limiting the duration of exposure by flushing with water immediately and continuously for 30 minutes, decreases the severity of toxicity. Sodium bicarbonate can be given to prevent or correct metabolic acidosis. Since fluoride-induced hyperkalemia cannot be reversed effectively, removal of potassium, as well as fluoride by hemodialysis or hemoperfusion, may need to be considered (43). To avoid local damage and reduce systemic absorption, calcium gluconate gel 2.5% to 5% can be applied (40). Eye exposure may be treated by irrigation with 1% calcium gluconate drops after immediate and copious irrigation with water for at least 30 min (7).

If ingestion was recent, a source of calcium, such as milk, calcium chloride, or lime water, should be given orally and/or by gastric lavage. Calcium will react with fluoride within the GI tract to form calcium fluoride, a relatively insoluble, nonabsorbable complex, and thus, reduce systemic toxicity.

Calcium gluconate is administered to prevent rapid depletion of plasma calcium or to replace it (60,62). Aggressive fluid replacement is necessary to increase renal clearance of the ion, and counteract losses from burns, vomiting, and diarrhea and to counteract hypocalcemic-induced vasodilation. Whitford et al (66) demonstrated in rats that administration of sodium bicarbonate, to induce metabolic alkalosis, reduces fluoride toxicity.

Boric Acid

At one time boric acid (H_3BO_3) was recommended for more than 40 medical uses. It is a weak bacteriostatic compound with great potential for causing toxicity. Boric acid is an excellent insecticide for roaches and other crawling insects. It can be mixed with flour or sugar and water and is formed into clumps, which are put where insects congregate. Borates (e.g., as sodium tetraborate) are widely used as cleaning aids. Despite the eventual decrease in use of boric acid for its alleged medical purposes, the incidence of poisoning will probably not decline.

Ingestions of boric acid solution are reported in individuals who have accidentally used boric acid in place of Epsom salt (magnesium sulfate). Boric acid solutions have been mistakenly used in the preparation of baby formula, resulting in several deaths (14,15,63, 69). Boric acid readily penetrates abraded, but not intact skin (16,26,56,57). Problems are encountered when a boric acid solution or powder is applied to a wound, especially with occlusion. Absorption causes significant systemic effects.

Boric acid is cytotoxic. Its greatest danger is in tissues where it concentrates, such as the kidney. The fatal dose in adults is estimated to be 15 to 20 g, and in infants 5 to 6 g, but as little as one gram has been fatal (63,68).

After exposure, the signs and symptoms listed in Table 10.5 may be seen. A characteristic feature of boric acid poisoning is a severe erythematous rash (*boiled lobster rash*) that is seen on the palms, soles, and buttocks. The immediate cause of death is usually CNS depression. If the patient survives the acute poisoning event, complications, such as hepatic fatty necrosis, cerebral edema, or renal failure, may appear.

Treatment of poisoning is nonspecific and symptomatic. A fatality rate of 50% of those who ingest a toxic dose has been reported. In ingestion, gastric evacuation should be used.

TABLE 10.5. *Characteristics of boric acid poisoning*

Skin: erythematous ("boiled lobster") rash, blistering, desquamation, excoriation
Lethargy, weakness
CNS[a] depression, collapse, coma
Cardiovascular collapse
Twitching, tremors, convulsions
Hyperpyrexia
Hypotension
Cyanosis
Jaundice
Renal failure

[a] CNS, central nervous system.

Removal of boric acid or borates from blood can be accomplished by peritoneal dialysis or hemodialysis (3,69).

Phenol

Phenol (carbolic acid), one of the oldest disinfectants/deodorizers, is still used alone, and as an ingredient in many commercial products. Phenol is a significant cause of poisoning.

Intoxication can occur after absorption through intact skin, or by ingestion. Most poisonings are accidental. Phenol has a strongly characteristic odor and its presence can be readily detected on the breath.

Phenol is a protein precipitant that induces strong corrosive actions (22). It is a cellular depressant and causes a variety of signs and symptoms (Table 10.6). Death immediately after poisoning usually occurs from respiratory depression. Survival beyond a day or two is often met with renal damage that eventually leads to death. Although esophageal stricture is rare, it is a long-term complication that may develop. The adult lethal dose is estimated at 10 to 30 g (22).

Immediate emesis or lavage after phenol ingestion is important to consider, but are contraindicated in esophageal injury. Egg whites, milk, or gelatin solution, which serve as protein sources to interact with phenol remaining in the stomach, may be given. Activated charcoal, followed by a cathartic, may be preferred to ipecac-induced emesis or lavage in decontamination of the GI tract and preventing systemic absorption of phenol.

ALKALI

Alkaline substances are chemicals that have a pH of 11.5 or higher. The label of an alkaline product is sometimes misleading when trying to determine the degree of alkalinity. A reported pH value of a product that is intended to be diluted before use may refer either to the concentrated or diluted form. The user may be misinformed if the label is only casually read. Careful reading of labels is always necessary.

One way to report the degree of alkalinity of a product is to list potency as a percent of sodium hydroxide. Some household alkaline products contain this information, and a concentration of sodium hydroxide greater than 1% can cause tissue damage (49). The degree of injury as a result of alkali exposure is related to the quantity, concentration, length of exposure, and type of alkali. With most alkali solutions, concentration is more critical than volume.

In the United States, the greatest number of injuries from corrosive substances involves ingestion of alkali, rather than acids. The reason is probably related to the wider availability of alkaline household products. Also, the toxic potential of many alkali products is not universally recognized. Although the term "acid" is a common household term, "alkali" or "base" is less common. As a result, alkaline substances, such as dishwasher detergents and nonphosphate detergents, are stored carelessly in areas where children have easy access to them.

Most damage from ingested alkali occurs primarily to the esophagus (see Table 10.2), with gastric involvement reported in about 20% of cases. Seventy-five percent of all caustic injury to the esophagus in children under 5 years results from sodium hydroxide. Eighty-

TABLE 10.6. *Characteristics of phenol (carbolic acid) poisoning*

Nausea, vomiting, bloody diarrhea, abdominal cramping
Sweating (profuse)
Cyanosis
CNS stimulation, hyperactivity, convulsions, followed by CNS depression
Stupor
Hypotension
Increased respirations followed by depressed respirations
Pulmonary edema, pneumonia
Esophageal stricture
Hemolysis, methemoglobinemia
Jaundice
Renal failure
Cardiovascular collapse, shock
Skin: blanching, erythema, corrosion

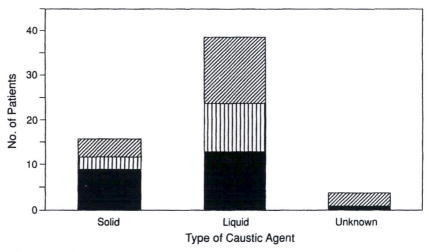

FIG. 10.2. Relation of the severity of esophageal injury to the type of caustic agent ingested. *Solid bars* represent first-degree burns, *hatched bars* second-degree burns, and *stippled bars* third-degree burns. The causative agent was known in 55 of 60 children with esophageal injuries. (From ref. 1.)

three percent of these victims are under 3 years, and 62% are males (6). Gastric acid is not sufficiently strong or present in sufficient quantity to neutralize even small quantities of strong alkali.

The physical form of an alkaline substance may determine the site and severity of caustic damage (Fig. 10.2). To illustrate, solid crystalline forms are not easily swallowed, nor are they readily spit out unless taken with lots of fluid. They adhere to the glossopharyngeal, palatal, and proximal esophageal mucosa to cause deep, irregular painful burns (28). Because of this adherence proximally, less damage is apt to occur distally. Liquid alkaline substances, on the other hand, pass freely through the esophagus and are considered to be more hazardous (22). Tissue damage will be more diffuse to the esophagus, as well as to the stomach (10,34,44,52). Suicidal adults often ingest alkaline products along with liquids so that they can ingest larger quantities. Deep esophageal and gastric damage, therefore, are seen commonly in these individuals (10,39,52).

Oral caustic burns cause much discomfort (see Table 10.3). A lack of dysphagia does not necessarily mean that esophageal injury is absent, and early management must still be initiated. Examining the mouth often confirms that an alkali substance was ingested. Sometimes a probable diagnosis can only be made from the child's obvious distress, along with discovery of an overturned or partially emptied alkaline-product container.

Mechanism of Toxicity

The initial reaction after contact of tissues with alkali is *saponification* (soap formation). Tissue damage resulting from alkali is a form of *liquefactive necrosis,* which destroys not only the surface epithelium, but also the underlying mucosal wall. This enhances its penetration into tissues (58). Consequently, systemic complications are common.

Characteristics of Poisoning

Esophageal damage after alkali injury occurs in stages (61). Initially, in the acute phase, which manifests within 3 to 5 days, there may be intramucosal or transmural damage involving the periesophageal tissues and structures in the mediastinum. Inflammation, edema, and congestion occur throughout the entire esophageal wall. In severe cases, the esophagus may perforate.

The second stage occurs over the next 5 to 12 days and is characterized by liquefactive necrosis resulting in intense inflammation and edema. This is the point at which the esophageal wall is most susceptible to ulceration, bleeding, and perforation. To illustrate the potential for damage, a 10-sec exposure of rabbit esophagus to 7N (22.5%) sodium hydroxide produces necrosis in all layers of the tissue (31). This phase is associated with deposition of fresh granulation tissue, which is eventually replaced by collagen fibers.

After the acute stage, healing and scarring begin. After 3 to 4 weeks, contraction and stricture are seen. Esophageal strictures are the most frequently observed complications of alkali ingestion. The usual incidence of strictures with granular or solid lye ingestion is 10% to 25% compared to approximately 100% for liquid lye (6,28).

Management of Poisoning

Skin and Eye Contamination

Skin and eye contamination should be flushed immediately and thoroughly with water for at least 15 to 20 min. Some treatment regimens suggest that severe alkali burns should be irrigated for at least 8 to 24 hr (58). All contaminated clothing and jewelry, and contact lenses if present, should be removed. As with acids, no medication should be placed on the lesion. Strong soap should not be used during or after the rinsing process.

Ingestion of Alkali

Ingestion of even a single granule of solid alkaline material or a milliliter or more of a liquid alkali warrants emergency consultation by qualified medical personnel. The extent of damage cannot be estimated from presenting symptoms. If a victim displays burns around the mouth and lips, then moderate-to-severe

toxicity may be suspected. However, even though the individual may not have observable burns in or around the mouth, this does not mean that severe esophageal damage has not occurred. Reflex swallowing of irritating substances is so quick that the substance is present in the mouth only for a short period.

As with acids, the treatment regimen for alkali ingestion is not standardized, and there are controversial points of view. Many precautions must be kept in mind. For example, emetics are contraindicated. Emesis reexposes the esophagus to the corrosive. Moreover, there is a possibility of aspiration of contents to cause severe edema, inflammation, ulceration of the glottis, and aspiration pneumonitis.

Gastric lavage is not universally recommended for alkali ingestion, but is occasionally performed only for large volumes of acid (50). Also, there is no great advantage to using activated charcoal since it adsorbs caustics poorly, and interferes with the endoscopy procedure used to determine extent of injury (29).

As a means of terminating exposure, dilution or neutralization after alkali ingestion has been questioned again. The general recommendation is to dilute with one or two glassfuls of cold milk or water. The objective is to minimize damage to the mouth, esophagus, and stomach.

Those who disagree with this approach contend that damage is instantaneous, and the resulting exothermic reaction increases the risk of further damage and vomiting (29,50). Also, it is difficult to persuade a small child to drink

TABLE 10.7. *Composition of Drano crystals and Clinitest tablets*

Drano crystals	
Sodium hydroxide	54.2%
Sodium nitrate	30.45%
Aluminum shavings	4.10%
Inert substances	11.25%
Clinitest tablets	
Sodium hydroxide	232.5 mg
Sodium carbonate	80.0 mg
Copper sulfate	20.0 mg
Citric acid	300.0 mg

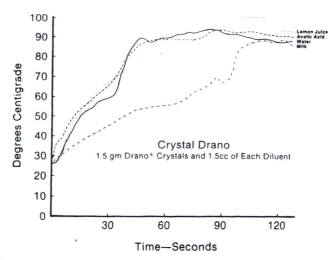

FIG. 10.3. The heat of reaction that occurs when various diluents are added to Crystal Drano. (From ref. 55.)

anything after ingestion of a corrosive because of the pain and tenderness experienced.

Rumack and Burrington (55) examined the neutralization/dilution question. In a series of *in vitro* experiments, a weighed quantity of crystal Drano or a Clinitest tablet (Table 10.7) was exposed to water, milk, lemon juice, or vinegar. The resulting temperature was determined and plotted as shown in Figs. 10.3 and 10.4.

It can be seen from these figures that the choice of diluent makes a difference in the amount of heat formed and its rate of formation. Milk appears to be the diluent of choice

for Clinitest tablets. Heat production was slower when milk was added to Drano. It is difficult to state with certainty that milk should be used to dilute Drano crystals since the temperature at the end of 2 min is similar as with the other diluents. Diluted solutions of vinegar or lemon juice (neutralizing agents) produce a significant increase in temperature, as compared to milk, and are not indicated in the management of ingested alkali.

If swallowing is possible, antacids and dairy products, such as ice cream and milk, are permissible. As long as the individual can swal-

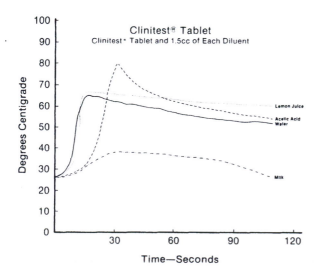

FIG. 10.4. The heat of reaction that occurs when various diluents are added to Clinitest tablets. (From ref. 55.)

low, all medications and clear liquids can be given orally and the diet increased progressively as tolerated.

Lesions may develop for 24 hr or more after ingestion. Patients must be observed closely for several days after ingestion. Endoscopic examination has proved to be useful in assessing esophageal damage after alkali ingestion (71).

When surgery is indicated it must be performed quickly. Early indications for surgery include mediastinal drainage after acute perforation, tracheostomy for laryngeal edema and respiratory distress, or a gastrostomy for feeding in acute severe injuries or extensive chronic strictures (6).

Occasionally the esophagus will require surgical reconstruction.

Steroids and Antibiotics

The rationale for use of glucocorticoids is to reduce fibrosis and esophageal rupture after alkali ingestion. It is based on animal studies (31,53). Using corticosteroids within the first 24 hr after corrosive alkali damage has been shown to decrease collagen formation, fibroplasia, and subsequent formation of scar tissue and stricture (20,64). Steroids are probably most effective in preventing stricture in cases of second-degree burns, are less effective in reducing damage in first-degree burns of the esophagus, and are questionable in treating third degree burns (8,23,25,61,65). On the other hand, steroids increase the possibility of infection. Antibiotics may be administered to reduce further complications from microbial invasion (45). Therapy with both agents must be initiated quickly to be effective. Some studies have shown steroids to be ineffective in decreasing development of esophageal stricture after ingested alkali in children, and development of stricture is related to the severity of the initial corrosive injury (1).

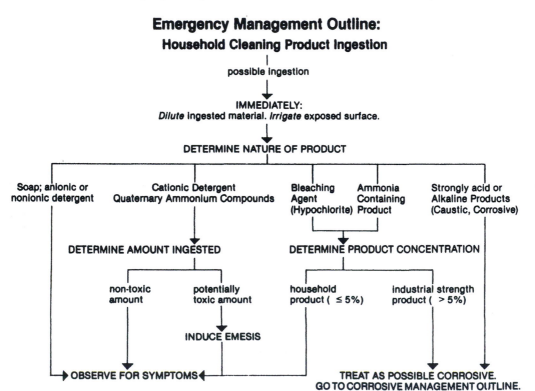

FIG. 10.5. Emergency management outline. Flow chart illustrating the steps involved in assessment and management of a victim of poisoning by a household product. (Reproduced with permission of the Soap and Detergent Association.)

Bougienage

With bougienage, a bougie (dilator) is passed through the esophagus to increase its caliber after stricture. Increasing the size of the dilator over a period of time aids in eventually widening the esophageal lumen. For severe strictures, bougienage may be required over many years.

Figure 10.5 presents a flow chart that illustrates important decisions and procedures in management of corrosive poisonings. This may be helpful when reviewing major treatment modalities discussed in this chapter.

SPECIFIC ALKALINE CORROSIVES

Disk Batteries

The use of small, flat disk-shaped (*button*) batteries has increased as the use of cameras, calculators, and other electronic gadgetry has increased in recent years. The incidence of ingestion of these batteries has increased proportionately (38). One estimate puts the number at 510 to 850 ingestions annually in the United States (36). A summary of 125 battery ingestions over an 11-month period revealed the location of the batteries before ingestion: 48.7%, loose or discarded; 34.4%, in the product; and 3.4%, in the manufacturer's package. Hearing-aid batteries were most commonly swallowed (33.9%), and 14 batteries were ingested by children after they removed them from their own hearing aids (37).

These batteries are constructed of a cathode can and anode cap separated by an electrode-soaked fabric (Fig. 10.6). Most often disk batteries are passed through the GI tract without incident (32,37). However, batteries have been known to become lodged within the esophagus and leak into the GI tract, resulting in severe corrosive toxicity and, sometimes, death.

Disk batteries may contain oxide salts of mercury, silver manganese, zinc, or cadmium; or lithium hydroxide. They also contain concentrated potassium or sodium hydroxide as a major ingredient.

In vitro studies have demonstrated that when the batteries come in contact with a moist environment they quickly begin to release their contents. In one study, batteries were immersed in normal saline in a 10 to 15:1 (vol:vol) ratio (64). The initial pH was 5.0. Bubbles were soon noted to emanate from the batteries, and a black-brown precipitate formed. The solutions quickly became alkaline and achieved a final pH between >10 to >12 by 2.5 hr. Even used or discarded (uncharged) batteries produced a pH of 8 to 9, accompanied by a brown-black precipitate.

Disc batteries may pass beyond the esophagus and are recovered in the stool within 48 to 72 hr. Those that lodge in the esophagus must be removed surgically (37,64). Activated charcoal is not indicated because of the small but real risk of airway obstruction (36). It is also uniformly unsuccessful as is ipecac-induced emesis (37). Cathartics are advocated to hasten removal of batteries that will reach

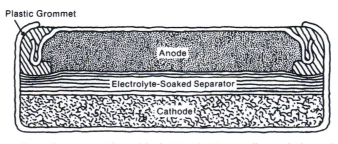

FIG. 10.6. Cross-section of a mercuric oxide button battery cell consisting of an amalgamated powdered zinc anode, a tightly compacted mercuric oxide and graphite cathode, an electrolyte-soaked felted fabric separator, and a plastic grommet, all contained in a steel can coated with nickel, and a steel top coated internally with copper and externally with gold and nickel.

the stomach or beyond, and H_2-antagonists and antacids are advocated to help reduce gastrointestinal bleeding. Benefit from these agents remains unproven. Metoclopramide may be given to hasten removal of batteries that demonstrate a persistent gastric position. The vast majority of battery ingestions are benign and do not require endoscopic or surgical intervention.

Soaps, Detergents, and Shampoos

Soaps and detergents constitute the largest class of household products found in greatest quantity around the household. Most soaps are relatively nontoxic and possess an emetic action that is possibly as effective as syrup of ipecac (Table 10.8). Soap-induced emesis is mediated through a direct effect on the GI tract, rather than systemic action (9). Ingestion of many soap products is not especially dangerous because soap is self-eliminating, and very few symptoms, other than upset stomach, will be experienced.

Bar soaps have a low order of toxicity. The most prominent symptoms produced by ingestion are usually nausea and vomiting, although diarrhea can appear and may become severe.

Although the same general statement about emetic action of soap is true, ingestion of strong detergents may cause a variety of reactions, depending on the specific product. Detergents contain a wide variety of inorganic and organic ingredients, among which are surfactants and wetting agents. Surfactants may be anionic, cationic, or nonionic. Most household detergents contain anionic or nonionic surfactants. Cationic detergents have a greater toxicity potential compared to anionic and nonionic detergents. The latter generally produce local irritation, whereas cationic detergents may incite severe irritation and possibly systemic effects.

Builders are added to detergents to improve cleaning action of the product, usually by inactivating calcium and other minerals. Commercially used builders may include carbonates, silicates, aluminosilicates, and sulfates. The use of phosphates as a builder was popular in previous years. Phosphates have been largely replaced in recent years because of the concern about their effect on the environment. The major problem of toxicologic concern from ingestion of most detergent products is the builder. Because of their high alkalinity, it may produce severe ocular irritation and oral and gastrointestinal burns (35).

Other ingredients including whitening agents, fabric softeners, suds-controlling agents, and enzymes are frequently added. These are usually of no toxicologic concern.

Granular soaps and detergents generally have a low order of toxicity. The exception is automatic dishwashing machine detergents, which are highly alkaline and produce corrosive action (30).

Shampoos have a low order of toxicity, although gastric irritation may cause a greater incidence of nausea and vomiting. Addition of "antidandruff agents" to shampoos generally increases the products' toxicity.

Management of soap, detergent, or shampoo ingestion should involve immediate dilution with water or milk. Spontaneous emesis should be expected; induction of emesis is seldom necessary. When highly alkaline prod-

TABLE 10.8. *Emetic action of household cleaning products in dogs*

Products	Mean emetic dose (g/kg)	Mean time for emesis (min)
Heavy-duty granular laundry detergent	0.02–0.05	1–4
Light-duty liquid detergent	0.3–1.5	15–45
General purpose liquid household cleaner	0.1–1.0	0.5–10
Bleach, liquid (sodium hypochlorite)	0.25	1–2
Toilet soap	5.0	30–60
Syrup of ipecac	0.1	30–50

ucts, such as automatic dishwasher detergents are ingested, management for a corrosive substance should be followed. If vomiting or diarrhea becomes prominent, symptomatic treatment and fluid replacement may be necessary.

Management of eye or skin exposure is the same as outlined previously for corrosives. The management outline for household soaps, detergents, and shampoos was given in Fig. 10.5.

Liquid hard-surface cleaners often contain pine oil or petroleum distillates. Although the quantity of such substances contained in these products is generally of little toxic concern, their chance for being aspirated during emesis is real. Consequently, victims who ingest one of these products should be kept as quiet as possible and not be made to vomit. (Refer to chapter 7).

Ammonia and Ammonium Solutions

Ammonia, oven cleaners, and drain cleaners are highly alkaline and extremely corrosive. Ammonia solution (household ammonia), *per se*, ranges from 5% to 10% ammonia, but an industrial strength solution greater than 50% is also available. Ammonia is used in a wide variety of products, and its corrosive action is seen on all cells. Ingestion of stronger solutions must be treated the same as any caustic substance.

Inhalation of ammonia gas produces irritation of the upper respiratory tract, often causing cough, dyspnea, and pulmonary edema. Contact with skin or eyes produces severe pain and corrosive damage. Ingestion of ammonia solution resembles that of a typical alkaline corrosive. Treatment is the same as for other alkaline corrosive substances.

A distinction must be made between ammonia, per se, and products advertised as *having ammonia*. These latter products contain small quantities of the substance and are usually of little toxic concern.

Bleach

Most bleach products are solutions of 3% to 6% sodium hypochlorite (NaOCl) in water.

The pH is approximately 11, which makes them highly alkaline. Bleach ingestion produces severe irritation and corrosion of mucous membranes with pain and inflammation. The amount of bleach actually ingested is usually small, probably due to its extremely bad taste, and bleach solutions are spontaneously vomited. Therefore, severe toxicity is often avoided. Two large clinical studies examined the outcome of ingestion of chlorine bleach. They found no esophageal strictures or perforations (33,51).

Management of bleach ingestion includes dilution with water or demulcents, such as milk or antacids. Neutralization with acidic solutions and ipecac-induced emesis are contraindicated. Hypochlorous acid is formed in the stomach when sodium hypochlorite reacts with hydrochloric acid. Hypochlorous acid is not toxic when absorbed in small quantities, since it is buffered by the blood. However, it is extremely irritating to mucous membranes of the esophagus and the GI tract.

Bleach should not be mixed with strongly acidic or alkaline cleaning agents in an unvented area, although this is apparently common practice in some households (see the case study at the end of this chapter). When bleach reacts with either acid or alkali, as shown in Fig. 10.7, either chlorine or chloramine gas may be released. Both can cause lacrimation and irritation to the mucous membranes and respiratory passages if inhaled in sufficient concentrations. In high concentrations, both could cause asphyxiation.

Some bleaches, especially the powdered ones, contain other oxidizing agents, such as peroxides or perborates. When present, ingestion of these types of bleaches must be treated more vigorously.

Iodine

The toxicity potential for iodine may be overstated and overemphasized. Deaths are rare (13). It is doubtful that the quantity contained in 0.5 to 1 ounce, which is the normal quantity found in most homes, would inflict

Sodium Hypochlorite + $\begin{cases} \text{Strong acid} & \rightarrow & Cl_2 \uparrow & + & NaOH \\ \quad (H^+) & & \text{(chlorine)} & & \\ \text{Strong alkali} & \rightarrow & NH_2Cl \uparrow & + & NaOH \\ \quad (NH_4^+) & & \text{(chloramine)} & & \end{cases}$

FIG. 10.7. Sodium hypochlorite (bleach) mixed with strong acid or strong alkali results in formation of chlorine or chloramine gas.

serious injury. Most fears of iodine or reasons for its bad image probably resulted from use in previous years of the 7% tincture, which is no longer used except in veterinary practice.

Iodine is a direct protein precipitant that is corrosive to mucous membranes. In the intestine, it is converted to the less toxic iodide, and rapidly deactivated by food in the GI tract. Furthermore, it causes a strong vomiting reflex, which removes much of the poison. All of these factors help minimize toxicity.

Major effects after ingestion of iodine (2%) involve the GI tract, with nausea, vomiting, diarrhea, and gastroenteritis being paramount. Hypotension, tachycardia, cyanosis, and other signs of shock may be apparent. Ingestion can be quickly recognized by the appearance of brown stains in the mouth or on the lips, or by brown-colored vomitus.

Iodine ingestion should be treated to reduce the extent of gastrointestinal damage. Dilution with milk or water is appropriate. A starch solution (1% to 10%) will absorb iodine. Gastric lavage, with soluble starch, is useful. Then, a 1% to 5% solution of sodium thiosulfate can be instilled to convert remaining iodine to iodide. Glucocorticosteroids should be administered as quickly as possible to reduce the chance of esophageal fibrosis, a complication that may occur later.

Death from massive ingestion usually occurs within 48 hr from circulatory collapse due to shock or from aspiration during emesis, which causes pulmonary edema (13).

Quaternary Ammonium Compounds

Quaternary ammonium compounds (QACs) are cationic surfactants used in a wide variety of products, such as disinfectants, bactericides, deodorants, and sanitizers. QACs are all potentially toxic. Toxicity varies with the specific compound, the concentration of prod-

uct, dose ingested, and the rate of administration. All QACs produce similar symptoms through a similar mechanism.

Concentrations above one-percent produce superficial necrosis of mucous membranes, causing GI tract erosion, ulceration, and hemorrhage. Edema of the glottis and brain has been reported, as well as damage to the heart, liver, and kidney.

All QACs cause disinfection only to chemically clean areas. In the presence of any trace of soap, they are inactivated. Thus, soap is a suitable means for preventing damage from QAC poisoning, from either skin contamination or oral ingestion. Ingestion of a cleaning agent greater than 5% to 10% of QACs should be treated as a corrosive alkaline ingestion.

SUMMARY

There is a wide variety of acids and alkali that have the potential to cause significant corrosive damage. Although acids and alkali differ in their pathophysiologic effects, precautions against exposures are similar. Table 10.9 lists some common household products that are rated based upon their relative toxicity.

Case Studies

CASE STUDY: CORROSIVE ALKALI TABLET INGESTION

History

A 38-year-old diabetic woman sought medical attention after ingesting 75 Clinitest tablets (see Table 10.7) approximately one week previously. She was nauseated immediately after ingestion and vomited everything she ate or drank. Still, she did not seek immediate medical attention. In the emergency room she

TABLE 10.9. *Summary of toxic household products*

Toxicity	Product	Toxic ingredient of effect	Treatment[a]
Soaps, Detergents, Cleaners, and Bleaches			
High	Electric dishwasher granules[b]	Caustic (may be severe)	Treat as caustic burn[b]
	Ammonia[b]	Caustic; coma and convulsions	As caustic[b]; supportive
	Bleach, commercial	Boric acid or oxalate poisoning	Milk, calcium; supportive
	Bleach, oxygen	Boric acid poisoning	Supportive
Medium	Bleach, chlorine	Gastrointestinal irritation, some causticity	Demulcents ± treat as caust burn
	Borax	Boric acid poisoning	Supportive
	Water softeners (soluble)[b]	Some caustic; hypocalcemia and acidosis possible	Milk; as for caustic[b]; supportive
	Liquid general cleaners:		
	Kerosene	Pneumonia, systemic toxicity	As for petroleum distillates
	Pine oil	Gastrointestinal and genitourinary irritation; depression and weakness	Supportive; demulcents
	Detergent granules[b] for laundry, dishes, and general use	Gastrointestinal irritation to causticity (some frankly caustic and have higher toxicity)	Demulcents; treat as caustic burn[b]
Low	Detergent powders[b]	Gastrointestinal irritation (causticity possible but unlikely)	Demulcents, soap; ± treat as caustic burn[b]
	Liquid detergents	Gastrointestinal irritation	Demulcents, soap
	Toilet soap	Gastrointestinal irritation	Demulcents
	Fabric softeners	None	None
	Window cleaners (liquid)	Alcohol	*See* footnote e
Inhalation hazard	*Chlorine bleach mixed with:*		
	Strong acid (bowl cleaner)	Chlorine gas (intense respiratory irritation)	Bicarbonate aerosol; oxygen
	Ammonia	Chloramine fumes (respiratory irritation, nausea)	Terminate exposure; supportive
Disinfectants and Deodorizers			
High	Naphthalene deodorizer (bathroom, toilet, garbage can)	Irritation, coma, convulsions, hemolysis, kidney damage	Supportive; alkalinize urine; transfuse as needed
	Acid disinfectant (boric, chloroacetic, formic, salicytic, etc.)	Corrosive, plus systemic effects of anion	Supportive; treat as caustic burn
	Phenolic disinfectant	Phenols; hexachlorophene (gastrointestinal irritation, shock, coma; corrosion or kidney damage possible)	Treat as caustic burn or anticipate renal failure
Medium to high[c]	Alkali disinfectant (sodium or ammonium hydroxides)	Potentially caustic	Demulcents; ± treat as caustic burn
	Benzalkonium and other QAC[d] disinfectants	Gastrointestinal irritation, convulsions, coma, respiratory distress, collapse	Supportive; demulcents; mild soap solution or milk
	Pine oil disinfectant	Gastrointestinal and genitourinary irritation; depression and weakness	Supportive; demulcents
	Halogen disinfectant	Hypochlorites or chlorinated hydrocarbons (irritation; excitation)	Demulcents; ± treat as caustic burn; sedation as needed
Medium	Wick deodorizer	Formaldehyde and hydrocarbons (gastrointestinal irritation, abdominal pain, shock, hematuria, coma, convulsions)	Supportive; demulcents
	Deodorizing cleanser	Pine oil or QAC	*See* above
	p-Dichlorobenzene or sodium bisulfate deodorizer (bathroom, toilet, garbage can)	Irritation, abdominal pain, narcosis; liver, kidney damage possible	Supportive; demulcents; sodium bicarbonate

TABLE 10.9. *Continued.*

Toxicity	Product	Toxic ingredient of effect	Treatment[a]
Low	Iodophor disinfectant	Detergent-iodine complex (gastrointestinal irritation)	Demulcents
Nil	Spray deodorizer	Variable	Symptomatic
	Refrigerator deodorizer	Charcoal (inert)	None
Cosmetics			
High	Permanent wave neutralizer	May contain either:	Supportive
		Perborate (boric acid poisoning)	For boric acid poisoning
		Bromate (irritation, collapse, hemolysis, kidney damage)	Sodium thiosulfate by mouth; demulcent; consider dialysis early
	Fingernail polish remover	Toluene; aliphatic acetates (irritation; central-nervous-system depression)	Supportive
Medium	Fingernail polish	Same as fingernail polish remover	Supportive
	Hair dye, metallic	Metal salts, pyrogallol (metal poisoning; corrosive)	For metal (if severe); demulcents
	Permanent wave lotion	Thioglycolate (irritation; possible hypoglycemia)	Supportive; demulcent
	Bath oil	Perfume; sulfated castor oil	Demulcent (milk)
	Shaving lotion	Alcohol	Supportive
	Hair tonic	Alcohol, others (variable)	Supportive[e]; demulcents
	Cologne; toilet water	Alcohol, essential oils	Supportive[e]; demulcents
Low	Perfume	Alcohol, essential oils (irritation; possible hypoglycemia)	Supportive[e]; demulcents
	Shampoo	Anionic detergent (irritation)	Demulcent (milk)
	Bubble bath	Sodium lauryl sulfate (gastrointestinal irritation)	Demulcent (milk)
	Depilatory	Thioglycolate (*see* above)	Supportive; demulcent
	Hair straightener	Glycols and alcohols; may be caustic	Supportive ± as for caustic
	Hair dye, oxidation	Various amines, etc. (gastrointestinal irritation; ?methemoglobinemia)	Demulcent; methylene blue for severe methemoglobinemia
	Deodorant	Alcohol; aluminum or zinc salts (gastrointestinal irritation; possible hypoglycemia)	Supportive[e]; demulcents
	Shaving cream	Soaps	Demulcent (milk)
	Bath salts	Polymeric phosphate; borax	For causticity or boric acid poisoning
Nil	Makeup, liquid		
	Eye makeup		
	Hair dye, vegetable (henna, indigo)		
	Cleansing or conditioning cream	None	None
	Hair dressing (nonalcoholic)		
	Hand lotion or cream		
	Lipstick, tube rouge		

[a] In addition to evacuation of stomach (except with caustic burn) or removal from skin, when indicated.
[b] Products threatening caustic effects will be identified with a *caution* label.
[c] Depending on constitution and concentration.
[d] QAC, quaternary ammonium compounds.
[e] Ethyl alcohol, in addition to being a depressant, may produce hypoglycemia in young children. Related alcohols, with the exception of methanol, have qualitatively similar effects; none of the above contains methanol.

was in hypoglycemic coma. She received intravenous glucose, and was soon discharged.

Several days later, she was seen again in the emergency room for hypoglycemic coma and severe abdominal cramping. It was at this time that she admitted to ingesting the Clinitest tablets.

Physical examination was unremarkable except for epigastric tenderness. Esophagoscopy of the distal half of the esophagus showed white plaques with erythematous mucosa and ulceration surrounding them.

The endoscope was not advanced into the stomach until a week later. At that time, stricture of the distal esophagus and esophagitis were observed. Three weeks later, pathologic changes in the antral portion of the stomach included contraction and ulceration. Further studies revealed esophagitis and food retained in the stomach. The duodenum appeared normal.

The constricted esophagus was dilated with bougienage. Eventually a hemigastrectomy and gastroduodenotomy were performed. On examination of the removed tissue, a benign gastric ulcer with severe adjacent fibrosis and inflammation was noted. (See ref. 39.)

Discussion

1. After ingestion of 75 Clinitest tablets, why were symptoms delayed? What are some of the reasons you think helped this patient to survive?
2. What was the purpose of the bougienage?
3. The endoscopic examination was undertaken quite slowly (e.g., only the proximal half of the esophagus was examined initially, with the next portion examined a week later). Discuss the reason for this delay.
4. Define the terms *endoscopy, hemigastrectomy* and *gastroduodenotomy*.

CASE STUDY: TOXICITY TO ALKALINE BATTERY INGESTION

History

A 16-month-old girl presented to an emergency facility as an alert, irritable, tachypneic child. Vital signs included temperature, 102.2°F; pulse, 172 beats/min; respirations, 52/min; and blood pressure, 118/80 mm Hg. She was estimated to be 10% dehydrated.

Previous to admission, she experienced a vomiting episode and developed a fever. It was not until she became progressively irritable and developed abdominal distension and tachypnea that she was brought to the hospital.

During examination, chest X-ray films revealed a round radiopaque foreign body lodged in the upper thoracic region. At this time, the parents remembered that an alkaline battery for their camera flash attachment had been missing for about 3 days. There was no other information the family could provide.

Laboratory results were all within the normal physiologic limits.

Treatment began with a thoracostomy, which resulted in removing about 100 mL of a straw-colored fluid mixed with black particulate matter. After an esophagoscopy, a flat alkaline camera battery measuring approximately 22 mm × 5 mm was recovered. There was marked black discoloration and necrosis of the surrounding esophagus. It was felt that the esophagus was probably perforated.

The victim was given clindamycin hydrochloride intravenously, and fluid replacement. She remained stable after surgery, but was later sent back to the operating room to have the mediastinum drained and a feeding gastrostomy inserted.

Approximately 2 hr later she died from cardiopulmonary arrest. A large amount of blood was removed from her stomach during resuscitation attempts.

Postmortem examination revealed that death occurred from hemorrhage by perforation. Microscopic examination revealed liquefactive necrosis which extended through the mucosa and submucosa layers of the esophagus. (See ref. 44.)

Discussion

1. The outstanding major point with regard to this case is that an object, about the thick-

ness of three stacked quarters was swallowed and caused death, not from suffocation but from esophageal perforation. Why do you think this smooth flat object became lodged in the esophagus, and did not enter the stomach?

2. It is estimated that batteries contain a 45% potassium hydroxide solution, that is on the order of 8N KOH. Describe the type of corrosive injury that occurs with a caustic substance of this magnitude.

CASE STUDY: BATTERY ACID INGESTION

History

A 49-year-old man who owned an automotive garage ingested an undetermined quantity of battery acid (concentrated sulfuric acid) in an apparent suicide attempt. On admission to the emergency room he complained of burning in his mouth and dysphagia. He later vomited. A frothy, blood-tinged secretion was observed in his mouth and pharynx. The mucosa of the hypopharynx appeared white and the uvula were swollen. Coarse rhonchi were present bilaterally. His abdomen was tender on touch; bowel sounds were minimal. Laboratory results are shown in Table 10.10.

Abdominal roentgenography showed a large radiopaque mass in the region of the stomach.

Treatment consisted of intravenous penicillin and hydrocortisone acetate. Approximately 12 hr postadmission, the patient experienced respiratory distress and a tracheostomy was

TABLE 10.10. *Laboratory findings*

WBC	=24,000 mm³
Hct	=51%
PTT	=100 sec
PT	=40% (16.8 sec)
pH	=7.32
pO₂	=79 mm Hg
pCO₂	=33 mm Hg

WBC, white blood cells; Hct, hematocrit; PTT, partial thromboplastin time; PT, prothrombin time.

performed. A gastrostomy was planned. However, upon close examination, blood was found in the abdominal cavity. A gastrectomy was, therefore, performed instead.

Three days later, the patient was readmitted to surgery for further examination and possible reassessment. At that time, 1,500 mL of fresh blood was found in the abdominal cavity and a gangrenous portion of the ileum was removed.

The patient was followed closely and on the 11th hospital day, upper gastrointestinal bleeding from an erythematous esophagus developed. There was no esophageal stricture. A vigorous antacid regimen was prescribed.

By the 16th hospital day, the man was drinking fluids. He was discharged 19 days after ingestion, and a high-protein diet prescribed. Six months later he showed complete recovery, weight gain, and no signs of esophageal stricture. (See ref. 12.)

Discussion

1. Did the ingestion of battery acid by this man produce the expected type of injury with respect to site and extent of damage?
2. What was the purpose of treating this patient with an antibiotic and steroid?
3. Although a gastrostomy was originally planned, a gastrectomy was performed instead. Of what value would this later procedure have considering the extent of gastric damage?

CASE STUDY: HYDROCHLORIC ACID INGESTION

History

The patient, a 13-year-old boy, attempted suicide by drinking approximately 60 mL of a liquid toilet bowl cleaner (15% HCl) and 3.250 mg acetaminophen. When he arrived at the emergency department he was lethargic, vomiting, and had gastric pain. He also had tachycardia.

Esophagogastroduodenoscopy revealed mucosal ulceration with hemorrhage and clotting in the antrum, body, and fundus of the stomach. The esophagus and duodenum were spared. The patient was placed on a liquid diet, antidepressants, and ranitidine.

On the 11th day he complained of anorexia and vomiting. He had lost 12 lb over the previous two weeks and was able to accept only one ounce of liquid at a time.

An upper gastrointestinal series was performed 14 days postingestion. It revealed an antral ulcer and prepyloric stricture. The patient received total parenteral nutrition (TPN) through a central line, small amounts of oral liquids, and antacids. Ranitidine was continued.

He was transferred to a psychiatric unit for the next four weeks. A second upper gastrointestinal examination was performed 10 weeks postinjury, and revealed multiple ulcers on the greater curvature of the stomach. He was readmitted, complaining of anorexia and vomiting. Endoscopy disclosed multiple ulcers, diverticula, and prepyloric stenosis. He was now able to tolerate a liquid diet, and was taken off TPN and sent home.

He gained 5 lb over the next six weeks, despite the fact that his appetite was poor. By four months postinjury, the ulcer size had decreased.

By 11 months postingestion, the boy was asymptomatic, and had gained 17 lb. An upper gastrointestinal examination revealed that the ulcers healed, obstruction was no longer present, and he had normal peristalsis. At 15 months all signs and gastrointestinal symptoms had resolved, and he returned to school. (See ref. 28.)

Discussion

1. Of the two substances ingested by this patient, which one is considered to be of greater concern: (a) 60 mL of the liquid toilet bowl cleaner or (b) 3.25 g of acetaminophen? Give reasons to support your answer.
2. This case is interesting because the victim did not require gastric resection. Many similar ingestions would have required it.

Physicians managing this case reported that they specifically delayed early surgery because of the boy's psychiatric illness. What reasoning did they use to arrive at this decision?
3. Comment on the type of drugs used. What is their mechanism of action, and were they needed?

CASE STUDY: HYDROFLUORIC ACID POISONING

History

A petroleum refinery operator was working in the plant's alkylation unit. This unit used hydrofluoric acid under pressure as a catalyst to produce high octane gasoline components. At the time of the accident, the unit was shut down and neutralization of the acid was almost completed.

The operator attempted to remove a plug and was splashed in the face with anhydrous hydrofluoric acid. He was wearing protective clothing which consisted of a hard hat with safety visor, neoprene boots, gloves, and jacket. After approximately 10 min, he was washed with water, and a magnesium oxide preparation was applied to the exposed area.

The patient was transported to an emergency facility, arriving with stable vital signs: blood pressure, 130/88 mm Hg; pulse, 88 beats/min; and respirations, 32/min. There were third-degree burns throughout the lower quarter of his forehead, both eyelids and cheeks, and his nose and upper lip. His pharynx was red and he had trouble swallowing. Some keratoconjunctivitis was reported, but no corneal damage. Also, dysphagia was evident, but breath sounds were clear.

The patient's treatment consisted of injecting the burn area with 40 mL of 10% calcium gluconate and intubation of the airway to assess respiratory function. Morphine 10 mg subcutaneously was given for pain; Pontocaine drops were instilled into the eyes to reduce irritation. Laboratory findings are shown in Table 10.11.

TABLE 10.11. *Laboratory findings*

pH	=7.21
pO_2	=68 mm Hg
pCO_2	=38 mm Hg
HCO_3^-	=15 mEq/L
O_2 saturation	=88%
Serum Ca^{2+}	=3.5 mg/dL

The patient was later taken to the operating room for excision of the eschar and debridement of the burn area. He appeared to be progressing satisfactorily. However, in the recovery room, he developed ventricular fibrillation, which was converted successfully. He subsequently died from a series of ventricular fibrillation episodes, the last one resulting in asystole.

Postmortem examination revealed intense congestion of the upper respiratory mucosa and pulmonary edema. His serum fluoride concentration was 0.3 mg/dL. (See ref. 60.)

Discussion

1. What type of systemic toxicity does hydrofluoric acid manifest?
2. Why was the victim's serum calcium so low? What was the probable relationship between the serum calcium concentration and the cause of death?
3. Usually, tetany is a clinical manifestation of hypocalcemia. In this patient, what was the sign (aside from the laboratory report) that indicated a decreased serum calcium concentration?

CASE STUDIES: ACUTE SODIUM FLUORIDE TOXICITY

History: Case 1

A 25-year-old man who intentionally ingested a commercially available rat poison was admitted to the emergency room 2.5 hr later. An unmarked box containing a finely textured blue powder was also brought along.

It was thought at the time to contain arsenic. Later, it was shown to be sodium fluoride.

Physical examination was unremarkable except for tachycardia (160 beats/min) and gallop rhythm. The stool was positive for occult blood. Cyanosis was not apparent. Laboratory values are shown in Table 10.12.

An ECG recording revealed tachycardia with a QT interval of 0.45 sec. Blood and urine toxicologic analyses were negative for drugs and arsenic.

Treatment consisted of 300 mg dimercaprol intramuscularly, since the initial diagnosis was arsenic poisoning. A nasogastric large-bore tube was inserted. Gastric lavage was performed using 3 L milk. After a while, there was profuse drainage of bright red blood from the nasogastric tube. Fluid replacement consisted of saline and dextrose.

The patient developed ventricular fibrillation about 1 hr after admission. The arrhythmia continued despite defibrillation procedures and treatment with lidocaine. He died after 30 min of unsuccessful resuscitation.

Postmortem findings showed severe congestion of the lungs and liver, along with enlargement of the left ventricle. The stomach and esophagus had marked hyperemia, and the lumen of the stomach contained about 50 mL of a purplish-brown fluid that tested positive for fluoride. (See ref. 4.)

History: Case 2

A 2.5 year-old girl ingested an undetermined amount of commercial grade laundry powder that was intended for use as a *whitener*. The major ingredient was sodium silicofluoride, although this information was not

TABLE 10.12. *Laboratory findings*

Na^+	=148 mEq/L
K^+	=4.3 mEq/L
Cl^-	=105 mEq/L
CO_2	=47 mEq/L
Hct	=48%
Hb[a]	=16.4 g%

[a] Hb, hemoglobin.

TABLE 10.13. *Laboratory findings*

Na$^+$	=138 mEq/L
K$^+$	=6.7 mEq/L
HCO$_3^-$	=mEq/L
Cl$^-$	=107 mEq/L
+2 protein in urine	
BUN[a]	=31 mg/dL
Ca^{2+}	=3.4 mg/dL

[a] BUN, blood urea nitrogen.

made available to emergency room personnel for some time after admission. She was brought to the emergency facility because of progressive vomiting and lethargy that had been evident for about 6 hr. She experienced respiratory distress and periods of ventricular tachycardia and fibrillation for the next 2 days.

She presented in a coma with respirations of 6 to 8/min. Other vital signs were normal. Generalized twitching and nystagmus were also present. Chvostek's and Trousseau's signs were not present. She responded only to deep pain. Gastric lavage was performed yielding a yellowing viscous material.

Laboratory findings were unremarkable for hematology, blood glucose, and supine fluid analysis. Other values are shown in Table 10.13.

The electrocardiogram showed a normal sinus rhythm and QT interval of 0.52 sec.

Nine hours after admission, peritoneal dialysis was initiated with calcium chloride added to the dialysate. The patient received a continuous infusion of calcium, and was also given 0.1% calcium hydroxide (lime water) orally. Ventricular tachycardia was controlled with lidocaine and eight separate courses of electrical cardioversion.

Nine hours after peritoneal dialysis was initiated, she became responsive and was fully conscious 2 days later. No other major problems were noted, aside from a bout of viral pneumonitis. (See ref. 70.)

Discussion

1. In both cases, there was a prolonged QT interval. Discuss the mechanism of fluoride-induced cardiotoxicity.

2. What is the mechanism of fluoride-induced pulmonary toxicity?
3. Are there any specific antidotes for fluoride toxicity? If so, what are they?
4. Patient 1 tested positive for fecal occult blood. How does this relate to the pathogenesis of fluoride toxicity?

CASE STUDY: CHRONIC BORAX INTOXICATION

History

A 4 1/2-month-old boy had experienced seizures since age 2 months. At 3 months of age, he was diagnosed as having epilepsy and treated with phenobarbital. Seizures continued despite the use of anti-epileptic medication. On admission to the hospital, he appeared pale and irritable and had patchy, dry erythema over the scalp, trunk, and limbs. The results of a physical examination were generally unremarkable.

Laboratory values were mainly within normal limits, but a hypochromic normocytic anemia was detected.

During examination the patient was quite irritable and began to cry. In order to appease the child, his mother dipped a pacifier into a small brown bottle she carried in her purse. When she gave the baby the pacifier coated with this thick yellow-brown liquid, he immediately stopped crying.

The bottle was labeled ''Borax and Honey.'' Listed ingredients were: borax 10.5 g, glycerin 5.25 g, and honey to 100 g. Apparently she had learned this practice from her own mother who had used this preparation on all her children. The child had received approximately 1 ounce per week since he was 1 month old.

With this information, blood and urine samples were analyzed for boric acid content (Table 10.14).

After the borax-honey-pacifier *therapy* was discontinued the child had no further seizures, and the EEG recording returned to normal after 1 week. Phenobarbital therapy was discontinued.

TABLE 10.14. *Laboratory findings*

Measurement	mg/dL	
	Blood	Urine
Borax	14.5	12.3
Boric acid	9.44	7.95

The infant was discharged, but therapy with iron supplements was initiated. After several months, the blood profile became normal. (See ref. 21.)

Discussion

1. How does acute borax poisoning differ from chronic borax intoxication as seen in this case study?

CASE STUDIES: CHLORINE BLEACH POISONINGS

History: Case 1

A 2-year-old girl drank several ounces of household bleach (5.4% sodium hypochlorite). She vomited almost immediately, and was given milk and olive oil. She presented to the emergency room with burns of the lips, tongue, and hard and soft palate. Esophagoscopy was delayed because the child had pneumonia. The course of treatment consisted of antibiotics and corticosteroid therapy.

It was necessary to begin parenteral feeding because of increased difficulty in swallowing. Hematemesis and fecal occult blood were noted on the 4th hospital day. It was not until 3 weeks after admission that an esophagoscopy could be performed. At that time it revealed a severely burned esophagus with a 4 to 5 cm area of narrowing. At the end of 1 month there was no change in the size of stricture, despite several attempts at dilation. The following week a gastrostomy was performed. She was discharged 2.5 months after admission. (See ref. 19.)

History: Case 2

An 83-year-old diabetic woman was cleaning her bathtub with undiluted Clorox (5.2% sodium hypochlorite). The stain was *stubborn* to remove, even with soap, so she added almost a full can of Sani-Flush (80% sodium bisulfate). Almost immediately she experienced an intense burning sensation around the mouth, nose, throat, and eyes. Though she began coughing, she persisted in cleaning the area. She finally left the small unventilated room when her breathing became extremely difficult, approximately 3 to 4 min after coughing began.

She presented at the emergency room with symptoms of severe, near-fatal pulmonary edema.

Treatment consisted of oxygen, morphine, rotating tourniquets, prednisone, and a diuretic. She recovered completely within 10 days and was discharged. (See ref. 27.)

History: Case 3

A 31-year-old man injected 0.3 mL of 5.25% sodium hypochlorite (Clorox) into a right antecubital vein and then injected approximately the same amount into a left antecubital vein using a 1.0-mL insulin U-100 syringe. He experienced immediate left-sided chest pain and several episodes of vomiting and was taken to the emergency department by ambulance.

On arrival, his vital signs were normal except for blood pressure of 162/98 mm Hg. He was alert, awake, and in no apparent distress. He had tenderness in the right lower quadrant of his abdomen, and his liver edge was 3 to 4 cm below the coastal margin. There was erythema on both antecubital areas.

The ECG, urinalysis, serum electrolytes, arterial blood gas, and serum glucose were normal. His urine toxicology screen was negative. The blood ethanol concentration was 135 mg/dL. Measured serum osmolality was 324 mOsm/kg; calculated osmolality, 288 mOsm/kg; and osmolar gap, 36 mOsm/kg.

The patient said that he felt depressed and had given himself the bleach injections while watching a movie. This was the patient's first suicide attempt.

Emergency medical personnel applied warm compresses to each antecubital area and observed him for six hours, during which he experienced neither further chest pain nor vomiting. After psychiatric consultation and treatment with multivitamins, folate, and thiamine, he was discharged after arranging outpatient follow-up. He continued to do well three days later. (See ref. 48)

Discussion

1. Is a solution of sodium hypochlorite acidic or basic?
2. Is the site of injury consistent with the chemical classification of this poison?
3. What happens when bleach is mixed with gastric juice?
4. What is a gastrostomy, and why was it performed on the patient in case 1?

CASE STUDY: BENZALKONIUM CHLORIDE POISONING

History

Two and one-half month old twins (one each boy and girl) were brought to a hospital. They had fever, dehydration, circumoral erythema, and numerous oral and pharyngeal grayish-white lesions. Both infants also had a red, dry, scaly diaper rash. The boy had been diagnosed the day before as having candidiasis, and benzalkonium chloride (1:50,000) was prescribed to be applied topically.

The mother had a prescription filled and had been applying the medication to the mouth of both children. But whenever the drug was applied, immediately the children would salivate profusely and cry. This was followed by a period of anorexia, irritability, and fever. It was at this point the twins were brought to the hospital.

Direct laryngoscopy showed no lesions.

TABLE 10.15. *Laboratory findings*

Measurement	Male infant	Female infant
WBC	22,700 mm^3	24,800 mm^3
Serum uric acid	12 mg/dL	9.2 mg/dL
Alkaline phosphatase	350 IU/L	240 IU/L
SGOT[a]	40 IU/L	20 IU/L

[a] SGOT, serum glutamate oxaloacetic transaminase.

Drooling and an intermittent cough were noted. The boy also had evidence of pneumonitis, which cleared within 4 days. Laboratory results are shown in Table 10.15.

Information was later obtained from the pharmacist who dispensed the benzalkonium prescription that a 17% stock solution had been diluted incorrectly to its prescribed concentration. Instead, it was diluted two parts to one part water (resulting in an 11% solution) and was dispensed.

The girl stayed 1 week, but the boy remained in the hospital for 2 weeks. (See ref. 67.)

Discussion

1. How is benzalkonium chloride classified, and what is its toxicity rating?
2. What toxic effects are produced by this type of product?
3. What is considered a *safe* or recommended dose of benzalkonium chloride for topical use?
4. How would the clinical manifestations of acute ingestion of this compound differ from the present case study?
5. On admission, the boy had a fever; the girl did not. What was the probable cause?

Review Questions

1. Poisoning with a *rust remover* will most likely involve which of the following substances?
   A. Hydrochloric acid
   B. Sulfuric acid

C. Oxalic acid

D. Ascorbic acid

2. Electric dishwasher detergents are highly:

A. Acidic

B. Alkaline

3. Strongly acidic substances are all strongly corrosive.

A. True

B. False

4. With which of the following blood electrolytes does sodium fluoride react to cause major deficiency problems?

A. Potassium

B. Manganese

C. Chloride

D. Calcium

5. Poisoning by muriatic acid indicates that treatment is required for which of the following acids?

A. Hydrochloric

B. Sulfuric

C. Oxalic

D. Tartaric

6. In the United States, which is the more common cause of poisoning?

A. Acids

B. Alkali

7. Laundry bleach contains a 3% to 6% concentration of:

A. Sodium hypochlorite

B. Carbon tetrachloride

C. Oxalic acid

D. Carbolic acid

8. Which of the following is a true statement?

A. Soap causes emesis through stimulation of the chemoreceptor trigger zone (CTZ).

B. On the average, detergents are more toxic than soap.

C. Enzymes in some soap and detergent products are of toxic concern.

D. Shampoo ingestion should be treated as a toxic emergency.

9. Erythema, reported as a *boiled lobster rash* is a symptom of toxicity with:

A. Phenol

B. Boric acid

C. Oxalic acid

D. Benzalkonium chloride

10. A major and early symptom of oxalic acid intoxication is:

A. Hyponatremia

B. Hypernatremia

C. Hypokalemia

D. Hyperuricemia

E. None of the above

11. Which of the following is a manifestation of iodine toxicity: corrosive action on membrane protein (I), circulatory collapse and shock (II), or stimulation of respiratory secretions (III)?

A. I only

B. II only

C. III only

D. I and II only

E. II and III only

F. I, II and III

12. The most appropriate treatment for strong acid spilled on the skin is to treat the lesion with:

A. Vinegar solutions

B. Mineral oil

C. Water

D. Sodium bicarbonate solution

13. A "button battery" that is lodged in the esophagus for more than 24 hours should be removed.

A. True

B. False

14. Outline the procedures to follow when managing bleach ingestion.

15. Cite the advantages and disadvantages of diluting ingested corrosives with (a) water, (b) milk, and (c) carbonated beverages.

16. A particular danger exists when an ingested acid or corrosive substance is *neutralized in vivo* with another chemical agent. Describe the potential problem.

17. Describe the toxic reaction expected from ingesting Clinitest tablets.

18. Ingested acids and alkali cause tissue necrosis that is characteristic for each type of corrosive, based on its site and description of damage. Fill in the blanks:

	Site of damage	Type of damage
Acid	_____	_____
Alkali	_____	_____

19. A patient presents at the ER with fine material in the stomach that is described as *coffee grounds* in consistency. What is the most likely source of this material?

20. It is often stated that no creams or ointments should be placed on skin that has been severely damaged by an acid or alkali, if the victim is to be transported to a emergency facility. Why is this so?

21. Outline the procedure for managing acid or alkali burns to the eye.

22. Compare and contrast use of the terms *caustic* and *corrosive*.

23. Corticosteroids and antibiotics are often given after ingestion of corrosive substances. Why?

24. Discuss the specific action of sodium thiosulfate in treating iodine ingestion.

References

1. Anderson KD, Rouse TM, Randolph JG. A controlled trial of corticosteroids in children with corrosive injury of the esophagus. *N Engl J Med* 1990;323:637–640.

2. Ashcraft KW, Padula RT. The effect of dilute corrosives on the stomach. *Pediatrics* 1974;53:226–232.

3. Baliah T, MacLeish H, Drummond KN. Acute boric acid poisoning: report of an infant successfully treated by peritoneal dialysis. *Can Med Assoc J* 1969;101:166–168.

4. Baltazar RF, Mowers MM, Reider R, et al. Acute fluoride poisoning leading to fatal hyperkalemia. *Chest* 1980;78:660–663.

5. Brown MG. Fluoride exposure from hydrofluoric acid in a motor gasoline alkylation unit. *Am Ind Hyg Assoc J* 1985;46:662–669.

6. Buntain WL, Cain WC. Caustic injuries to the esophagus: a pediatric overview. *South Med J* 1981;74:590.

7. Caravati EM. Acute hydrofluoric acid exposure. *Am J Emerg Med* 1988;6:143–150.

8. Cardona JC, Daly JF. Current management of corrosive esophagitis: an evaluation of results in 239 cases. *Ann Otol Rhinol Laryngol* 1971;80:521–527.

9. Carter RO, Griffith JF, Weaver JE. The household products manufacturer's role in poison prevention. *Clin Toxicol* 1969;2:238–294.

10. Cello JP, Fogel RP, Boland CR. Liquid caustic ingestion. *Arch Intern Med* 1980;140:501–504.

11. Chernick WS. The ions: potassium, calcium, magnesium, fluoride, iodide, and others. In: DiPalma JR, ed. *Pharmacology in medicine.* 4th ed. New York: McGraw-Hill; 1971:940–957.

12. Chodak GW, Passaro E. Acid ingestion: need for gastric resection. *JAMA* 1978;239:225–226.

13. Clark MN. A fatal case of iodine poisoning. *Clin Toxicol* 1981;18:807–811.

14. Connelly JP, Crawford JD, Soloway AH. Boric acid poisoning in an infant. *N Engl J Med* 1958;259:1123–1125.

15. Done AK. Borates. In: Haddad LM, Winchester JF, eds. *Clinical management of poisoning and drug overdose.* Philadelphia: WB Saunders; 1983:929–931.

16. Ducey J, Williams B. Transcutaneous absorption of boric acid. *J Pediatr* 1953;43:644–651.

17. Edmonson MB. Caustic alkali ingestions by farm children. *Pediatrics* 1987;79:413–416.

18. Foster DE, Barone JA. Rectal hydrofluoric acid exposure. *Clin Pharm* 1989;8:516–518.

19. French RJ, Tabb HG, Rutledge LJ. Esophageal stenosis produced by ingestion of bleach. *South Med J* 1970;63:1140–1143.

20. Goldman LP, Weigert JM. Corrosive substance ingestion: a review. *Am J Gastroenterol* 1984;79:85–89.

21. Gosselin RE, Smith RP, Hodge HC, eds. *Clinical toxicology of commercial products.* 5th ed. Baltimore: Williams and Wilkins; 1984:III-245–246.

22. Haddad LM, Dimond KA, Schweistris JE. Phenol poisoning. *J Am Coll Emerg Physicians* 1979;8:267–269.

23. Hawkins DB, Demeter MJ, Barnett TE. Caustic ingestion—controversies in management—review of 214 cases. *Laryngoscope* 1980;90:98–109.

24. Hodgson JH. Corrosive stricture of the stomach: case report and review of the literature. *Br J Surg* 1958;44:358–361.

25. Howell JM, Dalsey WC, Hartsell FW, Butzin CA. Steroids for the treatment of corrosive esophageal injury: a statistical analysis of past studies. *Am J Emerg Med* 1991;10:421–425.

26. Johnstone DE, Basila N, Glaser J. A study of boric acid absorption in infants from the use of baby powder. *J Pediatr* 1955;46:160–167.

27. Jones FL. Chloride poisoning from mixing household cleaners. *JAMA* 1972;222:1312.

28. Kirsh MM, Ritter F. Caustic ingestion and subsequent damage to the oropharyngeal and digestive passages. *Ann Thorac Surg* 1976;21:74–82.

29. Knopp R. Caustic ingestions. *J Am Coll Emerg Physicians* 1979;8:329–336.

30. Krenzelok EP, Clinton JE. Caustic esophageal and gastric erosion without evidence of oral burns following detergent ingestion. *J Am Coll Emerg Physicians* 1979;8:194–196.

31. Krey H. Treatment of corrosive lesions in the esophagus. *Acta Otolaryngol Suppl (Stockh)* 1952;102:1–49.

32. Kulig K, Rumack CM, Rumack BH, Duffy JP. Disk battery ingestion. *JAMA* 1983;249:2502–2504.

33. Landau GD, Saunders WH. The effect of chlorine bleach on the esophagus. *Arch Otolaryngol* 1964;80:174–176.

34. Leape LL, Ashcraft KW, Scaepelli DG, Holder TM. Hazard to health—liquid lye. *N Engl J Med* 1971;284:578–581.

35. Lee JF, Simonowitz D, Block GE. Corrosive injury of the stomach and esophagus due to non-phosphate detergents. *Am J Surg* 1972;123:6529.

36. Litovitz TL. Button battery ingestions: a review of 56 cases. *JAMA* 1983;249:2495–2500.

37. Litovitz TL. Battery ingestions: product accessibility and clinical course. *Pediatrics* 1985;75:469–476.

38. Litovitz T, Schmitz BF. Ingestion of cylindrical and button batteries: an analysis of 2392 cases. *Pediatrics* 1992;89:747–757.

39. Lowe JE, Graham DY, Boisaubin EV, Lanza FL. Corrosive injury to the stomach: the natural history and role of fiberoptic endoscopy. *Am J Surg* 1979;137:803–806.

40. MacKinnon MA. Treatment of hydrofluoric acid burns. *J Occup Med* 1986;28:804–806.

41. Maull KI. Liquid caustic ingestions: an *in vitro* study of the effects of buffer, neutralization, and dilution. *Ann Emerg Med* 1985;14:1160–1162.

42. McCutcheon RS. Toxicology and the law. In: Doull J, Klaassen CD, Amdur MO, eds. *Toxicology—the basic science of poisons*. 2nd ed. New York: Macmillan; 1980:727–733.

43. McIvor ME. Acute fluoride toxicity. *Drug Safety* 1990;5:79–85.

44. Messersmith JK, Oglesby JE, Mahoney WD. Gastric erosion from alkali ingestion. *Am J Surg* 1970;119:740–741.

45. Middlekamp JN, Cone AJ, Ogura JH, et al. Endoscopic diagnosis and steroid and antibiotic therapy of acute lye burns of the esophagus. *Laryngoscope* 1961;21:1354–1362.

46. Middlekamp JN, Ferguson TB, Roper CL. Ingestion of liquid drain cleaner. *GP* 1969;40:86–89.

47. Mitchell GA. The management of fluoride poisoning. In: Maddad LM, Winchester JF, eds. *Clinical management of poisoning and drug overdose*. Philadelphia: WB Saunders; 1983:690–697.

48. Morgan DL. Intravenous injection of household bleach. *Ann Emerg Med* 1992;21:1394–1395.

49. Muhlendahl KE, Oberdisse U, Krienke EG. Local injuries by accidental ingestion of corrosive substances by children. *Arch Toxicol* 1978;39:299–324.

50. Penner GE. Acid ingestion: toxicology and treatment. *Ann Emerg Med* 1980;9:374–379.

51. Pike DG, Peabody JW Jr, Davis EW, Lyons WSA. Re-evaluation of the dangers of Clorox ingestion. *J Pediatr* 1963;63:303–305.

52. Ritter FN, Newman MH, Newman DE. A clinical and experimental study of corrosive burns of the stomach. *Ann Otol Rhinol Laryngol* 1968;77:830–841.

53. Rosenberg N, Kunderman PJ, Uroman L, Moolten SE. Prevention of experimental lye strictures of the esophagus by cortisone. *Arch Surg* 1951;63:147–151.

54. Roy CC, Silverman A, Cozzetto FJ. *Pediatric clinical gastroenterology*. St Louis: CV Mosby; 1975.

55. Rumack BH, Burrington JD. Caustic ingestions: a rational look at diluents. *Clin Toxicol* 1977;11:27–34.

56. Siegel E, Wason S. Boric acid toxicity. *Pediatr Clin North Am* 1986;33:363–367.

57. Skipworth GB, Goldstein N, McBride WP. Boric acid intoxication from "medicated talcum powder." *Arch Dermatol* 1976;95:83–86.

58. Stewart CE. Chemical skin burns. *Am Fam Physician* 1985;31:149–157.

59. Stremski ES, Grande GA, Ling LJ. Survival following hydrofluoric acid ingestion. *Ann Emerg Med* 1992;21:1396–1399.

60. Tepperman PB. Fatality due to acute systemic fluoride poisoning following a hydrofluoric acid skin burn. *J Occup Med* 1980;22:691–692.

61. Tewfik TL, Schloss MD. Ingestion of lye and other corrosive agents—a study of 86 infant and child cases. *J Otolaryngol* 1980;9:72–77.

62. Trevino MA, Herrmann GH, Sprout WL. Treatment of severe hydrofluoric acid exposures. *J Occup Med* 1983;25:861–863.

63. Valdes-Dapena MA, Arey JB. Boric acid poisoning—three fatal cases with pancreatic inclusions and a review of the literature. *J Pediatr* 1962;61:531–546.

64. Votteler TP, Nash JC, Rutledge JC. The hazard of ingested alkaline disk batteries in children. *JAMA* 1983;249:2504–2506.

65. Webb WR, Kontras P, Ecker RR. An evaluation of steroids in caustic burns of the esophagus. *Ann Thorac Surg* 1970;9:95–98.

66. Whitford GM, Reynolds KE, Pashley DH. Acute fluoride toxicity: influence of metabolic alkalosis. *Toxicol Appl Pharmacol* 1979;50:31–39.

67. Wilson JT, Burr IM. Benzalkonium chloride poisoning in infant twins. *Am J Dis Child* 1975;129:1206–1207.

68. Winther LK. Accidental corrosive burns of the esophagus. *J Laryngol Otol* 1978;92:693.

69. Wong DC, Heimback MD, Truscott DR. Boric acid poisoning: report of 11 cases. *Can Med Assoc J* 1964;90:1018–1023.

70. Yolken R, Konecny P, McCarthy P. Acute fluoride poisoning. *Pediatrics* 1976;58:90–93.

71. Zargar SA, Kochhar R, Nagi B, et al. Ingestion of strong corrosive alkalis: spectrum of injury to upper gastrointestinal tract and natural history. *Am J Gastroenterol* 1992;87:337–341.

11 | Plants

Plant ingestion is a common cause of poisoning exposures in children under age 5 in the United States, and a significant cause of toxicity in adults (Table 11.1) (22). Each year more than 15,000 Americans are poisoned by plant ingestion (16). The incidence of calls into Poison Control Centers in the United States concerning plant ingestions is estimated to be in the range of 5% to 10% of all calls (21).

The incidence of plant-induced poisoning is also reported to be increasing. As more and more adults forage through the countryside in search of *nature's foods*, poisonous plants can be mistaken for edible ones. Also, as the nation's awareness for self-care and self-medication grows, many are exploring the use of herbs and natural products for disease prevention or self-treatment of various maladies. Studies have shown that many products of plant origin are available in numerous retail outlets and these are potentially toxic if misused (1). Moreover, children often see the bright berries of many plants and, perhaps believing they are fruits or confections, consume

them. Sometimes the green, leafy foliage of some plants are used in salads, or with other nontoxic food items growing in the family garden. Both adults and adolescents may experiment with plants that they believe have hallucinogenic properties.

In some cases, an actual plant part may not need to be ingested. Drinking water from a vase containing plant stems may be sufficient to cause serious toxicity. In other instances, plants that are considered to be harmless have been treated with toxic insecticides, herbicides, or fertilizers may be consumed (22).

Although plant ingestions are commonplace, they rarely cause serious toxicity or death. In most instances, a victim of plant ingestion experiences little more than localized irritation, such as pain or edema in and around the mouth. Some plants, however, can cause serious toxicity and possibly death. Any ingestion of plant material of unknown identity should be treated as potentially toxic ingestion until it can be classified otherwise.

Of the approximately 30,000 species of plants growing in North America, both cultivated and wild, only a surprisingly few are responsible for most poisonings (Table 11.2). In one year, 12 species represented over 30% of all toxic ingestions (13). Fewer than 50 species, of the approximately 700 to 1,000 toxic plants growing in the United States, cause over 95% of all poisonings.

Defining exactly what constitutes a poisonous plant is not easy. Almost any plant can cause nausea and vomiting or intestinal cramping when enough of it is ingested. Separating scientific reality from folklore and myth, when it concerns plant toxicity, is extremely difficult. However, a suitable definition is that poisonous species are those that contain specific components that, when small quantities are ingested, cause specific biochemical alterations or physiologic symptoms. According to this definition, jimsonweed and foxglove are poisonous plants because small quantities of their components can produce significant toxic effects, even death.

Not all parts of some poisonous plants are toxic, and the toxic principle(s) may be pres-

TABLE 11.1. *Substances most frequently involved in human exposure*

Substance	Number	%[a]
Cleaning substances	191,830	10.4
Analgesics	183,013	10.0
Cosmetics	153,424	8.3
Plants	112,564	6.1
Cough and cold preparations	105,185	5.7
Bites/envenomations	76,941	4.2
Pesticides (including rodenticides)	70,523	3.8
Topicals	69,096	3.8
Antimicrobials	64,805	3.5
Foreign bodies	64,472	3.5
Hydrocarbons	63,536	3.5
Sedatives/hypnotics/antipsychotics	58,450	3.2
Chemicals	53,666	2.9
Alcohols	50,296	2.7
Food poisoning	46,482	2.5
Vitamins	40,883	2.2

From ref. 24.
Despite a high frequency of involvement, these substances are not necessarily the most toxic, but often represent only ready availability.
[a] Percentages are based on the total number of human exposures rather than the total number of substances.

TABLE 11.2. *Frequency of plant exposures by plant type*

Botanical name	Common name	Frequency
Philodendron spp.	Philodendron	6,407
Dieffenbachia spp.	Dumbcane	4,242
Capsicum annuum spp.	Pepper	3,687
Euphorbia pulcherrima	Poinsettia	3,289
Ilex spp.	Holly	2,839
Phytolacca americana	Pokeweed, Inkberry	2,349
Crassula spp.	Jade plant	2,244
Spathiphyllum spp.	Peace lily	1,969
Brassaia & *Schefflera* spp.	Umbrella tree	1,878
Epipremnum aureum	Pothos, Devil's ivy	1,735
Toxicodendron radicans	Poison ivy	1,735
Saintpaulia spp.	African violet	1,509
Taxus spp.	Yew	1,452
Pyracantha spp.	Fire thorn	1,265
Rhododendron spp.	Rhododendron, Azalea	1,192
Chlorophytum comosum	Spider plant	1,034
Ficus benjamina	Weeping fig tree	1,030
Chrysanthemum spp.	Chrysanthemum	990
Solanum dulcamara	Climbing nightshade	989
Quercus spp.	Oak	932

From ref. 24.

ent in the plant only during certain seasons or stages of growth. Slight variations in methods used to prepare plants for intentional consumption may make a tremendous difference in whether or not the final preparation is safe or toxic. The specific plant or plant parts ingested, therefore, must be identified before one can formulate an opinion on its toxicity and the best way to manage the ingestion.

MANAGEMENT OF THE PLANT-POISONED PATIENT

Several important rules dictate what should be done when a person is the victim of a potentially toxic plant ingestion. Figure 11.1 is a guide to the procedures most commonly used.

All plant ingestions must be considered potentially toxic until shown otherwise. Identi-fication of the plant is often the most difficult task. The parent of a child who has ingested a plant part may be completely unaware of its identity, or where the child found it. The name of a plant used by the parent may or may not be an accurate description. Frequently *nicknames* or family or trivial nomenclature for plants are used and often the correct botanical name is not known. Also, different names may be applied to the same plant, depending on the region of the country. In certain areas, poison dogwood refers to a species of *Cornus*, whereas in other regions it refers to poison sumac. The name *elephant's ears* may refer to *Caladium*, *Colocasia*, or *Dieffenbachia* species, to mandrake, or to several other plants.

The first task is to try to identify the plant. Table 11.3 provides some helpful information used to describe plants. Time is usually to the victim's advantage. Since the toxic principles of most plants must first be leached out of the plant leaf, stem, etc., there is usually sufficient time to properly identify the plant.

The first point of contact should be the local or regional Poison Control Center. Poison Control Centers are equipped with a variety of information retrieval systems and they represent countless hours of experience in the management of plant ingestions. If the Poison Control Center cannot positively identify the plant, it may suggest other centers in the country that specialize in phytotoxicology. Alternatively, nurserymen are usually very knowledgeable in botanical plant names and common names when a specific plant is described to them. Wild plants are best identified by a botanist, or local agricultural extension agency. For mushrooms, a mycologist may need to be contacted for proper identification of some species.

For most plant ingestions, management consists of demulcent therapy. Many plants contain constituents that are extremely irritating to the oral mucous membranes, but not damaging to other tissues. Ice cream, milk, or a frozen confection will soothe most irritations of the GI tract associated with plant ingestions. The victim should be observed closely over the next 12 to 24 hr to assure that no

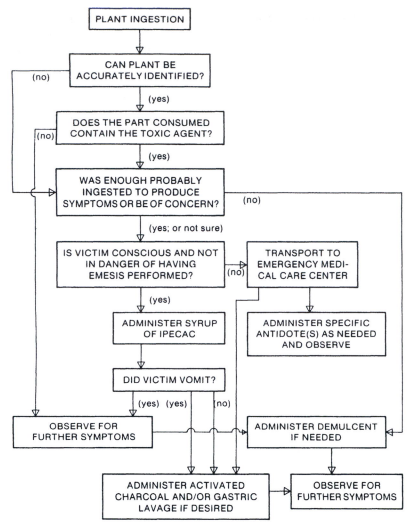

FIG. 11.1. Flow chart illustrating the steps involved in assessment and management of a victim of poisoning by a plant.

additional symptoms appear as a result of delayed absorption or delayed toxic effects.

If the plant in question has been identified as toxic or has toxic potential or enough of a plant has been ingested to cause concern, gastric decontamination should be considered. Ipecac-induced emesis is the preferred method. All regurgitated material should be carefully examined for assessment as to the nature of the plant parts that were ingested.

Many plants have a powerful emetic action of their own that may cause profuse, spontane-

ous vomiting. If this occurs, the vomitus should be examined. Demulcents may be given at this time if needed. If the plant is poisonous, or, if after vomiting the victim displays symptoms that suggest toxicity, medical assistance will be necessary.

Gastric lavage is limited in value for decontaminating the stomach after a plant ingestion. Most undigested plant parts will not fit through the opening of even the largest orogastric tube. However, after ipecac-induced emesis, gastric lavage may be performed to wash out any remaining poison and may be

TABLE 11.3. *Aids to help identify a potentially poisonous plant*

Specific site where plant was growing, including whether in sunny or shady area, moist or dry soil. Is this a house plant, cultivated variety, or wild-growing weed?

Shape and texture of leaves including description of edges, arrangement on stalk, and vein structure.

Color, size, texture, and shape of seeds, fruits, berries or flowers, including their arrangement and grouping.

Plant's dimensions, both above and below the soil.

Nature of plant (e.g., free-standing plant, bush, or tree, vine, ground cover)

Common and botanical names

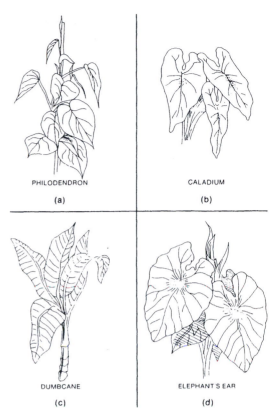

(a) PHILODENDRON (b) CALADIUM

(c) DUMBCANE (d) ELEPHANT'S EAR

FIG. 11.2. Common household plants of the Arum family that cause poisoning.

useful as long as ingestion occurred within the past 5 to 6 hr.

Activated charcoal is generally not an acceptable alternative to syrup of ipecac in gastrointestinal decontamination of a poisonous plant. Adsorption of the toxic principles onto activated charcoal is dependent on these components existing as a fine powder or in solution. A leaf, berry, or other coarse plant part that contains toxic principles probably will not release them until it is sufficiently digested. It is better to remove the entire plant part, if at all possible. Activated charcoal may be given after ipecac-induced emesis or gastric lavage to adsorb residual poison.

Saline cathartics may be given to hasten removal of ingested plants and after administration of a slurry of activated charcoal.

COMMON POISONOUS PLANTS

As pointed out above, there are many poisonous plants. However, most poisonings occur from a relatively small number of species of both cultivated and wild plant varieties.

Arum-Family Plants

Of all the houseplants, those of the Arum family (Fig. 11.2a–d) are responsible for most frequently encountered plant ingestions or exposures. These plants include caladium or *fancy-leaf* (*Caladium bicolor*), dumbcane

(*Dieffenbachia picta*) and *D. sequine*, elephant's ear (*Colocasia antiquorum*), and philodendron (*Philodendron* spp.). Table 11.4 lists others.

These plants all possess large leaves that contain tiny needle-sharp crystals of calcium oxalate, arranged parallel in compact bundles called *raphides* or in starlike clusters called

TABLE 11.4. *Plants of the Arum family*

Common name	Botanical name
Alocasia	*Alocasia* spp.
Caladium	*Caladium* spp.
Dumbcane	*Dieffenbachia* spp.
Elephant ears	*Colocasia* spp.
Jack-in-the-pulpit	*Arisaema triphyllum*
Philodendron	*Philodendron* spp.
Skunk cabbage	*Symplocarpus foetidus*
Swiss-cheese plant	*Monstera* spp.

Toxic components: calcium oxalate, bradykinin-like substances, enzymes.

druses. Biting into a leaf results in pain as these crystals pierce the sensitive membranes of the mouth and lips. A second bite is usually avoided, and significant systemic toxicity is rare.

Crystalline raphides, containing calcium oxalate, exist in specialized cells called idoblasts, and were once thought to be the cause of irritation resulting from biting into a piece of dieffenbachia (11). Early investigations implicated a substance that caused smooth muscle contraction and was inhibited by antihistamines (15). In other studies, edema and irritation seemed to result from a bradykinin-like substance or an enzymatic reaction (3,20).

Ingestion of plants from the Arum family results in localized edema, pain, and irritation. Occasionally, the tongue swells to the point that swallowing and speaking become difficult (hence, the origin of the term *dumbcane*). If swelling of the tongue, pharynx, or larynx becomes severe enough as to hamper breathing or induce choking, emergency medical treatment is necessary to maintain a patent airway. In one instance, a victim's tongue swelled so much that it protruded through his mouth for three days (31). Dermal exposure may result in localized dermatitis, particularly when the skin comes in contact with the sap from within the plants.

Management of ingestions of Arum family plants is supportive and symptomatic. Demulcents and cold packs may be helpful.

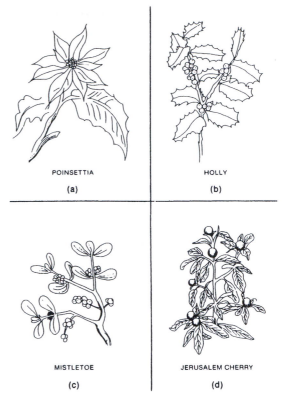

FIG. 11.3. Common "Christmas" plants; **b–d** cause poisoning.

Christmas Plants

Another group of houseplants reported to entice children includes a variety of plants commonly seen around the holidays such as poinsettia, holly, mistletoe, and Jerusalem cherry (Fig. 11.3a–d and Table 11.5).

Jerusalem cherry (*Solanum pseudocapsicum*) has bright orange cherry-like ornamental berries that contain the extremely toxic substance *solanine*. Solanine is a glycoalkaloid found also in the nightshade plants which produces intense gastrointestinal symptoms. The glycoalkaloid is hydrolyzed by gastric acid to alkamine, which has toxic action upon the cardiovascular and nervous system to cause circulatory collapse and respiratory distress, as well as fever, drowsiness, restlessness, and headache (10).

All ingestions of Jerusalem cherry or any other Solanaceae plant must be treated aggressively. Spontaneous vomiting will most likely occur. If it does not, however, gut decontamination, using syrup of ipecac, lavage, activated charcoal, and cathartics should be considered. In addition, good supportive and symptomatic care is required.

For years there has been a misconception that the poinsettia plant (*Euphorbia pulcherrima*) is toxic. There have been numerous published reports warning about its toxic potential. A report of a 2-year-old child who died after ingestion of poinsettia (33) is often quoted, even though its conclusion is not true.

TABLE 11.5. *Ornamental Christmas plants*

Common name	Botanical name	Toxic substance(s)	Signs and symptoms
Holly	*Ilex* spp.	Ilicin Saponins	Gastrointestinal irritation
Jerusalem cherry	*Solanum pseudocapsicum*	Solanine Solanidine Solanocapsine	Nausea, vomiting, abdominal pain, diarrhea, altered mental status, headache, hallucinations
Mistletoe	*Phoradendron flavescens*	Viscotoxin Phoratoxin Viscumin	Nausea, vomiting, abdominal pain, diarrhea, cardiac abnormalities (potential)
Poinsettia	*Euphorbia pulcherrima*	Latex sap	Nontoxic

Poinsettia is nontoxic. The milky sap may cause mild irritation to mucous membranes, resulting in oral discomfort from a bite (41).

Management, if necessary, would consist of a demulcent to reduce mouth pain. If any of the sap touches the skin, it should be washed off with soap and water.

White mistletoe berries (*Phoradendron flavescens*) or the bright red berries of Christmas holly (*Ilex opaca*) are potentially toxic. Rarely does systemic toxicity occur, since both berries cause severe gastrointestinal irritation resulting in nausea and vomiting. Also, the berries of mistletoe sold for decoration at Christmas will usually have been replaced with plastic spheres.

The toxicity of mistletoe is related to the presence of alkaloids, lectins, and cardiotoxins. The primary manifestations are gastrointestinal, causing abdominal pain, nausea, vomiting, and diarrhea. A recent assessment of toxicity to mistletoe reveals that ingestion of one to three berries or one or two leaves is unlikely to produce serious toxicity. If more than these amounts have been ingested, induction of emesis with ipecac is recommended, followed by a slurry of activated charcoal and a saline cathartic (17).

Holly contains saponins and triterpenes, which are responsible for intense gastrointestinal symptoms, including bloody vomitus.

Cardiotoxic Plants

Numerous plants cultivated in gardens and displayed as houseplants contain toxic substances that produce digitalis-like actions on the heart (Table 11.6). These plants include foxglove (*Digitalis purpurea*), oleander (*Nerium oleander*), lily-of-the-valley (*Convallaria majalis*) and star-of-Bethlehem (*Ornithogalum umbellatum*) (Fig. 11.4a–d).

Ingestion of foxglove or oleander resembles digoxin poisoning, with gastrointestinal and cardiac symptoms predominating. Intoxication requires serial monitoring of the electrocardiogram and serum potassium, since hyperkalamia may be present. Ingestion of even small quantities of these plants must be treated aggressively. Gastric decontamination with syrup of ipecac followed by serial doses of activated charcoal and supportive care is recommended.

Lilly-of-the-valley ingestions are less serious because only small amounts of convallatoxins are present. Large ingestions need to be treated, as above.

The ornamental hedge, yew (*Taxus canadensis*) contains the potent cardiotoxic toxins, *taxine A and taxine B*. Yew is a favorite ornamental evergreen shrub that grows in most areas of the Midwest and northeast and is of great toxicologic concern. The tiny red berries that adorn the stems are especially attractive and enticing to children. All portions of the yew plant, except the bright red fleshy part that caps the seeds, contain taxine alkaloids. A single chewed berry (containing the seed that harbors concentrated toxin) is potentially lethal to a child, but often larger quantities need to be ingested to produce toxicity.

Ingestion of these plants may produce se-

TABLE 11.6. *Plants containing cardiac glycosides*

Common name	Botanical name	Cardiotoxin	Signs and symptoms
Foxglove	*Digitalis purpurea*	Digoxin Digitoxin Gitoxin Others	Irritation of mouth and stomach, vomiting, abdominal pain, diarrhea, cardiac disturbances (ventricular ectopy, conduction block, cardiogenic shock, hyperkalemia)
Oleander	*Nerium oleander*	Oleandroside Oleandrin Nerioside	See Foxglove
Yellow oleander, tiger apple	*Thevetia peruviana*	Thevetin A & B Thevetoxin Peruvoside Ruvoside Neriifolin	See Foxglove
Lily-of-the-valley	*Convallaria majalis*	Convallatoxins	See Foxglove; but less likely to cause serious toxicity
Rhododendron, azalea, laurel	*Rhododendron* spp.	Grayanotoxins (andromedotoxin)	Nausea, vomiting, bradycardia, hypotension, hyperkalemia

vere gastrointestinal irritation, but the major concern is progressive decreased atrioventricular (AV) nodal conduction, which may lead to severe bradycardia. Treatment is aimed at gastric evacuation, correction of electrolyte imbalance, and maintaining cardiac function.

Rhododendron, azaleas, and laurel contain several toxins. Grayanotoxins (formerly andromedotoxin) are of special concern since they structurally resemble cardiac glycosides and Veratrum alkaloids. However, intoxication is more likely to be associated with bradycardia and hypotension than with arrhythmias. Human poisonings are more likely to occur from honey made from the nectar of grayanotoxin-containing plants than from ingestion of plant parts. Gastrointestinal decontamination is required for large ingestons of plant parts.

Castor Bean

Seeds of the castor plant (*Ricinus communis*) are among the most toxic of all the cultivated plants that grow in the United States The plant (Fig. 11.5a) is grown for its oil and as an ornamental shrub. Castor beans (seeds) are quite attractive to children, and ingestion of a single chewed seed may be fatal. Unchewed seeds often pass through the GI tract without causing clinical problems (32).

Castor beans contain the deadly phytotoxin *ricin*. Ricin consists of two polypeptide chains, one of which binds to intestinal cells and the other is an inhibitor of protein synthesis. Ordinarily inactivated by heat during production of castor oil, ricin may cause gastrointestinal hemorrhage. The primary target organs for inhibition of protein synthesis include the kidney, liver, and pancreas.

Symptoms of poisoning include intense gastrointestinal irritation, with burning in the mouth and throat. Muscle weakness, general malaise, reduced reflexes, convulsions, and dyspnea are also reported. Blood pressure remains normal until 2 to 3 hr before death, at which time it falls (5). The cause of death is usually cardiovascular collapse and decreased respiratory functions. Onset of all symptoms, other than localized irritation, may be delayed for 12 to 18 hr or more. Consequently, close observation of the victim throughout this period is required.

Ingestion of castor beans, even if not chewed, or of any part of the castor plant, must be treated as a potential emergency. Again, spontaneous vomiting may remove most of the plant parts from the GI tract. Activated charcoal and cathartics should follow emesis, and the victim must be observed for at least 24 hr. Symptoms appearing during this period

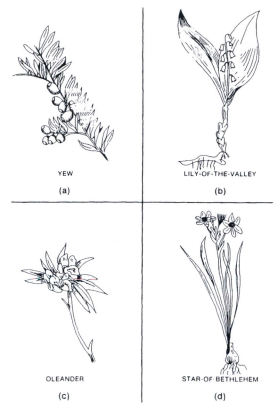

FIG. 11.4. Common outdoor ornamental plants that cause poisoning.

Symptoms of oxalic acid poisoning include nausea and vomiting, weakness, and muscle cramps.

Ingestions should be treated with emesis, followed with milk (a source of calcium) or calcium hydroxide solution (lime water). Calcium combines with oxalic acid in the GI tract to form insoluble calcium oxalate. Calcium salts may be administered intravenously to replace calcium that might be lost from the blood. Intravenous fluids are given to help prevent accumulation of the precipitate in the renal tubules.

Nightshade

Three nightshade species, bittersweet or woody nightshade (*Solanum dulcamara*), black or common nightshade (*Solanum nigrum*), and the deadly nightshade (*Atropa bel-*

should be treated appropriately (e.g., convulsions with diazepam). Urinary alkalinization with sodium bicarbonate may aid in elimination of absorbed ricin.

Rhubarb

The leaf, but not the stem, of the rhubarb plant (*Rheum rhaponticum*) (Fig. 11.5b) contains oxalic acid. The leaf is occasionally used to embellish salads, or cooked as a side dish. Heating does not destroy the toxic principle. Once absorbed, it combines with calcium from the blood to form the insoluble substance calcium oxalate, which may crystallize in the renal tubules. If severe, this precipitate may block the tubules to cause acute renal failure. A single bite of rhubarb leaf is usually not sufficient to cause systemic toxicity, but multiple bites may be.

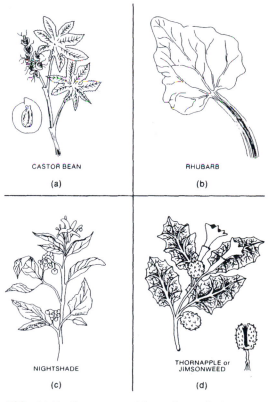

FIG. 11.5. Common outdoor plants that cause poisoning.

TABLE 11.7. *Nightshade species*

Common name	Botanical name	Toxic substances	Signs and symptoms
European bittersweet, woody nightshade, climbing nightshade	*Solanum dulcamara*	Solanine Chaconines	Nausea, vomiting, diarrhea, abdominal pain, drowsiness, tremor, difficulty in breathing
Black nightshade, common nightshade	*Solanum nigrum*	Solanine Chaconines	See above
Deadly nightshade, belladonna	*Atropa belladonna*	Tropane alkaloids Atropine Hyoscamine	Anticholinergic

ladonna) all belong to the Solanaceae family (Fig. 11.5c). The woody nightshade is reported to be one of the most commonly ingested plants in the United States (24). It is not considered lethal in quantities normally ingested, and usually produces little more than gastrointestinal irritation. Ingestion of several berries may be serious. Berries of the black nightshade are as noxious as those of the woody nightshade (Table 11.7).

Deadly nightshade (*Atropa belladonna*) is the plant to seriously avoid. Atropine, at a concentration of 0.25% to 0.5%, is found in this species, and can be lethal if ingested in sufficient quantity (38).

Symptoms of poisoning and their management are the same as for jimsonweed, discussed below. Fortunately, intoxication with deadly nightshade is rare in the United States, because the plant does not grow well here.

Jimsonweed

Jimsonweed (*Datura stramonium*), also known as thorn apple, locoweed, and angel's trumpet, is commonly encountered throughout most of the United States (Fig. 11.5d). It is often seen growing wild among rows of crops (Fig. 11.6). Unilateral mydriasis has been reported in farmers working with harvesting equipment, indicating poisoning. Children have been fatally poisoned by eating the flowers, and teenagers by ingesting a concoction made from infusing seeds in water (27).

The fruit pods that appear in the fall each contain 50 to 100 brown-black seeds. It is these seeds that are most toxic, with 10 seeds

containing approximately 1 mg atropine. Other alkaloids include hyoscyamine and hyoscine, present throughout the plant in varying proportions. As little as 4 to 5 g of the leaves or seeds can be fatal (39).

Intentional ingestions of jimsonweed concoctions have increased in frequency over recent years (25,36). During a six-year period, 73 jimsonweed exposures were reported to one regional Poison Control Center (19). This incidence will undoubtedly increase even more in future years, as licit drugs become

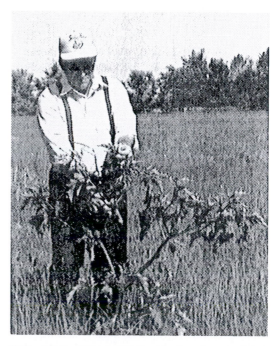

FIG. 11.6. Jimsonweed growing in a wheat field. Plant size may exceed 3 feet tall.

TABLE 11.8. *Symptoms and signs of jimsonweed ingestion*[a]

Signs and symptoms	No. of patients	% of patients	Not recorded
Hallucination	26	100	3
Disorientation	27	100	2
Mydriasis	29	100	—
Dry mucous membranes	16/17	94	12
Flushed face	11/13	85	16
Combative state	20	74	2
Tachycardia	21	72	—
Blood pressure alterations	15	52	—
Temperature >38.2°C	3	10	—

From ref. 36.
[a] Total number of patients = 29.

more commonly abused, and illicit drug items become more difficult to obtain.

Symptoms of jimsonweed poisoning include typical manifestations of anticholinergic poisoning, including blurred vision, CNS stimulation, euphoria, delirium, terrifying hallucinations, tachycardia, hyperthermia, and coma. A study involving 29 patients who ingested jimsonweed revealed the composite symptoms noted in Table 11.8 (36). Especially vivid were the hallucinations. Most were visual, e.g., insects on the wall, persons being chased by sharks, etc. Disorientation to time, place, or person was also prevalent.

Jimsonweed intoxication must be treated quickly. After gastric decontamination, physostigmine salicylate is given intravenously. Physostigmine is a reversible cholinesterase inhibitor that promotes accumulation of endogenous acetylcholine. This neurotransmitter competes with the poison for muscarinic receptor sites, and reverses the toxic symptoms. Although other cholinesterase inhibitors (e.g., neostigmine) may benefit the victim by increasing acetylcholine concentration at peripheral sites, they are quaternary amines and, consequently, do not enter the CNS in sufficient concentration. Thus, they are not effective in reversing the CNS component. Physostigmine, a tertiary amine, does penetrate into the CNS.

Hospitalization of the poisoned patient is indicated since a deranged mental state and sensorium may persist for several days. Even days after apparent recovery, victims of jimsonweed poisoning have been known to wander aimlessly into barren areas and die of exposure, or into a lake or pond and drown.

Pokeweed

Boiled shoots of the pokeweed (*Phytolacea americana*) (Fig. 11.7) are considered delicacies and are processed and canned for use in the home. However, pokeweed can be extremely dangerous if it is improperly prepared. Its clumps of shiny purple berries (*inkberries*) are attractive to children who may associate them with grapes or other fruits. The berries, although poisonous in large numbers, do not usually cause severe toxicity in the amounts normally ingested unless they are macerated into *grape juice* and this liquid is consumed. Pokeweed roots are the most toxic part of the plant, and are occasionally mistaken for horseradish or parsnips, or used to brew herbal teas. They contain toxic substances that have not yet been identified.

Pokeweed induces a variety of symptoms that include burning in the mouth, nausea and vomiting, visual disturbances, weak pulse, and respiratory difficulties.

Poisoning is best treated by removing all

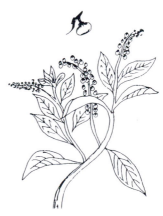

POKEWEED or INKBERRY

FIG. 11.7. Pokeweed.

traces of the plant from the stomach, then administering sequential doses of activated charcoal and a saline cathartic. Specific symptoms are treated as necessary.

Cyanogenic Plants

Several plants contain cyanogenic glycosides, such as *amygdalin, prulaurasin*, and *prunasin*, in their leaves, stems, bark, and seed pits, but not in their pulpy, edible fruits. Common examples of such plants are listed in Table 11.9. When ingested, the glycosides are hydrolyzed in alkaline medium to hydrocyanic acid. Cyanide-containing plants may induce all of the symptoms discussed for cyanide in chapter 6 and treatment is identical to that for cyanide poisoning. Mild ingestions may require only gastric decontamination and support care.

Herbal Intoxication

Herbal remedies were once the mainstay of treating most illnesses of Colonial Americans. With the development or importation and eventual refining of commercial medicinal

TABLE 11.9. *Common cyanogenic plants*

Apple (*Pyrus sylvestris*)
Apricot (*Prunus armeniaca*)
Cherry (*Prunus cerasus*)
Peach (*Prunus persica*)
Wild black cherry (*Prunus serotina*)
Cherry laurel (*Prunus caroliniana*)
Choke cherry (*Prunus virginiana*)

TABLE 11.10. *Psychoactive substances used in herbal preparations*

Labeled ingredient	Botanical source	Pharmacologic principle	Reported effects
African yohimbe bark; yohimbe	*Corynanthe yohimbe*	Yohimbe	Mild hallucinogen
Broom; Scotch broom	*Cytisus* spp.	Cytisine	Strong sedative-hypnotic
California poppy	*Eschscholtzia californica*	Alkaloids and glucosides	Mild euphoriant
Catnip	*Nepeta cataria*	Nepetalactone	Mild hallucinogen
Cinnamon	*Cinnamomum camphora*	?	Mild stimulant
Damiana	*Turnera diffusa*	?	Mild stimulant
Hops	*Humulus lupulus*	Lupuline	None
Hydrangea	*Hydrangea paniculata*	Hydrangin, saponin, cyanogenes	Stimulant
Juniper	*Juniper macropoda*	?	Strong hallucinogen
Kavakava	*Piper methysticum*	Yangonin, pyrones	Mild hallucinogen
Kola nut; gotu kola	*Cola* spp.	Caffeine, theobromine, kalonin	Stimulant
Lobella	*Lobella inflata*	Lobeline	Mild euphoriant
Mandrake	*Mandragora officinarum*	Scopolamine, hyoscyamine	Hallucinogen
Mate	*Ilex paraguayensis*	Caffeine	Stimulant
Mormon tea	*Ephedra nevadensis*	Ephedrine	Stimulant
Nutmeg	*Myristica fragrans*	Myristicin	Hallucinogen
Passion flower	*Passiflora incarnata*	Harmine alkaloids	Mild stimulant
Periwinkle	*Catharanthus roseus*	Indole alkaloids	Hallucinogen
Prickly poppy	*Argemone mexicana*	Protopine, bergerine, isoquinilines	Narcotic-analgesic
Snakeroot	*Rauwolfia serpentina*	Reserpine	Tranquilizer
Thorn apple	*Datura stramonium*	Atropine, scopolamine	Strong hallucinogen
Tobacco	*Nicotiana* spp.	Nicotine	Strong stimulant
Valerian	*Valeriana officinalis*	Chatinine, velerine alkaloids	Tranquilizer
Wild lettuce	*Lactua sativa*	Lactucarine	Mild narcotic-analgesic
Wormwood	*Artemisia absinthium*	Absinthine	Narcotic-analgesic

From ref. 37.

remedies, the use of herbs in health care began to decline. This apparent decrease in the use of home remedies persisted until fairly recently when the emphasis on health care once again began to change. Many Americans now have renewed interest in herbal remedies. Although many herbal remedies are safe and may even be pharmacologically worthwhile, many others can be lethal if misused (4,7,8,29).

The range of potential toxic action is widespread. One specific toxic concern involves the psychoactive effects that occur with a large number of herbs. Many of these herbs are rolled into cigarettes, boiled into tea, or taken in capsule form. Table 11.10 lists a variety of psychoactive substances, along with their reported effects. Unfortunately, many of the users may be unprepared for these effects. They may not even suspect that these effects can occur, since herbs are often viewed as food rather than as drugs.

Mushrooms

Poisonous mushrooms account for 50 to 100 of the nearly 5,000 species that grow in the United States (18). Poisoning by mushrooms is unpredictable, since different species may produce variable symptoms and require various treatment. Some are poisonous only if eaten raw, and others only if ingested during certain stages of growth. Even differences in soil composition may significantly influence the potential to cause toxicity. The problem is compounded further because poisonous mushrooms may grow next to nonpoisonous varieties. The rule of thumb is that no wild mushroom should ever be consumed unless accurate identification is possible.

Almost all cases of mushroom poisoning in this country are caused by members of the *Amanita* genus, especially *A. muscaria* and *A. phalloides* (Death Cap) (Fig. 11.8a,b). As little as one-third of a cap of *A. phalloides* may be fatal to a child, and one-half of a cap fatal to an adult. Most fatal poisonings are from *A. phalloides*, and it is responsible for over 95% of all deaths from mushroom poisoning (2).

Amanita mushrooms contain a mixture of thermostable cyclopeptides, including phalloidin, phalloin, and amanitin congeners (40). Muscarine is the toxin in *Clitocybe* and *Inocybe*, and provokes symptoms of toxicity within a few minutes to hours. Onset of symptoms from phalloidin, phalloin, or amanitin is characteristically delayed up to 24 hr. Fatal cases of Amanita poisoning reported in one study revealed a latent period average of 10.3 hr, whereas survivors had an average latent period of 12.6 hr (14). It is generally accepted that the amatoxins (primarily alpha-amanitin) (Fig. 11.9), more than the phallotoxins, are responsible for the lethality of *A. phalloides* mushrooms (14). They initiate cellular destruction by inhibiting nuclear RNA polymerase II, which blocks protein synthesis, leading to cell death. Primary action is seen on the gastrointestinal mucosa, hepatocytes, and renal tubular cells (18). Hepatic cells are especially susceptible to damage because of their rapid uptake of the toxin (30).

Characteristics of Mushroom Poisoning

Symptoms of poisoning vary widely among various species of mushrooms (Table 11.11). Delayed onset of symptoms usually means that ingestion of *A. phalloides* is likely. Most nonlethal mushrooms produce symptoms early after ingestion. Because the patient may remain asymptomatic for up to 24 hr after ingestion, the victim or physician may not suspect that symptoms are due to mushroom poisoning.

The characteristics of cyclopeptides in *A. phalloides* can be described in three stages. In the early stage, 6 to 24 hr, there is generally an abrupt onset of severe abdominal pain associated with profuse, cholera-like diarrhea and emesis. The next 24 to 48 hr is usually marked by a period of apparent recovery. During this time, cellular destruction of the kidney and liver is ongoing. The third phase occurs about 3 to 5 days postingestion, and is characterized by hepatocellular damage and renal insufficiency. Circulatory failure manifests later,

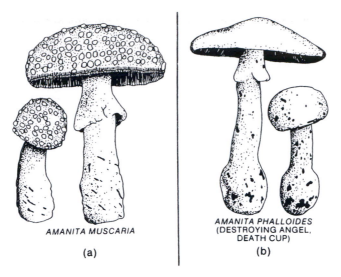

FIG. 11.8. Toxic mushroom species.

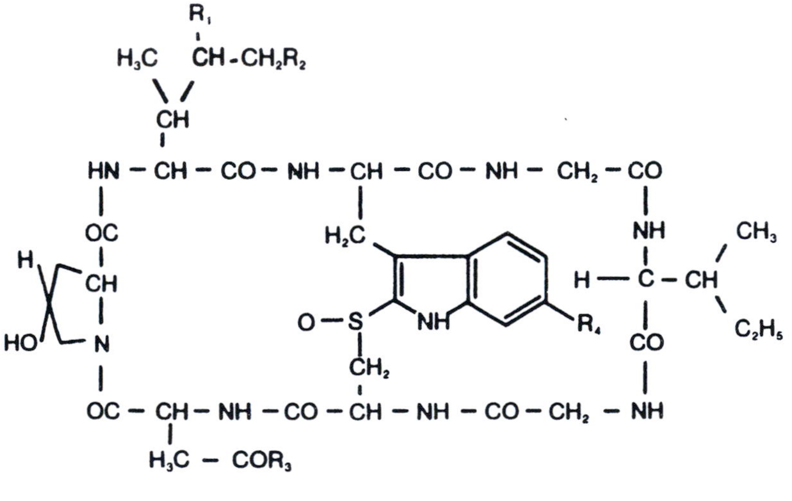

R₁ CH-CH₂R₂ structure (amatoxin core)

	R₁	R₂	R₃	R₄
α-Amanitin	OH	OH	NH₂	OH
β-Amanitin	OH	OH	OH	OH
γ-Amanitin	H	OH	NH₂	OH
ε-Amanitin	H	OH	OH	OH
Amanin	OH	OH	OH	H

FIG. 11.9. The amatoxins.

TABLE 11.11. *Comparative features of mushroom toxicity*

Group	Toxin	Mushroom	Target organs	Onset	Clinical manifestations	Treatment
I	Cyclopeptides —Amanitin —Phalloidin	*Amanita* *A. phalloides* *A. galerina*	Gastrointestinal tract, blood, liver, kidney	Delayed	Nausea, vomiting, diarrhea, abdominal pain, jaundice, renal failure, coma, death	Supportive care (thioctic acid, penicillin)
II	Gyromitrin —monomethylhydrazine	*Gyromitra*	Gastrointestinal tract, blood, liver, kidney	Delayed	Nausea, vomiting, bloody diarrhea, renal & liver failure, convulsions, coma, death	Pyridoxine
III	Muscarine	*Clitocybe* *Inocybe*	Autonomic nervous system	Rapid	Cholinergic crisis: SLUD, blurred vision, hypotension, constricted pupils	Atropine
IV	Coprine	*Coprinus*	Autonomic nervous system	Rapid	Antabuse-like reaction with ethanol: severe headache, facial flushing, orthostatic hypotension, tachycardia, diaphoresis, arrhythmias	Supportive care
V	Ibotenic acid —Muscimol	*Amanita* *A. muscaria*	Central nervous system	Rapid	Dizziness, ataxia, euphoria, muscle twitches, mydriasis, convulsions, coma	Supportive care; physostigmine, only if severe anticholinergic signs & symptoms are present
VI	Psilocybin Psilocin	*Psilocybe* *Panaeolus*	Central nervous system	Rapid	Hallucinations, blurred vision, mydriasis, convulsions, coma	Supportive care

with the victim showing signs of becoming jaundiced and lapsing into a hepatic coma within a week. Death occurs in 4 to 7 days of mushroom consumption (18).

Management of Mushroom Poisoning

Management of poisonous mushroom ingestions should consist of good supportive care, including fluid replacement and correction of metabolic disturbances. The death rate from poisoning by *A. phalloides* is reported to be 50% to 90% of untreated victims (18,30). With good management, however, this rate may be reduced to approximately 20% to 25% (14) or less (28).

For *A. muscaria*, if ingestion is suspected, administer ipecac and observe for signs and symptoms for at least three hours. Early manifestations are primarily CNS depression. Supportive care is usually sufficient (6). For *A. phalloides*, if the time since ingestion is less than 4 hr, ipecac-induced emesis may be beneficial. Since signs and symptoms are delayed, it is unlikely to detect poisoning before 4 hr. Activated charcoal and cathartics have been recommended.

A variety of potential antidotes have been suggested to treat *A. phalloides* poisonings.

None has demonstrated a significant outcome (14).

Thioctic acid (alpha-lipoic acid) is a Krebs cycle coenzyme used experimentally for treatment of poisoning by *Amanita* or the rare *Galerina* species. Thioctic acid exerts a direct protective effect against hepatocellular damage by a yet unknown mechanism. It must be given early after ingestion of the toxic mushroom.

Penicillin G and corticosteroids have also been used. Given intravenously, they may limit hepatotoxicity by competing with amanitin for binding on serum proteins, thereby leaving more toxin free for renal excretion (18). Cimetidine has been used to protect mice against *Amanita* poisoning in limited experiments. The toxin caused severe mitochondrial damage, although animals that received cimetidine were protected (35). The clinical usefulness of these antidotes is yet to be determined.

TABLE 11.12. *Nontoxic houseplants*

Common name	Botanical name
African violet	*Saintpaulia ionantha* or *Episcia reptans*
Aluminum plant	*Pilea cadierei*
Baby's tears	*Helxine soleirolii*
Begonia	*Begonia semperflorens*
Boston fern	*Nephrolepis exaltata*
Bridal veil	*Tradescantia*
Christmas cactus	*Schlumberga bridgesii*
Coleus	*Coleus blumei*
Fiddleleaf fig	*Ficus lyrata*
Gardenia	*Gardenia radicans*
Grape ivy	*Cissus rhombifolia*
Hawaiian ti	*Cordyline terminalis*
Hen and chicks	*Echeveria* spp.; *Sempervivum tectorus*
Jade plant	*Crassula argentea*
Mother-in-law tongue	*Sansevieria trifasciata*
Rubber plant	*Ficus elastica*
Sensitive plant	*Mimosa pudica*
Snake plant	*Sansevieria trifasciata*
Spider plant	*Chlorophytum comosum*
String of hearts	*Creopegia woodii*
Swedish ivy	*Plectranthus australis*
Umbrella plant (schefflera)	*Brassaia actinophylla*
Wandering Jew	*Tradescantia albiflora*; *Zebrina pendula*
Wax plant	*Hoya carnosa* or *H. exotica*
Weeping fig	*Ficus benjamina*
Zebra plant	*Aphelandra squarrosa*

It should be noted that several different species have identical common names. Some may cause diarrhea in infants.

SUMMARY

Poisoning may occur from a variety of plant ingestions. As we learned early in the chapter, most ingestions cause little more harm than irritating the mouth or stimulating nausea or vomiting. However, there are some very toxic plants, and their ingestion must be handled as any other toxic emergency. A list of nontoxic plants (Table 11.12) is given below.

To date, few medical problems have been reported from ingesting herbal remedies. The *medicinal teas* and other crude dosage forms of commerce are, for the most part, neither uniformly prepared nor assayed for purity. They consist of crudely prepared mixtures containing plant fibers, crystalline oxalates, and often pollen, mold spores, insect parts, and other allergy-causing substances. The potential for a toxic or allergic response to these preparations is always present.

Case Studies

CASE STUDY: *DIEFFENBACHIA* INGESTION

History

When brought to the emergency room, the 40-year-old woman was experiencing dysphagia, excessive salivation, and pain of the mouth and tongue. Six hours previously she had bitten into the stalk of a *Dieffenbachia* houseplant. She probably did not ingest any of the plant material because she reported that it caused her a great deal of oral pain and she quickly spat out the pulp and juices.

Physical examination revealed severe edema of the left side of the face, tongue, buccal mucosa, and palate. Salivation was profuse and she had extreme difficulty in speaking. All laboratory findings were within the normal limits. She was admitted for observation.

Treatment consisted of meperidine hydrochloride for pain, followed by oral administration of 30 mL of aluminum-magnesium hydroxide every 2 hr. During the observation period, there was no evidence of respiratory distress, muscular hyperactivity, or gastrointestinal disturbance. The following day she could swallow soft foods and liquids, but the extent of inflammation was unchanged from the time of admission.

She was discharged after 19 hr even though oral inflammation and edema remained unchanged. Pain continued in her face, and necrosis of the surface of the tongue and buccal mucosa was evident.

Eleven days later, the lesions were still observable, but the facial edema was reduced. Dietary intake by this period was almost back to normal. (See ref. 12.)

Discussion

1. This patient had no systemic complications. What are some of the reasons why systemic toxicity is not generally associated with ingestion of *Dieffenbachia*?
2. Why was aluminum-magnesium hydroxide suspension given?
3. What treatment is usually given to initially reduce oral swelling in the oral cavity?
4. Are antidotes available for plant ingestions involving the Arum family? If so, what are they?

CASE STUDY: JIMSONWEED POISONING

History

A 15-year-old boy was found nude with a flushed face, incoherent behavior, and symptoms of hallucinations. On admission to the emergency department, he was comatose, responding only to deep painful stimuli. Pupils were dilated and equal, but responded minimally to light. His skin was hot and dry. Doll's eye movements were intact. Hyperactive deep tendon reflexes were noted, and positive Babinski responses were obtained. He occasionally displayed episodes of myoclonic jerks.

Vital signs are listed in Table 11.13. Within 1 hr after admission, vital signs began to diminish. Because poisoning by an anticholinergic substance was suspected, 2 mg physostigmine salicylate were administered intravenously. Within 15 min he began to respond. He became more alert and responsive to verbal commands. He then admitted to ingesting *loco seeds*.

The patient was completely stabilized in 6 hr, although he continued to experience hallucinations. His neurologic status improved, and he was released by the 8th hospital day, without apparent neurologic damage. (See ref. 26.)

Discussion

1. What alkaloid is present in jimsonweed?
2. What is the botanical name for locoweed?
3. Discuss the mechanism of toxicity of jimsonweed. What is the usual prognosis of poisoning if the patient is (a) treated with physostigmine, or (b) not treated?
4. If physostigmine were not available, could neostigmine be given instead?
5. What do you suppose *Doll's eye movements* represents?

TABLE 11.13. *Vital signs*

Time	Blood pressure (mm Hg)	Respirations per min	Pulse per min	Temp (°C)
On admission	170/100	44	144	38.7
1 hr after admission	140/50	60	160	39.8
15 min after physostigmine	160/68	40	120	38.8

CASE STUDY: FATAL OLEANDER INGESTION

History

A 96-year-old woman with suicidal intentions ingested an undetermined quantity of oleander leaf. She had previously taken no medication except for occasional aspirin. Her family found her at home, weak and vomiting. She could barely talk, and within a few minutes after discovery her speech ceased.

On arrival at an emergency facility 15 min later, she experienced a transient generalized tonic seizure, which was followed by cardiopulmonary failure. Cardiopulmonary resuscitation was begun immediately. She was given 5% dextrose in sodium bicarbonate, epinephrine, lidocaine, atropine, phenytoin, calcium chloride, and isoproterenol. Despite the vigorous treatment, she died 40 min after arrival. The victim's laboratory findings are summarized in Table 11.14.

On autopsy, all coronary vessels were patent and showed no signs of thrombotic occlusion. A quantity of green vegetative material was found in the stomach.

At first, the digoxin value noted above was thought to be in error since the patient was not taking a digitalis product. Additional laboratory studies confirmed the value, however. Further studies showed that the lethal dose of oleander glycosides swallowed by this patient was approximately 200 times higher than the dose known to be lethal in animals. (See ref. 29.)

Discussion

1. What is the toxin present in oleander?
2. How does this toxin manifest toxicity?

TABLE 11.14. *Laboratory findings*

Na^+	=161 mEq/L
K^+	=8.6 mEq/L
Cl^-	=111 mEq/L
CO_2	=26 mEq/L
Digoxin	=5.8 ng/mL

Were this patient's symptoms compatible with information described within the text concerning oleander poisoning?
3. Why was a digoxin concentration of 5.8 ng/mL noted even though the patient was not taking any heart medication?
4. Would this patient have benefitted from the use of Digibind?

CASE STUDY: HOLLY BERRY INGESTION

History

Identical 2-year-old twin girls reportedly swallowed "a handful" of holly berries. Each child was given 15 mL of syrup of ipecac along with 120 mL water, at home. Each vomited in approximately 50 min after ingesting the berries. The vomitus of one child (A) had a more intense orange color than that of the other child (B). By 90 min postingestion, Twin A had vomited about 10 times and was markedly drowsy.

Twin A continued to vomit over the next hour, at which time she was taken to a physician for evaluation. She continued to vomit, totaling about 40 times over 6 hr. Each emesis consisted of a small volume of fluid. She did not appear dehydrated, and was sent home without specific treatment.

Twin B vomited only five times during the same period. Her mother reported that she did not become drowsy.

Around 20 hr postingestion, both children experienced an episode of "green" watery diarrhea. The day after berry ingestion, Twin A passed two green semisoft stools, and vomited three times. Twin B passed one similar stool. She did not vomit. Both girls were asymptomatic by 30 hr postingestion. (See ref. 34.)

Discussion

1. Why did Twin A react so much more profoundly than Twin B?

2. Were symptoms after ingestion of holly berries what you would expect?
3. What is the most logical cause of drowsiness in Twin A?

CASE STUDIES: MUSHROOM POISONING

History: Case 1

A 58-year-old man picked wild mushrooms that he cooked and ate. About 90 min later he became nauseated and diaphoretic. After another 30 min his family noticed that he was confused, so he was transported to a hospital.

On arrival 15 min later, he was vomiting and had profuse diarrhea. He was agitated and disoriented, and had visual hallucinations. His vital signs included blood pressure, 140/80 mm Hg; pulse rate, 84 beats/min; and temperature, 36.7°C. Physical examination showed generalized muscular fasciculations and pallor. Pupils were constricted.

Treatment consisted of intravenous fluids, gastric lavage, and activated charcoal. After 5 hr, gastrointestinal symptoms, confusion, and agitation had resolved. He reported paresthesia in his hands, and numbness in both hands and legs. These symptoms resolved over the next 24 hr and he had no further problems. The mushrooms were identified as *Amanita muscaria*. (See ref. 18.)

History: Case 2

A 59-year-old woman (patient A), who had picked and eaten wild mushrooms on many previous occasions, picked a batch and shared them with a 56-year-old male friend (patient B). Both cooked the mushrooms for their dinners. Patient A consumed 1 to 2 bites. Patient B consumed more, although the exact amount was not known.

Six hours after eating, patient A experienced nausea, vomiting, abdominal cramps, and diarrhea. Twelve hours after ingestion, patient B experienced similar symptoms. Patient A's symptoms were less severe than patient B's.

Patient B was taken to the hospital 48 hr after mushroom ingestion. Patient A did not seek assistance until 60 hr after consumption.

On admission, patient B was pale and diaphoretic. Vital signs included blood pressure, 86/60 mm Hg; pulse, 88 beats/min; and temperature, 36.9°C. He experienced constant vomiting and diarrhea, which tested positive for occult blood. He was awake and responsive, although lethargic.

Laboratory tests revealed an aspartate aminotransferase concentration of 5,210 IU/L (normal, <25 IU/L), alanine aminotransferase concentration of 4,120 IU/L (normal, <20 IU/L), and total bilirubin concentration of 1.6 mg/dL. Prothrombin time was 22.3 sec (normal, 12.2 sec).

A diagnosis was made of amanitin poisoning, based on symptoms and laboratory suggestion of liver damage. Therapy with thioctic acid, 400 mg/day intravenously in four divided doses, was begun and continued 13 days. The patient's prognosis remained guarded throughout his hospital stay due to complications including bacterial and fungal sepsis, respiratory distress that required ventilatory assistance, and acute renal failure that required dialysis. He was discharged eight weeks later.

Patient A experienced only mild abdominal distress, which largely dissipated by the time of her hospital examination 60 hr after mushroom ingestion. Signs and symptoms were not remarkable, and she was not hospitalized.

Patient A later identified the site where she had gathered the mushrooms. In the near vicinity were numerous specimens of *Amanita virosa*. (See ref. 18.)

Discussion

1. What factors might suggest the difference in intensity of symptoms for patients A and B in case 2?
2. Explain the temporal relationship between elevated aspartate aminotransferase, alanine aminotransferase, and bilirubin and a

probable diagnosis of liver damage for patient B in case 2.

3. What is the reason for rapid onset of symptoms of poisoning in case 1, and delayed onset of symptoms in case 2?

CASE STUDIES: POKEWEED POISONING

History: Case 1

A 43-year-old woman purchased some powdered poke root from a local health food store. About 30 min after consuming a cup of tea made from the powdered plant material (following mixing directions on the label), she became nauseated and vomited. She also experienced cramping, abdominal pains, and watery diarrhea. Later, she became very weak, and blood was found in the emesis and stool. Her husband brought her to an emergency facility.

She presented with hypotension and tachycardia. Gastric lavage was performed, followed by nasogastric suction.

Treatment consisted of volume expansion and electrolyte balancing. Nasogastric suction of a bloody material continued, and the diarrhea continued to reveal blood. She was stabilized in 24 hr and discharged the following day. (See ref. 9.)

History: Case 2

On one summer afternoon, 52 campers and counselors in a *nature group* were offered a salad made with leaves from the pokeweed plant. The young leaves had been picked, boiled, drained, and boiled again earlier that day. Within 0.5 to 5.5 hr after consuming the salad, 21 people developed the symptoms listed in Table 11.15.

Symptoms lasted 1 to 48 hr, with a mean duration of 24 hr. Eighteen persons were seen by local physicians or in a hospital emergency room. Four were admitted to the hospital for 24 to 48 hr because of protracted vomiting and dehydration. All survived. (See ref. 23.)

TABLE 11.15. *Symptoms of pokeweed plant poisoning*

No. patients with symptoms	Symptoms
18	Nausea, stomach cramps
17	Vomiting
11	Headache
10	Dizziness
8	Burning in stomach or mouth
6	Diarrhea

Discussion

1. What are the active components of pokeweed?
2. What are the major toxic actions of such compounds? Do these case studies correlate with the expected signs and symptoms of pokeweed toxicity?
3. Both of these reports of pokeweed toxicity would not have happened if certain obvious precautions would have been observed. What are the precautions?

CASE STUDY: BURDOCK ROOT TEA POISONING

History

A 26-year-old woman purchased a package of burdock root tea from a local health foods store. The tea was prepared by steeping the root product in water.

One morning, she drank one-half cup of tea that had been steeping for 1 1/2 days. Within 5 min she began to experience blurred vision and a dry mouth. Her husband noted that her speech and actions were bizarre, and she appeared to be hallucinating. She was brought to an emergency facility with symptoms of dry mouth, blurred vision, urinary retention, and bizarre behavior. Physical findings revealed blood pressure, 140/108 mm Hg; and pulse rate, 104 beats/min. Pupils were equally dilated and minimally reactive to light. Chest and heart auscultatory examinations were unremarkable. There was slight tenderness in the hypogastrium. Sensory and motor neuronal examination, as well as deep tendon reflexes, were normal.

Treatment with physostigmine salicylate was initiated since symptoms suggested poisoning by an anticholinergic substance. In addition, she was catheterized. (See ref. 8.)

Discussion

1. The toxic principle in the burdock root tea that was responsible for symptoms was atropine. Although we have not yet considered atropine toxicity in depth, do the symptoms this victim displayed represent what you would expect, based on your knowledge of the pharmacology of atropine?
2. What is the procedure used to establish or confirm anticholinergic poisoning?
3. Name three other toxic plants that are commonly ingested that contain atropine-like alkaloids.
4. Why was the patient catheterized?

Review Questions

1. A parent who states that his son was poisoned by dumbcane is referring to which of the following plants?
   A. Rhubarb
   B. Poinsettia
   C. Dieffenbachia
   D. Jimsonweed
2. Which of the following plant seeds contain ricin?
   A. Oleander
   B. Castor bean
   C. Mistletoe
   D. Yew
3. Symptoms of jimsonweed poisoning are:
   A. Muscarinic
   B. Antimuscarinic
4. Which of the following is a true statement?
   A. Rhubarb stems and leaves both contain the toxic principle.

   B. Jimsonweed seeds are also called *inkberries*.
   C. Poisoning by oleander induces symptoms that are most closely descriptive of atropine.
   D. The poisonous principle of yew is taxine.
5. Chronic intoxication by ingesting the toxic principle of rhubarb is most closely associated with dysfunction of the:
   A. Brain
   B. Liver
   C. Heart
   D. Kidney
6. Intoxication with oleander causes symptoms most closely associated with dysfunction of the:
   A. Brain
   B. Liver
   C. Heart
   D. Kidney
7. All of the following belong to the Arum family *except*:
   A. Dieffenbachia
   B. Poinsettia
   C. Caladium
   D. Philodendron
8. Plants that are considered to have a *caustic* component should not be vomited if ingested.
   A. True
   B. False
9. Which of the following is considered to be the toxic principle in "Death Cap" mushrooms?
   A. Solanine
   B. Taxine
   C. Amanitin
   D. Hyoscyamine
10. All of the following are true about jimsonweed *except*:
    A. Each seed contains approximately 10 mg atropine.
    B. The incidence of poisoning is increasing.
    C. Hallucinations caused by poisoning are mostly visual.
    D. It is also called locoweed.
11. Which of the following plants, if ingested,

would most likely have caused the symptoms listed below, early after its ingestion?

Eyes: miotic
Heart: BP normal; rate = 61/min
GIT: intense vomiting; intestinal spasm; rigid abdomen; no xerostomia or mouth pain
CNS: normal functions

A. Philodendron
B. Rhubarb
C. Jimsonweed
D. Taxus

12. Jimsonweed intoxication causes symptoms that are most closely related to toxicity by which of the following substances?
    A. Ethylene glycol
    B. Digitalis glycosides
    C. Scopolamine
    D. Physostigmine

13. Using the following key, identify the major toxic concern encountered with poisoning by each of the following plants:
    A. Hypertensive crisis
    B. Delirium; euphoria
    C. Acute renal failure
    D. Hepatitis
    E. Erythrocytic hemolysis
    Amanita mushrooms
    Jimsonweed
    Rhubarb
    Castor bean

14. What name is given to the bundles of calcium oxalate crystals arranged in a parallel arrangement?

15. Describe the two-fold beneficial effect milk provides when plant parts containing oxalic acid are ingested.

16. Thioctic acid is under investigation as a treatment regimen for what type of plant? Against what specific toxic action does it protect?

17. What are some of the reasons for the increased incidence of poisoning by plants?

18. Activated charcoal may be an effective adsorbent of the toxic principles of many plants. What are some of the limitations with using AC for poisonous plant ingestions?

19. Even in the absence of symptoms of toxicity after plant ingestion, the victim should be carefully observed over the next 12 to 24 hr. Cite the reasons.

20. List some reasons why gastric lavage may have limited value in treating plant poisoning.

21. Describe the expected outcome of poisoning from the deadly nightshade plant. What is the toxic component of this plant?

22. Discuss why gastric lavage may be a poor method of gastric decontamination after ingestion of castor seeds or taxus berries.

References

1. [Anonymous]. Toxic reactions to plant products sold in health food stores. *Med Lett* 1979;21:29–31.
2. [Anonymous]. Mushroom poisoning. *Lancet* 1980; 2:351–352.
3. Arditti J, Rodriquez E. *Dieffenbachia:* uses, abuses and toxic constituents—a review. *J Ethnopharmacol* 1982;5:293–302.
4. Bain RJI. Accidental digitalis poisoning due to drinking herbal tea. *Br Med J* 1985;290:1624.
5. Balint GA. Ricin: the toxic protein of castor oil seeds. *Toxicology* 1974;2:77–102.
6. Benjamin DR. Mushroom poisoning in infants and children—the *Amanita pantherina/muscaria* group. *Clin Toxicol* 1992;30:13–22.
7. Boyd EL, Tjolsen E. Are they safe? *J Pharm Technol* 1986;2:153–159.
8. Bryson PD, Watanabe AS, Rumack BH, Murphy RC. Burdock root tea poisoning. *JAMA* 1978;239:2157.
9. Centers for Disease Control. Plant poisoning—New Jersey. *MMWR Morb Mortal Wkly Rep* 1981;30:65–66.
10. Dalvi RR, Bowie WC. Toxicology of solanine: an overview. *Vet Hum Toxicol* 1983;25(1):13–15.
11. Dore WG. Crystalline raphides in the toxic houseplant *Dieffenbachia*. *JAMA* 1963;185:1045.
12. Drach G, Maloney WH. Toxicity of the common houseplant dieffenbachia. *JAMA* 1963;184:1047.
13. Ellis M, Robertson WO, Rumack B. Plant ingestion poisoning from A to Z. *Patient Care* 1979;13(12):86–140.
14. Floersheim GL. Treatment of human amatoxin mushroom poisoning myths and advancements in therapy. *Med Toxicol* 1987;2:1–9.
15. Fochtman FW, Manno JE, Winek CL, Cooper JA. Toxicity of the genus *Dieffenbachia*. *Toxicol Appl Pharmacol* 1969;15:38–45.
16. Geehr E. Common toxic plant ingestions. *Emerg Med Clin North Am* 1984;2:553–562.
17. Hall AH, Spoerke DG, Rumack BH. Assessing mistletoe toxicity. *Ann Emerg Med* 1986;15:1320–1323.
18. Hanrahan JP, Gordon MA. Mushroom poisoning: case reports and a review of therapy. *JAMA* 1984;251:1057–1061.

19. Klein-Schwartz W, Oderda GM. Jimsonweed intoxication in adolescents and young adults. *Am J Dis Child* 1984;138:737–739.
20. Kuballa B, Lugnier AA, Anton R. Study of *Dieffenbachia*-induced edema in mouse and rat hindpaw— respective role of oxalate needles and trypsin-like proteases. *Toxicol Appl Pharmacol* 1981;58:444–451.
21. Kunkel DB, Spoerke DG. Evaluating exposures to plants. *Clin Lab Med* 1984;4:603–614.
22. Lampe KF. Toxic effects of plant toxins. In: Klaassen CD, Amdur MO, Doull J, eds. *Toxicology—the basic science of poisons*. 3rd ed. New York: Macmillan; 1986:757–767.
23. Lewis WH, Smith PR. Poke root herbal tea poisoning. *JAMA* 1979;242:2759–2760.
24. Litovitz TL, Bailey KM, Holm KC, Schmitz BF. 1991 annual report of the American Association of Poison Control Centers National Data Collection System. *Am J Emerg Med* 1992;10:452–505.
25. Mahler DA. The jimson-weed high. *JAMA* 1975;31:138.
26. Mikolich JR, Paulson GW, Cross JC. Acute anticholinergic syndrome due to jimson seed ingestion. *Ann Intern Med* 1975;83:321–325.
27. Mitchell JE, Mitchell FN. Jimson weed poisoning in childhood. *J Pediatr* 1955;47:227–231.
28. Olson KR, Woo OF, Pond SM. Treatment of mushroom poisoning. *JAMA* 1985;252:3130–3131.
29. Osterioh J, Herold S, Pond S. Oleander interference in the digoxin radioimmunoassay in a fatal ingestion. *JAMA* 1982;247:1596–1597.
30. Plotzker R, Jensen DM, Payne JA. Case report. *Amanita virosa* acute hepatic necrosis: treatment with thioctic acid. *Am J Med Sci* 1982;283:79–82.
31. Pohl RW. Poisoning by dieffenbachia. *JAMA* 1961;177:162–163.
32. Rauber A, Heard J. Castor bean toxicity re-examined: a new perspective. *Vet Hum Toxicol* 1985;27:498–502.
33. Rock JF. The poisonous plants of Hawaii. *Haw Forest Agric* 1920;17:61.
34. Rodrigues TD, Johnson PN, Jeffery LP. Holly berry ingestion: case report. *Vet Hum Toxicol* 1984;26(21):157–158.
35. Schneider SM, Borochovitz D, Krenzelok EP. Cimetidine protection against alpha-amanitin hepatotoxicity in mice: a potential model for the treatment of *Amanita phalloides* poisoning. *Ann Emerg Med* 1987;16:1136–1140.
36. Shervette RE, Schydlower M, Lampe RM, Fearnow RG. Jimson "loco" weed abuse in adolescents. *Pediatrics* 1979;63:520–523.
37. Siegel RR. Herbal intoxication. *JAMA* 1976;236:473–476.
38. Trabattoni G, Visintini D, Terzane GM, Lechi A. Accidental poisoning with deadly nightshade berries: a case report. *Hum Toxicol* 1984;3:513–516.
39. Weintraub S. Stramonium poisoning. *Postgrad Med* 1960;28:364–367.
40. Wieland T. Poisonous principles of mushrooms of the genus *Amanita*. *Science* 1968;159:946–952.
41. Winek CL, Butala JH, Shanor SP, Fochtman FW. Toxicology of poinsettia. *Clin Tox* 1978;13:27–45

12 Analgesics, Antipyretics, and Anti-inflammatory Agents

Numerous products contain nonnarcotic (non-opioid) analgesics. They are used to treat a wide variety of clinical conditions, including pain, inflammation, and fever. Some are available without prescription, although others require the patient to be under the care of a licensed medical practitioner. Despite this plethora of products, there are three nonnarcotic analgesics that are most commonly used in the United States. These are aspirin, acetaminophen, and ibuprofen. Other nonsteroidal anti-inflammatory drugs (NSAIDs) may induce a variety of adverse effects, but they are not usually associated with acute toxic reactions. Ibuprofen, on the other hand, has been associated with many acute poisonings. Surprisingly, it has not caused severe toxicity in adults, in spite of its widespread availability and use. The salient features of toxicity of non-narcotic analgesics are summarized in this chapter.

SALICYLATES

Aspirin poisoning may affect people of all ages. Children are most susceptible and are usually the victims of accidental ingestions. Adult salicylate toxicity is normally due to chronic misuse or intentional ingestions of large quantities. Children present the greatest risk of developing serious toxic complications after salicylate poisoning.

The chance for a fatal outcome in children is enhanced if the child is febrile and/or dehydrated. Consider what may occur when a child with an upper respiratory tract infection or other minor affliction is given aspirin by a well-meaning parent. Since this child may also be lethargic and not eating or drinking adequately, the stage is now set for enhancement of toxicity. The child is given one dose followed by another and another. Within a short time after continuous therapy, the tissues become completely saturated with aspirin (2). At this point, serum concentrations increase geometrically. In other words, a 50% increase in the daily aspirin dose may cause the serum concentration to rise by 300% (37). Before it is realized, the child has been accidentally poisoned.

Although the Poison Prevention Packaging Act of 1970 set guidelines that have contributed to a reduction by approximately one-half in the incidence of accidental ingestions, and greatly decreased the number of aspirin-induced deaths, aspirin is still a serious cause of poisoning in children under 5 years of age (11). The concern for a possible association between it and Reye's syndrome may eventually reduce the overall incidence of aspirin poisoning in children even more (60).

Aspirin products may be referred to as *candy* by parents to encourage a child to ingest the necessary dose. The problem arises when a curious, unattended child finds a bottle or two of *candy-flavored* aspirin tablets, or even adult aspirin products. The dose of aspirin for children at which symptoms of toxicity are likely to occur is 150 mg/kg. In an otherwise healthy 20-kg child, it would be necessary for the child to ingest approximately an entire bottle of 36 children's aspirin (81 mg of salicylate/tablet). Ingesting only 9 adult-strength aspirin (325 mg each) would place the child in the same jeopardy (Table 12.1).

Methyl salicylate (Oil of Wintergreen) is another source of salicylate intoxication in children. Methyl salicylate is included in topical liniments, and is used alone as an analgesic rub, and in food flavoring. A child may find a bottle of methyl salicylate that smells like wintergreen candy, and the opportunity to taste it is difficult to refuse. Since methyl salicylate is a liquid it can be easily ingested. It has been shown that one teaspoonful (approximately one *swallow*) contains the equivalent of 7 g salicylate, or approximately 22 adult aspirin tablets. As little as 4 mL of methyl salicylate may be lethal to a child (24). The results of an interesting study that revealed the inconsistency in the literature of reported salicylate in methyl salicylate was presented in chapter 1. It may be helpful to review that section now.

Mechanism of Toxicity

Many of the pathophysiologic consequences of salicylate toxicity can be explained

TABLE 12.1. *Toxicity profile for salicylate ingestions*

Range of toxicity	Signs and symptoms	Blood concentration range (mg/dL)	Single oral dose ingested (mg/dL)	Approximate no. of tablets ingested by a child[a]		Approximate no. of tablets (325 mg) ingested by an adult[b]
				Children's aspirin (81 mg)	Adult aspirin (325 mg)	
Asymptomatic		<45				
Mild toxicity	Nausea Gastritis Mild hyperpnea Tinnitus	45–65	<150	<37	<9	<30
Moderate toxicity	Hyperpnea Hyperthermia Sweating Dehydration Marked lethargy Possible excitement	65–90	150–300	37–74	9–18	30–63
Severe toxicity	Severe hyperpnea Coma Convulsions Cyanosis Pulmonary edema Respiratory failure Cardiovascular collapse	90–120	300–500	74–123	18–30	63–105
Lethal	Coma Death	120	>500	>123	>30	>105

From ref. 14.
[a] Acetylsalicylic acid (ASA) tablets ingested by a 20-kg child.
[b] ASA tablets ingested by a 68-kg adult.

by CNS stimulation and interference with the uncoupling of oxidative phosphorylation within the electron transport system. It may be helpful to follow these events outlined in Fig. 12.1.

The respiratory center is stimulated directly by salicylates, and indirectly by an increase in pCO_2 production. Salicylates enhance oxygen consumption by increasing the cellular metabolic rate. This results in hyperthermia with accumulation of CO_2, which then causes hyperpnea (increased depth of respiration). Also, toxic doses of salicylate stimulate the respiratory center directly, producing both hyperpnea and tachypnea (increased rate of respiration). The increased respiration rate causes a greater than normal amount of CO_2 to be expired by the lungs. As a result, there is less plasma CO_2.

Recall the following reactions of the bicarbonate buffer system for maintaining blood pH:

$$H_2O + CO_2 \rightleftarrows H_2CO_3 \rightleftarrows H^+ + HCO_3^-$$

Since there is less CO_2 available, less carbonic acid $[H_2CO_3]$ is formed resulting in a deficit of carbonic acid with a subsequent decrease in hydrogen ion concentration $[H^+]$. Blood pH is dependent on the bicarbonate/carbonic acid ratio according to the Henderson-Hasselbalch equation:

$$pH = 6.1 - \log \frac{[HCO_3^-]}{[H_2CO_3]}$$

The concentration of HCO_3^- in plasma and extracellular fluid is normally 27 mEq/L, and the concentration of carbonic acid is 1.35

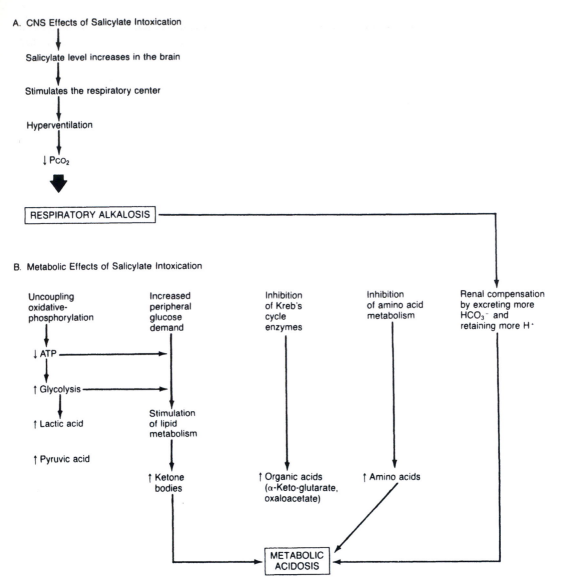

FIG. 12.1. Pathophysiologic consequences of salicylate intoxication.

mEq/L. The pH of plasma is dependent on the HCO_3^-/H_2CO_3 ratio of 20/1. At this ratio the pH of blood is 7.4. Therefore, as the Pco_2 and H_2CO_3 concentrations decrease, the HCO_3^- concentration is the same and the ratio of HCO_3^-/H_2CO_3 increases, resulting in elevation of blood pH.

The kidney attempts to compensate for the acid-base imbalance by excreting more HCO_3^-, and retaining H^+ and nonbicarbonate anions. Usually this mechanism operates to

correct the acid-base imbalance and return the ratio to 20/1. However, as can be seen in Fig. 12.1, in salicylate toxicity this may add to the latent metabolic acidosis.

The second action of salicylate intoxication results from uncoupling of oxidative phosphorylation, which ultimately produces metabolic acidosis with a high anion gap (31). Again, it may be useful to follow these events in Fig. 12.1.

The electron transport chain and oxidative

phosphorylation were previously discussed in chapter 6 in response to cyanide-induced cellular anoxia. It should be remembered that mitochondria are organelles whose preliminary function is production of an energy source, ATP. Hydrogen atoms and electrons from glycolysis and the Krebs cycle are transferred, via a series of oxidation-reduction reactions of the cytochrome system of the electron transport chain, to molecular oxygen, forming water. During these reactions, inorganic phosphate becomes coupled with ADP to form ATP. The process of electron donor to acceptor with resultant production of ATP is termed *oxidative phosphorylation.*

Uncoupling of oxidative phosphorylation results in a decrease in ATP production. Cells attempt to compensate by increasing glycolysis. However, only 2 moles of ATP are produced by substrate phosphorylation during glycolysis. In addition to a less efficient energy pathway, increased glycolysis also results in production of lactic and pyruvic acids. The body also uses its glycogen stores to obtain energy. Eventually, these are depleted and the body switches to lipid metabolism to meet energy demands. Although this is an efficient mechanism, it leads to excessive free fatty acid in the liver, producing increased ketone bodies, which can cause ketoacidosis.

Other contributing factors, which lead to metabolic acidosis as a result of salicylate toxicity, include (1) inhibition of dehydrogenase enzymes of the Krebs cycle, causing an accumulation of alpha-ketoglutarate and oxaloacetate and (2) inhibition of amino acid metabolism, resulting in accumulation of amino acids. The culminating result of biochemical actions of salicylate is metabolic acidosis with a high anion gap (Fig. 12.1).

Salicylates also interfere with normal blood glucose concentration. There may be an initial increase in blood glucose because of the utilization of muscle glycogen stores and mobilization of fats to free fatty acids and ketones. Eventually, however, there is depletion of glucose stores with resultant hypoglycemia. Hypoglycemia may be of greater significance in chronic salicylism, or during the latter stages of acute salicylate toxicity. It has been shown in animal studies that, even with normal blood glucose concentrations, there may be a significant decrease in brain glucose (63).

Ingesting high doses of salicylate results in switching salicylate metabolism from first-order to zero-order kinetics. That is, the rate of degradation is independent of dose, and an increase in dose results in a greater than expected increase in serum and tissue salicylate concentrations. After an acute overdose of salicylate, there is an increase in apparent volume of distribution with increasing amount ingested and absorbed. This is a result of decreased plasma protein binding of salicylate at high doses (38). The practical implication is that higher drug concentrations produce disproportionately higher concentrations of drug in tissues, especially the CNS (60).

Characteristics of Poisoning

Clinical manifestations of salicylate toxicity are presented in Table 12.1. They are arranged in increasing order of severity and related to amount ingested and blood salicylate concentration.

The major early toxic manifestations of salicylate poisoning result from stimulation of the CNS. These may include nausea, vomiting, tinnitus, headache, hyperpnea, and neurologic abnormalities, such as confusion, hyperactivity, slurred speech, and generalized convulsions. The severity of CNS toxicity is related closely to the brain salicylate concentration (23). As previously mentioned, salicylate-induced CNS stimulation results in hyperventilation, decreased Pco_2, and respiratory alkalosis. In subtoxic quantities, renal compensation proceeds to counteract the respiratory alkalosis. Compensated respiratory alkalosis is accomplished by renal excretion of bicarbonate, resulting in lowering of the blood pH toward normal. In adults and children older than 4 years of age who have ingested a mild-to-moderate dose of salicylate (see Table 12.1), the acid-base disturbance at this point tends to correct. Young children develop metabolic acidosis rapidly.

In the discussion of mechanism of toxicity, several metabolic abnormalities have been identified. Increased glycolysis, gluconeogenesis, and lipid metabolism result in depletion of glucose from peripheral tissues, accumulation of organic acids in the blood, and an increase in ketone bodies (see Fig. 12.1). Two other factors also contribute to metabolic acidosis: the vasomotor depressant effect related to toxic quantities of salicylate which impair renal function, and the dissociation of salicylate at plasma pH contributing to lowering of the plasma pH. The severity of metabolic acidosis is dose-related and occurs more frequently in infants and very young children after chronic salicylate therapy for some febrile conditions (62). In adults, salicylate toxicity usually results from accidental or intentional ingestion of a large single dose of salicylate; metabolic acidosis is normally delayed (18,62).

Dehydration is another serious consequence of salicylate toxicity. There are several contributing factors. First, increased heat production from salicylate-induced glucose and lipid metabolism results in hyperpyrexia and diaphoresis. Also, hyperventilation occurs as a result of CNS stimulation, and there is increased pulmonary fluid loss. Renal-compensated respiratory alkalosis results in the loss of HCO_3, followed by sodium, potassium, and an equiosmolar quantity of water. Metabolic acidosis adds to the increased urinary output and electrolyte loss. The severe dehydration described above is more common in children, and usually associated with moderate-to-severe salicylate toxicity (60).

A useful way to evaluate the degree of potential toxicity after acute oral ingestion is to correlate blood salicylate concentrations with the patient's clinical status. Several factors have been included in Table 12.1 to aid in predicting the extent of toxicity after an acute overdose.

Blood salicylate concentration ranges were selected from the Done nomogram (Fig. 12.2). This nomogram is valuable when evaluating *acute* salicylate poisoning, provided the approximate time of ingestion is known and a

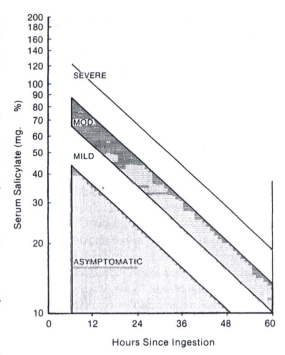

FIG. 12.2. Done nomogram for assessing the extent of salicylate poisoning. (From ref. 14.)

single oral dose has been ingested. It is recommended that serial salicylate determinations be made, beginning at least within 6 hr postingestion. The nomogram is not useful in cases of chronic salicylate toxicity, multiple ingestions, or ingestion of enteric-coated tablets (66).

If a 6-hr postingestion blood salicylate concentration is less than 40 mg/dL, it is unlikely that serious toxic effects will be observed. This correlates with salicylate ingestions of less than 150 mg/kg. The patient is generally asymptomatic and can usually be managed easily at home.

It has been estimated that in up to 50% of suicide attempts involving aspirin, the medication was ingested in combination with other drugs such as anticholinergics, narcotics, isoniazid, or aluminum hydroxide (3). Some salicylate-intoxicated patients may, therefore, present with a variety of signs and symptoms not generally related to salicylate toxicity alone.

Poisoning by methyl salicylate proceeds in

a manner similar to aspirin. Symptoms appear earlier, partly because methyl salicylate causes higher blood concentrations more rapidly. Prevalent early symptoms include CNS excitement, hyperpnea, and hyperpyrexia.

For salicylic acid, symptoms are similar to aspirin, but it causes greater gastrointestinal irritation. Salicylic acid is an infrequent cause of poisoning.

Management of Poisoning

Salicylate poisoning from acute oral ingestions of large quantities requires prompt medical attention. Treatment is multifaceted and largely supportive. Results are not always satisfactory. Management strategies involve removal of aspirin from the GI tract, and correction of metabolic acidosis, dehydration, hyperthermia, hypoglycemia, and hypokalemia.

The general sequence for managing salicylate toxicity should begin with gastric decontamination. In children, emesis is easier to accomplish and probably more effective.

After ingestion of large amounts of salicylate, time to peak concentration is delayed, and absorption may continue over a period of 8 to 12 hr due to decreased gastric emptying and decreased drug dispersion in the GI tract (36). Also, overdoses with enteric-coated or sustained-release salicylate preparations may result in delayed peak concentrations greater than 24 hr (66). Therefore, measures to prevent absorption, such as ipecac-induced emesis, gastric lavage, and activated charcoal, may be helpful even several hours postingestion (47). There are no data, however, to support the use of either multiple-dose activated charcoal or irrigation as a means to enhance excretion of salicylates (43).

Evacuation of the stomach should be followed by administration of activated charcoal to adsorb any remaining drug. Salicylate binding to activated charcoal has been shown in one study to be reversible over a 24 hr period by 15% to 20% (15). This is another reason to emphasize the use of a cathartic after activated charcoal to prevent the development of intestinal obstruction and enhance the transit time of charcoal through the GI tract. Data from studies with volunteers demonstrated that sorbitol with activated charcoal was superior to charcoal alone in preventing salicylate absorption when the combination was administered within 1 hr after ingestion (5,29,30).

Dehydration is common in salicylate poisoning and appropriate fluid replacement is critical. This may be managed by administering oral fluids. When toxicity is within the moderate-to-severe range, dehydration is usually treated with parenteral fluids. At this point rehydration, not correction of acid-base imbalance, is the major consideration. It is important to keep the patient hydrated so that kidney function is maintained. Salicylates are largely excreted by the kidney.

Replacement of lost fluid and electrolytes is essential, but the CNS and metabolic actions of salicylate toxicity are not reversed until salicylate concentrations fall below 50 mg/dL. Therefore, it is important to concentrate on ways to improve salicylate excretion, since there are no specific antidotes available.

Sodium bicarbonate is given to help correct metabolic acidosis associated with moderate-to-severe toxicity, and to produce an alkaline urine that will promote movement of salicylate from intracellular sites to plasma to enhance excretion by the kidney. Glucose is added to correct hypoglycemia and ketosis. Potassium chloride is added to correct hypokalemia and help prevent alkalosis from sodium bicarbonate administration. Alkaline diuresis is only effective in removing salicylate from the body when potassium depletion is corrected. During potassium replacement, serum potassium concentrations should be closely monitored because either hypokalemia or hyperkalemia may cause cardiac arrhythmias.

Enhancing elimination of salicylate by forced alkaline diuresis was encouraged previously (45). However, forced alkaline diuresis (infusion of large volumes of sodium bicarbonate and furosemide) has produced complications, such as pulmonary and cerebral edema, and electrolyte and acid-base disturbances. Consequently, this procedure has not been recommended. Furthermore, the use of sodium bicarbonate alone has been shown to be equally as effective and probably safer for reducing plasma salicylate concentrations after salicylate poisoning (47).

Hyperthermia is common with moderate-to-severe salicylate toxicity. Fever can be reduced by cold or tepid water (*not* alcohol) sponging. Other symptomatic treatment includes diazepam for seizures, calcium supplements for hypocalcemic tetany, and vitamin K_1 (phytonadione) for coagulation defects.

In cases of severe salicylate toxicity, especially in cases involving renal failure, consideration may be given to using an extracorporeal procedure (hemodialysis or charcoal hemoperfusion) to enhance drug elimination.

OTHER NONSTEROIDAL ANTI-INFLAMMATORY DRUGS

NSAIDs are among the most widely prescribed drugs. One NSAID, ibuprofen, can also be purchased in low doses (200 mg tablets) in the United States without prescription. In spite of the large number of people taking NSAID therapy, toxic overdose is rare (6,12,64).

A comparison of adverse drug reactions reported for NSAIDs is shown in Table 12.2. It can be seen that, next to aspirin, ibuprofen was the most widely used NSAID. Ibuprofen also has the lowest incidence of fatal and nonfatal adverse reactions (48). The remaining discussion of NSAIDs in this chapter will concentrate on ibuprofen. For a comprehensive evaluation of the toxicity of individual NSAIDs, the reader is referred to the review by Smolinske et al (59).

Ibuprofen

Ibuprofen can be predicted to be safe. After absorption it is quickly metabolized with an elimination half-life of approximately 2 hr. A single 400-mg dose results in a peak plasma concentration of 29 μg/mL 90 min after ingestion, decreasing to 3 μg/mL at 8 hr. Blood concentrations are not detectable at 12 hr (6). A single therapeutic dose is completely eliminated within 24 hr (21). An acute overdose does not prolong the elimination half-life of ibuprofen (21).

Mechanism of Toxicity

The mechanism of ibuprofen-induced toxicity after acute overdose is obscure. Acute renal

TABLE 12.2. *Summary of reported adverse drug reactions (ADR) for NSAIDs per million prescriptions*

NSAID	Millions of Rx (or units)	Fatal ADR (cases/10^6 Rx)	Nonfatal ADR (cases/10^6 Rx)
Phenylbutazone	2.81	4.99	25.29
Diflunisal	2.50	4.00	93.31
Piroxicam	7.53	2.66	91.16
Sulindac	5.47	2.01	46.61
Fenoprofen	3.26	1.84	24.85
Indomethacin	9.02	1.66	25.39
Tolmetin	2.57	1.55	59.05
Meclofenamate	1.80	1.11	47.72
Naproxen	11.86	0.67	20.75
Ibuprofen	20.45	0.44	10.22
Aspirin	241.0[b]	NA	NA

From ref. 48.
NSAID, nonsteroidal anti-inflammatory drug.
[a] Period: August 1983 to August 1984.
[b] Number of 100-tablet units sold $\times 10^6$.

failure is believed to result from decreased production of intrarenal prostaglandins. This, in turn, decreases the renal blood flow and glomerular filtration rate (35).

Characteristics of Poisoning

In most reported cases of ibuprofen overdose, patients have either no symptoms, or mild manifestations of gastrointestinal irritation, such as nausea and vomiting. Gastric erosions and hemorrhage are not commonly cited with acute overdoses. Metabolic acidosis, hypotension, and renal dysfunction are reported only rarely. CNS toxicity is rare. Drowsiness, lethargy, and mild coma have been reported, but generally resolve in 24 hr even with large doses (10,22). Adults and children have ingested overdoses of ibuprofen that resulted in blood concentrations 20 or more times greater than therapeutic concentrations with few adverse effects.

A survey was undertaken to document the extent of ibuprofen-induced toxicity during a two-year period. The relationship between ingested dose and symptoms is shown in Table 12.3.

Seventeen children who ingested up to 2.4 g were asymptomatic. Two other children experienced only mild symptoms with ingestions up to 3.6 g. Doses between 1.4 and 24 g caused no ill effects in 13 adults. Seven others reported mild symptoms, most commonly nausea and vomiting. An elderly male ingested between 9.6 and 16 g, that resulted in elevated plasma urea and creatinine concentrations. The remaining two victims ingested other drugs besides ibuprofen. To illustrate, a 70-year-old man took 12 g ibuprofen along with an unknown quantity of diazepam and chlorpheniramine. He became hypotensive, was comatose for about 12 hr, but recovered fully. The single fatality was a 67-year-old woman who ingested an unknown amount of ibuprofen and salicylate. She became hypotensive and comatose and died after cardiac arrest (12). Two antemortem plasma ibuprofen concentrations gave values of 440 mg/L and 170 mg/L. Salicylate concentration was 240 mg/L.

Management of Poisoning

Treatment of acute overdoses of ibuprofen and similar NSAIDs should consist of basic poison management, including symptomatic and supportive care. Seventy-three percent of the patients in Table 12.3 received an emetic or gastric lavage. Another 20% were given oral fluids. The remainder required no treatment. To date there have been no studies to evaluate the efficacy of either ipecac-induced emesis or gastric lavage in reducing NSAID toxicity. Activated charcoal will ad-

TABLE 12.3. *Symptoms of ibuprofen reported[a]*

Age	Severity	Total patients for age group	Symptoms	Alleged dose of ibuprofen (g)
Children	None	17	None	0.2–2.4
	Mild	2	Drowsiness, sweating	Up to 3.6
Adults	None	13	None	1.4–2.4
			Abdominal pain, nausea, vomiting, drowsiness, nystagmus, double vision, headache, tinnitus	
	Severe	2	Raised plasma urea and creatinine conc.	9.6–16
			Coma and hypotension	12 (+other drugs)
	Fatal	1	Initially vomiting, confusion, hyperventilation; 41-hr after admission, collapsed, cold sweating, cardiac arrest	Unknown (+other drugs)

From ref. 12.
[a] Period 1980–1981.

sorb mefenamic acid, phenylbutazone, and tolfenamic acid. It is probable that it will also adsorb other NSAIDs, including ibuprofen (64).

No CNS or other significant toxicity is usually seen with ingestions of ibuprofen less than 3 g (22). Renal function tests do not seem to be indicated unless 6 g to 20 g or more of ibuprofen has been ingested (22). A nomogram to predict the outcome of acute ibuprofen poisonings has been devised and revised (Fig. 12.3), but its clinical utility is limited

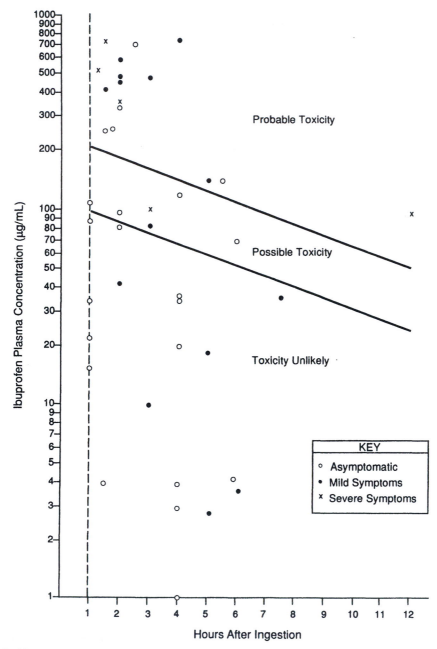

FIG. 12.3. Nomogram relating plasma ibuprofen level to severity of intoxication. (From ref. 59.)

since treatment is largely symptomatic and based on clinical findings (21,22).

ACETAMINOPHEN

Acetaminophen (paracetamol) now surpasses aspirin as a major cause of poisoning. For many years acetaminophen was not generally recognized in the United States as an important source of poisoning. With increasing use over the past decade, an increase in toxic events has been reported (55). In fact, use of salicylates in children has decreased over the past decade, due to concern with Reye's syndrome. This has promoted increased use of acetaminophen, as well as increased acetaminophen poisonings. In a recent survey, analgesics ranked second highest in frequency of all poisoning exposures reported during 1991, but ranked first in the category of substances causing the largest number of deaths (41). The report also indicated that acetaminophen was involved in approximately 60% of all analgesic exposures, and acetaminophen was involved 4.5 times more often than salicylates. Children are able to tolerate toxic ingestions better than adults since a dose almost 10 times the therapeutic dose is required before toxicity becomes a potential threat (54).

Acetaminophen, like aspirin, is safe when taken as directed. In acute overdose, unlike aspirin, acetaminophen does not cause early neurologic or other warning signs of toxicity (e.g., tinnitus). Patients present in otherwise good health, and by the time the potential for toxicity is realized (by either the victim or attending physician), irreversible liver damage may have already occurred. Furthermore, there is a phase of apparent recovery when symptoms subside. If this is interpreted as an emergence from danger and one fails to seek medical assistance, permanent hepatic damage may occur.

Mechanism of Toxicity

The most serious toxic consequence from acetaminophen poisoning is hepatic necrosis.

Acetaminophen is absorbed rapidly from the stomach and upper GI tract. Most of the drug is metabolized by conjugation with glucuronide and sulfate (Fig. 12.4). Anotherpathway, normally of minor importance, involves the cytochrome P_{450}-dependent mixed-function oxidase system. Approximately 4% of a therapeutic dose is metabolized bythis route.An intermediate metabolite formed via this system is a highly reactive arylating compound, N-acetyl-p-benzoquinoneimine (NAPQI). NAPQI binds covalently to hepatocyte proteins causing hepatocellular necrosis. At therapeutic doses, glutathione inactivates NAPQI by conjugation and subsequent transformation to acetaminophen-3-mercapturic acid, which is readily excreted. When a massive overdose is ingested, liver enzymes are saturated and the supply of glutathione is inadequate to detoxify NAPQI. The concentration of toxic metabolite, therefore, increases and can bind covalently to sulfhydryl groups of hepatic cellular proteins, resulting in centrilobular necrosis.

A dose of 15 g for adults, or 4 g for children, is normally sufficient to cause significant hepatotoxicity (8,25). On the basis of animal experiments, this amount of acetaminophen can deplete liver glutathione concentrations by 70% in a 70-kg man (56). The threshold dose for producing hepatotoxicity is 250 mg/kg; absorption of less than 125 mg/kg usually produces no significant hepatotoxicity (51). Estimates of the amount of acetaminophen ingested are often unreliable, and predictions of hepatotoxicity should be based on serum acetaminophen concentrations (1).

The incidence of hepatotoxicity in children is significantly lower with blood acetaminophen concentrations that would be potentially toxic in adults (49,55). In a study of 417 children less than 6 years of age, only three had aspartate transaminase (AST) values greater than 1,000 IU/L. Animal studies suggest there is an age-dependent rate of glutathione turnover and that younger animals can tolerate higher doses of acetaminophen (34,42,44). In humans, reduced toxicity in children may be attributed to early spontaneous emesis

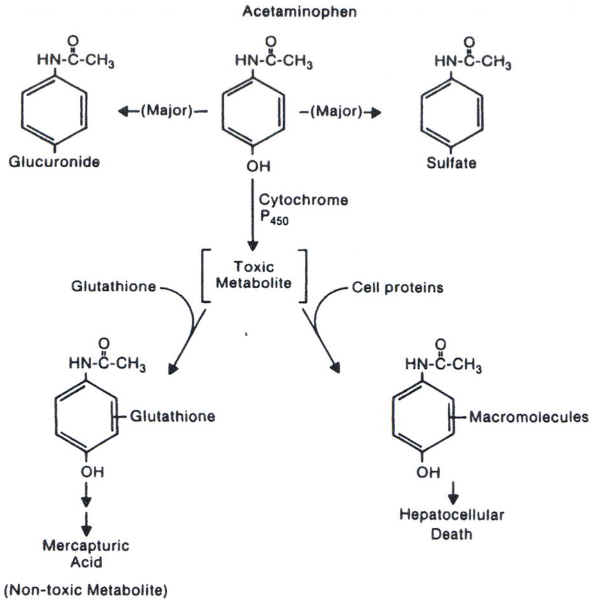

Acetaminophen

HN-C-CH$_3$

←(Major)—   —(Major)→

Glucuronide   OH   Sulfate

Cytochrome P$_{450}$

Glutathione   Toxic Metabolite   Cell proteins

HN-C-CH$_3$ HN-C-CH$_3$

Glutathione   Macromolecules

OH   OH

Mercapturic Acid   Hepatocellular Death

(Non-toxic Metabolite)

FIG. 12.4. Scheme for acetaminophen metabolism.

or differences in acetaminophen metabolism (44,54).

Toxicity after acute overdoses may be more severe in patients with chronic alcoholism or in patients taking drugs, such as phenobarbital or phenytoin, which induce liver microsomal enzymes (32,58,65). In fact, chronic alcoholics are prone to serious hepatotoxicity while taking therapeutic doses of acetaminophen. Inhibition of the cytochrome P$_{450}$ system (e.g., with cimetidine) without interfering with glucuronidation and sulfation of acetaminophen would be potentially useful in reducing acetaminophen hepatotoxicity (53). The clinical usefulness of cimetidine as an antidote for acetaminophen overdose is still investigational (13).

Characteristics of Poisoning

Except for signs of hepatotoxicity that may not appear for days after ingestion, acetaminophen causes few remarkable signs or symptoms. Clinical manifestations are divided into three phases, with a fourth phase of resolution of symptoms if the patient survives hepatotoxicity. Signs and symptoms show a consistent pattern and are reported in Table 12.4.

Stages of Poisoning

The ultimate outcome is not correlated directly with intensity of the initial symptoms. As can be seen in Table 12.4, symptoms of acute toxicity are those of gastrointestinal distress. Stage I may appear quickly and persist 24 hr or more. If acetaminophen is ingested alone, it is not likely that there will be serious CNS depression. Most patients exhibit initial symptoms and recover.

The real danger is that symptoms may subside quickly and the patient progresses to Stage II, a period of relatively quiescence with apparent recovery. If the individual fails to seek medical assistance during this period, thinking that the most serious events have occurred and that no further damage is possible, prognosis can be grave. Destruction of hepatocytes is inevitable during this phase. As noted by increased serum glutamic-oxalacetic transaminase (SGOT, AST) in Fig. 12.5, liver damage has already begun. The figure also shows

TABLE 12.4. *Stages of acetaminophen poisoning*

Stage I	0.5–24 hr	Within a few hours after ingestion patients experience anorexia, nausea, pallor, vomiting, and diaphoresis. Malaise may be present. Patient may appear normal.
Stage II	24–48 hr	Symptoms of Stage I are less severe, and patient may think everything is normal. A period of "perceived recovery." Right upper quadrant pain may be present due to hepatic damage. Blood chemistry becomes abnormal with elevations of liver enzymes and bilirubin, Prothrombin time prolonged. Renal function begins to deteriorate but BUN normally remains low as a result of decreased hepatic urea formation.
Stage III	72–96 hr	Starts 3–5 days after ingestion. Characterized by symptoms of hepatic necrosis. Coagulation defects, jaundice, renal failure, and myocardial pathology are all frequently present. Hepatic encephalopathy has been noted. Hepatic biopsy at this time reveals centrilobular necrosis. Nausea and vomiting may reappear. Death is due to hepatic failure; it is frequently preceded by anuria and coma.
Stage IV	4 days–2 weeks	If the damage done during Stage III is not irreversible, complete resolution of hepatic dysfunction will occur.

From ref. 40.

the anticipated outcome of acetaminophen toxicity. That is, during Stage I (nausea, vomiting, etc.) blood SGOT is within the normal range. However, during Stage II these serum enzyme concentrations are already rising, and other laboratory abnormalities may also be detected concurrently (e.g., elevated bilirubin, alkaline phosphatase, lactate dehydrogenase, and prothrombin time). The *solid line* in Fig. 12.5 represents the natural course of toxicity, the *dotted line* shows the outcome when the antidote, *N*-acetylcysteine (NAC), is given; and the *dotted-dashed line* shows expected outcome for patients with severe toxicity. If results of liver function tests are still normal after the second day, there will probably be no significant liver damage. If survival is to be assured, treatment with *N*-acetylcysteine must be initiated before Stage II begins.

Stage III may manifest within 72 to 96 hr after ingestion. It is characterized primarily by elevated plasma lactic dehydrogenase (LDH), SGOT, and bilirubin. Prothrombin time may be increased, and case reports have described hemorrhagic tendencies after acetaminophen toxicity.

Eventually the liver damage may cause jaundice and other sequelae depicted in Table 12.4. Myocardial tissue damage and renal failure have been reported. These effects are less predictable and overall less devastating than the hepatic response.

Plasma acetaminophen concentrations are the most important predictor for assessing the probability of developing hepatic damage (1). Therapeutic, toxic, and lethal acetaminophen serum concentrations are listed in Table 12.5. Significant damage is likely with an acetaminophen concentration greater than 200 μg/mL at 4 hr postingestion, or above 50 μg/mL at 12 hr postingestion (57). These values were obtained from the Rumack-Matthew nomo-

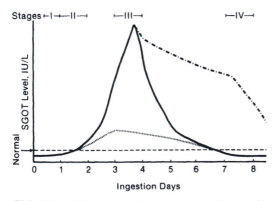

FIG. 12.5. Hepatotoxicity, as shown by an elevation of SGOT after toxic acetaminophen ingestion. The *solid line* is acetaminophen alone, the *dotted line* shows protection of liver damage with acetylcysteine, and the *dotted-and-dashed line* shows those individuals with a severe course. Notice that the solid line begins to rise early and peaks by stage III. (From ref. 56.)

TABLE 12.5. *Risk of toxicity associated with serum acetaminophen concentration*

Risk assignment	Predicted serum acetaminophen concentration (μg/mL)				
	4-hr	or	8-hr	or	12-hr
Slight risk	≤ 120		≤ 60		≤ 30
Possible risk	>120 and <200		>60 and <100		>30 and <50
Probable risk	≥ 200		≥ 100		≥ 50

From ref. 56.

gram for acetaminophen poisoning (Fig. 12.6). Like the nomogram for salicylate poisoning, this graph should be used only for a single acute ingestion, and only when the approximate time of ingestion is known. Blood samples for analytical determination of acetaminophen should be drawn at least 4 hr postingestion to permit complete absorption and peak serum concentration. Then the patient's serum acetaminophen concentration can be plotted on the nomogram to assess the probability of hepatic damage.

Since the time of ingestion is difficult to establish in some poisonings, another way to assess the possibility of hepatic damage is to determine the patient's plasma half-life of acetaminophen. This is accomplished by measuring at least three plasma concentrations and plotting them to obtain a $t_{1/2}$ value. The normal serum acetaminophen half-life is 1 to 3 hr and will be prolonged after an overdose. When using this method as an indicator for potential liver toxicity, it is generally assured that if the plasma $t_{1/2}$ exceeds 4 hr, liver damage is likely to occur. If the half-life is greater than 12 hr, hepatic coma will probably ensue.

It is always hoped that acetaminophen-poisoned patients will survive the events of Stage III. If they do, then Stage IV, the period of resolution of hepatic injury, ensues, and liver function tests generally return to normal.

Management of Poisoning

Prompt diagnosis and early treatment are essential for assuring recovery from acute acetaminophen poisoning. Early in the management protocol, as soon as poisoning has become evident, gastric decontamination should be undertaken to reduce the quantity of acetaminophen present within the GI tract. Decontamination includes ipecac-induced emesis, lavage, activated charcoal, and a cathartic. The appropriate choice should be based on time since ingestion, physical findings, and presence of co-ingestants (39). For example, if serum acetaminophen concentrations can be determined within 8 hr postingestion, gastric decontamination may not be necessary. Ipecac-induced emesis or gastric lavage may not be beneficial in reducing absorption in potentially toxic doses of acetaminophen if used more than 4 hr postingestion.

There is increasing evidence for effective use of activated charcoal after acetaminophen ingestions. It still remains a controversial subject.

Although recent studies have shown that

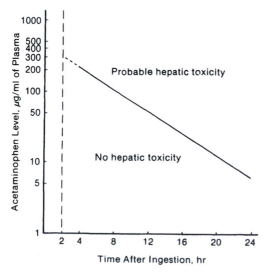

FIG. 12.6. Rumack and Matthew nomogram for assessing the extent of acetaminophen toxicity. (From ref. 56.)

activated charcoal effectively adsorbs acetaminophen and reduces absorption, there are other factors to consider. Since activated charcoal is a nonspecific adsorbent, it will adsorb almost any chemical in the GI tract, including the specific antidote for acetaminophen, *N*-acetylcysteine (57). If *N*-acetylcysteine is adsorbed onto activated charcoal, it cannot be absorbed sufficiently into the blood and its effectiveness will be diminished. This may be of more theoretical than practical importance. In many instances, by the time *N*-acetylcysteine is administered, several hours have already elapsed since activated charcoal was given. As long as the initial dose of *N*-acetylcysteine is given within the first 10 to 16 hrs after ingestion of acetaminophen, the regimen should be beneficial. Also, not all studies show that activated charcoal significantly reduces *N*-acetylcysteine blood concentrations and, thus, concomitant use of activated charcoal and *N*-acetylcysteine may be effective (46,52).

As stated earlier, hepatotoxicity is not due to acetaminophen, *per se*, but to a chemically reactive toxic metabolite, NABQI, which accumulates when the amount of glutathione is inadequate to convert NABQI to acetaminophen-3-mercapturic acid. The greatest potential for hepatotoxicity occurs when blood acetaminophen concentrations are in the area above the line in the nomogram shown in Fig. 12.6. The logical response would be to simply administer glutathione. Unfortunately, glutathione does not enter hepatocytes and is, therefore, useless as an antidote. The next choice is to administer a substance that will penetrate hepatocytes and act as a substitute for glutathione or increase its synthesis.

Several sulfhydryl-containing protective agents have been studied, including methionine, cysteamine (mercaptamine), dimercaprol, and D-penicillamine (16,26). Methionine has also been shown to be effective in the treatment of acetaminophen poisoning in humans. *N*-acetylcysteine and methionine afford antidotal activity mainly by restoring intracellular glutathione concentrations. Both compounds require prior conversion to cysteine

(17). Besides enhancing synthesis of glutathione, *N*-acetylcysteine and methionine also serve as a source of inorganic sulfur. This may promote increased conversion of acetaminophen to its sulfate metabolite, as well as reduce formation of other metabolites including the toxic intermediate, NAPQI-NAPQI (19).

Within the first 10 to 16 hr after poisoning, a loading dose of 140 mg/kg of *N*-acetylcysteine is given orally, followed by 70 mg/kg every 4 hr for 17 to 18 doses (72 hr total). In the event that the patient vomits the loading dose or any of the maintenance doses within 1 hr of administration, a replacement dose is given immediately and the patient continues on the same schedule. When persistent vomiting occurs, *N*-acetylcysteine can be instilled through a nasogastric tube.

Oral administration is, at least theoretically, better than intravenous dosing (50). Arguments in favor of giving the antidote orally stress that substances that are absorbed from the GI tract are transported immediately to the liver. Moreover, if *N*-acetylcysteine is injected intravenously, less will be delivered initially to the liver because it is distributed throughout the body. It should be pointed out that a solution for intravenous use is available in Canada and Europe, and studies confirm that it is also effective (9).

The importance of beginning *N*-acetylcysteine therapy early cannot be overemphasized. Table 12.6 summarizes data from a study that examined the effect on blood SGOT concentrations for *N*-acetylcysteine given at different times after acetaminophen ingestion. The data

TABLE 12.6. *Effect of* N-*acetylcysteine on blood SGOT[a] concentrations at different times after acetaminophen ingestion*

Initiation of treatment (time)	No. of patients	Mean maximum SGOT (IU/L)
<10 hr	57	229
10−16 hr	52	1,557
16−24 hr	39	2,695

From ref. 56.
[a] SGOT, serum glutamate oxaloacetate transaminase.

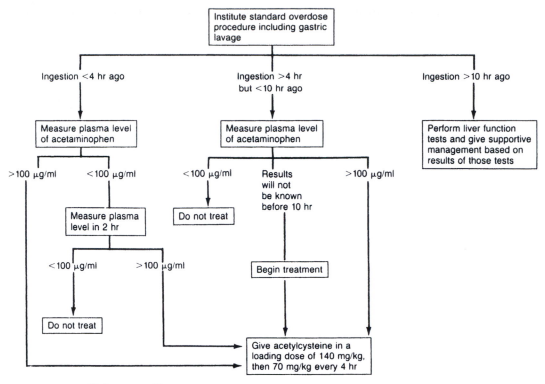

FIG. 12.7. Flow chart for management of acetaminophen poisoning.

clearly substantiate a correlation between the time treatment is initiated and increases in SGOT concentrations, which should indicate a relative degree of hepatotoxicity.

Throughout treatment, the patient is monitored constantly for vital signs, blood chemistry, and hepatic function. The basic management protocol is summarized in Fig. 12.7.

SUMMARY

Non-narcotic analgesics are commonly used for minor pain management. They are also a source of accidental and intentional overdose. This chapter demonstrates that the benign actions of this class of drugs are replaced by significantly toxic outcomes when large quantities are ingested. In addition, the toxicokinetic profiles are much different from the pharmacokinetic features of these drugs. Nomograms have been constructed to aid in the clinical assessment of the toxicity potential for this class of drugs, but they are useful only for acute ingestions.

Case Studies

CASE STUDIES: SALICYLATE TOXICITY IN CHILDREN

History: Case 1

An 18-month-old boy weighing 10 kg was brought to a local hospital because of fever, irritability, hyperventilation, and hematemesis. He had been treated for the past 2 days for an upper respiratory infection. His parents said they gave him only one baby aspirin tablet every 4 to 6 hr. Because aspirin poisoning was nevertheless suspected, a blood salicylate test was ordered. When the blood salicylate concentration was found to be 55 mg/dL, he was transferred to a larger medical center for further assessment.

TABLE 12.7. *Laboratory findings*

Na$^+$	=148 mEq/L
K$^+$	=7.2 mEq/L
HCO$_3^-$	=11 mEq/L
Glucose	=87 mg/dL
BUN	=158 mg/dL
Creatinine	=3.9 mg/dL
WBC	=16,000/mm^3
PT	=elevated
PTT	=elevated
pCO$_2$	=20 mm Hg
pH	=7.34
Blood salicylate	=168 mg/dL

BUN, blood urea nitrogen; WBC, white blood cells; PT, prothrombin time; PTT, partial thromboplastin time.

On arrival at the second hospital, the patient was lethargic, but arousable. Physical examination revealed signs of moderate dehydration and temperature of 40.5°C. Systolic blood pressure was 90 mm Hg, pulse was 220 beats/min, and respirations were 70/min. Laboratory values are listed in Table 12.7.

Treatment consisted of volume expansion with saline, dextrose, and sodium bicarbonate. Fifty grams of albumin per liter were added to the intravenous fluid. The patient underwent lavage with normal saline, and activated charcoal and magnesium sulfate were added through the nasogastric tube. He was given 100% oxygen and placed on a ventilator.

Due to onset of renal failure and persistence of elevated serum salicylate concentrations, peritoneal dialysis was initiated, using 1.5% Impersol solution containing 5% albumin. Twenty-four hours later, the serum salicylate concentration had decreased to 40 mg/dL and the BUN was reduced to 34 mg/dL. After 48 hr, the serum salicylate concentration was only 4 mg/dL and kidney function was markedly improved. Dialysis was discontinued, and the boy was showing signs of improvement until 12 hr later when he became hypotensive and signs of septic shock appeared (WBC = 5,400 mm^3 with a severe shift to the left). A diagnosis of disseminated intravascular coagulation (DIC) was made. Blood cultures grew *Escherichia coli*. The victim died on the 4th hospital day, despite antibiotics and additional supportive measures. (See ref. 7.)

History: Case 2

Twelve hours before admission to an emergency facility, an otherwise healthy 5-year-old boy complained to his mother of stomach pain, and vomited. This was followed later by difficult, rapid breathing. He complained further of *ringing* in his ears. His mother found an empty bottle of adult aspirin tablets and brought him to the hospital.

On arrival, he was lethargic but arousable. There were signs of dehydration. Physical examination revealed rectal temperature, 102°F; blood pressure, 110/65 mm Hg; pulse rate, 120 beats/min; and respirations, 45/min. Laboratory values are listed in Table 12.8.

Overall, this patient's condition was largely unremarkable, and he survived after supportive therapy. (See ref. 61.)

Discussion

1. Patient 1 was given albumin by intravenous infusion. What was its purpose?
2. Comment on the dose of aspirin the victim in case 1 supposedly received. Is this probably all the aspirin he ingested? If so, what were the complicating factors that caused his serum salicylate concentration to rise so high?
3. The victim in case 2 may have taken a larger dose of aspirin than the victim in case 1, but his serum salicylate concentration was lower. Is this possible? If so, why?
4. Was either patient in metabolic acidosis? How does this correlate to your under-

TABLE 12.8. *Laboratory findings*

Serum salicylate	=61 mg/dL
Blood glucose	=160 mg/dL
pCO$_2$	=25 mm Hg
pH	=7.30
HCO$_3^-$	=15 mEq/L
Urine	=scanty; pH 5.3, 3$^+$ ketonuria

standing of the mechanism of salicylate toxicity?

5. Patient 1 had a normal blood glucose concentration, whereas patient 2 had a blood glucose concentration that was above normal. What are the factors that likely influenced this value, and what accounted for the difference?

CASE STUDY: SALICYLATE TOXICITY IN AN ADULT

History

A 22-year-old woman who was feeling depressed the night before she was admitted to an emergency facility consumed a full glass of vodka. She vomited throughout the night. The following morning her husband tried unsuccessfully to awaken her; he even immersed her in a cold bath.

He then brought her to the hospital where physical examination revealed an unresponsive woman with blood pressure, 128/90 mm Hg; pulse, 140 beats/min; temperature, 102°F; and respirations, 40/min. She occasionally exhibited spontaneous movements of her extremities. Other physical findings were unremarkable. Laboratory findings are included in Table 12.10. Information later revealed that the patient had ingested approximately 250 aspirin tablets (325 mg each) during the previous night.

Treatment consisted of hydration and forced alkaline diuresis. As shown in Table 12.9, the serum salicylate concentration de-

creased to below the toxic level after approximately one day. (See ref. 27.)

Discussion

1. Does the initial serum salicylate concentration correspond to the amount of aspirin tablets reportedly ingested as listed in Table 12.9? If not, can you state reasons for the discrepancy?

2. Would the glassful of vodka have caused her clinical state? If she weighed 125 pounds, what would her maximum blood alcohol level (BAC) have been? (See chapter 4.)

3. Explain why this patient presented to the emergency room in an alkalotic state.

CASE STUDY: ATTEMPTED POISONING WITH ENTERIC-COATED ASPIRIN

History

The patient was a 25-year-old woman with a history of psychiatric disease and multiple suicide attempts. She was taking tranylcypromine sulfate, a monoamine oxidase inhibitor. Approximately 4 hr before admission to a hospital, she took 90 to 100 tablets of an enteric-coated aspirin preparation, each containing 325 mg aspirin. She vomited several times before admission, bringing up remnants of the ingested tablets.

The patient was lethargic on admission.

TABLE 12.9. *Serum salicylate concentrations and stage of consciousness, blood gases, and pH*

Hr after admission	Level of consciousness	Serum salicylate concentration (mg/dL)	pO$_2$ (mm Hg)	pCO$_2$ (mm Hg)	HCO$_3^-$ (mEq/L)	pH
0	Comatose	140	113	21	17.5	7.54
4	Semicomatose	110	162	20	22	7.65
9	Awake-drowsy	94	121	22.5	19	7.55
15	Awake-drowsy	68	82	26	21	7.52
23	Awake-drowsy	46	91	29	24	7.53
32	Awake-alert	34				

From ref. 26.

TABLE 12.10. *Laboratory findings*

Na$^+$	=141 mEq/L
Cl$^-$	=112 mEq/L
K$^+$	=3.2 mEq/L
BUN	=80 mg/L
Glucose	=1,230 mg/L
pCO$_2$	=20 mm Hg
pO$_2$	=123 mm Hg
Total CO$_2$	=17 mEq/L
pH	=7.52

Blood pressure was 180/90 mm Hg; heart rate, 100 beats/min; and respirations, 28 to 34/min. Her chest was clear. Laboratory values are listed in Table 12.10. These values were consistent with respiratory alkalosis and metabolic acidosis. She also developed tinnitus and hyperthermia.

Treatment was initiated with intravenous saline and potassium chloride. Serial blood specimens were drawn for serum salicylate determinations.

Salicylate concentration 6 hr after ingestion was 30 mg/dL. The rise in serum salicylate was slow, with peak concentration being reached after 24 hr. This remained elevated for more than 3 days. Regular adult aspirin tablets would have resulted in higher blood salicylate concentrations at 6 hr, with peak concentration reached in less than 24 hr post-ingestion. Serum salicylate concentrations were plotted on Done's nomogram, and the extent of severity of intoxication could not be predicted. Based on the 6 hr concentration of 30 mg/dL, one might have erroneously predicted an asymptomatic event if it had been assumed that she ingested regular aspirin tablets. The patient actually developed moderately severe symptoms. (See ref. 33.)

Discussion

1. Did the rate of rise of serum salicylate occur as you would predict, based upon what you know about enteric-coated tablets?
2. List other factors that might have contributed to the slow increase in serum salicylate concentrations.

CASE STUDY: SALICYLIC ACID OINTMENT INTOXICATION

History

A 42-year-old man suffering from psoriasis used a 40% salicylic acid ointment to cover his hands and feet, and covered the treated areas with an occlusive polyethylene covering. A 2% salicylic acid ointment was used to treat affected areas on the rest of his body.

After the fourth application, all within 24 hr, the patient developed malaise associated with deafness, flushing, and sweating. Serum salicylate concentration was 72 mg/dL, and other laboratory results revealed metabolic acidosis. He had used a total of 300 g of 40% and 150 g of 2% salicylic acid ointment.

The patient received forced alkaline diuresis. He recovered without further incident. (See ref. 2.)

Discussion

1. List the substances that could be used to promote forced alkaline diuresis. Outline how alkalinization of urine assists in promoting salicylate excretion?
2. Discuss the advantages and disadvantages of forced alkaline diuresis, as opposed to alkaline diuresis alone.

CASE STUDIES: POISONING WITH ACETAMINOPHEN

History: Case 1

A 19-year-old woman ingested a bottle of 30 Tylenol Extra Strength tablets (500 mg acetaminophen/tablet). Sixteen hours after ingestion she was brought to an emergency facility. She presented with nausea, vomiting, and dizziness while standing. Her physical examination was unremarkable. She indicated she had taken no other medicine and her health was good. Serum acetaminophen concentration was 32 μg/mL. Other laboratory findings are shown in Table 12.11.

TABLE 12.11. *Laboratory values associated with an acute acetaminophen overdose*

Measurement	Days after ingestion								
	1	2	3	4	5	6	8	13	18
Prothrombin time (sec, patient/control)	15/12	24/12	47/12	29/12	17/12	14/12	13/12	11/12	11/12
SGOT (U/mL)	197	910	3,000				50	30	40
SGPT (U/mL)	190	800	11,720	5,500			1,170	178	64
Alkaline phosphate (U/mL)	97								
LDH (U/mL)	261								
Bilirubin (mg/dL, total/direct)	2.5/1.5	4.2[a]	4.9[a]		3.6				
Creatinine (mg/dL)		0.7	1.0	N.D.[b]	6.0	8.1	11.3	3.5	1.2
BUN (mg/dL)	7	5	7		46	59	79	31	23
Sodium (mEq/L)	145					134	138	145	151
Potassium (mEq/L)	4.2					2.8	3.4	4.4	4.5
Chloride (mEq/L)	109					92	104	110	112
CO$_2$ (mEq/L)	12					13	9	20	23
Hemodialysis performed (X)							X		

From ref. 28.
SGPT, serum glutamate pyruvic transaminase; LDH, lactate dehydrogenase.
[a] Total bilirubin only.
[b] Quantity of blood not sufficient for test.

At this point, approximately 20 hr postingestion, an *N*-acetylcysteine antidote protocol was initiated. Liver enzyme levels rapidly returned to normal. She continued to complain of abdominal discomfort and cramping.

Four days later there were signs of kidney failure (see Table 12.11). She became lethargic, and urine output was diminished. Hemodialysis was started on the 7th hospital day because of signs of increased metabolic acidosis and azotemia. Two days later she entered the diuretic phase of acute tubular necrosis. Serum creatinine concentrations decreased over the next few days.

The patient was discharged about two weeks after hospitalization. (See ref. 28.)

History: Case 2

A 3-year-old girl was in otherwise good health except for a slight cough. Her mother administered a single dose of cough preparation containing dextromethorphan hydrobromide. The next day the child told her mother she had taken some acetaminophen (Tylenol) tablets. She appeared in good health except for slight weakness and unsteadiness while walking, and went to bed as usual. No other medications were given to the child.

The next morning the child awakened and complained of a headache. She vomited four times. She was pale and very lethargic.

On admission to a hospital she was described as shaky, vomiting, lethargic, and sleepy. She also had decreased consciousness. Hepatomegaly was present, but there were no signs of liver disease, jaundice, or hepatitis. Physical examination revealed normal pulse rate, blood pressure, and temperature. A presumptive diagnosis of Reye's syndrome was made and she was transferred to a larger medical center.

Physical examination confirmed the previous findings. Laboratory results showed a hemoglobin content of 10.5 g/dL and WBC count of 10,800 mm^3 with 80% banded neutrophils. Serum electrolytes, BUN, calcium, phosphate, and albumin levels were all within normal limits. Blood glucose was 150 mg/dL and ammonia concentration was 88 μg/dL.

A toxicology drug screen showed the presence of salicylate at 4.8 mg/dL and acetamino-

TABLE 12.12. *Laboratory values indicating the degree and time course of toxicity associated with acute acetaminophen intoxication*

Time after ingestion (days)	Acetaminophen (μg/mL)	SGOT (IU/mL)	SGPT (IU/mL)	LDH (IU/mL)	Prothrombin time (min)	Total bilirubin (mg/dL)
1	96	617	557	497	1.3	1.0
2	26	—	—	—	—	—
3		20,376	13,303	11,640	1.6	1.3
4		2,967	5,772	533	1.3	1.1
5		761	4,093	300	0.8	0.9
50		52	30	234		

From ref. 4.

phen at 96 μg/mL. Table 12.12 lists the significant response observed with the liver enzymes, and prothrombin time for this patient until she was released on the 7th hospital day. The parents estimated that she had probably ingested about 35 acetaminophen tablets (325 mg each).

The patient received intravenous fluids with glucose and hydrocortisone added. *N*-acetylcysteine was not given.

This case is especially interesting from two standpoints. First, the liver enzyme concentrations (Table 12.12) were reported to be the highest ever reported by the hospital. Second, the young girl did not receive the standard treatment protocol, and survived without apparent sequelae. On further examination, approximately 7 weeks after discharge, all hepatic enzymes were within normal limits. (See ref. 4.)

History: Case 3

A 6-week-old boy was admitted to a hospital. He had a 2 hr history of extreme lethargy and unresponsiveness. For the past 48 hr he was irritable and had a slight fever. He had a history of intermittent vomiting and diarrhea since birth, but these worsened over the past 48 hr. A parent had been administering acetaminophen drops (Tempra), 0.3 mL every 4 hr, and acetaminophen drops (Tylenol), 0.6 mL every 4 hr, during that time. On the morning of admission the boy was lethargic, but arousable.

Physical examination revealed a completely unresponsive child. Respirations were normal at 40/min; pulse, 132 beats/min; and rectal temperature, 36.1°C. The infant appeared to be well nourished, and was not dehydrated. The only physical abnormality was a palpable liver edge at 4 cm below the right costal margin.

Laboratory values showed blood glucose, 5 mg/dL; prothrombin time, 53 sec (control: 28 sec); SGOT, 2,350 IU/L; SGPT, 825 IU/L; lactic dehydrogenase, of 3,000 IU/L, alkaline phosphatase, 380 IU/L; and total bilirubin, 1.1 g/dL. Plasma acetaminophen concentration was 119 mg/L.

The infant received intravenous glucose and consciousness improved rapidly. At 4 hr he was fully responsive to stimuli. He was started on the standard 17-dose protocol of *N*-acetylcysteine.

Clinical improvement overall was rapid and progressive. Liver function returned to near normal by the 5th hospital day. The child was discharged on the 11th hospital day in good condition. A follow-up visit was scheduled for 2 weeks. The parent failed to keep the appointment, and the child was unavailable for further examination. (See ref. 20.)

Discussion

1. In case 1, there seemed to be more renal toxicity than hepatic damage. The antidote was not even administered for 20 hr after ingestion. Is there any special reason for this?

2. Were the blood acetaminophen concentrations in the three cases within the toxic or nontoxic range?

3. Would you have suspected hepatic coma to develop in case 2?

4. Based on information presented in the histories, did all patients show signs and symptoms of all the phases usually described for acetaminophen toxicity?

5. In case 3, the infant received two preparations of acetaminophen concurrently. The parent reportedly gave one for irritability, and the other for fever. How can health professionals reduce the chance of this from happening?

CASE STUDY: ACETAMINOPHEN HEPATOTOXICITY IN AN ALCOHOLIC

History

A 39-year-old male alcoholic was hospitalized with submandibular infection after a fracture. On admission, laboratory values for aspartate aminotransferase (AST), alanine aminotransferase (ALT), and lactic dehydrogenase were 5640 IU/L, 354 IU/L, and 655 IU/L, respectively. Bilirubin was 16.5 mg/dL, and alkaline phosphatase, 386 IU. Prothrombin time was 21 sec (control 10.6 sec). Because these laboratory values were not consistent with alcoholic liver disease, the patient was questioned for other causes. He admitted to ingesting 3.8 g acetaminophen (approximately 21 g total) each day for the past week.

The patient was treated with hemoperfusion because of incipient hepatic encephalopathy. By day 4, AST and ALT values were 925 and 647 IU/L, respectively. Bilirubin was 35 mg/dL, and the prothrombin time, 16.1 sec (control: 10.9 sec). Hemoperfusion was stopped. His condition improved slowly during the next several days and he was discharged without sequelae. (See ref. 58.)

Discussion

1. This patient ingested approximately 21 g acetaminophen over a week, which is hardly a toxic dose in normal individuals. Suggest reasons why he became intoxicated from this dose.

2. Review the procedure for hemoperfusion. Do you think hemodialysis would have been as effective? Why or why not?

CASE STUDY: IBUPROFEN-INDUCED COMA

History

A comatose woman, age 50, was brought to an emergency facility. She was last seen conscious by her family 12 hr earlier. She had a history of cardiovascular disease and was taking warfarin, furosemide, digoxin, captopril, and potassium supplementation.

The patient's pulse was 112 beats/min, with respirations 16/min, and temperature 32°C. Neurologic examination revealed that she was completely unresponsive to verbal stimuli. Extremities moved without purpose to noxious stimuli. Muscle tone was increased in all extremities, and deep tendon reflexes were normal. Pupils were constricted, yet reactive, and the corneal reflex was present. Laboratory values were unremarkable; arterial blood pH was 7.2 Toxicologic screening was negative for ethanol. Acetaminophen concentration was less than 10 μg/L, salicylate concentration was 2.4 mg/dL, and serum digoxin was 1.1 ng/mL. All other drugs screened for were negative.

She was resuscitated with endotracheal intubation and mechanical ventilatory support. Naloxone, 0.8 mg, was given without response. Mannitol was administered. A CT scan ruled out traumatic brain injury as a cause of coma.

She regained consciousness shortly and admitted taking 40 to 60 ibuprofen tablets (600 mg each) shortly after her last family visit, in a suicide attempt.

Four hours postadmission she was able to respond to verbal stimulation. By 7 hr, she was alert and oriented, and therefore, was extubated. She experienced gastrointestinal bleeding and her hematocrit fell from 42% to 36%, but stabilized at 36% without transfusion by the second day. Renal assessment revealed nonoliguric renal failure with mild deterioration in renal function. Her increased creatinine level returned to baseline within 4 days. She recovered without adverse sequelae, and was discharged later. (See ref. 10.)

Discussion

1. This case illustrates that toxic symptoms of ibuprofen overdose are quickly reversed with only supportive treatment. Discuss the major reason(s) for this quick response.
2. Ibuprofen is bound to plasma protein to the extent of 99%. Comment on the validity of using alkaline diuresis, hemodialysis, or hemoperfusion to increase drug elimination in ibuprofen overdoses.

Review Questions

1. All of the following statements about aspirin-induced toxicity are true *except*:
   A. Salicylates increase oxygen consumption by increasing cellular metabolic rate.
   B. Metabolic acidosis occurs, in part, when oxidative phosphorylation is uncoupled.
   C. Hyperglycemia is the usual outcome of chronic salicylism.
   D. The kidney attempts to compensate for decreasing H_2CO_3 levels by excreting HCO_3^-.
2. After ingestion of a toxic acetaminophen dose, at which of the following periods does hepatocellular toxicity begin?
   A. Stage I
   B. Stage II
   C. Stage III
   D. Stage IV
3. Activated charcoal reduces the systemic absorption of acetaminophen.
   A. True
   B. False

4. Which of the following is a logical treatment for ibuprofen overdose: Syrup of ipecac (I); acetylcysteine (II); potassium chloride (III)?
   A. I only
   B. II only
   C. I and II only
   D. I, II and III
5. Which of the following is contraindicated in treating a toxic dose of acetylsalicylic acid?
   A. Syrup of ipecac
   B. Oral fluids
   C. Saline cathartics
   D. None of the above
6. Salicylate blood concentrations are considered to be lethal at the point when which of the following concentrations is exceeded?
   A. 45 to 64 mg/dL
   B. 65 to 90 mg/dL
   C. 90 to 120 mg/dL
   D. Greater than 120 mg/dL
7. Tinnitus is an early warning signal of aspirin and acetaminophen toxicity.
   A. True
   B. False
8. Which of the following can be given to treat acetaminophen toxicity: Glutathione (I), *N*-acetylcysteine (II), methionine (III)?
   A. II only
   B. I and II only
   C. II and III only
   D. I, II and III
9. At which of the following blood salicylate concentrations are most patients considered to be asymptomatic?
   A. 25 mg/dL
   B. 55 mg/dL
   C. 65 mg/dL
   D. 75 mg/dL
10. Early toxic manifestations of salicylate poisoning are due to an action on which of the following target organs?
    A. CNS
    B. Heart
    C. Liver
    D. Kidney

11. The elimination half-life of ibuprofen is closest to which of the following?
    A. 0.5 hr
    B. 1 hr
    C. 2 hr
    D. 4 hr

12. Which of the following is true about oil of wintergreen?
    A. One teaspoonful contains approximately 4 g of salicylate.
    B. One teaspoonful is a potentially lethal dose to a child.
    C. Both A and B are true.
    D. Neither A nor B are true.

13. Conversion of acetaminophen to its toxic metabolite via the cytochrome P_{450} mechanism is an example of what specific type of enzymatic conversion?
    A. Glucuronide formation
    B. Sulfate formation
    C. Oxidation
    D. Reduction

14. Concerning salicylate intoxication, which of the following is correct?
    A. Moderate toxicity usually appears when a single oral dose of 200 mg/kg is ingested.
    B. Blood salicylate concentrations less than 40 mg/dL usually correlate with an asymptomatic episode; except in the case of chronic salicylism.
    C. Children under five years are at greatest risk of acute toxicity and usually display metabolic acidosis.
    D. All of the above are correct.
    E. A & B are correct.

15. Ethanol potentiates acetaminophen toxicity because it:
    A. Inhibits reductase enzymes
    B. Stimulates reductase enzymes
    C. Inhibits oxidase enzymes
    D. Stimulates oxidase enzymes

16. Explain why a patient is in greater danger of serious damage from a toxic dose of acetaminophen if he has been using alcohol or barbiturates.

17. Discuss the reasons why potassium chloride is sometimes given to persons treated for aspirin intoxication.

18. Cite at least two reasons why the chance for lethal toxicity is more potentially severe with acetaminophen than with aspirin.

19. Discuss the physiologic event known as *compensated respiratory alkalosis,* which occurs after a toxic ingestion of aspirin.

20. Discuss the factors that lead to salicylate-induced ketoacidosis. Would you expect the anion gap to be normal or increased?

21. Discuss the probable mechanism associated with ibuprofen-induced toxicity.

22. List all the reasons why ibuprofen is claimed to be relatively safe when taken in overdosage.

23. If the time since ingestion of acetaminophen is unknown, how can one estimate the probability of hepatic damage?

24. Outline the role of cimetidine in treating toxic acetaminophen ingestion.

References

1. Amber J, Alexander M. Liver toxicity after acetaminophen ingestion: inadequacy of the dose estimate as an index of risk. *JAMA* 1977;238:500–501.
2. Anderson JAR, Ead RD. Percutaneous salicylate poisoning. *Clin Exp Dermatol* 1979;4:349–351.
3. Anderson RJ, Potts DE, Gabrow PA, et al. Unrecognized adult salicylate intoxication. *Ann Intern Med* 1976;85:745–748.
4. Arena JM, Rourk MH, Sibrack CD. Acetaminophen: report of an unusual poisoning. *Pediatrics* 1978;61:68–72.
5. Barone JA, Raia JJ, Huang YC. Evaluation of the effects of multiple-dose activated charcoal on the absorption of orally administered salicylate in a simulated ingestion model. *Ann Emerg Med* 1988;17:34–37.
6. Barry WS, Meinzinger MM, Howse CR. Ibuprofen over-dose and exposure *in utero:* results from a post-marketing voluntary reporting system. *Am J Med* 1984;77:35–39.
7. Bender KJ. Salicylate intoxication. *Drug Intell Clin Pharm* 1975;9:350–360.
8. Black M. Acetaminophen hepatotoxicity. *Ann Rev Med* 1984;35:577–593.
9. Bronstein AC, Linden CH, Hall AH, et al. Intravenous *N*-acetylcysteine for acute acetaminophen poisoning. *Vet Hum Toxicol* 1985;27:316.
10. Chelluri L, Jastremski MS. Coma caused by ibuprofen overdose. *Crit Care Med* 1986;14:1078–1079.
11. Clarke S, Walton WW. Effect of safety packaging on aspirin ingestion by children. *Pediatrics* 1979;63:687.
12. Court H, Streete P, Volans GN. Acute poisoning with ibuprofen. *Hum Toxicol* 1983;2:381–384.

13. Critchley JA, Scott AW, Dyson EH, Jarvie DR. Is there a plan for cimetidine or ethanol in the treatment of paracetamol poisoning? *Lancet* 1983;2:1375–1376.

14. Done AK. Salicylate intoxication: significance of measurements of salicylate in blood in cases of acute ingestion. *Pediatrics* 1960;26:800–807.

15. Filippone GA, Fish SS, Lacontre PG, et al. Reversible absorption (desorption) of aspirin from activated charcoal. *Arch Intern Med* 1987;147:1390–1392.

16. Flanagan RJ. The role of acetylcysteine in clinical toxicology. *Med Toxicol* 1987;2:93–104.

17. Flanagan RJ, Meredith TJ. Use of *N*-acetylcysteine in clinical toxicology. *Am J Med* 1991;91:1315–1395.

18. Gabow PA, Anderson RJ, Potts DE, Schrier RW. Acid-base disturbances in the salicylate-intoxicated adult. *Arch Intern Med* 1978;138:1481–1484.

19. Galinsky RE, Levy G. Effect of *N*-acetylcysteine on the pharmacokinetics of acetaminophen in rats. *Life Sci* 1979;25:693–700.

20. Greene JW, Craft L, Ghishan F. Acetaminophen poisoning in infancy. *Am J Dis Child* 1983;137:386–387.

21. Hall AH, Smolinske SC, Conrad FL, et al. Ibuprofen overdose: 126 cases. *Ann Emerg Med* 1986;15:1308–1313.

22. Hall AH, Smolinske SC, Stover B, et al. Ibuprofen overdose in adults. *Clin Toxicol* 1992;30:23–37.

23. Hill JB. Salicylate intoxication. *N Engl J Med* 1973;288:1110–1113.

24. Howrie DL, Moriarty R, Breit R. Candy flavoring as a source of salicylate poisoning. *Pediatrics* 1985;75:869–871.

25. Jackson CH, MacDonald NC, Cornett JN. Acetaminophen—a practical pharmacologic overview. *Can Med Assoc J* 1984;131:25–33.

26. James SH, Martinak JF. Recovery following massive self-poisoning with aspirin. *NY J Med* 1975;75:1512–1514.

27. James J, Routledge PA. Recent developments in the management of paracetamol (acetaminophen) poisoning. *Drug Safety* 1992;7:170–177.

28. Jeffery WJ, Lafferty WE. Acute renal failure after acetaminophen overdoses: report of two cases. *Am J Hosp Pharm* 1981;36:1355–1358.

29. Keller RE, Schwab RA, Krenzelok EP. Contribution of sorbitol combined with activated charcoal in prevention of salicylate absorption. *Ann Emerg Med* 1990;19:654–656.

30. Kirshenbaum LA, Matthews SC, Sitar DS, Tenebein M. Does multiple-dose charcoal therapy enhance salicylate excretion? *Arch Intern Med* 1990;150:1281–1283.

31. Krause DS, Wolf BA, Shaw LM. Acute aspirin overdose mechanism of toxicity. *Ther Drug Monit* 1992;14:441–451.

32. Kumar S, Rex DK. Failure of physicians to recognize acetaminophen hepatotoxicity in chronic alcoholics. *Arch Intern Med* 1991;151:1189–1191.

33. Kwong TC, Laczin J, Baum J. Self-poisoning with enteric-coated aspirin. *Am J Clin Pathol* 1983;80:888–890.

34. Lanterburg BH, Vaishnaw Y, Stillwell WG, et al. The effects of age and glutathione depletion on hepatic glutathione turnover *in vivo* determined by acetamin-

ophen probe analysis. *J Pharmacol Exp Ther* 1980;213:54–58.

35. Lee CY, Finkles A. Acute intoxication due to ibuprofen overdose. *Arch Pathol Lab Med* 1986;110:747–749.

36. Levy G. Clinical pharmacokinetics of aspirin. *Pediatrics.* 1978;69[Suppl]:867–872.

37. Levy G, Tsuchiya T. Salicylate accumulation kinetics in man. *N Engl J Med* 1972;287:430–432.

38. Levy G, Yaffe SF. Relationship between dose and apparent volume of distribution of salicylate in children. *Pediatrics* 1974;54:713–714.

39. Lewis RC, Paloucek FP. Assessment and treatment of acetaminophen overdose. *Clin Pharm* 1991;10:765–774.

40. Linden C, Rumack BH. Acetaminophen overdose. *Emerg Med Clin North Am* 1984;2:103–119.

41. Litovitz TL, Bailey KM, Holm KC, Schmitz BF. 1991 Annual report of the American Association of Poison Control Centers National Data Collection System. *Am J Emerg Med* 1992;10:452–505.

42. Mancini RE, Sonaware BR, Yaffe SJ. Developmental susceptibility to acetaminophen toxicity. *Res Commun Chem Pathol Pharmacol* 1980;27:603–606.

43. Mayer AC, Sitar DS, Tenebein M. Multiple-dose charcoal and whole-bound irrigation do not increase clearance of absorbed salicylate. *Arch Intern Med* 1992;152:393–396.

44. Miller RP, Roberts RJ, Fischer LJ. Acetaminophen elimination kinetics in neonates, children, and adults. *Clin Pharmacol Ther* 1976;19:284–294.

45. Morgan AG, Polak A. Excretion of salicylate in salicylate poisoning. *Clin Sci* 1971;41:475–484.

46. North DS, Peterson RG, Krenzeick EP. Effect of activated charcoal administration on acetylcysteine serum levels in humans. *Am J Hosp Pharm* 1980;38:1022–1024.

47. Notarianni L. A reassessment of the treatment of salicylate poisoning. *Drug Safety* 1992;7:292–303.

48. Paulus HE. FDA Arthritis Advisory Committee meeting: postmarketing surveillance of nonsteroidal anti-inflammatory drugs. *Arthritis Rheum* 1985;28:1168–1169.

49. Peterson RG, Rumack BH. Age as a variable in acetaminophen overdose. *Arch Intern Med* 1981;141:390–393.

50. Prescott LF. Treatment of severe acetaminophen poisoning with intravenous acetylcysteine. *Arch Intern Med* 1981;141:366–369.

51. Prescott LF. Paracetamol overdose—pharmacological considerations and clinical management. *Drugs* 1983;25:290–314.

52. Renzi F, Donovan J, Marten T, et al. Concomitant use of activated charcoal and *N*-acetylcysteine. *Ann Emerg Med* 1985;14:568–572.

53. Ruffalo RL, Thompson JF. Cimetidine and acetylcysteine as antidote for acetaminophen overdose. *South Med J* 1982;75:954–958.

54. Rumack BH. Acetaminophen overdose in young children. *Am J Dis Child* 1984;138:428–433.

55. Rumack BH, Peterson RG. Acetaminophen overdose: incidence, diagnosis, and management in 416 patients. *Pediatrics* 1978;62:898–903.

56. Rumack BH, Peterson RC, Koch GG, Amara IA. Acetaminophen overdose: 662 cases with evaluation

of oral acetylcysteine treatment. *Arch Intern Med* 1981;141:380–385.

57. Rybolt TR, Burrell DE, Shults JM, Kelley AK. *In vitro* coadsorption of acetaminophen and *N*-acetyl-cysteine onto activated carbon powder. *J Pharm Sci* 1986;75:904–906.

58. Seeff LB, Cuccherini BA, Zimmerman HJ, et al. Acetaminophen hepatotoxicity in alcoholics. *Ann Intern Med* 1986;104:399.

59. Smolinske SC, Hall AH, Vandenberg SA, et al. Toxic effects of nonsteroidal anti-inflammatory drugs in overdose. *Drug Safety* 1990;5:252–274.

60. Snodgrass WR. Salicylate toxicity. *Pediatr Clin North Am* 1986;33:381–391.

61. Snodgrass W, Rumack BH, Peterson RG, Holbrook ML. Salicylate toxicity following therapeutic doses in young children. *Clin Toxicol* 1981;18:247–259.

62. Temple AR. Acute and chronic effects of aspirin toxicity and their treatment. *Arch Intern Med* 1981;141:364–369.

63. Thurston JH, Pollock PG, Warren SK, et al. Reduced brain glucose with normal plasma glucose in salicylate poisoning. *J Clin Invest* 1970;49:2139–2145.

64. Vale JA, Meredith TJ. Acute poisoning due to nonsteroidal anti-inflammatory drugs: clinical features and management. *Med Toxicol* 1986;1:12–31.

65. Wootton FT, Lee WM. Acetaminophen hepatotoxicity in the alcoholic. *South Med J* 1990;83:1047–1049.

66. Wortzman D, Grunfield A. Delayed absorption following enteric-coated aspirin overdose. *Ann Emerg Med* 1987;16:434–436.

13 ‖ Opioids

When considering overdoses of opioids (narcotics), heroin (diacetylmorphine) is probably the first drug that comes to mind, and we picture users as long-term habitual drug abusers of low socioeconomic status. This association is actually unjustified, since victims of opioid overdose may be any age and represent all social and economic levels, and the drug may be obtained by illicit means or legally obtained by prescription (18).

It does appear that, even though the number of opioid abusers (estimated at 500,000 Americans) is high, the overall frequency of emergency department visits involving these agents has reached a plateau (26). Newer semisynthetic and synthetic opioids have gained popularity as drugs of abuse. For example, the surge of *T's and blues* abuse that began in the late 1970s involves the combination of pentazocine (Talwin) and tripelennamine (Pyribenzamine). Another example of *street* pharmacology is the use of a combination of glutethimide (Doriden) and codeine, known as *Loads* or *Sets*. By combining opioids and other centrally acting drugs, victims suffering from acute toxicity experience a greater array of effects. Additionally, propoxyphene, diphenoxylate, codeine, and methadone continue to be encountered in acute intoxication, both from accidental ingestion of drugs used legitimately, as well as from illicit use. An overdose involving any one of these *soft* drugs can be just as life-threatening as an overdose of morphine or heroin, and victims must receive the same treatment measures to assure their recovery.

Many attempts have been made to develop an analgesic that is as potent and effective as morphine, but lacks significant respiratory depression action and is less likely to produce physical dependence. It was first anticipated that drugs such as methadone, pentazocine, propoxyphene, and meperidine, would not cause as much dependency as morphine. Unfortunately, these synthetic analgesics contributed to the significant problem of chemical dependence and are implicated in many acute drug intoxications. Also, there is always the danger of accidental ingestion of toxic doses of these compounds. This is especially true for the children of parents who are participating in a methadone maintenance program (2).

Another menace to street use of pharmaceuticals is the increase in fraudulent prescriptions and increase in thefts and burglaries of pharmacies and physicians' offices. Increased use of these drugs seems to be related to the supply and potency of heroin. In 1978, the purity of heroin on the street plunged to a concentration reported as low as 2%. Although this is not the all-time low reported for street heroin potency, there was definitely a concurrent increase in the use of other substances, such as pentazocine, hydromorphone, and meperidine.

The differences between naturally occurring opioid alkaloids and semisynthetic and synthetic opioids are minimal when dealing with an acute toxic episode. Differences are related primarily to individual pharmacokinetic properties of the drugs. There are very few differences in characteristic signs and symptoms of acute overdose within this class of drugs. However, there are significant differences among the various opioids. Concerning treatment, naloxone (Narcan) is a pure antagonist that can reverse the effects of all opioid intoxications. The variability of effectiveness of this antagonist is a function of the pharmacokinetic properties of the toxic substance.

The naturally occurring and semisynthetic opioid alkaloids are derivatives of phenanthrene. Structural differences are noted in Table 13.1. The natural opium alkaloids have been used for centuries. The familiar dried exudate of the unripened seed pod of the Asian poppy plant, *Papaver somniferum*, contains at least 25 different alkaloids. The phenanthrene derivatives, morphine and codeine, are the two major naturally occurring opioids.

Acetylation of morphine at the C-3 and C-6 positions produces one of the most potent semisynthetic opioid alkaloids, heroin. Other semisynthetic derivatives of morphine include the morphons, e.g., hydromorphone (Dilaudid); oxymorphone (Numorphan); codons, e.g., hydrocodone (Hycodan); and oxycodone (Percodan), formed by oxidation of the alco-

TABLE 13.1. *Naturally occurring and semisynthetic opiate alkaloids and antagonists*

Phenanthrene nucleus

	R_1	R_2	R_3	7,8
Morphine	—OH	—OH	—H	Present
Methylmorphine (Codeine)	—O—CH$_3$	—OH	—H	Absent
Hydrocodone (dihydrocodeinone)	—O—CH$_3$	=O	—H	Absent
Oxycodone	—O—CH$_3$	=O	—OH	Absent
Oxymorphone	—OH	=O	—OH	Absent
Hydromorphone	—OH	=O	—H	Absent
Diacetylmorphine (heroin)	—O—C(=O)—CH$_3$	—O—C(=O)—CH$_3$	—H	Present
Naloxone[a]	—OH	=O	—OH	Absent

[a] C$_{17}$—CH$_2$—CH$_2$=CH$_2$.

holic hydroxyl at the C-3 position to a keto group and saturation of the double bonds between C-7 and C-8 (8,9). It is interesting to note that substituting an allyl group at the C-17 position produces *N*-allyl-normorphine, an antagonist to morphine and other opioids.

MECHANISMS OF TOXICITY AND CHARACTERISTICS OF ACUTE OPIOID POISONING

Although this chapter includes various groups of drugs, all opioid derivatives have the potential to produce severe toxicity that is dependent on the dose and route of administration. The mechanisms by which they produce their toxic effects are similar. To understand them, their pharmacologic effects will be reviewed briefly.

It has been postulated that toxic effects are related to different actions of these drugs at various opiate receptors in the CNS (33). A listing of some opioids and their associated receptor sites is shown in Table 13.2. Clinical responses of analgesia, euphoria, respiratory depression, and miosis are believed to result from occupation of the μ-receptors. A dif-

ferent type of analgesia results when the κ-receptors are involved, and the psychogenic effects, such as dysphoria, delusions, and hallucinations, result from opioid action at the σ-receptors (11,28,29).

Acute opioid toxicity may result from a variety of situations. These include intentional, accidental, or therapeutic overdose of prescribed medications. Whatever the reason, the toxicologic effects are basically the same. However, trying to generalize the outcomes from acute opioid overdose is difficult since there is significant individual variability to these drugs and rapid production of tolerance. The most common characteristics of acute opioid toxicity are listed in Table 13.3.

Signs and symptoms associated with acute opioid overdose usually begin within 20 to 30 min after oral ingestion and within minutes after parenteral administration. The most significant effects involve opioid action on the CNS. Nausea and vomiting are also among the first symptoms noted. Vomiting results from stimulation of the chemoreceptor trigger zone (CTZ) and is less likely to occur if the victim is kept in the recumbent position.

The most obvious and severe toxic effect

TABLE 13.2. *Opioid receptors for possible toxic action*

Receptor	Opioid	Clinical effect
mu	Morphine-like analgesics	Analgesia Euphoria Respiratory depression Miosis
kappa	Pentazocine Nalorphine Cyclazocine (morphine-like analgesics may have some kappa activity) Levallorphan	Analgesia Sedation Miosis
sigma	Pentazocine Cyclazocine Nalorphine	Dysphoria Delusions Hallucinations

of opioid poisoning is central depression. The victim is usually asleep or in a stuporous condition. The extent of CNS depression and its duration will vary according to the opioid involved, the quantity, and route of administration. For a large overdose, the victim rapidly lapses into coma and is not arousable by verbal or painful stimuli.

It is believed that when these drugs bind to specific opiate receptors there is an alteration in the release of central neurotransmitters from afferent nerves, which are sensitive to noxious stimuli. The highest concentration of receptors appears to be in the limbic system (38). This interaction with opioids on the limbic system produces euphoria, tranquility, and other mood alterations. The site of sedative/hypnotic action is the sensory area of the cerebral cortex.

In acute overdose, respiration will be severely depressed to a rate as low as 2 to 4 per min. Cyanosis becomes apparent and many

victims have a frothy pulmonary edema. In humans, death from an acute opioid overdose is almost always from respiratory arrest. When there is high concentration of drug in the medulla and brainstem, there is decreased sensitivity of the brainstem respiratory centers to increases in carbon dioxide, and, in the medulla, there is depression of the rhythm of respiration (9,44).

Respiratory depression with acute overdose is further complicated by bradycardia and hypotension. There are two possible explanations for the decrease in heart rate. One theory suggests that opioids stimulate the vagal centers. The other suggests that there is selective depression of the supramedullary centers which can lead to suppression of autonomic reflexes. During acute poisoning, blood pressure is normally not greatly affected. Hypotension usually occurs in the later stages of poisoning and results from hypoxia (9).

Pinpoint pupils (miosis) are usually considered to be the classical sign of narcotic poisoning. Tolerance to miosis does not occur. In some overdoses, however, the pupils may not be constricted, due to asphyxial changes resulting from decreased pulmonary oxygen exchange. Therefore, the pupils relax and dilate. When mydriasis occurs, the victim's prognosis is grave.

The body temperature usually decreases and the skin feels cold and clammy. This is due to suppression of the hypothalamic heat-regulating mechanisms. Skeletal muscles also

TABLE 13.3. *Characteristics
of opioid toxicity*

CNS[a] depression—coma
Respiratory depression
Pulmonary edema
Hypothermia
Miosis
Bradycardia
Hypotension
Decreased urinary output
Decreased gastrointestinal motility

[a] CNS, central nervous system.

become flaccid and sometimes the jaw relaxes. The tongue may even fall back to block the airway. There is decreased urinary output, which can be related to release of antidiuretic hormone (ADH).

Gastric motility and tone of both small and large intestines may be decreased, resulting in severe constipation. In the case of massive overdose, convulsions may occur due to stimulation of the cortex.

Death, even in an addict, is almost always due to respiratory failure, complicated by such factors as pneumonia, shock, and pulmonary edema. The usual triad of coma, pinpoint pupils, and depressed respiration strongly suggests an opioid overdose, but accurate diagnosis also depends on the individual's history and evidence of prior drug misuse.

MANAGEMENT OF TOXICITY

Opioid ingestions frequently delay gastric emptying. Thus, in acute overdose, as long as the patient is alert, emesis should be performed. If the patient is obtunded, gastric lavage is indicated.

Since victims of opioid overdoses are often comatose with depressed respiration, the major treatment objective is to support and maintain vital functions. Therefore, the first step is to provide adequate respiratory assistance and cardiovascular support.

Opioid overdoses are treated readily with an ideal direct antagonist. The use of an antagonist brings about dramatic improvement in respiration within minutes. Overall, the antagonist will reverse CNS depressant, analgesic, convulsant, psychotogenic, and dysphoric actions of opioids (35,43).

Levallorphan is an opioid antagonist, but it has partial agonist action. Major disadvantages to its use are with semicomatose or comatose individuals, in whom CNS depression is not due to an opioid, or in whom depression is partially due to some other CNS depressant, such as alcohol or barbiturates. In these cases, the partial agonistic activity may produce additive depressant effects. Mixed poisonings

are common. For this reason, a pure antagonist is preferred.

Naloxone was the first pure opioid antagonist, and it is considered the drug of choice for treatment of opioid intoxications. Dramatic improvement in respiration is seen within minutes after it is administered. Its purity as an antagonist, though, has been challenged. Limited data indicate that it may also possess some degree of agonist activity (12).

The recommended initial dose of naloxone is 0.4 mg for adults and 0.01 mg/kg for children. Several doses may be given at 2- to 3-min intervals. If CNS depression is due to an opioid, coma and respiratory depression will be resolved with 1 to 2 min. If it is not due to an opioid, naloxone will not worsen the existing condition. Since it has a short half-life of 60 to 90 min, and usually causes no ill effects in a patient without an opiate overdose, a 2-mg bolus may be given and, if necessary, repeated within 5 min. Twenty to 24 mg may be required for severe opioid intoxication.

Table 13.4 lists half-lives of representative opioids. It should be noted that for substances with long half-lives, larger doses of naloxone are frequently required. For example, acute oral ingestions of a toxic dose of a long-acting opioid, such as methadone or propoxyphene, will be managed better by continuous infusion of naloxone rather than by bolus administration (35). The reason for continuous infusion is based on the fact that respiratory depression may recur because of naloxone's short half-life.

Comatose patients must be aroused as quickly as possible. If hypoxia persists and adequate tissue oxygenation is not achieved quickly, capillary damage followed by shock is likely to ensue.

Patients with pulmonary edema are at special risk. Diuretics, digitalis, steroids, and antihistamines have all been recommended as supportive therapy. However, all have doubtful efficacy.

Respiratory depression lasts much longer than the antagonistic effects of naloxone. The patient must, therefore, be closely monitored for at least the next 24 to 48 hr. If depressed

TABLE 13.4. *Comparison of opioids*

Narcotic	Equianalgesic dose (mg)	Plasma half-life (hr)	Blood concentrations Therapeutic (μg/dL)	Toxic (μg/dL)	Lethal
Morphine	10	2.5–3	1–7	10–100	>400 μg/dL
Codeine	120	3–4	1–12	20–50	>60 μg/dL
Heroin	3–4	2.5–3	—	10–100	>400 μg/dL
Methadone	8–10	15 single dose 22–25 maintenance	30–100	200	>400 μg/dL
Propoxyphene	240	about 12	5–20	30–60	80–200 μg/dL
Meperidine	80–100	3–4	30–100	500	1–3 mg/dL
Pentazocine	30–50	2–3	10–60	200–500	1–2 mg/dL
Hydromorphone	1.5	2–4	0.1–3	10–200	>300 μg/dL
Oxycodone	15	—	1–10	20–500	—

respiration reappears, additional naloxone is necessary. Naloxone should ideally be used only to return respiration to normal. Other symptoms can usually be managed by other means. A victim of overdose who is breathing normally does not need naloxone.

NATURALLY OCCURRING OPIOIDS

Codeine

Codeine, or methylmorphine (see Table 13.1), possesses analgesic and antitussive properties. It is less potent than morphine, i.e., 120 mg of codeine produces the same degree of analgesia as 10 mg of morphine. Also, tolerance does not develop as rapidly with codeine compared to morphine.

Toxicity and death due to codeine alone are infrequently encountered. The lethal dose is between 500 mg and 1 g. Acute toxic ingestions of codeine produce the typical triad of symptoms seen with morphine: coma, miosis, and respiratory depression.

Codeine is usually taken in combination with other drugs, including analgesics, antihistamines, expectorants, or sedatives. When ingested concurrently with other agents, the toxic dose is lower (25). Besides the legitimate pharmaceutical preparations available, users of illicit preparations have also found that the combination of codeine with glutethimide taken orally may produce euphoria comparable to heroin, lasting about 6 to 8 hr.

SYNTHETIC OPIOIDS

Diphenoxylate

Diphenoxylate is a meperidine congener used in combination with atropine in an antidiarrheal preparation (Lomotil). The therapeutic dose is 20 mg daily (adults), and 3 to 10 mg daily (children). Despite the fact that diphenoxylate is not indicated for children under age 2, accidental and therapeutic intoxications are a problem (36). Unfortunately, most people do not view diphenoxylate products as extremely toxic, so they leave them carelessly unattended on bedroom tables or elsewhere where children have easy access to them.

There is an extremely narrow dose range between therapeutic and toxic blood concentrations (Therapeutic Index; See chapter 1) in children. Although part of the toxicity problem with diphenoxylate products in children is due to the opioid component, a large portion is due to the anticholinergic activity of atropine. This is discussed in further detail in chapter 15.

Acute intoxications, especially in children, are characterized primarily by anticholinergic effects. These may consist of hyperpyrexia, flushing of the skin, lethargy, hallucinations, urinary retention, and tachycardia. This phase is followed by miosis, respiratory depression, and coma due to the opioid activity. Symptoms are highly variable and dose dependent. The quantity of atropine contained in each Lomotil dose is subtherapeutic, although it will cause anticholinergic side effects, and these are magnified when taken in overdose.

Fentanyl (Sublimaze)

This is a synthetic opioid agonist that was initially introduced for short-term use as an anesthetic in 1968. As a prototype for this category of opioids, other fentanyl derivatives have been synthesized for medicinal uses; all have a much greater analgesic action than morphine. In 1980, a variety of fentanyl derivatives appeared on the street under the name *China White*. One derivative, 3-methylfentanyl, has been responsible for more than 100 overdose deaths in California alone since 1979, and in one county in Pennsylvania more recently (14,15).

Several fentanyl derivatives have surfaced on the illicit market as *designer drugs*. The term applies to synthetically modified controlled substances, such as fentanyl, meperidine, or amphetamine, using commonly available industrial chemicals in the manufacturing process to avoid the Federal Controlled Substances Act. Therefore, these drugs were temporarily *legal* (6). Alpha-methylfentanyl is 200 times as potent as morphine, and the minimum lethal dose is about 125 μg. 3-Methylfentanyl is 7,000 times as potent as morphine, and the minimum lethal dose is reported at 5 μg.

As with other opioids, the most significant acute toxic effect of fentanyl derivatives is respiratory depression, which is dose-dependent and may last up to 30 min. The hemodynamic effects include bradycardia and hypotension. The remaining characteristics of toxicity include chest wall rigidity, nausea, vomiting, hypothermia, and seizures.

Meperidine

Meperidine hydrochloride (Demerol) is a pure opioid agonist that was described initially in 1939 as an anticholinergic drug. It was the first synthetic opioid to be marketed. Today, it is one of the most commonly used opioid analgesics. Its structure is dissimilar to morphine, but similar to fentanyl (Table 13.5). Like other opioids, meperidine exerts pharmacodynamic actions by binding to opioid receptors, particularly the κ-receptor. A 75 to 100 mg dose of meperidine, given parenterally, will produce an equianalgesic response to 10 mg morphine. Since meperidine undergoes first-pass metabolism, oral administration produces less than one-half the total analgesic response compared to parenteral administration. When meperidine is prescribed for postoperative or chronic pain, it is often necessary to increase the dose to maintain the therapeutic response. However, a potential problem may result from cumulative doses of meperidine, which is related to its pharmacokinetic properties and described below.

Meperidine is metabolized in the liver by two pathways (31). The first involves hydrolysis by carboxyesterase to meperidinic acid. The other involves N-demethylation by microsomal enzymes to normeperidine, an active metabolite. Elimination half-lives for meperidine and normeperidine are 3 to 6 hr and 24 to 48 hr, respectively (40). Since normeperidine has a longer $t_{1/2}$, repeated administration of meperidine will result in elevated normeperidine/meperidine ratios.

Normeperidine has been shown to have one-half the analgesic activity, but two times the convulsant activity of meperidine (30). When meperidine is administered orally, the normeperidine/meperidine ratio is higher, compared to parenteral administration. This is related to the high first-pass effect, also (39). Normeperidine concentration also accumulates with impaired renal function and in cancer patients. Neurotoxicity of normeperidine is manifest by signs of CNS stimulation, including tremors, twitching, multifocal myoclonus and seizures. These signs can be correlated directly to normeperidine concentrations, and generally appear after several days of meperidine use (1,13,19). Unfortunately, normeperidine toxicity is often unrecognized, but should be considered in patients receiving large doses of meperidine.

TABLE 13.5. *Synthetic opiates: phenylpiperidine type*

	R_1		R_2	

	R_1	R_2 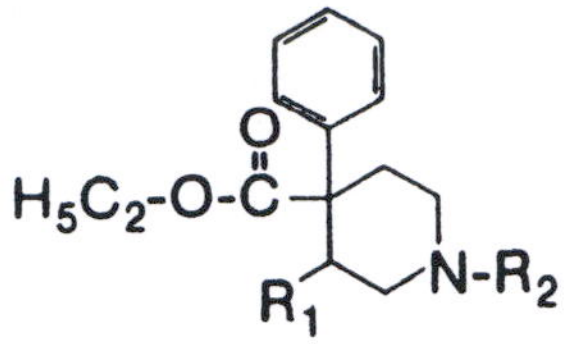
Meperidine	—H	—CH$_3$
Alphaprodine	—CH$_3$	—CH$_3$
Diphenoxylate	—H	—CH$_2$—CH$_2$—C—C≡N 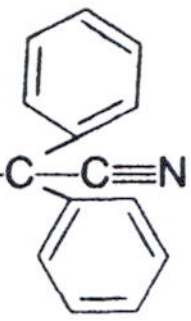
Fentanyl	—H	—CH$_2$—CH$_2$—C$_6$H$_5$

Treatment of normeperidine toxicity consists of discontinuing use of meperidine and giving a benzodiazepine derivative to reduce CNS excitation. Naloxone should be given carefully, if at all, because it may increase the incidence of seizures (19). Normeperidine toxicity may be prevented by avoiding prolonged administration of meperidine, especially in patients with impaired renal function (1).

A meperidine analog, 1-methyl-4-phenyl-1,2,5,6-tetrahydropyridine (MPTP) has appeared on the street among intravenous drug abusers. It was sold as a new synthetic heroin. Use of MPTP has been associated with a severe form of parkinsonism (33,41). It has been shown to cause selective destruction of the substantia nigra (7,23). All patients responded to therapy with a combination of L-dopa and carbidopa (Sinamet).

Pentazocine

Pentazocine (Fig. 13.1), a benzomorphan derivative that is 3 to 4 times less potent than morphine as an analgesic, was expected to possess little or no abuse potential when initially studied and marketed. Today, there is little question of its abuse potential. Reports of addiction and abuse among narcotic addicts began to appear shortly after it was introduced

into therapy (16). Its illicit use has continued to increase over the years (22).

The manufacturer of Talwin tablets introduced a new form of this oral medication early in 1983. Called Talwin-NX, pentazocine is combined with naloxone, an antagonist. The objective is to inhibit the action of pentazocine if the tablets are dissolved and injected. Naloxone is not normally absorbed from the GI tract, and when taken orally, exerts no antagonistic pharmacologic activity. However, when injected parenterally, it can cause withdrawal symptoms in opioid abusers. A parenteral dose of 30 to 45 mg provides the same analgesic action as 10 mg of morphine or 75 to 100 mg meperidine. Onset of clinical effects is 15 to 20 min after intramuscular or subcutaneous injection, but only 2 to 3 min after an intravenous injection.

Pentazocine exerts its major actions on the CNS and smooth muscles. CNS effects include analgesia, sedation, and respiratory depression at doses of 20 to 30 mg. Parenteral doses of 60 to 90 mg may produce psychiatric

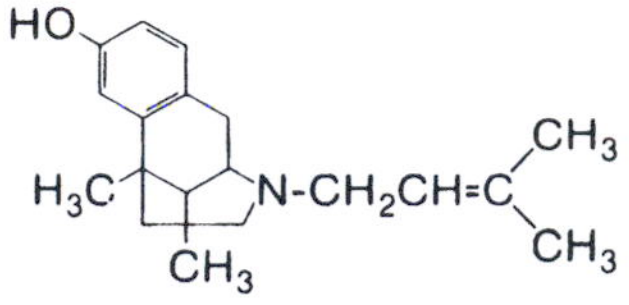

FIG. 13.1. Pentazocine structural formula.

disturbances, including dysphoria, depression, confusion, and hallucinations (20). The cardiovascular responses to pentazocine differ from other opioids in that high doses cause increased blood pressure and heart rate, flushing, chills, and sweating. These effects may occur because pentazocine increases blood concentrations of epinephrine and norepinephrine (42). Both tolerance and physical dependence have been reported with frequent and repeated use of pentazocine (17).

Chronic parenteral use of pentazocine may result in skin ulcerations, which appear as deep indurations distinguishable from dermal lesions commonly seen resulting from other abused drugs. Severe cellulitis, ulcerations, abscesses, and muscle necrosis are commonly found among users of T's and blues (8,37).

The antihistamine tripelennamine has a long history of use among street addicts. It was, therefore, not unexpected to see it combined with paregoric, heroin, or morphine in mixtures known on the street as *blue velvet* (34).

Tablets are dissolved in water, strained through cotton, and injected intravenously. There is an immediate *rush* (similar to that of heroin) that lasts about 5 to 10 min and is followed by dysphoria, which often results in the person injecting a second dose. After three or four injections, the rush may be followed by a feeling of well-being lasting about 4 to 6 hr (8,37).

One difficult-to-explain phenomenon is the pleasant experience some people report from combining tripelennamine with pentazocine-naloxone combination tablets (21,34). The naloxone would, theoretically, prevent these effects. It is possible that reports of pleasurable responses fail to include psychologic factors (21).

Propoxyphene

Propoxyphene (dextropropoxyphene) is a synthetic analog of methadone (Fig. 13.2) and, if taken in overdose, causes all the classic signs of opioid poisoning (24). Both the

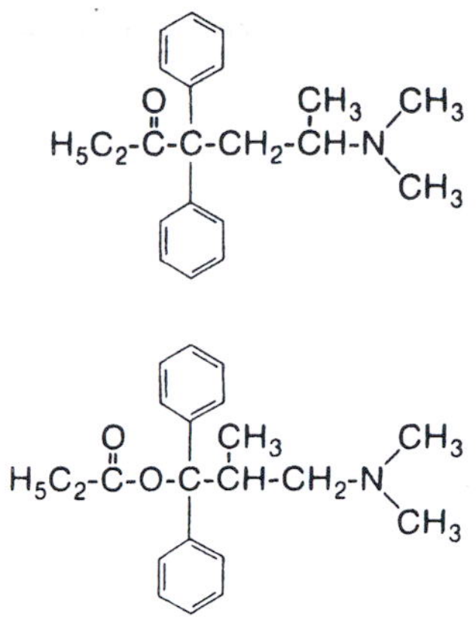

FIG. 13.2. Methadone (**top**) and propoxyphene (**bottom**) structural formulas.

hydrochloride and napsylate salts cause similar toxic problems. As with diphenoxylate-containing products, most people do not consider the toxic potential of propoxyphene to be great. Too frequently, large quantities are being used for trivial pain without advising the recipient of the potential for toxicity.

The majority of its victims are adults, and it is a means of committing suicide. Toxic doses for adults are stated to be 800 mg of the hydrochloride salt and 1,200 mg of the napsylate salt. Cardiac and respiratory arrest have been reported with doses of 35 mg/kg (3,10).

One special concern is ingestion of a product that also contains acetaminophen (24). Clinical symptoms caused by propoxyphene overdose may completely overshadow those of a toxic acetaminophen ingestion, leading to the sequel of events discussed in chapter 12. The problem is magnified when the victim has previously taken ethanol, a barbiturate, or other CNS depressants, as is frequently the case (24). These agents stimulate the hepatic mixed-function oxidase enzymes responsible for converting acetaminophen to its toxic intermediate metabolite. They also potentiate the CNS sedative action of propoxyphene. The influence that ethanol exerts on propoxyphene toxicity, as shown by blood concentrations of propoxyphene at the time of death, is illustrated in Table 13.6. In this study, fatalities

TABLE 13.6. *Blood concentrations of propoxyphene at the time of death with and without concurrent ethanol ingestion[a]*

Group	No.	Mean (mg/dL)	SD[b]
With ethanol	13	0.48	0.36
Without ethanol	22	0.72	0.39

From ref. 45.
[a] Blood concentrations represent total of drug plus its major metabolite, norpropoxyphene.
[b] SD, standard deviation.

associated with ethanol consumption occurred at significantly lower blood levels of propoxyphene than when alcohol was not present.

SUMMARY

Opiate use is centuries old. A significant number of Americans today use these substances for legitimate purposes. Because of this popularity, poisoning occurs at a high rate. Symptoms are characteristic and death is common in persons who have taken large doses. Important symptoms of poisoning can and often do appear because the victim has ingested a normal dose of opioid and has also taken another drug or chemical that potentiates the opioid effect.

A specific antagonist, naloxone, is available to treat opiates and opioids. No similar antagonist exists for symptomatic treatment of nonnarcotic depressants.

Case Studies

CASE STUDIES: OPIOID OVERDOSES

History: Case 1

A 19-year-old woman with a history of psychiatric illness, weighing 70 kg, ingested 200 tablets of Codenal (British dosage form), which contained a total dose of 2.3 g codeine base and 1.7 g phenobarbital. She arrived at an emergency facility in deep coma with miotic pupils and shallow respirations.

The patient was given two intravenous injections of naloxone, 0.4 mg each dose, after which there was significant improvement in her respiratory status and slight dilation of the pupils. The gastric contents were found to contain large amounts of codeine. There was no quantitative codeine analysis reported for blood or urine.

The patient was further treated with a continuous drip of nalorphine, 0.7 μg/kg/min, but after 36 hr there was no improvement in neurologic status. Naloxone was not available in the hospital in sufficient quantity, which accounted for the change in medication. A 6-hr hemodialysis was unsuccessfully tried.

The nalorphine drip was discontinued 5 days later and the patient's respiratory condition remained satisfactory. There were signs of brainstem damage. The patient died suddenly during a convulsive crisis 10 days after admission. (See ref. 5.)

History: Case 2

A 2-year-old girl was found playing with her father's briefcase at about 4:00 p.m. He usually kept a container of Lomotil tablets in the case for his spastic colitis. At this point there were no indications that the child had tampered with her father's medication or that she had ingested any.

The child went to bed for the evening at 7:00 p.m., and at that time appeared to be *dopey*. She awoke at 11:30 p.m., staggered into the living room with her arms and hands in a stiffened position, and collapsed. She turned blue, and it appeared she had stopped breathing.

She arrived at an emergency facility cyanotic with shallow, irregular respirations. Her temperature was normal, pupils constricted, reflexes brisk, and she displayed catatonic-like behavior.

Since there was the possibility that she had ingested Lomotil, she was given 1 mg nalorphine, after which she began to respond with normal respirations and disappearance of cyanosis. She later relapsed back into a comatose state and developed cyanosis. She was then given oxygen, and three additional 1-mg doses of nalorphine every half-hour. Again, she became conscious. A chest X-ray film showed a mild infiltrate in the right lower lobe, and she developed a fever of 102°F. She was placed on antibiotic therapy. The patient was discharged the second hospital day.

It was later determined that the girl ingested about 25 Lomotil tablets. Lomotil contains 2.5 mg diphenoxylate hydrochloride and 0.025 mg atropine sulfate per tablet. (See ref. 36.)

TABLE 13.7. *Laboratory findings*

Measurement	On admission	2 hr later
pCO_2	37 mm Hg	33 mm Hg
pO_2	72 mm Hg	40 mm Hg
O_2 saturation	92%	70%
pH	7.31	7.29

problems (her father was a known addict serving a jail term because of assault on her mother; the mother was also serving a jail term because of contempt of court), she was not discharged until 15 days after admission. As a side issue, the child was readmitted 2 weeks later for lead poisoning. (See ref. 2.)

History: Case 3

A 2-year-old girl ingested 20 mg methadone hydrochloride that she had found in her babysitter's purse. She was brought to the emergency department 3 hr after ingestion.

Physical examination revealed irregular respirations, 12/min; heart rate, 100 beats/min; and systolic pressure, 100 mm Hg. She was comatose; her pupils were constricted. Laboratory findings are given in Table 13.7.

Treatment consisted of intravenous nalorphine hydrochloride and gastric lavage. Over an 8-hr period, the patient was given the antagonist 7 times after bouts of CNS and respiratory depression. Each time nalorphine was given, there was prompt improvement in her respiration rate.

Eight hours after admission to the hospital, the child had spontaneous respirations. However, she then experienced respiratory problems and her breathing rate fell to 10/min. Again, she was given nalorphine and placed on a respirator. She was responsive within 10 min and her breathing rate increased to 18/min.

Bilateral infiltrates were noted on a chest X-ray film. A tracheal aspirate sample was cultured and grew a coagulase-positive *Staphylococcus aureus*. Antibiotic therapy was initiated.

The patient was alert and respirations were stabilized by the third day. Because of legal

History: Case 4

A 21-year-old woman who had a history of heroin abuse and was a participant in a methadone maintenance program was comatose when admitted to an emergency facility. On admission she was covered with vomitus. Needle marks were present on both arms, and her pupils were miotic, but responsive to light. Respirations were shallow, blood pressure was 86/30 mm Hg; and pulse, 144 beats/min. A chest X-ray film revealed pulmonary edema.

Laboratory results are given in Table 13.8.

Treatment consisted of oxygen, fluid replacement, insulin, and two ampules of naloxone hydrochloride (total of 0.8 mg) intravenously. The patient was alert almost immediately after injection of the antidote, but over the next 3 hr it was necessary to administer three additional bolus injections to maintain her responsiveness.

Later, she was given naloxone as an intrave-

TABLE 13.8. *Laboratory findings*

Na^+	=130 mEq/L
K^+	=5.1 mEq/L
Cl^-	=97 mEq/L
CO_2 combining power	=20 mEq/L
Glucose	=409 mg/dL
pCO_2	=49 mm Hg
pO_2	=47 mm Hg
O_2 saturation	=75%
pH	=7.24

nous infusion, 2.5 μg/kg/hr. It was necessary to continue this infusion for 30 hr. There was great improvement by the fifth hospital day at which time she was discharged. (See ref. 4.)

Discussion

1. In all four cases, does the necessity for repeated or continuous doses of the antagonist (Naloxone) correlate with the type of opioid involved?
2. What signs of opioid intoxication were evident in all the case studies? Give a pharmacologic reason for each of these signs.
3. In case 2, what was the approximate quantity of drug ingested? What effect would atropine have on the GI tract? How does this affect the opioid-poisoned patient?
4. In case 4, why was it necessary to administer naloxone by continuous intravenous infusion? Besides methadone, what other types of opioid overdose might require treatment in this manner?
5. Patient 1 ingested a large amount of codeine. Is it likely that her respiratory depression was due more to the phenobarbital than to the codeine she ingested? Why or why not?

CASE STUDIES: ABUSE OF PENTAZOCINE-NALOXONE AND TRIPELENNAMINE COMBINATION

History: Case 1

A 27-year-old man had a history of substance abuse since he was 12 years old. At that time he started using alcohol. For the most recent several years he also used marijuana, cocaine, heroin, and methylphenidate sporadically. Both biologic parents were alcoholics; his step-father was dependent on alcohol and heroin, and an uncle was dependent on alcohol and cocaine.

The subject was introduced to T's and blues (pentazocine-naloxone and tripelennamine) by a friend. He injected the combination and reported a rush followed by an alternating

speed and nod phenomenon that persisted for several hours. At one point he injected the pentazocine-naloxone combination without the tripelennamine, but he could not get the desired effect until the antihistamine was added. He continued to use these over the next several months.

He became worried about his use of drugs. When he tried to decrease his use, he experienced nausea, headaches, muscle aches, rhinorrhea, and diarrhea. He entered into a chemical-dependence program. While in the hospital, he showed no signs or symptoms of withdrawal. He was not given any drugs, and experienced no further problems. (See ref. 34)

History: Case 2

This 19-year-old man had a history of hyperactivity as a child. He began using alcohol at age 16, and marijuana a year later. Between ages 17 and 19 he abused codeine, heroin, diazepam, and methaqualone sporadically. Both parents and two brothers had a strong history of alcohol and substance abuse.

The subject was introduced to T's and blues. He used these drugs at the rate of 4 to 5 times a month for approximately two years. He noted a warm feeling after intravenous injection that lasted 5 to 10 min, and was followed by a calm and serene feeling for the next 3 to 4 hr. He indicated that the sensation was similar to that of heroin, but less intense.

He eventually became concerned about his use of drugs and stopped taking them. None of the symptoms of opioid withdrawal occurred. (See ref. 34.)

Discussion

1. Neither of the subjects experienced symptoms of opioid withdrawal after cessation of drug administration. Postulate the reasons for this.
2. Both subjects had a history of alcohol and substance abuse, as did other members of their families. What effect did these histor-

ies have on the responses the subjects reported to T's and blues administration?

3. Do you think the combination of pentazocine with naloxone would be more or less toxic than pentazocine alone, if taken in massive overdose? Give the reasons for your answer.

CASE STUDIES: PROPOXYPHENE POISONING ALONE AND COMBINED WITH ACETAMINOPHEN

History: Case 1

A 19-month-old girl ingested an unknown quantity of 65-mg propoxyphene capsules. She was brought to a local hospital 40 min later. On arrival the child was lethargic, rigid, and staring; her pupils were miotic. She experienced a generalized seizure and was given 2.5 mg diazepam, intramuscularly. She then experienced respiratory arrest, which required intubation. When she was given 0.2 mg naloxone, she awoke from the coma.

She was transferred to a larger medical center; at this time propoxyphene was detected in her urine, but not blood. From time to time there were signs of increasing CNS depression, but this was easily overcome by giving another intramuscular dose of naloxone (0.2 mg). Within 10 min of each dose, she showed clinical improvement in vital signs, and her pupils returned to normal. She completely recovered 12 hr after ingestion. (See ref. 27.)

History: Case 2

A 48-kg, 28-year-old woman, currently on a methadone maintenance program (80 mg methadone/day), stated that she had ingested about 90 tablets, each containing 100 mg propoxyphene napsylate and 650 mg acetaminophen. The patient went to bed but awoke after 10 hr and vomited five times. Nine hours later she was unresponsive, and was brought to a local emergency department.

On admission, she was comatose but could move her extremities in response to painful stimuli. Blood pressure was 100/70 mm Hg; pulse, 60/min; and rectal temperature, 88°F. Pupil size was 8 mm, and she was responsive to light. Coarse rhonchi were detected in both lungs. Laboratory evaluation of the urine revealed the presence of the following drugs: propoxyphene, methadone, phenobarbital, secobarbital, pentobarbital, methaqualone, and salicylic acid.

A bolus (2.8 mg) of naloxone was given without response. The stomach was lavaged with activated charcoal followed by magnesium citrate solution. Acetylcysteine was initiated 24 hr after drug ingestion and repeated five additional times.

Hemodialysis was initiated at 36 hr and continued for 4 hr. After this period, the patient awoke, appeared oriented, and was able to follow instructions. She was discharged 2 weeks after admission with no apparent residual hepatic or CNS involvement.

The admitting physician stated that the patient most likely absorbed the entire contents of the ingestion because she did not vomit for 10 hr after ingestion. Also, blood acetaminophen and propoxyphene concentrations were consistent with the massive ingestion reported by the patient. (See ref. 32.)

Discussion

1. When respiratory depression is complicated by seizures (i.e., as the victim in case 1 experienced), what is the additional problem encountered? Why was diazepam, rather than a barbiturate, given to control seizures?
2. Patient 2 survived in spite of all the reasons she should have succumbed. Comment on these factors (that is, the dose, presence of barbiturates, 24-hr lapse before N-acetylcysteine was given, lack of response to initial naloxone dose, etc.).
3. In patient 2 identify the clinical manifestations that were caused by acetaminophen and propoxyphene?

Review Questions

1. All of the following symptoms are characteristic of a heroin overdose *except*:
   A. Ataxia
   B. Hypertension
   C. Euphoria
   D. Miosis

2. Which of the following is true concerning opioid receptor sites?
   I. Respiratory depression results from stimulation of the κ-receptor.
   II. Hallucinations result from stimulant action of the μ-receptor.
   III. Dysphoria is an outcome of opioid action at the σ-receptor.
   A. II only
   B. III only
   C. I and II only
   D. II and III only
   E. I, II, and III

3. The reported toxic dose of propoxyphene hydrochloride is 500 mg.
   A. True
   B. False

4. Which of the following is a true statement?
   A. Deaths due to codeine toxicity are a common occurrence.
   B. The synthetic opioid derivatives are, as a general rule, less toxic than natural opiates.
   C. Propoxyphene is most closely related chemically and toxicologically to pentazocine.
   D. Pentazocine produces a lower incidence of perceptual disturbance than other opioids.

5. The most significant toxic effect from an opioid overdose is related to its action on the CNS.
   A. True
   B. False

6. Which of the following is a symptom of morphine overdose: respiratory depression (I), pinpoint pupils (II), or diarrhea (III)?
   A. II only
   B. III only
   C. I and II only
   D. II and III only
   E. I, II and III

7. Excessive administration of morphine has which of the following effects upon acid-base balance?
   A. Respiratory acidosis
   B. Respiratory alkalosis
   C. Metabolic acidosis
   D. Metabolic alkalosis

8. When treating a patient with heroin overdosage with the usual modalities, one should also be alert for development of:
   A. Acute renal failure
   B. Acute hepatic necrosis
   C. Acute myocardial infarction
   D. Acute pulmonary edema
   E. Acute cerebrovascular accidents

9. Which of the following represents the "triad" of opiate toxicity?
   A. Hypertension, tachycardia, dyspnea
   B. Diarrhea, sweating, tachycardia
   C. Flatus, halitosis, bromidrosis
   D. Coma, miosis, respiratory depression
   E. Constipation, mydriasis, coma

10. Which of the following should be used to monitor the pharmacologic response to naloxone?
    A. Pupil size
    B. Respiratory rate
    C. Urinary output
    D. Blood glucose levels
    E. Blood pressure

11. Why is naloxone sometimes given as an intravenous bolus and other times as an infusion? List each of the major opioids and indicate the appropriate method of antidote administration in case of overdose.

12. Emesis may or may not be indicated as a means to induce gastric evacuation in opioid intoxications. What is the major criterion used to determine when emesis is appropriate?

13. Ideally, when naloxone is used to treat opioid poisoning, it is intended to bring about a single physiologic response. What is that response?

14. A victim of opioid toxicity is reported to have dilated pupils. What is the origin of this response, and what is the person's probable prognosis?

15. Signs and symptoms of acute opioid overdose vary significantly depending on the specific agent responsible for the effect.
    A. True
    B. False

16. Several drugs available previously were advocated as opioid antagonists. Discuss the reasons why only naloxone has persisted and is still used.

17. A victim of severe opioid toxicity may receive diuretics and steroids as part of the treatment process. Cite the reasons why each would be given.

18. Discuss why toxic ingestions of propoxyphene-acetaminophen combination products present a greater health hazard than ingestion of toxic doses of either drug alone.

19. Pentazocine for oral administration is marketed with naloxone combined into the tablet formulation. Discuss why a manufacturer would market such a combination product.

20. An acute toxic ingestion of Lomotil causes symptoms of poisoning that are not generally seen with most other opioid drugs. What are the reasons for these symptoms?

References

1. Armstrong PJ, Bersten A. Normeperidine toxicity. *Anesth Analg* 1986;65:536–538.
2. Aronow R, Paul SD, Woolley PV. Childhood poisoning—an unfortunate consequence of methadone availability. *JAMA* 1972;219:321–324.
3. Bogartz LJ, Miller WC. Pulmonary edema associated with propoxyphene intoxication. *JAMA* 1971;215:259.
4. Bradberry JC, Roebel MA. Continuous infusion of naloxone in the treatment of narcotic overdose. *Drug Intell Clin Pharm* 1981;15:945–950.
5. Cardan E. Fatal case of codeine poisoning. *Lancet* 1981;2:1313.
6. Chesker G. Designer drugs, the "whats" and the "whys." *Med J Aust* 1991;153:157–161.
7. Chiba K, Trevor A, Castagnoli N. Metabolism of the neurotoxic tertiary amine, MPTP, by brain mono-

amine oxidase. *Biochem Biophys Res Commun* 1984;120:574–578.
8. DeBard ML, Jagger JA. "T's and B's"—Midwestern heroin substitute. *Clin Toxicol* 1981;18:1117–1123.
9. Eckenhoff JE, Dech SV. The effects of narcotics and antagonists upon respiration and circulation in man: a review. *Clin Pharmacol Ther* 1960;1:483–524.
10. Gary N, Maher JF, DeMyttevaere A, et al. Acute propoxyphene hydrochloride intoxication. *Arch Intern Med* 1968;121:453.
11. Gilbert PE, Martin LR. The effects of morphine and nalorphine-like drugs in the nondependent, morphine-dependent and cyclazocine-dependent chronic spinal dog. *J Pharmacol Exp Ther* 1976;196:66–82.
12. Gillman MA, Lichtigfeld FJ. The paradox of naloxone. *Br J Anaesth* 1986;58:572–577.
13. Goetting MG, Thirman MJ. Neurotoxicity of meperidine. *Ann Emerg Med* 1985;14:1007–1009.
14. Henderson GL. Designer drugs: past history and future prospects. *J Forensic Sci* 1988;43:569–575.
15. Hibbs T, Perper J, Winek CL. An outbreak of designer drug-related deaths in Pennsylvania. *JAMA* 1991;265:1011–1013.
16. Inciardi JA, Chambers CD. Patterns of pentazocine abuse and addiction. *NY State J Med* 1971;71:1727–1733.
17. Jasinski DR, Martin WR, Hoeldtke RD. Effects of short- and long-term administration of pentazocine in man. *Clin Pharmacol Ther* 1970;11:385–403.
18. Joynt BP, Mikhael NZ. Sudden death of a heroin body packer. *J Anal Toxicol* 1985;9:238–240.
19. Kaiko RF, Foley KM, Grabinski PY, et al. Central nervous system excitatory effects of meperidine in cancer patients. *Ann Neurol* 1983;13:180–185.
20. Kand FJ, Pokorny A. Mental and emotional disturbances with pentazocine (Talwin) use. *South Med J* 1975;68:808–811.
21. Lahmeyer HW, Craig RJ. Pentazocine-naloxone: an "abuse proof" drug can be abused. *J Clin Psychopharmacol* 1986;6:389–390.
22. Lahmeyer HW, Steingold RG. Medical and psychiatric complications of pentazocine and tripelennamine abuse. *J Clin Psychiatry* 1980;41:275–278.
23. Langston JW, Ballard P, Tetrud JW, Irwin I. Chronic Parkinsonism in humans due to a product of meperidine-analog synthesis. *Science* 1983;219:979–980.
24. Lawson AAH, Northridge DB. Dextropropoxyphene overdose: epidemiology, clinical presentation and management. *Med Toxicol* 1987;2:430–444.
25. Leslie PJ, Dyson EH, Proudfoot AT. Opiate toxicity after self-poisoning with aspirin and codeine. *Br Med J* 1986;292:96.
26. Levine DG. Alcohol and drug abuse. In: Schwartz GR, Safar P, Stone JH, Storey PB, Wagner DK, eds. *Principles and practice of emergency medicine.* Vol 2. Philadelphia: WB Saunders; 1978:1257–1272.
27. Lovejoy FH, Mitchell AA, Goldman P. The management of propoxyphene poisoning. *J Pediatr* 1974;85:765–768.
28. Martin WR. Naloxone. *Ann Intern Med* 1976;85:765–768.
29. Martin WR, Jasinski DR, Mansky PA. Naltrexone, an antagonist for the treatment of heroin dependence. *Arch Gen Psychiatry* 1973;428:784–791.

30. Miller JW, Anderson HH. The effect of *N*-demethylation on certain pharmacologic actions of morphine, codeine, and meperidine in the mouse. *J Pharmacol Exp Ther* 1954;112:191–196.

31. Plotnikoff NP, Way EL, Elliot HW. Biotransformation products of meperidine excreted in the urine of man. *J Pharmacol Exp Ther* 1956;117:414–419.

32. Pond SM, Tong TG, Kaysen GA, et al. Massive intoxication with acetaminophen and propoxyphene: unexpected survival and unusual pharmacokinetics of acetaminophen. *J Toxicol Clin Toxicol* 1982;19:1–16.

33. Portaghese PS. Some principles in the design of more selective pharmacological agents: application to multiple opioid receptors. *Am J Pharm Educ* 1987;51:1–7.

34. Reed DA, Schnoll SH. Abuse of pentazocine-naloxone combination. *JAMA* 1986;256:2562–2564.

35. Romac DR. Safety of prolonged, high-dose infusion of naloxone hydrochloride for severe methadone overdose. *Clin Pharm* 1986;5:251–254.

36. Rumack BH, Temple AR. Lomotil poisoning. *Pediatrics* 1974;53:495–500.

37. Showalter CV. T's and blues: abuse of pentazocine and tripelennamine. *JAMA* 1980;244:1224–1225.

38. Simon EJ, Hiller JM. The opiate receptor. *Ann Rev Pharmacol Toxicol* 1978;18:372–394.

39. Stambaugh JE, Warner IW, Sanstead JK. The clinical pharmacology of meperidine—comparison of routes of administration. *J Clin Pharmacol* 1976;16:245–256.

40. Street-drug contaminant causing Parkinsonism. *MMWR Morb Mortal Wkly Rep* 1984;33:351.

41. Szeto HH, Inturrisi EE, Houde R, et al. Accumulation of normeperidine, an active metabolite of meperidine, in patients with renal failure or cancer. *Ann Intern Med* 1977;86:738–741.

42. Tammisto T, Jaatela A, Nikki P, Takki S. Effect of pentazocine and pethidine on plasma catecholamine levels. *Ann Clin Res* 1971;3:22–29.

43. Tenenbein M. Continuous naloxone infusion for opiate poisoning in infancy. *J Pediatr* 1984;105:645–648.

44. Weil JV. Diminished ventilatory response to hypoxia and hypercapnia after morphine in normal man. *N Engl J Med* 1975;292:1103–1106.

45. Whittington RM, Barclay AD. The epidemiology of dextropropoxyphene (Distalgesic) overdose fatalities in Birmingham and the West Midlands. *J Clin Hosp Pharm* 1981;6:251–257.

14 | Central Nervous System Depressants

Numerous drugs possess CNS-depressant activity. These include many sedative-hypnotic agents (Table 14.1). Dozens of other drugs that are used for various pharmacologic purposes produce sedation as an adverse effect. Also, many chemicals cause drowsiness and CNS depression as a major component of toxicity. Thus, there are many categories of CNS depressants.

This chapter will be limited to drugs used for sedative (antianxiety) and hypnotic (sleep-producing) effects. Alcohols and opioids have been discussed in other chapters as examples of agents that produce CNS depression. Antipsychotic drugs (e.g., phenothiazines) and antidepressants (e.g., tricyclics) will be covered in chapter 15.

Medical uses for sedative-hypnotic drugs have changed over the years. At one time, sedative drugs were the agents to treat a wide variety of neurologic and psychologic disorders ranging from minor anxiety and pain, to epilepsy, hypertension, and psychosis. Initially, opioids, bromides, and alcohol were used, but were later replaced by barbiturates, chloral hydrate, meprobamate, and similar compounds. More recently, benzodiazepine derivatives have dominated the market. A newer hypnotic, zolpidem, has been marketed recently as an agent that has even less potential to cause toxicity in overdose.

Many of the older drugs are of historical interest only. Use of meprobamate, methyprylon, and ethchlorvynol has declined over the past decade, but they are still causes of occasional toxic overdoses. Today, most sedative-hypnotic drug-related poisonings are due to barbiturates or benzodiazepines. Whereas poisoning with a barbiturate requires intensive care, benzodiazepine intoxications do not normally require aggressive treatment for survival.

It cannot be disputed that Americans love to sedate themselves! Sedative-hypnotic drugs account for hundreds of million prescriptions written annually in the United States. If we add to this the many million doses of illicit depressants and the tens of millions of alcoholic drinks that are consumed each year, the magnitude of the potential toxicity becomes clearer. Poisonings from CNS sedative-hypnotics occur too frequently, and are responsible for a large number of deaths annually.

There are pharmacologic differences among various classes of sedative-hypnotic drugs. However, management of acute toxicity is based on similar general principles.

TABLE 14.1. *Representative CNS[a] depressants*

Barbiturates
  Amobarbital
  Butabarbital
  Pentobarbital
  Phenobarbital
  Secobarbital
Nonbarbiturate sedative/hypnotics
  Bromides
  Chloral hydrate
  Ethchlorvynol
  Glutethimide
  Meprobamate
  Methaqualone
  Methyprylon
  Paraldehyde
Benzodiazepines
  Alprazolam
  Chlorazepam
  Chlordiazepoxide
  Chlorazepate
  Diazepam
  Flurazepam
  Halazepam
  Lorazepam
  Midazolam
  Oxazepam
  Prazepam
  Temazepam
  Triazolam

[a] CNS, central nervous system.

SEDATIVE-HYPNOTIC DRUGS

A *sedative* is defined as a compound that calms anxious and restless individuals. *Hypnotics* cause drowsiness and facilitate sleep, which is close to the normal pattern. An *anesthetic* produces deep sleep, unlike natural sleep. A person who is asleep after a dose of a hypnotic-sedative can be aroused, but it is not possible with anesthesia-induced sleep.

In a practical sense, the major difference among these three pharmacologic classes is the degree of CNS depression produced, which is related to dose. However, large doses of many antianxiety drugs can cause anesthesia, and smaller doses of a general anesthetic may produce mild sedation.

All of these agents produce similar effects on mood and consciousness. The toxicity profile for CNS depressants is variable and depends not only on dose and duration of action, but also the mental state of the individual and the physical setting involved with the poisoning.

Barbiturates

By the advent of the 20th century, bromides were the most popular and widely used drugs to treat anxiety and insomnia. With synthesis of barbituric acid, bromides were soon replaced with a new class of drugs, the barbiturates. These drugs were divided into three groups based on latency of onset and duration of action. *Short-acting* barbiturates have a duration of action of 4 to 6 hr, and include pentobarbital and secobarbital. *Intermediate-acting* barbiturates produce sedation persisting 8 to 10 hr, and include amobarbital and butabarbital. *Long-acting* barbiturates, such as phenobarbital and barbital, have a duration of action of 12 to 24 hr. Differences in potency of various barbiturates are minor.

This classification scheme is for convenience only. The short duration of action of certain barbiturates cannot be equated with decreased toxicity potential. In fact, just the opposite is true. Shorter-acting barbiturates are more lipid soluble. Hence, they reach higher CNS concentrations and cause greater depression than phenobarbital. Furthermore, toxic blood concentrations of phenobarbital are more readily decreased by hemodialysis and alkaline diuresis than similar blood concentrations of short-acting barbiturates.

Not long after these agents were introduced, their potential for abuse was realized and misuse became widespread. At the same time, there was an increase in acute poisonings with barbiturates. Today, barbiturate poisonings

are common in intentional (suicidal) poisonings, but less frequently encountered in accidental poisoning. Over 70% of suicides that occur annually are related to barbiturate overdose, either alone or with ethanol (9,21). Barbiturate overdose currently ranks as a leading cause of drug-related hospital admissions and death in the United States, as well as in many other countries around the world.

One of the reported contributing factors to barbiturate poisoning is *drug automatism*. To illustrate, assume that an individual consumes a prescribed dose of sedative and becomes drowsy. Later, not remembering that he has already taken a previous dose(s), he swallows another dose. This act may be repeated again and again until a potentially lethal quantity has been consumed. An interesting speculation is that the term *automatism* may be used conveniently to explain why a victim of barbiturate or other central sedative intoxication died, rather than admitting it was a suicide (22).

Mechanism of Barbiturate Toxicity

The most prominent toxic effect of barbiturate overdoses is classic, progressive CNS depression. Even when taken in large anesthetic doses, peripheral effects are minimal. If barbiturate-induced coma persists, toxic sequelae, including cardiovascular, pulmonary, and other organ system complications may result.

Barbiturates depress the polysynaptic neuronal pathways primarily, with monosynaptic pathways affected to lesser extent. This action is believed to be due to a direct gamma-aminobutyric acid (GABA)-like effect, or to stimulation of GABA release. GABA is an inhibitory neurotransmitter within the CNS. When released, central depression is noted. The effect of barbiturates on GABA appears similar to that of benzodiazepines, except that not all barbiturate actions can be explained by this action. Other mechanisms include an interaction with norepinephrine and acetylcholine. Evidence for the significance of these actions in poisoning by barbiturates is not as convincing as for interaction with GABA.

Respiratory depression is the major toxic event that follows barbiturate ingestion and usually causes early death. At a dose approximately three times greater than needed for hypnosis, the body's neurogenic driving force for breathing is eliminated (14). Hypoxic and chemoreceptor forces are also depressed. Therefore, the driving force is diverted to the carotid and aortic bodies. With increasing doses of barbiturates, the hypoxic driving force becomes even less responsive and the remaining driving forces eventually fail to operate. This, then, contributes to acid-base imbalances characteristic of barbiturate poisoning.

Hypothermia is another potentially serious problem that follows toxic ingestions of barbiturates. Lowered body temperature results from direct depressant action on the thermoregulatory center. It potentiates acidosis, hypoxia, and shock.

Sympathetic ganglia are depressed with larger doses. This may help explain why toxic barbiturate doses reduce the blood pressure. Normal doses do not cause significant cardiovascular effects, but only slight decreases in blood pressure and heart rate, as would be expected during sleep. High concentrations have direct myocardial suppressant actions, causing decreased force of contraction with reduced cardiac output (31). This, along with the effect on the sympathetic nervous system and developing anoxia from depressed respiration, helps explain the origin of shock that results from large doses.

Other significant clinical features of barbiturate toxicity include decreased gastrointestinal motility and tone, which may lead to increased drug absorption. Bullous lesions on the fingers, buttocks, and around the knees have been reported in about 6% of all patients with acute barbiturate poisonings and may be helpful in differential diagnosis of an unconscious patient. These lesions are not seen exclusively with barbiturates, however.

Recovery from barbiturate toxicity is usually complete after a prescribed treatment protocol. Complications, including hypostasis pneumonia, bronchopneumonia, lung abscesses, pulmonary and cerebral edema, circulatory collapse, irreversible renal shutdown, and neurologic lesions, may result (28). Such complications are the usual cause of delayed death.

Characteristics of Barbiturate Poisoning

Barbiturates can produce a wide range of CNS effects varying from sedation to hypnosis, to anesthesia, and eventually to complete paralysis of central voluntary and involuntary functions. Extent of paralysis is dependent primarily on dose. Consequently, severity of CNS depression after barbiturate overdose is also a function of dose.

Barbiturate poisoning can be expected to occur when 5 to 10 times the normal hypnotic dose is ingested. The normal hypnotic and, therefore, toxic doses for the classes of barbiturates varies because of differences in duration of action and lipid solubility. For example, short-acting barbiturates are highly lipid soluble and potentially more toxic than long-acting barbiturates, which are less lipid soluble. Lethal doses of short-acting barbiturates produce death in a short period of time. In suicides, victims are often found dead at the scene or they die shortly thereafter. In contrast, patients who overdose on long-acting barbiturates generally die later in the hospital. The normal hypnotic doses for barbiturates, pertinent pharmacokinetic parameters, and therapeutic, toxic, and lethal blood concentrations are given in Table 14.2. Tolerance to barbiturates or other depressants, if present, may modify the anticipated toxicity profile and should be taken into consideration.

Caution should be exercised when attempting to relate reported blood concentration data to degree of poisoning. It must be remembered that these are not absolute values. They represent a range of blood concentrations indicating therapeutic, toxic, or lethal levels. Severity of barbiturate intoxication is better determined by the victim's clinical manifestations. Barbiturate blood concentrations are usually used to confirm the initial

TABLE 14.2. *Barbiturate classification system*

Characteristics	Short-acting		Intermediate-acting		Long-acting	
	Pentobarbital	Secobarbital	Amobarbital	Butabarbital	Phenobarbital	Barbital
Trade name	Nembutal	Seconal	Amytal	Butisol	Luminal	Veronal
Duration of action (hr)	6–8	4–6	8–10	8–10	12–24	12–24
Plasma half-life (hr)	23–40	20–28	14–42	34–42	24–140	—
Detoxification	Hepatic	Hepatic	Hepatic/renal	—	Renal	Renal
Hypnotic dose (mg)	50–100	100–200	50–200	100–200	100–200	300–500
Therapeutic drug concentration (mg/dL)	0.01–0.10	0.01–0.10	0.10–0.50	0.10–0.50	1.5–3.9	1.0
Toxic drug concentration (mg/dL)	0.70–1.0	0.70–1.0	1.0–3.0	1.0–3.0	4.0–6.0	6.0–8.0
Lethal drug concentration (mg/dL)	1.0 and >	1.0 and >	3.0 and >	3.0 and >	8.0–15.0 and >	10.0 and >
pKa	7.85–8.03	7.90	7.75	7.7	7.24	7.8

diagnosis. If the clinical features indicate signs of severe CNS depression, but laboratory results still show low blood barbiturate concentrations, this may indicate that one or more additional CNS-depressant drugs are involved. The most likely offender is ethanol.

Drug concentrations can be used to identify the specific barbiturate involved, which aids in predicting the extent and duration of toxic effects. Progress of the poisoned patient can be monitored by determining drug concentrations. To illustrate, elimination kinetics for barbiturates after acute overdose or even chronic abuse is not the same as with therapeutic doses. Serial drug concentrations can be used to determine if elimination kinetics have changed.

Table 14.3 lists various states of consciousness and responses of the poisoned patient. Blood barbiturate concentrations generally parallel clinical manifestations. However, the same precautions must be exercised when interpreting the data.

Benzodiazepines

Because of inherent dangers common to therapeutic and toxic doses of barbiturates and older nonbarbiturate sedative-hypnotic compounds, drugs that are as pharmacologically effective as barbiturates, but possess a wider margin of safety, are constantly being devel-

oped. One of the outcomes of research is a class of drugs known as benzodiazepines.

Thousands of benzodiazepine derivatives have been synthesized and hundreds tested for CNS-depressant effects. Characteristics of those that are currently used are summarized in Table 14.4. They represent the single most widely used group of sedative drugs. Current research is directed toward further refinement of this class. It is doubtful that they will be replaced as a group for many years.

Benzodiazepines have a high therapeutic index (see chapter 1) and are the safest of all sedative-hypnotic drugs. In other words, the range between therapeutic dose and toxic or lethal dose is extremely wide. Increasing dosage, even to massive amounts, will not cause general anesthesia, as opposed to other sedative drugs (14). Consequently, their overall potential for toxicity is low, and patients with benzodiazepine overdose present with fewer problems.

Mechanism of Benzodiazepine Toxicity

Most toxic effects of benzodiazepines result from their sedative action on the CNS. At extremely high doses, neuromuscular blockade may occur. Also, after intravenous injection, peripheral vasodilation causes a fall in blood pressure, and shock may result.

Within the CNS, benzodiazepines are selec-

TABLE 14.3. *Clinical manifestations of acute barbiturate intoxication*

Stage of consciousness	Degree of intoxication	Short-acting barbiturate (blood concentration, μg/mL)
Alert	No signs of CNS depression	<6
Drowsy	All degrees of CNS depression between alert and stuporous	8
Stuporous	Markedly sedated but responsive to verbal or tactile stimuli	14
Coma 1 (stage 1)	Responsive to painful stimuli but not to verbal or tactile stimuli; no disturbance in respiration or blood pressure	18
Coma 2 (stage 2)	Unconscious, not responsive to painful stimuli; no disturbance in respiration or blood pressure	22
Coma 3 (stage 3)	Unresponsive or abnormally responsive to painful stimuli; slow, shallow, spontaneous respirations with low but adequate blood pressure	26
Coma 4 (stage 4)	Unresponsive or abnormally responsive to painful stimuli; apnea and inadequate respirations; inadequate blood pressure	34

From ref. 23.

tive for polysynaptic pathways. They inhibit presynaptic transmission by stimulating the inhibitory neurotransmitter, GABA. This action is believed to occur because the drugs antagonize a specific protein that normally inhibits binding of GABA to its receptor site. This effect is also generalized, occurring throughout the CNS. Although there is experimental evidence to suggest that benzodiazepines also stimulate or inhibit other central neurotransmitters, there are more supportive arguments for its effect on GABA.

TABLE 14.4. *Properties of representative benzodiazepine derivatives*

Drug	Oral dosage range	Peak oral plasma concentrations (hr)	Half-life (hr)	Major active metabolites (half-life in hr)	Elimination rate
Anxiolytics					
Diazepam (Valium)	6–40 mg/day	1–2	20–50	desmethyldiazepam (30–60)	slow
Chlordiazepoxide (Librium, Libritabs, various other)	15–100 mg/day	2–4	5–30	desmethylchlordiazepoxide, demoxepam, desmethyldiazepam	slow
Chlorazepate (Tranxene)	15–60 mg/day	—	30–60	desmethyldiazepam	slow
Prazepam (Centrax)	20–60 mg/day	6	78	3-hydroxyprazepam, desmethyldiazepam	slow
Halazepam (Paxipam)	60–160 mg/day	1–3	7	n-3-hydroxyhalazepam, desmethyldiazepam	slow
Oxazepam (Serax)	30–120 mg/day	1–2	5–10	None	rapid to intermediate
Lorazepam (Ativan)	2–6 mg/day	2	10–20	None	intermediate
Alprazolam (Xanax)	0.75–4 mg/day	0.7–1.6	12–19	α-hydroxyalprazolam	intermediate
Hypnotics					
Flurazepam (Dalmane)	15–60 mg	—	50–100	desalkylflurazepam (50–100)	slow
Temazepam (Restoril)	15–30 mg	2–3	9–12	None	intermediate
Triazolam (Halcion)	0.125–0.5 mg	0.5–1.5	2.3	α-hydroxytriazolam	rapid

TABLE 14.5. *Characteristics of benzodiazepine toxicity*

Mild	Moderate	Severe
Ataxia	Responds to verbal stimuli	Responds only to deep pain
Drowsiness	Coma stage 0–1	Respiratory depression (rare)
		Hypotension (rare)
		Coma stage 1–2

Respiration is not markedly affected, even with hypnotic doses of most benzodiazepines. Some derivatives may decrease alveolar ventilation (decreased Po_2, increased Pco_2) and induce CO_2 narcosis in persons with preexisting compromised respiratory functions (e.g., chronic obstructive pulmonary disease) (32). Benzodiazepines potentiate the respiratory depressant effect produced by other sedative drugs when taken concomitantly (2,14). Most deaths associated with benzodiazepine overdose after oral ingestion have actually occurred in persons who ingested ethanol or another CNS depressant concurrently. Intravenous dosing has greater associated risk of life-threatening hypotension and respiratory depression leading to death (3,10,30).

Characteristics of Benzodiazepine Poisoning

Signs and symptoms of benzodiazepine overdose are presented in Table 14.5. Effects on motor performance are more prominent than cognition. On occasion, severe paranoia, psychosis, hallucinations, and hypomanic behavior are noted (27).

Even in large doses, benzodiazepines cause little more than Stage 0 or Stage I coma (see chapter 3). The patient can still be aroused. When not arousable, or when cardiovascular and respiratory functions are severely depressed, other depressants may have been ingested (10,26). Serum benzodiazepine concentrations do not correlate well with toxic signs and symptoms. For diazepam, toxic blood concentrations are between 0.5 and 2.0 mg/dL.

Tolerance to benzodiazepines can occur after chronic ingestion. There may be cross-tolerance to barbiturates, methaqualone, and ethanol, also (14).

OTHER DEPRESSANTS

Another half-dozen or more CNS depressant drugs constitute the remaining ones that are still reported to be occasional causes of poisoning. Toxicity reports have declined in recent years.

Chloral Hydrate

Chloral hydrate, as well as chloral betaine and triclofos sodium, are potent CNS sedatives. Chloral hydrate is converted to its active metabolite, trichloroethanol. Chloral betaine and triclofos are converted to chloral hydrate and trichloroethanol, respectively. Chloral hydrate and metabolites of chloral betaine and triclofos are lipid soluble and readily enter the CNS. Poisoning resembles barbiturate intoxication. The LD_{50} for chloral hydrate in rats is 200 to 500 mg/kg. Significant toxicity occurs with doses >2 g. Lethal doses are between 5 and 10 g.

Chloral hydrate and ethanol in combination are referred to as the infamous *Mickey Finn*. Whether intense CNS depression that results is additive or synergistic to the depressants is not known. It has been suggested that each drug inhibits the metabolism of the other (14). If this is true, the overall effect may be more than additive. The corrosive action of chloral hydrate may cause gastritis, nausea, and vomiting. In addition, it has been shown to be nephrotoxic and hepatotoxic.

Glutethimide, Ethchlorvynol, and Methyprylon

Like other nonbarbiturate CNS depressants, glutethimide, ethchlorvynol, and methyprylon (the "GEM" sedatives) produce toxic symptoms similar to barbiturate poisoning. These depressants have unique characteristic features. For example, they produce significant fluctuations in the depth of coma, and the duration of coma is markedly prolonged. Severe hypotension, respiratory depression, bradycardia, hypothermia, and pulmonary edema occur to greater extent than typically noted with barbiturate poisoning. This probably occurs from direct action on the vasomotor center. Complications include hypovolemia, secondary to decreased peripheral resistance and persistent acidosis.

In addition, glutethimide has significant anticholinergic actions, resulting in mydriasis, blurred vision, dry mouth, constipation, and hyperthermia (after initial hypothermia).

The cyclic fluctuation in depth of coma and wakefulness after overdose with glutethimide may be due to recycling through the enterohepatic circulation (7), or formation and accumulation of an active metabolite, 4-hydroxy-2-ethyl-2-phenyl-glutaramide. This metabolite has a long half-life, and is at least two times more potent than the parent compound (13). Another factor unique to glutethimide is that its anticholinergic activity can reduce gastric motility significantly, permitting the already absorbed drug to be metabolized. After a time, bowel activity returns, more drug is absorbed, and the cycle continues.

Meprobamate

With introduction into medicine in the 1950s, meprobamate was an alternative to barbiturates for reducing anxiety. For nearly two decades, until the advent of benzodiazepines, meprobamate and its derivatives were the most commonly used nonbarbiturate antianxiety drugs.

Symptoms of meprobamate overdose are similar to those of barbiturates. Coma has been associated with blood concentrations between 10 and 20 mg/dL. The dosage range for severe toxicity is varied and probably due to individual differences in the rate of metabolism. Death results from irreversible shock, respiratory depression, and pulmonary edema. Twelve grams was fatal in one instance, whereas other patients have survived doses as high as 40 g (1,16,36). An interesting case study of meprobamate toxicity is presented at the end of this chapter.

Methaqualone

Methaqualone is a drug with abuse potential. Users of illicit methaqualone report that it increases interpersonal relations and has aphrodisiac activity.

Its precise mechanism of toxicity is unknown. Depressant action is believed to be similar to that of barbiturates. However, because methaqualone does produce sensual effects that differ from barbiturates, at least part of their activity differs. Mild toxic effects include hangover, headache, stupor, restlessness, dry mouth, and blurred vision. Severe overdoses, which are usually consistent with blood concentrations exceeding 3 mg/dL, generally produce coma accompanied by pyramidal signs, such as hypertonia, hyperreflexia, myoclonus, and convulsions. These effects are usually not observed in other sedative-hypnotic overdoses. Severe hypotension and pulmonary edema are usually absent with methaqualone intoxication, but hemorrhagic tendencies, due to inhibition of platelet aggregation and peripheral neuropathies, are frequently observed.

Antihistamines

With introduction of antihistamines in the late 1940s, it was realized quickly that these drugs produced a variety of effects centered around CNS depression. Sedation is the most common side effect of most antihistamines in

TABLE 14.6. *Characteristics of antihistamine toxicity*

CNS effects		Anticholinergic effects
Children	Adults	
Excitement	Disorientation	Dilated pupils
Tremors	Ataxia	Blurred vision
Hyperactivity	Dizziness	Tachycardia
Hallucinations	Sedation	Warm skin
Hyperreflexia	Coma	Dry mouth
Convulsions		Diminished bowel sounds
		Urinary retention

adults (Table 14.6). In overdose, CNS depression leading to coma may result. However, additional symptoms that resemble anticholinergic actions may also be present, and may be more significant than the degree of depression. These include mydriasis, flushing, fever, dry mouth, and blurred vision. Children usually experience central stimulation, hallucinations, tonic-clonic convulsions, and hyperpyrexia, rather than depression (15,33). Interesting case studies illustrating signs and symptoms of antihistamine overdose are presented at the end of chapter 15.

MANAGEMENT OF CNS-DEPRESSANT DRUG OVERDOSE

Management of any CNS-depressant drug overdose follows the same basic principles. Most clinical experience has accumulated with management of barbiturate intoxications. Therefore, management of barbiturate poisoning will serve as a model for the other CNS depressants discussed in this chapter.

Survival after CNS depressant overdose is very good. Fewer than 2% of victims succumb.

In the 1930s and 1940s, the primary treatment was directed toward heroic decontamination by gastric lavage followed by generous doses of activated charcoal. This practice was replaced in the late 1940s and early 1950s with a protocol that called for administration of large doses of CNS stimulants (analeptics). Morbidity and mortality rates with this treatment often ran into the 40% to 50% range. Analeptic drugs stimulated respiration sufficiently, but also increased the brain's demand for oxygen. Added to this was an increased chance for convulsions and cardiac arrhythmias. Today, analeptics are not part of the conventional treatment protocol.

Vasopressors were formerly given to elevate blood pressure. They can reduce blood volume significantly. If the patient is already hypotensive, the chance for survival is reduced. They are no longer recommended. Rather, cautious fluid replacement and inotropic agents, such as dopamine and dobutamine, are preferred.

In the 1960s the *Scandinavian Method* for treating barbiturate intoxication was developed because it was recognized that the two most significant pathophysiologic effects of CNS-depressant toxicity were hypoxia and shock. The protocol (Fig. 14.1) originated with Scandinavian physicians. It stressed support of physiologic functions, good nursing care, and no analeptic or vasopressor therapy. Basic elements of the approach are still retained.

Support vital functions
   Consciousness
   Airway
   Blood pressure

Prevent further absorption
   Emesis
   Lavage
   Activated charcoal and
     catharsis

Increase elimination of drug
   Forced diuresis
   Alkalinization of urine
   Dialysis, hemoperfusion

Conservative management with good
   nursing care
Symptomatic and continued
   supportive care

Evaluate for appropriate detoxification
or psychiatric aftercare

FIG. 14.1. Management of acute barbiturate poisoning.

The highest priority in treating any victim of depressant poisoning is to stabilize respiration and correct anoxia. If the brain suffers damage from insufficient oxygenation, other procedures will be of little benefit.

Oxygen should be given and the patient ventilated mechanically if needed. A cuffed endotracheal tube should be used in Stage 4 coma to decrease risk of aspiration pneumonia during lavage. To help prevent hypostatic pneumonia, the victim should be turned frequently. Prophylactic antibiotic treatment was thought to be beneficial. Now, it is considered unnecessary and can lead to superinfection.

Since circulatory collapse is a major threat after ingestion of massive doses of CNS depressants, cardiovascular function must be assessed quickly and deficiencies corrected. The treatment of choice in circulatory shock is volume expansion with a fluid challenge followed by appropriate pressor agents (e.g., dopamine).

Renal failure is the cause of one-sixth of all deaths (14). Therefore, kidney function must be monitored constantly. Signs of uremia may be an indication for hemoperfusion or hemodialysis.

Once supportive measures have been established, blood and urine samples should be obtained for toxicologic analysis. Results of analysis can aid diagnosis and evaluation of effectiveness of treatment.

Prevent Further Absorption of the Poison

If no contraindication exists, ipecac-induced emesis should be considered. In a comatose individual, gastric lavage is appropriate. Activated charcoal adsorbs barbiturates and most other common CNS-depressant drugs. A slurry can be instilled into the stomach through a nasogastric tube. Studies have shown repeated activated charcoal treatment significantly decreases their plasma half-life (34). In some cases, this procedure works as well as hemodialysis and hemoperfusion (4,5,24,29). A cathartic should be given to enhance elimination of the remaining drug.

Increase Excretion of Absorbed Drug

Increased excretion of the absorbed drug may be accomplished by repeated doses of activated charcoal, diuresis, dialysis, or hemoperfusion.

Barbiturates are weak acids, varying from pKa 7.2 for phenobarbital, to 8.1 for secobarbital. Thus, alkalinization will promote ionization of at least half the drug in the glomerular filtrate and cause it to be excreted more readily. Only long-acting barbiturates, which are eliminated primarily via the kidney, are readily eliminated by alkalinization. Urinary alkalinization is ineffective for short- and intermediate-acting barbiturates, or for any of the other CNS depressants presented in this chapter.

Neuvonen and Elonen (25) have shown that multiple doses of activated charcoal starting 10 hr after phenobarbital ingestion in healthy individuals significantly reduce blood concentrations. Whereas controls had a phenobarbital half-life of 110 hr, activated charcoal reduced this to 20 hr. Since phenobarbital undergoes enterohepatic circulation, it is possible that activated charcoal may interfere with barbiturate reabsorption. Others have shown similar results with nasogastric administration of activated charcoal (8).

Peritoneal dialysis increases elimination of some CNS depressants, but this procedure appears to be of low efficiency and is no longer recommended. Hemodialysis is variably effective in removing significant amounts of CNS depressants from blood in cases of toxic/lethal ingestions, or when the patient is in severe hemodynamic or renal compromise, and prolonged coma is likely. Hemoperfusion has been shown to effectively remove significant amounts of any of the CNS depressants discussed.

In some cases, greater efficacy may have been shown using charcoal hemoperfusion over resin hemoperfusion. Even though these extracorporeal measures reduce blood drug concentrations *in vitro*, their clinical significance may be questioned. Many of the drugs discussed in this chapter are either highly protein-bound or

TABLE 14.7. *Effectiveness of procedures to enhance drug elimination in CNS drug poisonings*

Drug	FD	PD	HD	CH	RH
Barbiturates					
Short-intermediate	Ineffective	—	+/−	++	+++
Long-acting	++	—	+	++	+++
Benzodiazepines	Not indicated	Not indicated	Not recommended	Not recommended	Not recommended
Chloral hydrate	Not recommended	Not recommended	+/−	++	++
Ethchlorvynol	Not recommended	Not recommended	+	++	+++
Glutethimide	Not recommended	Not recommended	+	+++	+++
Methyprylon	Ineffective	+/−	++	+++	?
Meprobamate	Not recommended	+/−	++	+++	+++
Methaqualone	Not recommended	Not recommended	+/−	+	+
Antihistamines	Ineffective	—	—	Not recommended	Not recommended

FD, forced diuresis; PD, peritoneal dialysis; HD, hemodialysis; CH, charcoal hemoperfusion; RH, resin hemoperfusion.
−, ineffective or no data; +/−, may be effective; +, effective; ++, good effectiveness; +++, excellent effectiveness.

have a large volume of distribution that limits the effectiveness of these procedures. Table 14.7 summarizes the effectiveness of various procedures used to increase the elimination of CNS depressant overdoses.

Benzodiazepine Antidote

Flumazenil (Mazicon), 1,4-imidazobenzodiazepine (Fig. 14.2), is an antagonist that can reduce or terminate the sedative, anxiolytic, anticonvulsant, ataxic, anesthetic, and muscle relaxant effects of benzodiazepines in a dose-dependent manner (6,18). Despite its short half-life, small doses (0.2 to 1.0 mg) of flumazenil are usually effective in reversing the sedative action of benzodiazepine poisonings.

Flumazenil is generally well tolerated. Adverse effects are usually mild, consisting mainly of nausea and vomiting. The appearance of a withdrawal syndrome is possible due to displacement of the agonist from the receptor site, but the incidence is low (19).

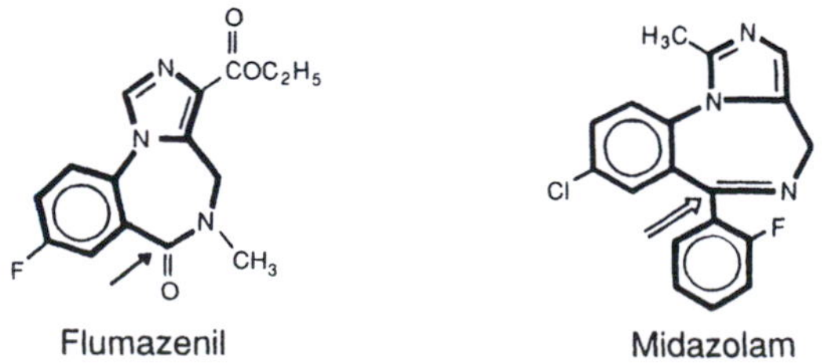

SUMMARY

Intoxication with CNS depressants causes a series of predictable effects highlighted by respiratory failure and cardiovascular collapse. Although certain depressant drugs may produce other characteristic symptoms, none take precedence over these two symptoms.

Treatment should be directed toward maintenance of vital functions, prevention of further absorption, and reduction of blood levels of absorbed drug. Good nursing care is an important component of therapy. There are no specific antidotes for most sedative-hypnotic drugs.

FIG. 14.2. Structural formulae showing flumazenil and midazolam.

Case Studies

CASE STUDIES: BARBITURATE OVERDOSE

History: Case 1

A 55-year-old woman was found in deep coma after ingesting an estimated 30 capsules of a sedative preparation, each containing 100 mg pentobarbital sodium and 260 mg carbromal. On admission to a hospital, blood pressure was 80/60 mm Hg; pulse, 80 beats/min; and respirations, 20/min and shallow. Pupils were dilated and fixed, no reflexes were present, and the patient was totally unresponsive to commands or stimuli. She was intubated and kept on a respirator. Large vesicles and bullae containing a clear fluid were present on the dorsal surface of her hands, around both knees, and on her heels.

Her initial serum barbiturate blood concentration was 4.3 mg/dL. Because her condition was deteriorating and respiratory acidosis appeared, hemodialysis was instituted. After two sessions of 8 to 9 hr each, she awoke on the third hospital day. At this point she was able to breathe without aid of a respirator. She made an uneventful recovery and was released about 2 weeks after admission.

At the time of this patient's discharge, the skin lesions were healed. Physicians who reported on this case observed that barbiturate was present in these blisters, and implied that the drug had irritated the skin's capillaries to cause vesicle formation. Similar blister formation has also been noted after poisoning with a variety of other sedative drugs and chemicals, including carbon monoxide. It thus appears that this is nonspecific and should not be used to differentiate one drug from another when attempting to define the nature of the poison. (See ref. 12.)

History: Case 2

A 22-year-old woman, with a history of generalized seizures and schizophrenia, ingested an undetermined quantity of phenobarbital. She had also been taking fluphenazine hydrochloride and benztropine mesylate for her medical conditions. She presented to the emergency department in coma, responding only to painful stimuli. Her vital signs included: blood pressure, 110/60 mm Hg; pulse, 102 beats/min; and rectal temperature, 37.3°C. Intravenous fluids were instituted. Respiration was supported artificially.

She was intubated with an endotracheal tube and lavaged. With the nasogastric tube in place, 40 g activated charcoal was administered followed by 20 g sodium sulfate. Activated charcoal (40 g) and magnesium citrate (60 mL) were administered every 4 hr for five additional doses.

Toxicologic analysis of blood for alcohol and other drugs was negative except for phenobarbital. The initial blood phenobarbital concentration of 141 μg/mL dropped to 47 μg/mL within 24 hr, during which time her clinical condition rapidly improved. (See ref. 8.)

Discussion

1. Mydriasis (dilated pupils) is a common sign of severe intoxication with sedative drugs. This was reported for patient 1. Why do you think mydriasis occurs? When present, what is the patient's probable prognosis?
2. The bullous skin lesions present in patient 1 contained barbiturate. Why is this not surprising?
3. Patient 2 received an initial dose of sodium sulfate, and magnesium citrate every 4 hr. What was the purpose of this treatment, and was it successful?

CASE STUDY: UNEXPECTED DEATH FROM MEPROBAMATE

History

A 51-year-old woman was found unconscious by her husband after she supposedly ingested 50 meprobamate tablets (400 mg each). She was a known alcoholic and had attempted suicide previously. She was also an asthmatic, and her medications included prednisone, bronchodilators, and multiple tranquilizers. When she arrived at the hospital she was unconscious, all reflexes were absent, and she responded only to deep pain. Her blood pressure was 110/60 mm Hg.

Gastric lavage was initiated immediately.

Three liters of fluid were necessary before the returned solution failed to show the presence of a white cloudy substance. Gastric lavage was repeated again on two separate occasions, and both procedures resulted in negligible return of ingested drug.

Further treatment was supportive. Ten hours after she was found unconscious, she was able to speak clearly, deep-tendon reflexes were normal, and blood pressure was 140/90 mm Hg.

Toxicologic analysis revealed an initial blood meprobamate concentration of 14.4 mg/dL. It was later learned that she had actually ingested 95 meprobamate tablets, or approximately 38 g.

She continued to show improvement throughout the second hospital day and at midnight was resting comfortably. Blood pressure was 140/80 mm Hg. However, at 1:30 a.m., she was found unconscious and cyanotic, with no pulse or respiration. Attempts to revive her were unsuccessful.

Postmortem findings initially provided no evidence or pathologic explanation for her death, or why she revealed a moderate degree of pulmonary edema and visceral congestion. Postmortem meprobamate concentrations included: blood, 18 mg/dL; brain, 14 mg/dL; kidney, 50 mg/dL; liver, 30 mg/dL; and total stomach contents, 25 g. It was then that a large white mass was found in her stomach. (See ref. 17.)

Discussion

1. This patient was doing fairly well until she was found unconscious and cyanotic in the hospital. How can you explain these events? Why did this patient die?
2. What was the white mass found in her stomach? Could you have predicted that this clumping of meprobamate would occur? (Hint: What did you learn in chapter 3 concerning concretions of ingested drugs?)

CASE STUDY: METHYPRYLON INTOXICATION

History

A 57-year-old woman was admitted to the hospital after she ingested 22.5 g of methyprylon, 2 to 12 hr previously. She was deeply comatose and not responding to painful stimuli. All reflexes were absent, except for a weak pupillary response to light. Vital signs included blood pressure, 60/32 mm Hg; and pulse 68 beats/min. Respirations were slow and shallow.

Treatment was instituted with gastric lavage, during which time systolic pressure dropped to 30 mm Hg and respirations ceased. She was intubated rapidly, and breathing maintained with a respirator. Blood pressure returned to normal with metaraminol bitartrate (Aramine).

To initiate forced diuresis, hypertonic mannitol and furosemide were given. Intravenous fluids consisting of 5% dextrose and 0.45% saline with potassium chloride were continued.

Four hours after admission, hemodialysis was instituted and, within 2 hr after dialysis, the patient's corneal and deep-tendon reflexes showed signs of responding. Dialysis was continued for another 6.5 hr when slight muscular twitching movement was noted. She was given phenytoin and diazepam to control these myoclonic movements. She also began to breathe and move spontaneously.

The initial methyprylon blood concentration was 20.9 mg/dL. Five hours later it had dropped to 9.2 mg/dL, and after dialysis, to 3.0 mg/dL. The quantity of drug recovered by gastric lavage was 4.3 g, or about 20% of the ingested dose. It was also estimated that the amount eliminated during the 8.5-hr dialysis period was 3.6 g, which accounted for another 20% of the ingested dose. Approximately 600 mg were excreted in the urine, which accounted for less than 5% of the ingested dose.

By 18 hr after admission, the patient was fully awake, aware of her environment, and attempting to talk. Over the next few days she was confused, but this gradually cleared, and she was discharged on the 12th hospital day. (See ref. 20.)

Discussion

1. This patient, recovering from poisoning induced by a CNS sedative, was given diazepam, another sedative. Comment on the use of such a therapeutic measure.

CASE STUDIES: MASSIVE DIAZEPAM OVERDOSE

History: Case 1

A 61-year-old woman was admitted to a hospital approximately 8 hr after ingestion of 450 to 500 mg diazepam. She was receiving chemotherapy for multiple myeloma and imipramine for depression. Her drug overdose was an attempted suicide. On admission, blood pressure was 110/80 mm Hg; heart rate, 75 to 80 beats/min; and respirations, 20/min. She was visibly depressed and responsive only to noxious stimuli. Laboratory test results were within normal limits.

The cause of intoxication was not initially apparent. Symptoms did not implicate imipramine as the source.

Treatment began with administration of naloxone hydrochloride (Narcan), 0.4 mg, and 50% dextrose. She showed no improvement. She was therefore placed under constant monitoring, and further treatment was nonspecific. Fluid administration continued. Other than an isolated incidence of mild hypotension (90/50 mm Hg) that soon resolved, there were no major changes in her clinical state.

She was fully alert and responsive 24 hr after admission and was discharged the following day with no apparent complications. (See ref. 11.)

History: Case 2

A 28-year-old man was brought to the hospital approximately 10 hr after ingesting 2,000 mg diazepam. Vital signs included: blood pressure, 100/60 mm Hg; heart rate, 68 beats/min; and respirations, 16/min. He was responsive to verbal stimuli, and oriented to time, place, and person.

All laboratory test results were within normal physiologic limits. Initial blood diazepam concentration was approximately 20 μg/mL, which is at least 40 times the minimal effective drug concentration. Blood diazepam concentrations remained elevated well above the normal therapeutic concentration for approximately 4 to 5 days.

The patient's initial treatment consisted of intravenously administered 50% dextrose and naloxone hydrochloride, 0.4 mg. His condition did not improve. He was then placed under observation and vital signs monitored. He was responsive and fully alert within 2 days after ingestion, at which time he was transferred to a psychiatric ward for further evaluation. (See ref. 11.)

Discussion

1. Does it seem strange that both patients survived these otherwise massive doses of drug? If you disagree, explain why. In neither case did spontaneous emesis occur, nor was it induced. Thus, both victims probably did absorb most of what they ingested.
2. Why was naloxone used in the initial treatment of both patients? Why was dextrose given?
3. Even though recovery was rapid for patient 2, diazepam blood concentrations remained elevated well above the therapeutic range for several days. Why was he fully recovered long before blood concentrations were in the therapeutic range (that is, what factor may account for this discrepancy)?

CASE STUDY: CLONAZEPAM POISONING

History

A 4-year-old boy was found by his mother on the living room floor. On the floor in an adjoining room were several opened and spilled bottles of his mother's anticonvulsant medication, clonazepam, a benzodiazepine. The mother last saw the boy about 5 hr earlier. At that time he was behaving normally. Now, the boy was not arousable.

He was transported to a hospital where he was awakened easily. He received syrup of ipecac, which produced a clear vomitus. Because it was assumed that (a) he did ingest a large quantity of clonazepam, and (b) the tablets had dissolved and he apparently absorbed the medication, he was taken to a larger medical center.

On admission, vitals included pulse, 80 beats/min; blood pressure, 80/56 mm Hg; respirations, 18/min; and temperature, 36°C. He responded to vocal commands, but made no spontaneous movements, and did not vocalize. Pupils were miotic, and equal. Deep tendon reflexes were brisk and symmetrical. Laboratory findings are shown in Table 14.8.

The boy was placed on a cardiac monitor in the ICU. A test dose of 0.4 mg naloxone produced no change in his condition. Gastric lavage brought up no tablet fragments. He was then given magnesium sulfate (5 g) and activated charcoal (5 g) via nasogastric tube. A charcoal stool was passed in 3 hr.

During the first 24 hr of hospitalization, seven distinct cycles ranging from alert agitation to unresponsive coma with miotic pupils were noted. Abdominal X-ray failed to disclose a concretion. By 5 hr postadmission, bowel sounds were markedly hypoactive. A second dose of magnesium sulfate returned bowel activity to normal.

By 24 hr postadmission (36 hr postingestion) the boy was alert, active, and behaving

TABLE 14.8. *Laboratory findings*

Na$^+$	=138 mEq/L
K$^+$	=4.8 mEq/L
Glucose	=125 mg/dL
BUN	=6 mg/dL
SGOT	=17 U/L

BUN, blood urea nitrogen; SGOT, serum glutamate oxaloacetate transaminase.

normally. He was kept for 7 days, at which time physical examination was normal.

A blood sample taken shortly after admission was sent out for analysis. It revealed a clonazepam blood concentration of 69 ng/mL. A typical oral therapeutic dose in an adult, measured 8 hr postingestion, would give a blood concentration of 4.2 to 9.6 ng/mL. (See ref. 35.)

Discussion

1. Explain the phenomenon of CNS cycling and explain how this shifting of neurologic response is illustrated in this case.
2. When the boy's pupils were described as miotic and equal, what does this mean as far as a diagnostic feature?
3. Why was naloxone administered? When the patient did not respond to naloxone, what conclusions could be made concerning the possible ingestion of benzodiazepine?
4. Why does clonazepam cause diminution of bowel sounds?

CASE STUDY: FLUMAZENIL FOR THE REVERSAL OF REFRACTORY BENZODIAZEPINE-INDUCED SHOCK

History

A 76-year-old woman arrived at an emergency facility complaining of weakness. She had a long history of progressive orthopnea, leg edema, and progressive cough. She had a long-term smoking habit, but denied any known, related medical problems.

The woman was alert. Respirations (labored) were 40/min; pulse was regular, 117 beats/min; blood pressure, 180/80 mm Hg. Pertinent physical findings included the presence of rales in the right lower half of her left chest. Mild to moderate pedal edema was observed. A chest X-ray film showed multiple masses in the right lung and large left pleural effusion.

Oral tracheal intubation was performed and

diazepam 10 mg given over 3 min when the patient developed respiratory failure. One minute later the patient became bradycardic (40 beats/min), hypotensive (systolic pressure 40 mm Hg), and she required ventilatory assistance. This deterioration was thought to be due to the benzodiazepine.

The patient received 1 mg atropine and a dopamine infusion of 20 μg/kg/min. These interventions increased her pulse to 50 beats/min and systolic blood pressure to only 60 mm Hg after 5 min.

She then received flumazenil 1 mg intravenously. Within 2 min, her pulse increased to 74 beats/min, systolic pressure improved to 100 mm Hg, and the benzodiazepine-induced CNS and respiratory depression were completely reversed. The dopamine infusion was rapidly discontinued with no change in the patient's condition.

The patient was admitted to the ICU and a diagnosis of adenocarcinoma of the lung was confirmed. Several days later she again developed agitation for which she received lorazepam 1 mg, intravenously. She again exhibited bradycardia and hypotension. She was unresponsive to standard therapy. The deterioration of her cardiovascular status was not treated and her vital signs returned to normal by 90 min. After a prolonged hospital course the patient succumbed to her cancer. (See ref. 6)

Discussion

1. Outline the mechanism of action of flumazenil in reversing diazepine-induced pharmacologic effects. The patient did not receive flumazenil after an adverse reaction to lorazepam. Would it have reversed this benzodiazepine's action had it been administered?

2. A 10 mg intravenous dose of diazepam is not normally toxic. Outline the factors that may have contributed to this patient's adverse response to diazepam.

Review Questions

1. Which of the following is a true statement?
   A. Most barbiturate poisonings occur by accidental ingestion.
   B. Barbiturates work by blocking GABA release within the brain.
   C. Hypothermia from low-dose barbiturate poisoning occurs by direct peripheral action on arterioles.
   D. Barbiturate intoxication occurs when 5 to 10 times the therapeutic dose is ingested.

2. Hemodialysis would have the greatest effect on reducing blood levels of which of the following?
   A. Secobarbital
   B. Pentobarbital
   C. Butabarbital
   D. Phenobarbital

3. Phenobarbital overdose is best treated by:
   A. Alkaline diuresis
   B. Acidic diuresis

4. Which of the following CNS depressants has the highest therapeutic index?
   A. Methaqualone
   B. Meprobamate
   C. Diazepam
   D. Glutethimide

5. A victim of barbiturate intoxication who is unconscious and not responsive to pain, but has no disturbance in respiration or blood pressure, is classified as Stage _____ coma?
   A. 1
   B. 2
   C. 3
   D. 4

6. All of the following statements are true about benzodiazepines *except*:
   A. They are the single most widely used group of CNS sedatives.
   B. Benzodiazepines selectively depress polysynaptic pathways within the CNS.
   C. Effects of benzodiazepine overdose

are more prominent on cognition than on motor function.

D. Cross-tolerance with ethanol and barbiturates may occur.

7. Someone poisoned with a *Mickey Finn* has ingested a combination of ethanol and:
   A. Meprobamate
   B. Phenobarbital
   C. Chloral hydrate
   D. Methaqualone

8. Which of the following depressants has significant anticholinergic activity that may require separate treatment when the drug is taken in toxic overdose?
   A. Meprobamate
   B. Methaqualone
   C. Glutethimide
   D. Pentobarbital

9. All of the following are true statements *except*:
   A. Prophylactic antibiotic therapy is part of the treatment for barbiturate poisoning.
   B. Repeated doses of activated charcoal after phenobarbital will help lower the blood barbiturate concentration.
   C. Hypothermia of 30°C may be treated by immersing the patient in water warmed to 40°C.
   D. Saline catharsis is beneficial in treating CNS depressant toxicity.

10. Which of the following treatments has no therapeutic benefit in management of barbiturate poisoning?
    A. Emesis/lavage
    B. Hemodialysis/hemoperfusion
    C. Analeptics
    D. Oxygen

11. In patients given sodium bicarbonate because of phenobarbital intoxication, urinary drug excretion is increased because the:
    A. Acid urine decreases the amount of ionized drug
    B. Acid urine increases the amount of ionized drug
    C. Alkaline urine increases the amount of ionized drug

D. Alkaline urine decreases the amount of ionized drug

12. Which of the following is most likely to produce central stimulation, hallucinations, tonic-clonic convulsions, and hyperpyrexia in children if present in toxic amounts?
    A. Meprobamate
    B. Midazolam
    C. Phenobarbital
    D. Diphenhydramine
    E. Chloral hydrate

13. All of the following are true of benzodiazepines *except*:
    A. Benzodiazepines antagonize the action of GABA.
    B. Benzodiazepines demonstrate cross-tolerance with alcohol and barbiturates.
    C. Therapeutic properties of benzodiazepines include anxiolytic, hypnotic, anticonvulsant, and anesthetic actions.
    D. Flumazenil (Mazicon) is a benzodiazepine antagonist used for benzodiazepine toxicity.
    E. Benzodiazepines can produce physical and psychologic dependence and have significant abuse potential.

14. Which of the following is *not* rational emergency toxicologic treatment in managing an overdose of phenobarbital?
    A. Alkalinizing the urine with $NaHCO_3$ to enhance renal elimination of phenobarbital
    B. Administration of analeptics to reverse the respiratory depression
    C. Activated charcoal via nasogastric tube
    D. Gastric lavage

15. Flumazenil is related chemically most closely to which group of CNS depressant drugs?

16. The short-acting barbiturates are said to be more potentially toxic than the long-acting ones. Cite the reasons why this is true.

17. Define the role of GABA in CNS-depressant intoxications. How is GABA classed physiologically and chemically?

18. Discuss the reliability in using blood levels of barbiturates as a predictor for determining severity of poisoning.
19. Identify the disadvantages of giving analeptic drugs to CNS-depressed-intoxicated patients.
20. Cite the advantages and disadvantages of using multiple doses of activated charcoal after a toxic barbiturate ingestion.

References

1. Allen MD, Greenblatt DJ, Noel BJ. Meprobamate overdosage: a continuing problem. *Clin Toxicol* 1977;11:501–515.
2. Ascione FJ. Benzodiazepines with alcohol. *Drug Ther* 1978;9:58–71.
3. Baker AB. Induction of anesthesia with diazepam. *Anesthesia* 1969;24:388–394.
4. Berg M, Berlinger W, Goldberg M, et al. Acceleration of the body clearance of phenobarbital by oral activated charcoal. *N Engl J Med* 1982;307:642–644.
5. Boldy DAR, Vale JA, Prescott LF. Treatment of phenobarbitone poisoning with repeated oral administration of activated charcoal. *Q J Med* 1986;235:997–1002.
6. Coates W, Evans TC, Jehle D, et al. Flumazenil for the reversal of refractory benzodiazepine-induced shock. *Clin Toxicol* 1991;29:537–542.
7. Decker WJ, Thompson HL, Arnesson LA. Glutethimide rebound. *Lancet* 1970;1:778–779.
8. Goldberg MJ, Berlinger WG. Treatment of phenobarbital overdose with activated charcoal. *JAMA* 1982;247:2400–2401.
9. Goldfrank L, Osborn H, Howland MA. Barbiturates. In: Goldfrank LS, ed. *Toxicologic emergencies.* New York: Appleton-Century-Crofts; 1986:391–397.
10. Greenblatt DJ, Allen MD, Noel BJ, Shader RI. Acute overdosages with benzodiazepine derivatives. *Clin Pharmacol Ther* 1977;21:497–514.
11. Greenblatt DJ, Woo E, Allen MD, et al. Rapid recovery from massive diazepam overdose. *JAMA* 1978;240:1872–1874.
12. Groschel D, Gerstein AR, Rosenbaum JM. Skin lesions as a diagnostic aid in barbiturate poisoning. *N Engl J Med* 1970;283:409–410.
13. Hansen AR, Kennedy KA, Ambre JJ, Fisher LJ. Glutethimide poisoning: a metabolite contributes to morbidity and mortality. *N Engl J Med* 1975;292:250–252.
14. Harvey SC. Hypnotics and sedatives. In: Gilman AG, Goodman LS, Rall TW, Murad F, eds. *The pharmacological basis of therapeutics.* 7th ed. New York: Macmillan; 1985:339–371.
15. Hays DP, Johnson BF, Perry R. Prolonged hallucinations following a modest overdose of tripelennamine. *Clin Toxicol* 1980;16:331–333.
16. Hilstand EC. Overdosage with meprobamate. *Ohio State Med J* 1956;52:1306–1307.
17. Jenis EH, Payne RJ, Goldbaum LR. Acute meprobamate poisoning: a fatal case following a lucid interval. *JAMA* 1969;207:361–362.
18. Karvokiros KA, Tsipis GB. Flumazenil: a benzodiazepine antagonist. *DICP—Ann Pharmacother* 1990;24:976–981.
19. Kulka PJ, Lauven PM. Benzodiazepine antagonists—an update of their role in emergency care of overdose patients. *Drug Safety* 1992;7:381–386.
20. Mandelbaum JM, Simon NM. Severe methyprylon intoxication treated by hemodialysis. *JAMA* 1971;216:139–140.
21. Matthew H. Barbiturates. *Clin Toxicol* 1975;8:495–513.
22. Matthew H, Lawson AH. *Treatment of common acute poisonings.* 4th ed. New York: Churchill Livingstone; 1979.
23. McCarron MM, Schulze BW, Walberg CB, et al. Short-acting barbiturate overdosage: correlation of intoxication score with serum barbiturate concentration. *JAMA* 1982;248:55–61.
24. Neuvonen PJ. Clinical pharmacokinetics of oral activated charcoal in acute intoxications. *Clin Pharmacokinet* 1982;7:465–489.
25. Neuvonen PJ, Elonen E. Effect of activated charcoal on absorption and elimination of phenobarbitone, carbamazepine and phenylbutazone in man. *Eur J Clin Pharmacol* 1980;17:51–57.
26. Palmer GC. Use, overuse, misuse, and abuse of benzodiazepines. *Ala J Med Sci* 1978;15:383–392.
27. Pfefferbaum B, Butler PM, Mullins D, Copeland DR. Two cases of benzodiazepine toxicity in children. *J Clin Psychiatry* 1987;48:450–451.
28. Plum F, Swanson AG. Barbiturate poisoning treated by physiological methods with observations on effects of betamethylethylglutarimide and electrical stimulation. *JAMA* 1957;163:827–835.
29. Pond S, Olson K, Osterloh J, Tong T. Randomized study of the treatment of phenobarbital overdose with repeated doses of activated charcoal. *JAMA* 1984;251:3104–3108.
30. Prensky AL, Raff MC, Moore MJ, Schwab RS. Intravenous diazepam in the treatment of prolonged seizure activity. *N Engl J Med* 1967;276:779–784.
31. Price HL. General anesthesia and circulatory homeostasis. *Physiol Rev* 1960;40:189–218.
32. Rao S, Sherbaniuk RW, Prasad K, et al. Cardiopulmonary effects of diazepam. *Clin Pharmacol Ther* 1973;14:182–189.
33. Schuller DE, Turkewitz D. Adverse effects of antihistamines. *Postgrad Med* 1986;79:75–86.
34. Veerman M, Espejo MG, Christopher MA, et al. Use of activated charcoal to reduce elevated serum phenobarbital concentration in a neonate. *Clin Toxicol* 1991;29:53–58.
35. Welch TR, Rumack BH, Hammond K. Clonazepam overdose resulting in cyclic coma. *Clin Toxicol* 1977;10:433–436.
36. Woodward MG. Attempted suicide with meprobamate. *Northwest Med* 1957;56:321–322.

15 | Anticholinergics, Phenothiazines, and Tricyclic Antidepressants

Numerous drugs and chemicals produce action on the autonomic nervous system as primary symptoms of toxicity. Some examples include plant toxicity (e.g., jimsonweed—anticholinergic effects; mushrooms—cholinergic stimulant or anticholinergic effects) and organophosphorus insecticides (cholinergic stimulation). Amphetamine-like drugs that stimulate the adrenergic system are discussed in chapter 16.

Stimulation or blockade of various neuronal pathways within the autonomic nervous system can bring about a variety of physiologic events. If sufficiently severe, many can be lethal.

ANTICHOLINERGICS

Anticholinergic (antimuscarinic, cholinergic-blocking) activity is one of the most common adverse actions associated with numerous drugs (Table 15.1). This adverse effect frequently overshadows many other pharmacologic actions, especially with the tricyclic antidepressants and many antipsychotics.

Anticholinergics competitively inhibit action of the neurotransmitter, acetylcholine, at central and peripheral receptor sites. Both muscarinic and nicotinic sites are vulnerable to blockade, depending on the dose of the compound and its chemical characteristics. Quaternary derivatives do not gain access to the CNS to the same extent as nonquaternary derivatives. Consequently, their action is directed more toward peripheral, rather than central, receptor sites. Thus, a variety of clinical problems may manifest depending on the particular agent.

Today, poisoning by drugs that are classed pharmacologically as anticholinergics per se is less common than it was in former years. Reports of toxicity to scopolamine, an anticholinergic that has potent CNS sedative activity, is reported to be on the increase, however (21). These cases frequently involve illegitimate use of the drug (8). Whether these reports are generalized, or represent illicit uses confined to isolated geographic areas, remains unknown at this time.

TABLE 15.1. *Representative substances that contain anticholinergic activity*

Antihistamines (H$_1$-antagonists)
  Brompheniramine
  Chlorpheniramine
  Cyclizine
  Dimenhydrinate
  Diphenhydramine
  Meclizine
  Orphenadrine
  Promethazine
  Pyrilamine
  Tripelennamine
Antiparkinsonian agents
  Benztropine
  Biperiden
  Ethopropazine
  Procyclidine
  Trihexyphenidyl
Antipsychotic agents
  Acetophenazine
  Chlorpromazine
  Chlorprothixene
  Perfenazine
  Promazine
  Triflupromazine
Tricyclic antidepressants
  Amitriptyline
  Desipramine
  Doxepin
  Imipramine
  Nortriptyline
  Protriptyline
  Trimipramine
Gastrointestinal anticholinergic/antispasmodic agents
  Anisotropine
  Atropine
  Belladonna tincture
  Glycopyrrolate
  Homatropine
  Hyoscyamine
  Methantheline
  Propantheline
  Scopolamine
Ophthalmic products
  Atropine
  Cyclopentolate
  Scopolamine
Plants
  See chapter 11

The reason for the decline in toxicity from legitimately used anticholinergics is that these drugs are not used as frequently in drug therapy. Until just a few years ago, the mainstay for treatment of peptic ulcer disease, hyperacidity conditions, and hyperspastic disorders was the belladonna alkaloids and related atropine-like drugs. These agents have been replaced with a different class of less toxic drugs, the histamine-2 (H_2)-antagonists (e.g., cimetidine, ranitidine), and other agents without appreciable anticholinergic effects. Atropine, hyoscyamine, and similar drugs were formerly included in numerous proprietary cold and asthma remedies, and antidiarrheals. Their use in medical management of these afflictions has been shown recently to be not only ineffective, but also potentially dangerous. Consequently, they are no longer used for these purposes. The former heyday of anticholinergic drug therapy has been modernized with newer, safer, and more effective medications.

Despite the decline in popularity of classic anticholinergics, poisoning from drugs that have a potent anticholinergic component continues to be reported. These drugs include antihistamines, phenothiazines, and the tricyclic antidepressants. Among these, the greatest potential for serious toxicity involves tricyclic antidepressant overdoses.

Infants and children are especially vulnerable to anticholinergic drug action (3,51). Toxicity has been reported after absorption of drugs from ophthalmic dosage forms.

TRICYCLIC ANTIDEPRESSANTS

Tricyclic antidepressants (Table 15.2) have been used in drug therapy since the late 1950s. Today, they represent the largest group of drug agents used for treatment of depression. They are referred to as *tricyclic* compounds because of their chemical structures, which contain three rings. A newer compound, maprotiline, is a *tetracyclic* (four rings) compound. It possesses the same degree of anticholinergic activity as imipramine, and a greater degree of CNS-sedative activity. For simplicity, all of the drugs, whether 3-ringed or 4, are referred to as tricyclics, tricyclic antidepressants, or TCAs.

Most reported toxicities occur with amitriptyline (20,38). In a review of 165 persons with tricyclic poisonings admitted to one hospital in a two-year period, 62% involved amitripty-

line, 15% doxepin, 10% imipramine, 8% desipramine, and the rest represented other tricyclic antidepressants. Toxicities result from both accidental and deliberate overdoses. Unlike poisoning with antipsychotic drugs, toxicity with tricyclics is potentially life-threatening. Furthermore, most poisonings involve multiple ingestions with at least one other drug (often ethanol), diazepam, propoxyphene, or codeine. Thus, there may be potentiated symptoms and additional problems encountered in treatment (20).

It should be remembered that many patients who take tricyclics and/or antipsychotic medications have a high risk for suicide (35). The margin of safety for antipsychotics is relatively high. For tricyclics, the margin is much less favorable. A rule of thumb is that the quantity of tricyclic antidepressants dispensed should be limited to a one-week supply (3). The same applies to using antipsychotic medications. In reality this rule is seldom followed.

Tricyclic antidepressant drug toxicity has increased to serious proportions in the United States, and around the world. It is reported that in some areas, tricyclics have surpassed CNS depressants as a major cause of poisoning (44). In one study, they were implicated in 10.8% and 6.7%, respectively, of acute poisonings in 1983 and 1984. They also were present in 29.5% and 21.4%, respectively, of poisoning-related deaths in the same years (24). Toxicity is compounded because of rapid absorption, tight binding to plasma proteins and tissues, enterohepatic recycling, and their low therapeutic margin. As with anticholinergic drugs per se, children are particularly sensitive to cardiovascular complications and seizure activities (3).

Large variations exist in adult toxic doses. Death has occurred (in adults) with 500 mg imipramine; others have survived doses exceeding 1,000 mg (22). It is probably of greater significance to consider the variable physiologic conditions of patients (Review the factors that influence toxicity, chapter 2). For example, a patient with preexisting heart disease will probably experience severe cardiac

TABLE 15.2. *Tricyclic antidepressant drugs*

Drug	Neurotransmitter uptake blocking activity		$t_{1/2}$	Time to reach steady state (days)
	Norepinephrine	Serotonin		
Secondary amines				
Amoxapine	+++	++	8	2–7
Nortriptyline	++	+++	18–28	4–19
Desipramine	++++	+++	14–62	2–11
Protriptyline	+++	—	55–124	10
Tertiary amines				
Amitriptyline	++	++++	31–46	4–10
Imipramine	++	++++	6–20	2–5
Doxepin	+	++	8–24	2–8
Trimipramine	+	+	7–30	2–6
Tetracyclic				
Maprotiline	++	+	21–25	6–10
Triazopyridine				
Trazodone	0	+++	4–9	3–7

0, none; +, slight; ++, moderate; +++, high; ++++, very high.

toxicity compared with someone who has normal cardiovascular function.

Mechanism of Tricyclic Antidepressant Toxicity and Characteristics of Poisoning

Tricyclics decrease the action of acetylcholine centrally and peripherally. The majority of toxic symptoms can be explained by this action. Chorea, for example, is believed to result from an imbalance in acetylcholine and dopamine levels at receptor sites in the basal ganglia (11). Imipramine has a dual action—it depresses acetylcholine and enhances dopamine levels. Myoclonus is caused by reduced serotonin uptake with its resultant increase within the synapse. Respiratory dysfunctions and disturbances in body temperature result from direct action of tricyclics on the respiratory center in the medulla and the thermoregulatory site in the hypothalamus, in addition to anticholinergic effects, such as decreased sweating. Experimental evidence currently suggests a cholinergic component in the reticular activating system which is responsible for maintaining arousal. If this is true, then depression and coma from tricyclic overdosage can probably be explained.

The usual characteristics of tricyclic antidepressant toxicity are summarized in Table 15.3. Those attributed to the CNS include agitation, delirium, confusion, disorientation, ataxia, visual and auditory hallucinations, loss of short-term memory, seizures, respiratory difficulties, and coma. Their onset may be rapid, occurring within an hour of ingestion (28,38). Either hyperthermia or hypothermia may develop. Imipramine causes hyperthermia more commonly, whereas amitriptyline induces hypothermia, which is probably due to its CNS-depressant action. Maprotiline appears to have great potential to cause tonic-clonic seizures (41). Desipramine has relatively less effect on the seizure threshold (3).

There are quantitative differences among anticholinergic actions of various tricyclic antidepressants. Amitriptyline is reported to induce the greatest degree of anticholinergic blockade, whereas desipramine causes the least amount (7). The peripheral anticholinergic actions listed in Table 15.3 play a fundamental role in assessment of a tricyclic antidepressant overdose.

Cardiovascular Effects

Tricyclic antidepressant agents produce prominent pharmacologic action on the cardiovascular system, even in therapeutic doses. In toxic doses, major symptoms of clin-

TABLE 15.3. *Characteristics of acute tricyclic antidepressant poisoning*

CNS[a]	Cardiovascular	Anticholinergic
Hypothermia	Ventricular rate >120 beats/min	Mydriasis
Respiratory depression	QRS duration >100 msec	Blurred vision
Seizures	Arrhythmias	Tachycardia
Abnormal tendon reflexes	Bundle branch block	Vasodilation
Disorientation	Cardiac arrest	Urinary retention
Agitation	Hypotension	Decreased gastrointestinal motility
Myoclonic jerks	Circulatory collapse	Decreased bronchial secretions
Coma		Dry mucous membranes and skin
Pyramidal signs		

[a] CNS, central nervous system.

ical importance are those on the cardiovascular system. They include tachycardia, arrhythmias, intraventricular conduction disturbances, and hypotension or hypertension. Mechanisms for these cardiac actions result from anticholinergic activity on the heart and a quinidine-like myocardial depressant action, as well as inhibition of norepinephrine uptake at adrenergic synapses. These myocardial depressant actions can be visualized on ECG by prolongation of the QT interval, and widening of the QRS complex. Blood concentrations of 100 μg/dL or greater are associated with significant cardiac effects, which are often fatal (6,34).

Tricyclic antidepressants and other anticholinergic agents block the vagus nerve. Recall that vagal stimulation releases acetylcholine, which reduces heart rate. Blocking this action leaves the sympathetic drive unopposed. Tachyarrhythmias are the usual outcome and, indeed, the most common cardiovascular complication. Specific cardiovascular effects include atrial tachycardia, fibrillation, and flutter; atrioventricular block; and ventricular tachycardia. Tachycardia may cause numerous effects including decreased cardiac output and hypotension. The quinidine-like actions of tricyclic antidepressants cause decreased AV conduction velocity, and establish conditions favorable for re-entry ventricular arrhythmias. Complete heart block may follow toxic doses of tricyclic antidepressants.

Additionally, tricyclics prevent neuronal transport and reuptake of norepinephrine and/or serotonin into nerve terminals in the sympathetic nervous system (27,49). Uptake of these neurotransmitters normally terminates their action. Accumulation within the synaptic area for a longer period causes sympathetic tone to dominate.

Arrhythmias may occur secondarily to depressed respiration or metabolic acidosis. The effect on blood pressure is variable. Because tricyclics decrease neurotransmitter reuptake into sympathetic neurons, effects from both alpha- and beta-adrenergic stimulation may be present. Initially, alpha-adrenergic stimulation causes increased peripheral resistance and beta-stimulation increases heart rate. Both actions contribute to hypertension. Eventually, this excessive neurotransmitter is metabolized by catechol-*O*-methyl transferase and monoamine oxidase, but the major mechanism for inactivation is reuptake. Peripheral alpha-adrenergic blockade produces *hypo*tension. Unless the patient is treated shortly after ingestion, hypotension is the more common sequelae. Of special note is that the extent of cardiovascular toxicity cannot be predicted easily from severity of the patient's neurologic symptoms (36).

Management of Tricyclic Antidepressant Poisoning

Tricyclic antidepressant poisoning is a serious medical emergency. Tricyclic antidepressant poisoning poses a complex array of clinical characteristics and various management protocols have been advocated.

Observation in an ICU is critical. The patient must be constantly monitored for cardiovascular and respiratory functions. Cardiac resuscitation must be readily available. The most crucial period for cardiac arrhythmias is the first 12 hr after ingestion (10). Even after the coma phase is terminated and neurologic signs appear normal, the chance for delayed life-threatening cardiovascular toxicity, often unexpected, remains (16). Cardiovascular complications have been reported to onset as long as 6 days after ingestion, even after significant clinical improvement was noted (17,43).

Physostigmine can produce significant bradycardia and asystole, and is no longer recommended for routine tricyclic antidepressant poisoning. It has been reported to cause atrial fibrillation (33). Relative contraindications to physostigmine include asthma, cardiovascular disease, gangrene, and mechanical obstruction of the gastrointestinal or urogenital tract (42).

Phenytoin is indicated for most tricyclic antidepressant-induced cardiac arrhythmias. Phenytoin enhances AV conduction time, and reverses the quinidine-like action (16). Propranolol slows the heart rate by blocking beta-adrenergic (stimulant) effects on the myocardium and reducing myocardial susceptibility to ectopic foci. However, some controversy exists over the use of propranolol. It has been shown to increase tricyclic antidepressant-induced myocardial toxicity in animal studies (37,47). The rationale for its use in tricyclic antidepressant poisoning is to reverse sympathomimetic actions. However, propranolol should be avoided or used with extreme caution in patients with asthma, congestive heart failure, or heart block (See chapter 18). Other antiarrhythmic drugs (e.g., quinidine and procainamide) should not be given because they can decrease AV nodal conduction.

If hypotension develops, a direct-acting sympathomimetic amine, such as dobutamine or dopamine, should be used cautiously. Indirectly acting pressor amines (such as mephentermine and metaraminol) that act by stimulating norepinephrine release are not indicated because their uptake into adrenergic neurons will be blocked by tricyclic antidepressants. Dihydroergotamine has been used safely to treat hypotension (3).

Animal data have shown that the incidence of cardiac arrhythmias increases when the pH is between 7.2 and 7.3 (43,44). Alkalosis decreases the chance for arrhythmia development (26). Alkalinization also promotes movement of potassium into cardiac muscle (50). Potassium narrows the width of the QRS complex of the ECG.

Once the patient has been stabilized, gastric decontamination should be undertaken to reduce the possibility of further drug absorption. Ipecac-induced emesis is preferred, if ingestion was recent. Gastric lavage is recommended even if it has been several hours since the time of ingestion due to the anticholinergic effects.

Activated charcoal effectively adsorbs tricyclic antidepressants and their metabolites, many of which are active (46). Activated charcoal has been shown to interrupt the enterohepatic circulation of tricyclic antidepressants, and for this reason, may be administered in multiple doses (39,46).

Diuresis, hemodialysis, and peritoneal dialysis do not benefit the tricyclic-poisoned patient significantly due to tight plasma protein binding, large volume of distribution, and limited water solubility. Hemoperfusion has been studied inadequately to date, but in severe intoxication when the prognosis is poor, it may be attempted (34).

Hyperthermia and fever can be treated with ice-water sponging or immersion in cooled water. Phenothiazines should not be used because their own anticholinergic action may potentiate that of the poison. Seizures are usually controlled adequately with diazepam.

ANTIPSYCHOTIC DRUGS

Several drugs used to treat severe psychotic disorders are commonly involved in overdoses. In addition to their use in mental diseases, they are also used as antiemetics, tranquilizers, and cough suppressants. These

TABLE 15.4. *Representative antipsychotic drugs*

Antipsychotic drugs	CNS	EPS	ANS
Phenothiazines			
Aliphatic	++++	++	++++
Chlorpromazine			
Promazine			
Triflupromazine			
Piperidine	++	+	+++
Mesoridazine			
Thioridazine			
Piperazine	+	++++	+
Perphenazine			
Fluphenazine			
Prochlorperazine			
Trifluoperazine			
Butyrophenones	+	+++	+
Haloperidol			
Thioxanthenes			
Chlorprothixene	+++	++	++
Thiothixene	+	++	+
Other			
Loxapine	+	++	+

CNS, central nervous system; EPS, extrapyramidal system; ANS, autonomic nervous system.

Plus system indicates greatest or least activity at a particular site: +, slight; ++, moderate; +++, high; ++++, very high.

drugs (Table 15.4) are known as antipsychotics, antipsychotophrenics, neuroleptics, major tranquilizers, psychototropics, and ataractics. The term *antipsychotics* will be used throughout this chapter.

Antipsychotic overdoses are common. Serious morbidity and mortality to pure antipsychotic overdoses are low (15). However, many antipsychotic drug poisonings represent mixed poisonings, involving a combination of different drugs.

There are many reasons for the large number of poisonings. First, antipsychotic drugs are widely prescribed. Mental patients who would have previously been institutionalized receive these drugs as outpatients. Therefore, antipsychotic drugs are widely available.

These drugs have been nothing short of revolutionary in permitting many patients to lead fairly normal lives. However, the average patient is a poor drug complier. Also, psychotic patients are at greater risk than the general population for suicidal or self-destruction gestures (5). Many of the tablet preparations resemble smooth-coated candy confections and therefore are attractive to children. Accidental poisoning in young people continues to be a special problem with these dosage forms. The situation is further compounded since psychotic patients often take a variety of other medications (e.g., TCAs, lithium, benzodiazepines). The CNS sedative effect produced by antipsychotics is at least additive to the sedation caused by other depressants (e.g., barbiturates, benzodiazepines). The anticholinergic actions of antipsychotics and TCAs are additive, and can be fatal.

Although drugs listed in Table 15.4 differ from one another in potency, they share a similar pharmacologic profile and mechanism of action. Likewise, they cause similar toxic effects. However, there are important differences among individual members, which will be indicated when appropriate.

Mechanism of Antipsychotic Drug Toxicity and Characteristics of Poisoning

The mechanism of antipsychotic toxicity is by inhibiting dopamine receptors in the limbic system and basal ganglia. Receptor blockade results in decreased neuronal cell firing. Synthesis of catecholamines in the CNS may also be inhibited.

Central effects of antipsychotics include sedation, muscle relaxation, lowering of seizure threshold, anxiolytic activity, and depression of vasomotor reflexes (3,30). Phenothiazines also produce significant peripheral actions, including blockade of alpha-adrenergic receptors, anticholinergic and antihistaminic properties, and adrenergic action secondary to inhibition of neurotransmitter reuptake.

Overdoses of antipsychotic drugs cause a variety of signs and symptoms that involve actions on the central, extrapyramidal, and autonomic nervous systems, and the cardiovascular system. Each of these will be considered separately.

Central Nervous System

All levels of the CNS are affected in antipsychotic overdoses, particularly the limbic system, hypothalamus, and basal ganglia. The limbic system is believed to be responsible for controlling behavior and mood. Antipsychotic activity is thought to be due to blockade of dopamine. The amygdala, which is part of the limbic system, may be stimulated by large doses of antipsychotics, and results in lowering of the seizure threshold. This outcome is such that the discharge pattern shown on an EEG recording resembles epilepsy (32). The response is most prominent with aliphatic phenothiazines and least with piperazine derivatives and thioxanthenes.

Overall activity of the CNS is closely regulated by the reticular activating system (RAS). The RAS essentially controls wakefulness. Antipsychotic drug overdose depresses the RAS, resulting in sedation, usually occurring within an hour of ingestion.

Coma is common in acute overdoses in children, but occurs rarely in adults. Coma characteristics differ from those caused by barbiturates. Instead of causing a flaccid appearance, the patient frequently displays episodic restlessness, tremors, spasms, and dystonic reactions.

The RAS of the brainstem also helps modulate respiration. Whereas therapeutic doses do not significantly affect respiration rate, overdoses of antipsychotic agents may cause significant depression. Whyman (52) described an unusual case of a middle-aged woman who, after being rapidly tranquilized with chlorpromazine, died suddenly from respiratory arrest. There were no other observable signs or symptoms of imminent toxicity that preceded death. Other cases involving respiratory complications, especially in children, have been reported. Kahn and Blum (29) announced their findings on infants who died with the sudden infant death syndrome (SIDS). The majority of babies admitted to a hospital with a history of SIDS had taken a phenothiazine-containing syrup prescribed for nasal congestion and/or cough. Li reports acute pulmonary edema in schizophrenia patients often ingesting large doses (2 to 4 g) of phenothiazines (31).

The hypothalamus modulates a multitude of physiologic functions, including control of the vasomotor and temperature regulating systems. Antipsychotic drugs inhibit these regulatory centers, resulting in vasodilation and orthostatic hypotension. Either hypo- or hyperthermia may result and can be fatal (4,5). Temperature elevations as high as 41°C have been reported (40). Haloperidol has been shown to cause hypothermia (3).

Extrapyramidal System

Dopaminergic receptors in the striatum within the basal ganglia are blocked by antipsychotic drugs. This blockade results in appearance of characteristic effects on the extrapyramidal system (EPS) (Table 15.5) that are often seen with therapeutic doses, but become prominent in overdose. Ten percent of all antipsychotic drug-intoxicated patients will experience these effects (29). More importantly, severity cannot be correlated with dosage or the patient's probable extent of poisoning. Some EPS effects include involuntary movements, such as tremors, tics, athetosis, widespread impairment of voluntary movement, or akinesia, and changes in muscle tone including muscle rigidity and dystonia.

Dystonia (uncoordinated spastic movements) is an extrapyramidal effect that is often reported and readily reversible. However, limited studies have shown that it may be persistent (2,14). In two cases, young children with a history of brain disease ingested phenothiazine medications. The dystonic reactions that subsequently developed did not remit over time. One explanation is that individuals with brain damage may be predisposed to permanent drug-induced neurologic damage.

Autonomic Nervous System

Antipsychotic drugs produce potent anticholinergic activity and alpha-adrenergic blockade. Anticholinergic potency is variable. Thioridazine has the greatest cholinergic blocking action; chlorpromazine, an intermediate action; piperazine derivatives and

TABLE 15.5. *Characteristics of phenothiazine toxicity*

Degree of toxicity	CNS	EPS	ANS
Mild	Sedation Ataxia Slurred speech Hypothermia or hyperthermia	Minimal	Orthostatic hypotension Miosis Constipation Blurred vision Urinary retention
Moderate	Coma stage 1, 2 Decreased seizure threshold Decreased vasomotor reflexes	Dystonia Akathisia Akinesia Tardive dyskinesia	As above, plus Quinidine effect Increased QT & PR intervals
Severe	Coma stage 2, 3	Laryngospasm Hypersalivation Dystonia Stiffness of extremities	As above, plus Hypotension Shock Arrhythmias Conduction block Renal failure

haloperidol, the least. Likewise, a difference can be shown for alpha-adrenergic blocking effects. These can be rank-ordered as: triflupromazine > chlorpromazine > thioridazine > fluphenazine > haloperidol > trifluoperazine (46). Thus, antipsychotic drug overdoses produce atropine-like signs (dry mouth, constipation, blurred vision, etc.) and alpha-adrenergic blocking effects such as orthostatic hypotension with reflex tachycardia.

Cardiovascular System

The cardiovascular effects of antipsychotic drug toxicity are related to peripheral and central mechanisms. Orthostatic hypotension ensues from central blockade of the vasomotor center, as well as from inhibition of alpha-adrenergic receptors (46).

Cardiac abnormalities result from a quinidine-like action. There is decreased AV nodal conduction leading to heart block and ventricular arrhythmias. ECG recordings show numerous abnormalities including prolonged PR and QT interval, blunted T wave, and depressed ST segment. Thioridazine produces the greatest incidence of T-wave abnormalities.

Children are more susceptible to cardiotoxic effects of antipsychotics. Those at greatest risk are patients with hypokalemia and/or preexisting cardiovascular disease. Most deaths are attributed to ventricular fibrillation or cardiac arrest (1,13,23). This action may be rapid, with death reported within 3 to 5 hr of poisoning.

Management of Antipsychotic Drug Poisoning

Antipsychotic drugs have a relatively wide therapeutic margin (3,25). In adults, daily therapeutic doses may range from 25 mg to 5,000 mg for chlorpromazine and 0.5 to 30 mg for haloperidol. Toxic doses are also spread over a wide range. A survey that reviewed 100 cases of chlorpromazine toxicity revealed that the average dose for minimally severe intoxication was 1.4 g. The average dose for severe intoxication was 6.2 g. However, survival of 10 g and even 30 g by adults has been reported (9,18).

Patients who have taken toxic overdoses of antipsychotic drugs must be assessed immediately for severity of clinical symptoms and monitored constantly for unexpected changes in condition (40). Stabilization of vital signs is the first priority. Severe hypotension may have produced shock. Elevation of blood pressure and maintenance of normal blood flow should receive immediate attention. After fluid challenge, norepinephrine or dopamine will assist in maintaining an adequate cardiac output. Dopamine is preferred over norepinephrine because of its selective cardiac actions.

Phenothiazines are radiopaque. Both whole and partial tablets can be visualized in the GI tract. Therefore, this allows for quick determination if necessary for differential diagnosis.

Phenytoin or lidocaine control phenothiazine-induced arrhythmias because they decrease automaticity and increase conduction velocity. Quinidine and procainamide are contraindicated. In addition, phenytoin may be beneficial in treating moderate seizure activity. If seizures are not controlled, diazepam should be added. Short-acting barbiturates (e.g., pentobarbital and secobarbital) were formerly considered to be a mainstay in controlling convulsant activity. Their respiratory suppressant action makes them less than ideal.

Physostigmine is a drug of choice for treating anticholinergic toxicity. Physostigmine should not be used routinely, but may be used in patients with hemodynamically unstable supraventricular tachycardia who are unresponsive to cardioversion. Also, it may be useful in ventricular dysarrhythmias unresponsive to phenytoin, lidocaine, or cardioversion. It should only be used during and after good supportive care (30). Atropine should be available to treat symptoms associated with physostigmine overdose.

Decrease Absorption of the Drug

Once the patient's immediate needs are satisfied, additional measures should be undertaken to reduce further drug absorption. Both emesis and lavage are suitable, with preference dependent on the patient's overall picture (i.e., whether or not consciousness or seizures are present, etc.). Some references state that emesis is not effective in removing antiemetic agents from the GI tract. Recent evidence points to the contrary. Emetics will induce vomiting in a significant number of persons intoxicated with antiemetic medications (see chapter 3).

Antipsychotic drugs are not water soluble and thus, not rapidly absorbed from the stomach. Furthermore, their anticholinergic action delays gastric emptying. Procedures for removing unabsorbed drug from the GI tract may, therefore, be effective even if not undertaken for several hours after ingestion (5). A saline cathartic will hasten elimination from the intestine.

After emesis or lavage, activated charcoal should be given to adsorb remaining traces of drug. Additionally, these drugs, as with tricyclic antidepressants, are cycled via the enterohepatic circulation. Repeated administration of activated charcoal over the next 24 to 48 hr may be instituted to effectively hasten elimination of drug from the blood.

Increase Excretion of Absorbed Drug

Forced diuresis is not successful for increasing elimination of antipsychotic drugs (53). Approximately 70% of a dose is taken up by the liver and, as stated earlier, excreted via bile.

Dialysis and hemoperfusion have, likewise, failed to show that intoxicated patients are benefitted significantly (53). Phenothiazines are highly protein-bound and have a high volume of distribution.

SUMMARY

Poisoning by drugs and plants that cause anticholinergic toxicity is common. Although the use of drugs classed pharmacologically as anticholinergics has declined in recent years, other drugs with anticholinergic activity still continue to cause problems. This certainly holds true for tricyclic antidepressants and antipsychotic drugs.

Tricyclic antidepressants induce a wide variety of toxic effects that includes cholinergic blockade, as well as other mechanisms. Poisoning is a medical emergency.

Antipsychotic drug toxicity is commonplace and can be severe. Symptoms of overdose are varied and often unpredictable. On the other hand, they can usually be managed if principles of therapy are followed.

Case Studies

CASE STUDY: ANTICHOLINERGIC POISONING

History

A 33-year-old woman was brought to the emergency room after being found in her apartment bound and gagged. On admission she was alert, but could remember only her name. Vital signs included blood pressure, 150/100 mm Hg; pulse, 115 beats/min; respirations, 16/min; and rectal temperature, 100°F.

The patient showed no signs of trauma. Pupils were dilated (8 mm) and not reactive to light. Heart and lung sounds and chest X-ray film were all normal. ECG showed sinus tachycardia at a rate of 120 beats/min, PR interval of 0.18 sec, QRS of 0.08 sec, and QTc interval of 0.30 sec.

Examination of the abdomen indicated there were no bowel sounds. Abdominal muscles were relaxed and the abdomen distended. The remainder of the physical examination was unremarkable. Laboratory results are summarized in Table 15.6.

Therapy consisted of oral 50% dextrose in water and 50 g activated charcoal.

It was obvious that the woman had been poisoned, but the identity of poison could not be determined. She showed no improvement over the next several hours. However, about 12 hr later, her mental status began to improve.

TABLE 15.6. *Laboratory findings*

Na⁺	=146 mEq/L
K⁺	=4.3 mEq/L
Cl⁻	=109 mEq/L
HCO₃⁻	=22 mEq/L
BUN[a]	=7 mg/dL
Glucose	=97 mg/dL
Creatinine	=0.07 mg/dL

[a] BUN, blood urea nitrogen.

It was then revealed that she had been drinking wine from a glass that was contaminated very likely with an anticholinergic drug by a guest, who drugged, then robbed her. Toxicologic analysis of the patient's blood and urine failed to disclose the presence of any drug, although a wine glass found in her apartment contained traces of scopolamine.

The source of scopolamine was never discovered. Scopolamine tablets would have imparted a disagreeable taste to the wine, and would have left a noticeable residue on the side of the glass. Scopolamine powder is not readily available. Ophthalmic drops (0.25%) can contain 2.5 mg scopolamine per mL. In a separate toxicity report, a dose of 0.45 mg scopolamine (i.e., 4 drops of 0.25% scopolamine ophthalmic solution) caused intense psychosis that persisted for 4 days. (See ref. 21.)

Discussion

1. In chapter 11, a case report of jimsonweed poisoning was described. With respect to symptoms of toxicity, how did that case compare with this one?
2. This patient apparently ingested a toxic but sublethal dose of scopolamine. Had she not improved as quickly as she did, what specific drug therapy would she have received?
3. Calculate the amount of scopolamine that would be contained in a 5-mL container of product that contained scopolamine, 0.25%.

CASE STUDIES: ANTICHOLINERGIC INTOXICATION FROM ANTIHISTAMINES

History: Case 1

A 13-year-old boy ingested 12 to 15 tablets of cyclizine, 50 mg each, to achieve a *euphoric* experience. He began to feel sick, was tremulous and hallucinating. He was therefore brought to an emergency facility.

At that time he was excitable and combative. He had the usual anticholinergic symptoms: dry mouth and dry, hot skin. He was disoriented to time and place, and experiencing auditory and visual hallucinations. Vitals included blood pressure, 140/90 mm Hg; heart rate, 134 beats/min; respirations, 22/min; and temperature, 36.8°C.

He was treated with activated charcoal and magnesium sulfate. Blood pressure increased to 140/110 mm Hg by evening. By the second day, he was no longer tremulous. His thoughts did continue to be disorganized and illogical. On the third day he was oriented to name, place, and time. He was discharged the next day in apparently good health. (See ref. 54.)

History: Case 2

A 16-year-old girl ingested 30 to 36 Dramamine (dimenhydrinate) tablets, 50-mg each, early in the evening. She swallowed them at the suggestion of a sister who took 42 tablets because she wanted to get *high*. The girl retired to bed, but slept restlessly and hallucinated throughout the night. She was taken to a hospital the next morning.

On examination, the patient was not oriented to time or place. Her mouth was dry. She was anxious and experiencing auditory and visual hallucinations. Vitals included heart rate, 120 beats/min; respirations, 24/min; and temperature, 36.5°C. Pupils were dilated. She complained of a feeling of having things on her, and picked at imaginary bugs. An ECG showed premature atrial contractions, and a PR interval of 0.14 to 0.16.

The patient did not require medical treatment. She was discharged the following morning. (See ref. 54.)

Discussion

1. These two victims of poisoning consumed antihistamines; toxic reactions were clearly those of anticholinergic actions. Summarize signs and symptoms to expect after a toxic dose of an anticholinergic drug. What is tremulousness?
2. Both patients were teenagers. What effect, if any, would their age have made on the way they responded to the drugs compared to a 35-year old person?
3. Patient 1 received a dose of magnesium sulfate. What is the common (i.e., household) name for this substance? Why was it given?

CASE STUDY: DIMENHYDRINATE POISONING

History

The patient was a 4.5-month-old boy who exhibited seizure activity of all four extremities. On admission to a hospital he was noted to be well developed and well nourished. His systolic blood pressure was 80 mm Hg; apical rate was 130 beats/min; respirations, 50/min; and temperature, 37.9°C. Pupils were 4 to 5 mm and responsive to light. He had diffusely increased tone and was unresponsive.

He was intubated and an IV was started. Diazepam 2.5 mg, phenytoin 3.8 mg/kg, and sodium bicarbonate 5 mEq were administered intravenously. Seizures responded to phenobarbital 2.5 mg IM.

On arrival at the pediatric I.C.U. he had continued seizure activity that responded to lorazepam 1 mg.

A tracing of his heart monitor showed first degree AV block with bigeminy. A 12-lead EGG revealed a junctional tachycardia with evidence of left bundle block. An echocardiogram showed poor left ventricular function with an ejection fraction of 44% (normal, 65%) and a shortening fraction of 15% (normal, 36%).

An initial toxicology screen was positive for tricyclic antidepressants. The phenobarbital and diazepam were also identified.

Treatment consisted of Plasmanate, which maintained the central venous pressure at 15 mm Hg. Phenytoin 10 mg/kg was given parenterally. He was managed with mechanical ventilation, intravenous fluids, anticonvulsants and antibiotics. He was extubated after 3 days.

Later, the child's family said he had been fine when the mother left him at a care giver's home on the morning of admission. An unopened four ounce bottle of apple juice had been sent with him. The child's mother brought the apple juice to the hospital. On gross examination the juice was cloudy. It was later shown to contain diphenhydramine at a concentration of 8000 μg/mL. The caretaker later confessed to police that she had placed the drug in the child's juice. (See ref. 19)

Discussion

1. Classify dimenhydrinate as to its pharmacologic profile.
2. The child was intoxicated with dimenhydrinate, yet, he had toxic blood levels of diphenhydramine. What was the probable source of the latter?

CASE STUDIES: TRICYCLIC ANTIDEPRESSANT OVERDOSE

History: Case 1

A 46-year-old woman ingested eight Elavil (amitriptyline) tablets, 25 mg each, and 15 Sominex (scopolamine, methapyrilene, salicylamide) tablets. (Note: This product has since been reformulated.) She was brought to the emergency room comatose, responding only to painful stimuli. She was sweating profusely, was flushed, and respirations were increased above normal. She displayed occasional myoclonal activity. Pupils were dilated at 5 mm and reactive to light.

Vital signs on admission consisted of blood pressure, 140/105 mm Hg; pulse, 100 beats/min; respirations, 20/min; and temperature, 98°F. Laboratory values are shown in Table 15.7.

Treatment consisted of immediate gastric lavage with a 7-L return, oxygen, fluids, and diazepam. Because she showed occasional PVCs a lidocaine drip was started. Physostig-

TABLE 15.7. *Laboratory findings*

Na$^+$	=138 mEq/L
Cl$^-$	=104 mEq/L
K$^+$	=4.4 mEq/L
HCO$_3^-$	=2.6 mEq/L
BUN	=12 mg/dL
pH	=7.38
pO$_2$	=73 mm Hg
pCO$_2$	=58 mm Hg

mine salicylate, 2 mg intravenously, was administered about 7 hr after admission.

Almost immediately, the patient awoke and became alert and oriented. To maintain alertness and orientation, she required additional physostigmine, so doses were administered 4 hr later and again 3 hr later.

With each challenge of physostigmine, she became responsive within seconds. The following day, an additional 2-mg dose of physostigmine was used again because of the appearance of frequent junctional premature beats. By this time signs of cholinergic stimulation (e.g., nausea, vomiting, diarrhea, and salivation) appeared. She was discharged 5 days after admission with no apparent residual effects. (See ref. 10.)

History: Case 2

A 32-year-old woman was brought to an emergency facility 9 hr after ingestion of 1.0 to 1.5 g amitriptyline hydrochloride. On examination, she was stuporous, responding only to deep pain. Reflexes were normal. Vital signs included blood pressure, 120/80 mm Hg; pulse, 126 beats/min; and respirations, 16/min and shallow.

Physical examination revealed a very sick individual who groaned in agony, and thrashed her arms in response to pain. Treatment consisted of 2 mg physostigmine salicylate intravenously. Within 15 min she had fully awakened. Watery diarrhea occurred, for which she was given 0.4 mg glycopyrrolate. Her vital signs had stabilized by five hours, and she did not require further physostigmine treatments. She still remained sluggish mentally.

Because tremors increased over the next few hours and diarrhea and myoclonus persisted, at 9 hr after admission another 2-mg dose of physostigmine salicylate was given, along with 0.2 mg glycopyrrolate. These doses were repeated periodically over the next 8 hr for a total quantity administered of 12 mg physostigmine salicylate, and 1.2 mg glycopyrrolate. Eleven hours after admission, there was a significant decrease in urinary output, and the patient was catheterized.

The following morning, she was alert and tremulous. She was also oriented and responding somewhat better, and no further myoclonus was observed. At this time, physostigmine and glycopyrrolate were discontinued and there were no further problems with urinary retention. She recovered completely 36 hr after admission.

Toxicologic analysis of the patient's blood and urine at the time of admission showed a serum amitriptyline level of less than 0.1 mg/dL. Urine amitriptyline concentration was 3.8 mg/dL, with the presence of a metabolite. (See ref. 45.)

History: Case 3

A 38-year-old woman was admitted to a hospital 2 hr after ingesting an estimated 20 to 30 of her mother's 50-mg desipramine tablets. She had also consumed an unknown quantity of alcohol. The woman was alert, oriented, and able to communicate normally.

On admission vital signs were: blood pressure, 140/90 mm Hg; pulse rate, 125/min; and respirations, 28/min. Temperature was not recorded. Bowel sounds were present, but hypoactive. No traces of any other drug were found.

The patient received 30 mL of syrup of ipecac, which resulted in vomiting fragments of the tablets. Neither activated charcoal nor cathartics were administered.

Over the next 6 hr the patient remained stabilized. Blood pressure returned to 120/90 mm Hg and the ECG was normal. Only tachycardia was evidenced, and this gradually declined. Eight hours postingestion she was fully awake, alert, and able to walk unassisted. Because of this improvement, she was transferred to the psychiatric emergency department for assessment.

Two hours later (10 hr postingestion), her condition was noted to have worsened. Speech was slurred and she was apparently experiencing auditory hallucinations. She was visibly fearful and agitated. Respirations became labored, blood pressure was palpable at 60 mm Hg, and her pulse was weak and irregular.

Cardiac tracing showed asystole. Cardiopulmonary resuscitation was initiated but the patient failed to respond. She was pronounced dead 11 hr after drug ingestion. Postmortem analysis of a blood sample showed a desipramine concentration of 8.6 μg/mL. Plasma concentrations of 1.0 μg/mL have been associated with coma, cardiac arrest, and death. (See ref. 12.)

Discussion

1. Onset of cholinergic symptoms in patient 1 on the second hospital day marked an important event. What was it?
2. Outline the mechanism of activity for physostigmine when it is used to treat tricyclic antidepressant poisoning.
3. In patient 1, was the cardiovascular response to amitriptyline intoxication expected or unexpected? Outline the mechanism that caused this response.
4. The ingredients in Sominex tablets surely produced some toxic symptoms of their own. What would you have expected? Did they add to the amitriptyline effects, or partially prevent them from being worse?
5. What actually caused patient 2 to develop urinary retention? Was this to be expected?
6. Discuss why glycopyrrolate, instead of atropine sulfate, was given to patient 2 instead of atropine sulfate.
7. The patient in case 3 illustrates the fact that death can occur even after symptoms (which were trivial to start) have subsided. What specific measures could have been instituted to reduce the likelihood of death?

CASE STUDIES: PHENOTHIAZINE TOXICITY

History: Case 1

A 54-year-old woman with a 30-year history of manic depressive psychosis was admitted to the psychiatric ward of a hospital. Vital signs at that time were: temperature, 36.9°C; pulse, 72 beats/min; blood pressure, 136 mm Hg; and respirations, 20/min. She was disoriented and talkative. Physical examination was otherwise unremarkable except for a systolic murmur.

Treatment consisted of thioridazine, 200 mg four times a day; and chlorpromazine, 500 mg at bedtime. Her acute psychosis resolved within 2 weeks. However, during the course of treatment, she experienced sudden cardiopulmonary arrest while being attended to in the bathroom. After successful resuscitation, an ECG showed sinus tachycardia, notched broad T waves, and prolongation of the QT interval to 500 msec.

For some unknown reason, she received another 200 mg thioridazine, and two more episodes of ventricular arrhythmias developed within 4 hr. Both responded to lidocaine. However, on the following day she experienced five more incidences of ventricular tachycardia, even though she was maintained on a continuous lidocaine drip. To convert back to sinus rhythm, she needed seven 50-mg bolus doses of lidocaine and 250 mg procainamide every 3 hr. Three direct current cardioversions were also delivered.

Lidocaine was discontinued the following day with the QT interval shortening to 380 msec. Procainamide was discontinued 4 days later. Approximately 2 weeks after admission, she was discharged with no apparent cardiac complications. (See ref. 1.)

History: Case 2

A 29-year-old man with a history of chronic schizophrenia had been hospitalized periodically for the past 10 years. His medications

TABLE 15.8. *Laboratory findings*

pCO_2	=30 mm Hg
HCO_3^-	=18 mEq/L
pH	=7.40
Hb[a]	=12.7 g
BUN	=22 mg/dL
Cholesterol	=234 mg/dL
Bromsulphthalein	=19% retention in 45 min
Alkaline phosphatase	=18.2 U

[a] Hb, hemoglobin.

for the past 5 years included imipramine, 50 mg 4 times a day; trifluoperazine, 10 mg twice a day; and thioridazine, 200 mg 4 times a day. About 1 year before his latest hospitalization, he began to experience dyspnea on exertion, orthopnea, and paroxysmal nocturnal dyspnea. He gained 60 pounds.

On admission, blood pressure was 100/78 mm Hg; pulse was 100 beats/min and regular. Physical examination revealed bilateral basilar rales and mild pitting edema in the lower extremities. A sinus tachycardia of 120 beats/min and nonspecific T-wave changes were noted on an ECG recording. Laboratory results are shown in Table 15.8.

This patient's treatment consisted of discontinuing the phenothiazines, bed rest, a salt-restricted diet, and digitalis. He lost 34 pounds within a week.

He was discharged and then reevaluated 15 months later after taking chlorpromazine continuously for 12 months. At this time, signs of congestive heart failure were again present, as were gallop rhythm and cardiomegaly. Recovery this time was less dramatic than previously. (See ref. 48.)

Discussion

1. Patient 1 became intoxicated with antipsychotic medication as an inpatient. Based on the case history, what were the warning signs, if any, that should have contraindicated the use of this medication?
2. Comment on the congestive heart failure in patient 2. Do you suppose the digitalis he received contributed to his overall condition?

3. Explain why quinidine was not used to treat ventricular arrhythmias in case 1.

Review Questions

1. Which of the following chemical classes of phenothiazines is associated with the greatest incidence of extrapyramidal symptoms?
   A. Aliphatic derivatives
   B. Piperazine derivatives
   C. Piperidine derivatives
   D. Thioxanthine derivatives
2. Inability to regulate the body temperature after phenothiazine overdoses is a result of a toxic action on the:
   A. Limbic system
   B. Reticular activation system
   C. Hippocampus
   D. Hypothalamus
3. Discuss the rationale for administering each of the following drugs to a victim of tricyclic antidepressant intoxication.
   A. Sodium bicarbonate
   B. Potassium chloride
4. A victim of poisoning who presented with symptoms of dilated pupils, blurred vision, dry mouth, constipation, and tachycardia was most likely poisoned by a:
   A. Chlorinated hydrocarbon insecticide
   B. Organophosphorus insecticide
   C. Anticholinergic drug
   D. Lead salt
5. Physostigmine is used to treat overdoses of which of the following drugs?
   A. Alpha-adrenergic stimulants
   B. Alpha-adrenergic blockers
   C. Muscarinic stimulants
   D. Muscarinic blockers
6. Which of the following is a true statement?
   A. Coma is a common outcome of phenothiazine intoxication in children.
   B. SIDS describes a series of symptoms on the autonomic nervous system that results from overdoses of phenothiazine drugs.
   C. Antipsychotic medications stimulate vasomotor tone.

   D. Dystonia is a form of respiratory depression that results from phenothiazine overdoses.
7. Phenothiazines block dopaminergic receptors in the limbic system.
   A. True
   B. False
8. Discuss the rationale for administering each of the following drugs to a victim of phenothiazine intoxication.
   A. Phenytoin
   B. Diazepam
9. The most common cause of drug-induced mortality associated with antipsychotic agents and the tricyclic antidepressants is:
   A. Hypertensive crisis
   B. Respiratory depression
   C. Methemoglobinemia
   D. Cardiac arrhythmias
   E. Generalized convulsions
10. All of the following general classes of agents have significant potential for producing anticholinergic effects *except*:
   A. H_1-antagonists
   B. Organophosphorus insecticides
   C. Tricyclic antidepressants
   D. Gastrointestinal antispasmodic agents
   E. Antipsychotic agents
11. The blood pressure response to a tricyclic overdose is variable over time. Discuss the probable mechanism of this variability.
12. If a victim of a tricyclic antidepressant drug poisoning goes into shock, how should it be treated? What are the benefits and risks of administering epinephrine?
13. Phenothiazines cause a variety of effects on the heart that may lead to cardiac arrhythmias. List them and discuss their probable importance to the arrhythmic event.
14. Cite how it can be readily determined that an overdose of phenothiazine tablets has been taken, even before symptoms appear.
15. Discuss the dosing schedule for physostigmine when it is used to diagnose the probable cause of a poisoning.
16. List the major factors that contribute to

the large number of poisonings by antipsychotic medications.

17. Theoretically, castor oil should work better as a means to rid the GI tract of an overdose of tricyclic antidepressant medication than a saline cathartic. Explain the reasoning behind this statement.

18. Toxicity to the CNS from scopolamine differs in one important aspect from atropine. Name it.

References

1. Alexander CS, Nino A. Cardiovascular complications in young patients taking psychotropic drugs. *Am Heart J* 1969;78:757–769.
2. Angle CA, McIntire MS. Persistent dystonia in a brain-damaged child after ingestion of phenothiazine. *J Pediatr* 1968;73:124–126.
3. Baldessarini RJ. Drugs and the treatment of psychiatric disorders. In: Gilman AG, Goodman LS, Rall TW, Murad F, eds. *The pharmacological basis of therapeutics.* 7th ed. New York: Macmillan; 1985:387–445.
4. Bark NM. Heatstroke in psychiatric patients: two cases and a review. *J Clin Psychiatry* 1982;43:377–380.
5. Barry D, Meyskens FL, Becker CE. Phenothiazine poisoning: a review of 48 cases. *Calif Med* 1973;118:1–5.
6. Biggs JT, Spiker DG, Petit JM, Ziegler VE. Tricyclic antidepressant overdose. *JAMA* 1977;238:135–138.
7. Blackwell B, Stefoupolos A, Enders P. Anticholinergic activity of two tricyclic antidepressants. *Am J Psychiatry* 1978;135:722–724.
8. Brizer DA, Manning DW. Delirium induced by poisoning with anticholinergic agents. *Am J Psychiatry* 1982;139:1343–1344.
9. Brophy JJ. Suicide attempts with psychotherapeutic drugs. *Arch Gen Psychiatry* 1967;17:652–657.
10. Bryan CK, Ludy JA, Hak SH, et al. Overdoses with tricyclic antidepressants. *Drug Intell Clin Pharm* 1976;10:380–384.
11. Burks JS, Walker JE, Rumack BH. Tricyclic antidepressant poisoning: reversal of coma, choreoathetosis, and myoclonus by physostigmine. *JAMA* 1974;230:1405–1407.
12. Callahan M. Admission criteria for tricyclic antidepressant ingestion. *West J Med* 1982;137:425–429.
13. Crane GE. Cardiac toxicity and psychotropic drugs. *Dis Nerv Sys* 1970;31:534–539.
14. Dabbous IA, Bergman AB. Neurologic damage associated with phenothiazine. *Am J Dis Child* 1966;111:291–292.
15. Dahl SG, Strandjord RE. Pharmacokinetics of chlorpromazine after single and chronic dosage. *Clin Pharmacol Ther* 1977;21:437–447.
16. Davies DM, Allaye R. Amitriptyline poisoning. *Lancet* 1963;2:543.
17. Davis JM. Overdose of psychotropic drugs—tricyclic antidepressants. *Psychiatry Ann* 1973;3:6–11.
18. Douglas ADM, Bates TJN. Chlorpromazine as a suicidal agent. *Br Med J* 1957;1:1514.
19. Farrell M, Heinrichs M, Tilelli JA. Response of life threatening dimenhydrinate intoxication to sodium bicarbonate administration. *Clin Toxicol* 1991;29:527–535.
20. Foulke GE, Albertson TE, Walby WF. Tricyclic antidepressant overdose: emergency department findings as predictors of clinical course. *Am J Emerg Med* 1986;4:496–500.
21. Goldfrank L, Flomenbaum N, Lewin N, et al. Anticholinergic poisoning. *J Toxicol Clin Toxicol* 1982;19:17–25.
22. Gosselin RE, Smith RP, Hodge HH, eds. *Clinical toxicology of commercial products.* 5th ed. Baltimore: Williams and Wilkins; 1984.
23. Greenblatt DJ, Allen MD, Koch-Wesen J, Shader RI. Accidental poisoning with psychotropic drugs in children. *Am J Dis Child* 1976;130:507–511.
24. Hepler BR, Sutheimer CA, Sunshine I. Role of the toxicology laboratory in the treatment of acute poisonings. *Med Toxicol* 1986;1:61–75.
25. Hoffman AS, Schwartz HI, Novick RM. Catatonic reaction to accidental haloperidol overdose: an unrecognized drug abuse risk. *J Nerv Ment Dis* 1980;174:428–430.
26. Jackson JE, Bressler R. Prescribing tricyclic antidepressants. Part III: management of overdose. *Drug Ther* 1982;13:175–189.
27. Jefferson JW. A review of the cardiovascular and toxicity of tricyclic antidepressants. *Psychosom Med* 1975;37:160–179.
28. Jick H, Dinan BJ, Hunter JR, et al. Tricyclic antidepressants and convulsions. *J Clin Psychopharmacol* 1983;3:182–185.
29. Kahn A, Blum D. Possible role of phenothiazines in sudden infant death. *Lancet* 1979;2:364–365.
30. Knight ME, Roberts RJ. Phenothiazine and butyrophenone intoxication in children. *Pediatr Clin North Am* 1986;33:299–309.
31. Li C, Gefter WB. Acute pulmonary edema induced by overdosage of phenothiazines. *Chest* 1992;101:102–104.
32. Logothetis J. Spontaneous epileptic seizures and EEG changes in the course of phenothiazine therapy. *Neurology* 1967;17:869–877.
33. Maister AH. Atrial fibrillation following physostigmine. *Can Anaesth Soc J* 1983;30:419–421.
34. Marshall JB, Forker AD. Cardiovascular effects of tricyclic antidepressant drugs: therapeutic usage, overdose, and management of complications. *Am Heart J* 1982;103:401–414.
35. Molcho A, Stouley M. Antidepressants and suicide risk: issues of chemical and behavioral toxicity. *J Clin Psychopharmacol* 1992;12:13S–18S.
36. Nicotra MB, Rivera M, Pool JL, Noall MW. Tricyclic antidepressant overdose: clinical and pharmacological observations. *Clin Toxicol* 1981;18:599–613.
37. Nymark M, Rasmussen J. Effect of certain drugs upon amitriptyline induced electrocardiographic changes. *Acta Pharmacol Toxicol* 1966;24:148–156.
38. Pellimen TJ, Farkkila M, Heikkila J, Luomanmaki K. Electrocardiographic and clinical features of tricyclic

antidepressant intoxications. *Ann Clin Res* 1987; 19:12–17.

39. Preskorn SH, Irwin HA. Toxicity of tricyclic antidepressants—kinetics, mechanism, intervention: a review. *J Clin Psychiatry* 1982;43:151–156.

40. Price WA, Giannini AJ. A paradoxical response to chlorpromazine—a possible variant of the neuroleptic malignant syndrome. *J Clin Pharmacol* 1983; 23:567–569.

41. Rotblatt MD. Antidepressant and seizures. *Drug Intell Clin Pharm* 1982;16:749–750.

42. Rumack BH. Anticholinergic poisoning: treatment with physostigmine. *Pediatrics* 1973;52:449–451.

43. Sedal L, Korman MG, Williams PO, Mushin G. Overdosage of tricyclic antidepressants: a report of two deaths and a prospective study of 24 patients. *Med J Aust* 1972;2:74.

44. Skoutakis VA. Tricyclic antidepressants. In: Skoutakis VA, ed. *Clinical toxicology of drugs: principles and practice.* Philadelphia: Lea and Febiger; 1982: 127–152.

45. Snyder BD, Blonde L, McWhirter WR. Reversal of amitriptyline intoxication by physostigmine. *JAMA* 1974;230:1433–1434.

46. Swartz CM, Sherman A. The treatment of tricyclic antidepressant overdose with repeated charcoal. *J Clin Psychopharmacol* 1984;4:336–340.

47. Thorstrand C, Bergstrom J, Castenfors J. Cardiac effects of amitriptyline in rats. *Scand J Clin Lab Invest* 1976;36:7–15.

48. Tri TB, Combs DT. Phenothiazine induced ventricular tachycardia. *West J Med* 1975;123:412–416.

49. Vohra JK. Cardiovascular abnormalities following tricyclic antidepressant drug overdosage. *Drugs* 1975;7:323–325.

50. Vohra J, Burrows GD. Cardiovascular complications of tricyclic antidepressant overdosage. *Drugs* 1974; 8:432–437.

51. Weiner N. Atropine, scopolamine, and related antimuscarinic drugs. In: Gilman AG, Goodman LS, Rall TW, Murad F, eds. *The pharmacological basis of therapeutics.* 7th ed. New York: Macmillan; 1985: 130–144.

52. Whyman A. Phenothiazine death: an unusual case report. *J Nerv Ment Dis* 1976;163:214–216.

53. Winchester JF, Gelfand MC, Knepshield JH, Schreiner GE. Dialysis and hemoperfusion of poisons and drugs—update. *Trans Am Soc Artif Intern Organs* 1977;23:762–842.

54. Woo OF. Acute intoxication with nonprescription antihistamines. *Contemp Pharm Pract* 1981;4:257–259.

16 | Central Nervous System Stimulants

TABLE 16.1. *Drug compounds with CNS[a]-stimulant activity*

Amphetamine
  See Table 16.2
Anorexiants
  See Table 16.2
Analeptics
  Doxapram
  Methylphenidate
  Pentylenetetrazol
  Picrotoxin
  Strychnine
Xanthines
  Caffeine
  Theobromine
  Theophylline
Local anesthetics
  Camphor
  Cocaine
Psychotomimetics
  See chapter 17

[a] CNS, central nervous system.

Many drug classes cause CNS stimulation when ingested in toxic amounts (Table 16.1). Traditionally, drugs, such as amphetamine and strychnine, produce strong convulsant activity. However, other drugs may act as moderate CNS stimulants. Stimulants represent a diverse group of compounds that are chemically and pharmacologically dissimilar. When ingested in moderate to high doses, they cause a variety of effects related to central nervous system excitation. Overdoses of this group are treated in much the same manner, with a few exceptions.

Specific stimulants considered in this chapter include amphetamine and its derivatives, strychnine, theophylline and caffeine, cocaine and camphor. Some of the hallucinogenic stimulants [e.g., 3,4-methylenedioxyamphetamine (MDA), 2,5-dimethoxy-4-methylamphetamine (DOM)] will be covered in chapter 17. Understanding the manifestations of toxicity and management of these drugs, as outlined in this chapter, will form the basis for treating almost all other chemicals that cause CNS stimulation as a major effect.

Discussion of stimulant toxicity in this chapter is limited to acute effects and their management. Another area of study, the psychology of abuse of amphetamine, cocaine,

and other stimulants, and the physiologic effects of chronic use, are left for textbooks in appropriate disciplines.

AMPHETAMINE-LIKE DRUGS

Numerous derivatives of amphetamine have been used over the years to modify a variety of medical conditions, legitimate or otherwise. Today, approved uses include management of narcolepsy, hyperkinesis (hyperactivity) in children, and short-term treatment of obesity. Many states have officially banned the use of these drugs. Consequently, legal amphetamine use has declined significantly. Also, intravenous amphetamine use has decreased in the United States, compared to a few years ago (25). However, amphetamine abuse and toxicity is still a significant medical problem.

All of the drugs that have amphetamine-like activity can be classed together as a group and referred to simply as *amphetamine*. Some of the more common drugs are listed in Table 16.2. Not all drugs shown in this table are important causes of intoxication, but they are included for completeness. It may be speculated that as amphetamine and methamphetamine (Table 16.3) become more difficult to obtain, other drugs may emerge as important causes of acute toxicity.

Mechanism of Toxicity

Amphetamine induces CNS stimulation, mainly by causing release of catecholamines

TABLE 16.2. *Drugs with amphetamine-like activity*

Amphetamine
Benzphetamine
Chlorphentermine
Dextroamphetamine
Diethylpropion
Methamphetamine
Phendimetrazine tartrate
Phenmetrazine
Phentermine
Phenylpropanolamine

TABLE 16.3. *Chemical formulas for amphetamine and methamphetamine*

$$R_1-\langle\rangle-\underset{R_2}{CH}-\underset{R_3}{CH}-\underset{R_4}{NH}$$

Chemical name	Substitutions			
	R_1	R_2	R_3	R_4
Amphetamine	H	H	CH_3	H
Methamphetamine	H	H	CH_3	CH_3

(epinephrine, norepinephrine, dopamine) into central synaptic spaces and inhibiting their re-uptake into nerve endings (56). In this manner, endogenous neurotransmitters remain present within the synapses in higher concentration and for longer than normal time. All neurons that normally respond to stimulation are affected.

One problem frequently encountered by amphetamine users is tolerance to some of the central effects, such as the anorexiant and euphoric actions. Therefore, users may need to increase the dose, sometimes approaching several hundred milligrams daily. Tolerance does not occur to all central actions, however. Toxic psychosis may appear after months of continued use. If use is continued in these individuals, the convulsive threshold may actually be lowered, and fatalities become a greater problem (25).

Characteristics of Poisoning

Amphetamine causes a variety of dose-related signs and symptoms. Most toxic effects are extensions of pharmacologic actions. Table 16.4 lists some of the more prominent features and ranks them according to severity. Symptoms noted as 1+ and 2+ may be experienced even with therapeutic doses and are generally not causes of great concern. Conditions listed as 3+ and 4+ reflect severe CNS stimulation and require immediate attention.

Amphetamine-induced psychosis with euphoria and hallucinations is common. Euphoria may account for the widespread abuse potential of amphetamine. Hallucinations are generally perceived as unpleasant. These may be auditory in nature (mostly in patients using amphetamines chronically), or visual (more common after a single large dose). Tactile hallucinations are experienced occasionally. Psychosis generally disappears within a week after onset, with hallucinations remitting first.

Respiratory and cardiovascular functions are stimulated. Sympathomimetic effects include tachypnea, tachycardia, hypertension, flushing, and diaphoresis. This leads eventually to depression of both systems once the neurotransmitter has been depleted.

Hyperpyrexia may be significant, with temperatures above 109°F reported (30,48). Temperatures this high are incompatible with life and are a contributing cause of death. Therefore, hyperpyrexia may be a contributory factor to death resulting from excessive exercise and use of amphetamine. In one case, a bicyclist ingested 105 mg amphetamine before a race. He collapsed eventually from heat exhaustion. Despite aggressive emergency treatment, he died of cardiovascular collapse (7). Hyperpyrexia is believed to be caused by drug-induced peripheral vasoconstriction, but

TABLE 16.4. *Characteristics of amphetamine toxicity grouped by severity*

Signs and symptoms	Severity[a]
Restlessness, irritability, insomnia, tremor, hyperreflexia, sweating, mydriasis	1+
Hyperactivity, confusion, hypertension, tachypnea, tachycardia, mild fever, hyperpyrexia	2+
Delirium, mania, self-injury, intense hypertension, tachycardia, arrhythmias, hyperpyrexia	3+
All of the above plus convulsions, coma, circulatory collapse, and death	4+

From ref. 13.
[a] For explanation, see text.

whether fatal hyperpyrexia is produced centrally or peripherally is not known.

The lethal dose of amphetamine varies. Severe toxicity has occurred with doses of 30 mg. However, a nontolerant woman survived a 200-mg dose (21). The acute lethal dose in adults has been reported at 20 to 25 mg/kg, and in children, 5 mg/kg (4,63). Death from as little as 1.5 mg/kg in an adult has also been noted (63). Therapeutic, toxic, and lethal blood amphetamine concentrations are listed in Table 3 of the Appendix.

METHYLXANTHINE DERIVATIVES

Three methylxanthine alkaloids are commonly encountered from natural resources: theobromine, theophylline, and caffeine. Cocoa and chocolate contain theobromine and some caffeine. Tea contains caffeine and some theophylline. Coffee and many cola-flavored beverages are rich sources of caffeine. Folklore reports that these and other beverages and foods containing methylxanthine derivatives have been an important part of almost all cultures. People around the world still rely on the early-morning ritual of cocoa, tea or coffee to *get them started* in the morning, and to *keep them going* in the afternoon and early evening.

In addition to their presence in foods and beverages, theophylline and caffeine are used in drug therapy. Methylxanthines stimulate the CNS, induce diuresis, relax smooth muscle (notably bronchial muscle), and stimulate cardiac functions. Caffeine also augments the analgesic properties of salicylates and is contained in numerous analgesic products. Theobromine possesses similar, but weaker pharmacologic activity on the CNS and CVS. It is, therefore, not used in drug therapy (41). Because of widespread use and appeal of caffeine and theophylline, they commonly cause adverse and toxic effects (12,19,23,36,41). Fatalities with theophylline are common (59). Caffeine-related fatalities are rare (12), but nevertheless are reported occasionally (17,35).

There are no data to explain the occurrence of toxicity. Most likely, caffeine overdoses are a result of its use as a stimulant. One fad is the use of amphetamine *look-alike* products. These are designed to mimic prescription stimulants in appearance. They are sold through nonlegitimate channels, and can contain caffeine alone, or in combination with phenylpropanolamine, ephedrine, or other CNS stimulants (17). Reasons for theophylline intoxications are listed in Table 16.5.

Mechanism of Toxicity

Caffeine and theophylline are potent stimulants of the cardiovascular and central nervous systems. Most significant toxic sequelae result from overstimulation. In addition, theophylline causes severe irritation to the GI tract. Nausea and/or vomiting are hallmarks of theophylline overdose.

There have been numerous theories to explain the mechanism(s) of xanthine toxicity. Many of these reports have failed to differentiate between actions prevalent in therapeutic doses, and those associated with toxicity. The exact mechanism of toxic action has not been described completely. However, three proposed mechanisms have generated considerable interest: (a) increased calcium release from intracellular sites; (b) accumulation of cyclic nucleotides, especially cyclic AMP (cAMP); and (c) adenosine receptor blockade (41). Toxicity probably results from more than one mechanism. Direct stimulation of the che-

TABLE 16.5. *Circumstances surrounding theophylline toxicity*

Cause of poisoning	% of total cases[a]
Physician error	51
Pharmacy error	3
Parent error	11
Accidental ingestion	8
Suicide gesture	11
Respiratory tract infection	23
Erythromycin interaction	2

From ref. 3.
[a] n = 65 patients. Percentages total more than 100 because 5 patients had a respiratory tract infection as well as other causes for toxicity.

moreceptor trigger zone appears to cause the nausea and vomiting.

Characteristics of Poisoning

Therapeutic blood concentrations of caffeine are less than 1 mg/dL (17). Adverse effects are observed with doses around 1 g, but acute toxic doses appear to be between 5 and 10 g either intravenously or orally. These doses can produce effects on the CNS, including restlessness, excitement, and insomnia that can progress to delirium. Patients may see

flashes of light and hear ringing and other noises. Muscles become tense and spastic. Cardiovascular effects may include tachycardia, extrasystoles, tachypnea, ventricular fibrillation, and cardiopulmonary arrest. As toxicity progresses, convulsions, coma, and death due to shock are likely.

Theophylline has a narrow therapeutic margin, 10 to 20 μg/mL. Because numerous factors including other drugs can stimulate or depress theophylline clearance, maintaining therapeutic blood concentrations can be difficult. Within a short period, blood concentrations can be subtherapeutic (below 10 μg/mL)

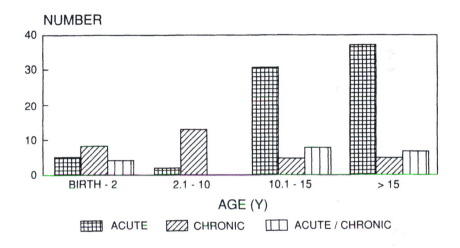

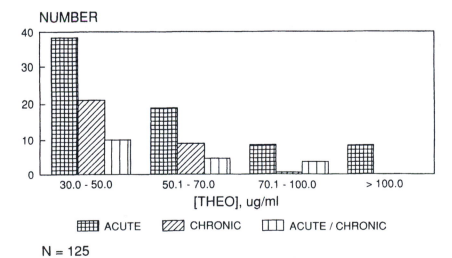

N = 125

FIG. 16.1. Profile of 125 patients who were poisoned with theophylline: age distribution by manner of intoxication (**top**) and peak recorded serum [THEO] by manner of intoxication (**bottom**). (From ref. 52.)

or toxic (above 20 μg/mL). Rapid intravenous administration of theophylline or aminophylline (theophylline ethylenediamine) can result in death due to cardiac arrhythmias.

Other manifestations of overdose include nausea and vomiting, headache, dizziness, palpitations and tachycardia, hypotension, and precordial pain. Also, patients have reported severe restlessness and agitation. Focal and generalized seizures may appear occasionally, even without other signs of toxicity. Seizures have occurred when plasma concentrations reached 25 μg/mL (24), although they usually do not appear until the concentration exceeds 40 μg/mL (41). Infants are reported to be more resistant to seizures. In sharp contrast to the above, an 11-month-old girl did not develop seizures, despite having a blood theophylline concentration of 180 μg/mL (49).

A 5-year prospective observational study of consecutive pediatric patients referred to a regional poison control center with a theophylline concentration of 30 or greater μg/mL was undertaken. The goal was to determine whether the method of intoxication influences the metabolic disturbances and pattern of life-threatening events that occur after theophylline intoxication in children (52).

As can be seen in Fig. 16.1, the method of intoxication has significant effects on the metabolic and clinical consequences of theophylline poisoning. Life-threatening events occur in those with acute theophylline intoxication at significantly higher theophylline than in those with chronic intoxication. After chronic intoxication, peak theophylline does not identify patients at risk for life-threatening events. Young age appears to be the primary risk factor. These findings potentially complicate the management of theophylline poisoning, given the difficulty of extracorporeal drug removal in young infants.

STRYCHNINE

Strychnine, in doses of 0.5 to 1.0 mg, was formerly used in a variety of medications intended for internal stimulant use. Although it is no longer used in medicine, some of these older remedies have remained in home medicine cabinets and pharmacies. Today, its legitimate use is mainly confined to pesticide products that are intended to control rodents. Strychnine is still an important cause of accidental poisoning in children and adults (62). Most poisonings result from suicidal ingestion of rodenticides (37).

Mechanism of Toxicity

Strychnine causes generalized stimulation of all portions of the CNS, both in the spinal column and brain, by depressing inhibitory pathways (15). This is seen only at postsynaptic sites. Therefore, excitatory neuronal activity is no longer checked by opposing inhibitory forces. In essence, strychnine converts normal reflex neural activity into explosive excitatory activity. The slightest sensory stimuli (e.g., tactile, auditory, visual) may induce convulsions.

Glycine is a postsynaptic inhibitory neurotransmitter in the brain and spinal cord. Strychnine inhibits glycine receptors competitively (26). This probably explains its convulsant activity. In fact, a rare disorder called nonketotic hyperglycinemia can sometimes be treated with strychnine (10,60). In this disorder, glycine is not metabolized and accumulates in the brain, resulting in severe neurologic deficiency. Because strychnine competes with glycine at the receptor site, it may produce a therapeutic effect, although its efficacy is limited.

Characteristics of Poisoning

The major effects of strychnine intoxication result from generalized stimulation of the CNS (Table 16.6). The victim of strychnine-induced convulsions assumes a characteristic pattern during seizure (Fig. 16.2), with the exact configuration defined by whichever of the body's muscles predominate. In other words, the stronger of a set of extensor/flexor muscles will be stimulated in tonic fashion.

This usually involves maximal extension. The back will be hyperextended and arched in a position termed *opisthotonos*. In this position, only the crown of the head and the feet may touch the ground.

After the tonic phase of seizure, a period of symmetrical extensor bursts occurs. This is followed by postictal depression in which the victim may sleep. This depends on the number of convulsive episodes, their intensity, and the dose ingested. Bursts of sensory stimulation may continue to initiate outbursts of repeated symmetrical thrashing.

Muscles of the face and neck are the first to become stimulated and contract. As they stiffen, the person's face assumes a characteristic grimace. The victim soon becomes generally hyperactive. A slight sensory stimulus can initiate symmetrical extensions, or in more advanced stages of poisoning, a full-blown convulsion. All voluntary muscle, including the diaphragm, abdominal and thoracic muscles, will be fully contracted. Consequently, respiration that is increased initially due to the central stimulant effect, ceases during the convulsive episode. Convulsive periods may recur with each episode, followed by increased depression. These contractions involve great energy expenditure. Also, since respiration ceases during convulsions, the cause of central hypoxia becomes obvious. Between episodes, the victim's muscles are extremely painful and consciousness is maintained.

Blood lactate may increase causing metabolic acidosis. Lactic acid is a by-product of muscular activity and is increased during periods of strenuous contraction. Heart rate and blood pressure are raised slightly during con-

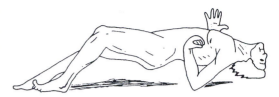

FIG. 16.2. Opisthotonos from a toxic overdose of strychnine. The body's weight in this example is supported entirely by the head and feet.

vulsive episodes as a result of sympathetic discharge.

A single large dose of strychnine may be sufficient to cause death from protracted convulsive episodes. Most victims, however, will sustain two to five convulsive episodes before death. Death is caused by medullary paralysis due to tissue hypoxia resulting from periods of severe muscle contraction. If a strychnine-poisoned patient is given a skeletal muscle relaxant to prevent seizures and is ventilated artificially, asphyxiation does not occur (54). The lethal dose of strychnine is reported to be approximately 15 mg for children and 30 to 100 mg for adults (15).

COCAINE

Cocaine may not be generally recognized as a central stimulant. However, central stimulation is one of its major pharmacologic and toxic actions. The euphoric effects of cocaine are caused by stimulation of the cerebral cortex. Even though cocaine has been used (abused!) for hundreds of years, use of cocaine has recently increased in the United States (28,40). There is no doubt that toxicity from overdose will continue to be a major problem for many years into the future.

Most cocaine use occurs by intranasal insufflation or inhalation of freebase cocaine, *crack*. A survey of cocaine users revealed that 61% were intranasal users, 21% smoked the freebase form, and 18% were IV users. Most fatalities follow intravenous use (40). Cocaine deaths have also been associated with *body packing*. In these cases, condoms or balloons filled with high purity cocaine have burst in-

TABLE 16.6. *Characteristics of strychnine toxicity*

Stiffness of facial and neck muscles
Hyperreactive reflexes
Lactic acidosis
Opisthotonos
Tetanic convulsions
Respiratory paralysis
Asphyxia
Death

side the GI tract while attempting to smuggle it out of or into a different country (61).

Mechanism of Toxicity

Cocaine interferes with reuptake of norepinephrine at adrenergic nerve endings. As a result, norepinephrine accumulates within the synaptic spaces and stimulates adrenergic receptors. Therefore, it produces sympathomimetic activity throughout the body. Cocaine has also been shown to block reuptake of dopamine and interfere with serotonin activity.

Characteristics of Poisoning

Signs and symptoms of cocaine toxicity are listed in Table 16.7. Feelings of euphoria or dysphoria may occur. Restlessness, excitement, and garrulousness can accompany euphoria. Motor coordination is not usually hampered at lower doses. With large doses, stimulation extends to the lower motor centers and cord reflexes. Muscular twitching is noted first and may be followed by clonic-tonic convulsions. Convulsions appear within 30 to 60 min after an acute oral toxic dose. The vom-

iting center may also be stimulated, and emesis is common.

As previously noted with other central stimulants, cocaine-induced convulsions are followed by central depression. Death from high doses is usually a result of medullary depression producing respiratory failure.

The sympathetic nervous system is stimulated both centrally and peripherally. Many CNS and cardiovascular effects listed in Table 16.7 are related to sympathomimetic activity. The most prominent cardiovascular feature is sinus tachycardia, which may produce ventricular arrhythmias. A direct toxic action on the myocardium has been shown occasionally after intravenous cocaine use (6,46).

Vasoconstriction is an outcome of sympathomimetic action on blood vessels. Vasoconstriction, combined with increased heart rate, produces hypertension. These initial effects are followed by hypotension and circulatory failure.

Hyperpyrexia may occur and be a contributory factor in cocaine death. It probably results from (a) increased body heat production as a result of increased muscular activity, (b) restricted heat loss due to vasoconstriction, or (c) direct stimulation of the heat-regulation center.

The effect of cocaine on the respiratory sys-

TABLE 16.7. *Characteristics of cocaine intoxication ("Caine reaction")*

Phase	CNA	Circulatory system	Respiratory system

Early stimulative	Excitement
	Apprehension
	Headache
	Nausea
	Vomiting
	Twitching of small facial
	  muscles, fingers
		Pulse variations; usually
		  will slow
		Blood pressure; elevation,
		  decrease
		Skin pallor
			Increased respiratory
			  rate and depth

Advanced stimulative	Seizures; tonic, clonic Hyperkinesis	Increased pulse Increased blood pressure	Cyanosis Dyspnea Rapid or irregular respiration
Depressive	Muscle paralysis Loss of reflexes Unconsciousness Loss of vital functions Death	Circulatory failure Death	Respiratory failure Cyanosis Death

tem follows the same progression: initial stimulation resulting in tachypnea, followed by dyspnea and respiratory failure.

CAMPHOR

Camphor-containing products are not generally considered by the laity to be toxic. Indeed, camphor has long been used externally as a rubefacient, mild analgesic, antipruritic, and counterirritant. As recently as the early 20th century, it was still listed in American and European literature as a cardiovascular stimulant (22). In the 1940s oral and subcutaneous uses were promoted to treat cardiac or respiratory collapse and fainting.

Internal and parenteral preparations of camphor are no longer available. However, the variety of proprietary products containing camphor (Table 16.8) attests to its continued popularity.

Over the years numerous reports of camphor poisoning have appeared. Overall incidence will decrease in the next few years, since the Food and Drug Administration imposed restrictions on sale of camphorated oil (180 mg camphor per mL) in the United States (14). Camphorated oil has been the largest single cause of camphor-related poisonings. Most poisonings have occurred because victims mistook it for castor oil, or other remedies that either sounded like or looked like camphorated oil, and ingested an unsuspected toxic dose (58).

One teaspoonful of camphorated oil may result in serious toxicity in adults, although recovery has occurred after ingestion of 1.5 ounces (16). Recall that the average volume of a swallow is 5 mL for a child, and 14 to 21 mL for an adult (27). A fatal dose, especially in a child, could easily be ingested with a single swallow.

Mechanism of Toxicity

The precise mechanism for inducing toxic symptoms is elusive. Camphor stimulates the brain at all levels. Necropsy of a 19-month-

TABLE 16.8. *Representative proprietary products that contain camphor*

Acne products
Komed
Analgesic (external) products
Absorbent Rub Relief Formula
Act-on-Rub
Analbalm
Banalg
Dencorub
Emul-O-Balm
Heet
Mentholatum
Mustarole
Panalgesic
Pronto Gel
Sloan's Liniment
Soltice Quick Rub
Antitussive; congestion products
Vicks VapoRub
Vicks Vapo Steam
Hemorrhoidal products
Pazo
Insect sting and bite products
Campho-Phenique
Chiggerex
Obtundia products
Poison ivy/oak products
Caladryl
Calamatum
Calamox
Ivarest
Ziradryl

old child who died from 1 g camphor revealed profuse dermal, bowel, stomach, and kidney hemorrhaging, and extensive degenerative changes in central neurons, especially in Sommer's section of the hippocampus (55). This neuronal damage could explain symptoms of severe CNS stimulation. The liver and kidney may show fatty degeneration.

Characteristics of Poisoning

Signs and symptoms of camphor poisoning may appear within 5 to 15 min after ingestion, or be delayed for several hours on a full stomach. Because it is highly lipid soluble, camphor enters the CNS quickly. Clinical manifestations of intoxication are listed in Table 16.9. Any odor of camphor on the breath or in urine should be considered positive for

TABLE 16.9. *Characteristics of camphor toxicity*

Nausea, vomiting
Burning in mouth, throat, and stomach
Dizziness
Dilirium, hallucinations
Dyspnea
Cold, clammy skin
Face alternately pale and flushed
Pulse rapid and weak
Irritation, excitement, convulsions
Depression following CNS stimulation
Muscle tremors and rigidity
Urinary retention, anuria
Transient hepatic damage

camphor poisoning. Death is from status epilepticus or postictal respiratory failure. If the victim survives, there are usually no residual problems extending beyond the initial encounter.

MANAGEMENT OF CNS STIMULANT TOXICITY

Treatment of CNS stimulant poisoning is directed primarily toward management of hyperthermia, convulsive episodes, normalization of blood pressure, and protecting against arrhythmia. Additionally, management should include gastrointestinal decontamination and methods to increase excretion (refer to chapter 3 for specific details). For most central stimulants, treatment is nonspecific and directed toward symptomatic care. However, in some cases, specific procedures may be beneficial. Table 16.10 summarizes many of the clinical manifestations associated with CNS stimulants, and Fig. 16.3 outlines procedures generally used in management of stimulant poisonings.

Amphetamines and Amphetamine-like Drugs

Amphetamine-poisoned patients often present with acute psychosis, delirium, or extreme anxiety. Phenothiazines have been recommended for treatment of amphetamine-in-duced psychosis, which is due to excess dopamine. Chlorpromazine has also been shown to reverse hyperthermia, convulsions, and hypertension associated with amphetamine toxicity without causing depression. The dose is repeated every 30 min as needed. Haloperidol has been advocated also since it produces less respiratory depression and reduced chance for sustained hypotension and reflex tachycardia (18). Both drugs are direct antagonists to amphetamine. Barbiturates antagonize amphetamine, but only when given in anesthetic doses.

Adverse effects of chlorpromazine and haloperidol include lowering the seizure threshold (see chapter 15). Their use in amphetamine poisoning can enhance toxicity, and should be avoided. Diazepam is preferred.

Convulsions are usually associated with increased body temperature. Management of hyperthermia may include use of a hypothermic blanket or placing the patient in a cool, quiet room. Salicylates may be helpful in temperature reduction.

Reduction of Absorption and Elimination Enhancement

Once the patient has been stabilized, gastric decontamination should be considered. Recall that emetics are contraindicated in patients experiencing seizures. A suggested management protocol for ingestion of a large amount of amphetamine that occurred within 4 hr includes emesis with syrup of ipecac. Gastric lavage is recommended when emesis is contraindicated. After 4 hr, activated charcoal is preferred over emesis. Renal clearance of amphetamine is enhanced by acidification of urine with ammonium chloride. In a study to demonstrate the effect of urine pH on amphetamine excretion, a pH value of 5.0 yielded 55% excretion of a dose of d-amphetamine within 16 hr, compared with 3% excretion at pH 8.0 (5).

Additional Measures

General measures of supportive and symptomatic care must be stressed. The victim

TABLE 16.10. *Summary of the clinical manifestations of CNS-stimulant toxicity*

Degree of toxicity	CVS[a]	CNS	Other
Mild	Tachycardia	Increased activity	"Goose bumps"
	Palpitations	Insomnia	Choreoathetoid movements
	Hypertension	Anxiety	Rapid shallow respirations
		Blank stare	Urinary retention
		Hyperthermia	Delayed gastric emptying
		Hyperreflexia	time
		Mydriasis	
		Blurred vision	
		Psychotic state	
Moderate	Pallor	Delirium	Diaphoresis
	Anginal pain	Confusion	
		Psychotic state	
		Pupils—dilated, sluggish	
		reaction to light	
		Nystagmus	
		Tremors	
Severe	Hypertensive crisis	Convulsions	Aspiration of vomitus
	Ventricular	Pupils—dilated,	Asphyxia
	fibrillation	nonreactive to light	Respiratory failure
	Circulatory collapse	Hyperthermia (>109°F)	Death
	Death	Coma	
		Death	

[a] CVS, cardiovascular system.

should be placed in a quiet environment, away from sensory stimulation, as this may precipitate further convulsions. Protection from self-inflicted harm using padded bed rails and physical restraints may be necessary. In severe

Correct life-threatening effects
CNS stimulation — chlorpromazine
Convulsions   — diazepam
Hypertension   — α-blocker, sodium
                              nitroprusside
Hyperthermia   — chlorpromazine

Prevent further absorption
Emesis   } (if seizures are absent)
Gastric lavage }
Activated charcoal
Saline cathartic

Enhance elimination
Forced acidic diuresis

Supportive and symptomatic care
Cool, quiet environment— to minimize external stimuli
Monitor electrolytes
Monitor vital functions
Obtain psychiatric consult

FIG. 16.3. Management of acute CNS stimulant poisoning.

toxicity, aggressive care to manage hypertension, tachycardia, seizures, and hyperthermia are given high priority.

Methylxanthine Derivatives

Management of caffeine or theophylline poisonings follows the same basic treatment procedures as described for other central stimulants (see Fig. 16.2). This includes gastric evacuation for large ingestions, and appropriate supportive and symptomatic care. Dialysis or hemoperfusion can lower toxic plasma concentrations significantly (51).

Theophylline

Seizures denote serious morbidity and grave prognosis. More than one-third of all patients who develop seizures from theophylline overdose will die or sustain severe neurologic sequelae (19). Therefore, seizures must be terminated quickly.

Theophylline-induced seizures are difficult to manage. In one cohort of 78 patients with seizure activity, more than 90% had intractable seizures despite receiving multiple anticonvulsants (19). Diazepam is often recommended as first-line therapy, but it often fails to control the problem (45,47). Still, diazepam should be given first. If it fails to control seizures, phenobarbital should be administered. If the patient has still not responded within 20 min, thiopental may be given (19). Such poor responders are definitely candidates for hemoperfusion.

Arrhythmias can usually be controlled with propranolol or verapamil. These block the SA and AV nodes, and also restore coronary blood flow by reversing theophylline-induced hypotension. These two actions decrease the overall myocardial demand for oxygen and correct minor myocardial ischemia induced by theophylline. The risk for arrhythmia is, therefore, reduced (8).

Of course, treatment may be complicated when propranolol is used. Beta-blockers can cause bronchospasm in asthmatic patients, which will magnify pulmonary pathology. Serum theophylline concentrations are helpful in management of acute overdoses.

Strychnine

Strychnine poisoning is managed in ways similar to other acute stimulant poisonings. All efforts at treatment must be directed toward prevention of convulsions. If the victim of strychnine poisoning is treated quickly, prognosis for complete, uneventful recovery is good (see the case study "Strychnine Poisoning," case 1, at the end of this chapter). The alkaloid is rapidly excreted through the kidney with 70% excretion reported within 6 hr (57). In fact, a patient theoretically can take two lethal doses in a 24-hr period without experiencing cumulative effects (15).

Diazepam provides superior control of tonic convulsions, without potentiating postictal depression. On occasion, a patient will experience depressed respirations with diazepam, but this is rare (29).

Keeping the victim quiet and away from all forms of sensory stimulation is extremely important. The slightest stimulation can evoke a seizure with opisthotonos.

Reduction of Absorption and Elimination Enhancement

Strychnine is rapidly absorbed from the GI tract. Seizure activity may occur within several minutes and tonic convulsions with 15 to 30 min. Therefore, measures to remove the alkaloid from the GI tract must be initiated shortly after ingestion. Before convulsant activity, emetics or lavage may be used. Activated charcoal also adsorbs strychnine. Forced diuresis or dialysis are probably of minimal value since strychnine is normally cleared rapidly from the blood.

Cocaine

Management of cocaine toxicity involves many of the same procedures described for amphetamine. The patient's condition must be quickly assessed and emergency measures undertaken to stabilize vital signs.

Diazepam is the drug of first choice to control cocaine-induced seizures. When seizure control is inadequate, phenobarbital may be substituted.

Cardiovascular effects must be treated aggressively. Propranolol, a beta-adrenergic blocking agent, will normally reverse and control hypertension and tachycardia (42–44). Intravenous doses will restore blood pressure and heart rate to normal within several minutes.

If the victim is in the depression stage of poisoning (hypotension), attention must be directed immediately toward raising the blood pressure. Intravenous fluids and vasopressors such as dopamine are indicated at this point.

Hyperthermia must also be controlled. Procedures discussed for amphetamine will be undertaken for victims of cocaine poisoning.

Cocaine-induced psychosis with hallucinations, paranoia, and hyperexcitability requires treatment. Neuroleptic agents have been used with success. More recently, lithium has been used (50).

Enhanced Elimination

Although some studies imply that forced diuresis with acidification of urine enhances cocaine excretion, neither procedure is accepted universally. Dialysis and hemoperfusion are generally ineffective for enhancing excretion.

Removal of cocaine-filled condoms or balloons from within the GI tract can usually be safely accomplished with oral cathartics. If unsuccessful, surgery may be required to remove them to prevent breakage (28).

Camphor

Camphor must be removed from the stomach as quickly as possible. Immediate emesis or gastric lavage is indicated (before convulsions and generalized stimulation occur). Activated charcoal should follow. Lavage should be continued until the odor of camphor is no longer detected. It has been suggested that whenever the quantity ingested is unknown, it should be assumed the amount was greater than 1 g, and the patient should be vigorously treated (53).

Barbiturates have long been used to control convulsions, but diazepam is generally preferred because it produces less respiratory depression. Hemodialysis will hasten removal of camphor from the blood. Succinylcholine may be used to help control muscular rigidity and spasm. As with any other CNS stimulant, the patient must be kept quiet and at minimum sensory input.

SUMMARY

A large number of drugs can cause stimulation of the CNS, leading to convulsions. Many of these drugs are well known as convulsants. Others are not generally recognized by the public as stimulants; their toxic potential is therefore greater.

Management of CNS stimulants is mostly nonspecific, directed toward controlling symptoms. Review these once again, following the steps outlined in Fig. 16.2.

Case Studies

CASE STUDIES: AMPHETAMINE TOXICITY

History: Case 1

A 16-year-old girl was taken to the emergency room an hour after confessing to her mother that she had ingested a large handful of what was supposedly mescaline tablets. Instead, she actually consumed an unknown amount of amphetamine. Gastric lavage was performed immediately and the victim admitted. Shortly, she became agitated, and experienced auditory hallucinations and insomnia that persisted for 2 days. She was discharged on the third day after showing constant improvement.

Two days later, she began experiencing auditory hallucinations again, this time with delusions. Moreover, she showed signs of stereotypic behavior by playing with the control dials on a television for 2 hr. She claimed to be conversing with deceased relatives, to have been appointed by God as a church elder, and that Satan had fathered her 16-month-old child.

She was readmitted to the hospital where she was treated with haloperidol, hydroxyzine, flurazepam, propoxyphene, and chlorpromazine at bedtime. Approximately 8 to 10 days later, she no longer experienced psychotic symptoms, and was discharged on the 14th hospital day. (See ref. 38)

History: Case 2

A 21-year-old man was brought to the Emergency Department after ingestion of an

TABLE 16.11. *Laboratory findings*

Hematocrit	=50%
WBCs[a]	=16,700/mm³
Na⁺	=151 mEq/L
K⁺	=5.8 mEq/L
Cl⁻	=108 mEq/L
Glucose	=95 mg/dL

[a] WBCs, white blood cells.

estimated 2.2 g amphetamine sulfate that he took in a suicide gesture.

On examination 1 hr after ingestion, he was fully oriented and agitated. He quickly became hyperkinetic and incoherent.

Physical findings included pulse, 168 beats/min; blood pressure, 160/80 mm Hg; rectal temperature, 108.4°F; and respirations, rapid and shallow at 48/min. His skin was blanched and slightly moist. Pupils were dilated to about 6 mm, and reacted minimally to light. The conjunctivae were edematous. It was not possible to move his head in any direction, but all extremities were moved easily and reflexes were normally reactive. Laboratory analysis revealed the information in Table 16.11.

Treatment consisted of vigorous gastric lavage, followed by chlorpromazine and pentobarbital. After chlorpromazine, the patient became hypotensive (60 mm Hg systolic) but resumed an adequate blood pressure when fluids were given. His temperature decreased to 101.6°F after immersion in an ice bath and massage. By 12 hr after admission, his temperature had returned to normal.

Twelve hours after admission, petechiae were noted over his lower extremities. His hematocrit fell 20 points over the next 5 days. He also developed acute renal failure. The patient responded slowly to all treatment, but eventually improved. He was discharged on the 37th hospital day. (See ref. 20.)

Discussion

1. When patient 1 was first brought to the hospital, the cause of intoxication was unknown. What specific laboratory test could have been performed to designate amphetamine as the probable cause of poisoning? What typical symptoms of amphetamine toxicity did this patient display?

2. Are hallucinations expected in all amphetamine overdoses? How should they be treated?

3. What are some of the reasons why patient 2 did not succumb to the dose of amphetamine he allegedly ingested?

4. Is reduction in hematocrit a typical finding in CNS stimulant overdose? What is the pathogenesis of low hematocrit in patient 2?

CASE STUDY: PHENYLPROPANOLAMINE INTOXICATION

History

An 18-year-old girl ingested eight diet tablets, each containing 50 mg phenylpropanolamine and 200 mg caffeine. She was seen approximately 2 hr later in an emergency facility. Blood pressure was 140/90 mm Hg, and pulse, 52 beats/min. Neurologic examination failed to disclose abnormalities. She was given atropine sulfate, and gastrointestinal decontamination with lavage. She was then discharged.

Shortly after discharge she experienced several generalized convulsions and was brought back to the emergency facility. She was lethargic, but awake and oriented. Her medical history revealed neurologic testing six years earlier to locate a possible cause of headaches. Test results were inconclusive; no pathology was found.

Within a couple hours, there was an abrupt decline in the patient's mental state. She lost all brainstem reflexes. Examination of spinal fluid revealed blood. She quickly deteriorated and died before further assistance could be given.

A postmortem examination revealed right intracerebral hematoma with rupture into the lateral ventricle and subarachnoid space. The brain was diffusely swollen. (See ref. 34.)

Discussion

1. Characterize the nature of phenylpropanol-amine and explain its pharmacologic actions. Postulate the role that caffeine had on the response to the stimulant, phenyl-propanolamine.
2. Why was atropine given during the first hospital admission?
3. Was there any way to predict this toxic event *a priori*, based upon the information presented?

CASE STUDY: METHYLPHENIDATE OVERDOSE

History

A 28-year-old woman walked into an emergency facility complaining of nausea and vomiting, shortness of breath, and intense anxiety. She indicated that she had recently given herself an intravenous injection of 40 mg methylphenidate (Ritalin). The drug source was Ritalin tablets, which she crushed, made into a "solution," and injected. She had used methylphenidate by this process on several previous occasions without problem.

Examination revealed needle tracks up to 6 inches in length along her left forearm. There was no evidence of other external injury.

Within 1 hr of arrival she became hypertensive. Shortly, she experienced cardiac arrest. The resuscitation attempt was unsuccessful, and she died.

At autopsy, the victim had an enlarged right ventricle and congested lungs. Microscopic examination of lung tissue revealed severe generalized granulomatoses and giant cells, with polarizable crystals. Analysis of blood revealed a methylphenidate concentration of 2.8 mg/L, more than 40 times greater than high therapeutic levels. There was 1.6 mg total drug in the stomach contents, even though she had not taken any drug orally. (See ref. 33.)

Discussion

1. One can speculate as to the cause of the abnormal pulmonary pathology. What do you think caused it?
2. Explain how the drug got into the stomach contents.

CASE STUDIES: FATALITIES FROM CAFFEINE-CONTAINING "LOOK-ALIKE" DRUGS

History: Case 1

A 23-year-old man, accompanied by his wife and brother, were drinking mixed drinks at a local pub. They left for home and shortly after arriving, the man's mother heard him coughing. She checked on him, and found he was experiencing respiratory difficulty. She also knew that the son and his wife had been experimenting with drugs, so she called the emergency medical service.

Arriving quickly, they found the man unconscious. He was transported to the hospital where he expired shortly thereafter.

The mother later indicated that the brother confessed that the deceased had taken "one-half of a pill" before leaving the pub. Also, the deceased's wife had flushed numerous pills down the toilet after the emergency medical service arrived! (See ref. 17.)

History: Case 2

This was a 21-year-old woman who, along with her husband, had been on a picnic the day before her death. She supposedly consumed 10 to 12 beers during the day, arrived home late, and retired between 3:00 and 4:00 a.m. The husband awoke at 5:00 a.m. and found his wife dead. He told the authorities that his wife had been purchasing diet pills from a magazine mail-order house, and had been taking only two a day. (See ref. 17.)

Discussion

Both victims were taking caffeine-containing nonprescription look-alike stimulant products. The amounts were not documented. Toxicologic analysis of blood samples revealed caffeine concentrations of 18.4 mg/dL (patient 1), and 25.1 mg/dL (patient 2). Both had large quantities of undissolved caffeine in their gastric contents. Both had blood alcohol concentrations around 0.1%. Neither had significant amounts of other drugs in their blood.

1. Discuss whether it is probable for toxicity, or death, to result from using these products at their recommended doses. What is the therapeutic blood concentration for caffeine?
2. What can be done to curtail availability and use of nonprescription look-alike products?
3. How much, if any, did the blood alcohol concentration in these cases contribute to the deaths?

CASE STUDY: CAFFEINE INTOXICATION

History

A 19-year-old woman had been riding her bicycle during the afternoon until she developed abdominal cramps and became ill. She retired early in the evening complaining of constant abdominal discomfort.

At 3:00 a.m., the father was awakened, and found her on the bathroom floor, doubled over at the waist. She was semicomatose and her breathing was irregular and shallow. He summoned a paramedical team and began mouth-to-mouth resuscitation on her. Paramedics found her in coarse ventricular fibrillation, and they attempted cardioversion. They then transported her to the hospital.

On arrival (3 hr after her father discovered her), she was unable to maintain a cardiac rhythm. Resuscitation attempts continued for 15 min, then were discontinued. She died without regaining consciousness, and before any vital signs or other laboratory values could be obtained.

Later, the family indicated that the girl had been in good health. A medical examination 6 weeks previously failed to reveal any abnormalities. She had been on a self-imposed diet over the past year and her weight had dropped from 180 to 100 pounds. She had a history of using OTC dietary aid products.

A toxicologic analysis of blood and stomach contents revealed she had been taking high doses of caffeine. A sample of heart blood contained a caffeine concentration of 18.1 mg/dL. Gastric contents contained approximately 18 g of caffeine. There was no further information that suggested a cause of death. (See ref. 35.)

Discussion

1. There are at least three clues in this case study that reveal the probable cause of this patient's death. What are they?
2. Speculate on what might have happened if this person had arrived at the hospital earlier in the evening. Describe the supportive treatment she probably would have received.

CASE STUDY: THEOPHYLLINE TOXICITY AS A RESULT OF ALTERED METABOLISM

History

A 66-year-old woman was admitted to the hospital with dyspnea on exertion, pleuritic chest pain, orthopnea, fever, and palpitations. A permanent pacemaker had been implanted 4 years previously. She was taking furosemide, digoxin, potassium chloride, and levothyroxine at the time of admission.

She was prescribed theophylline 200-mg slow-release capsules, to be taken twice a day. By the second hospital day she improved. All laboratory values, including drug levels, were within the normal range.

On day 3, the patient complained of severe

nausea. Neither dimenhydrinate nor prochlorperazine relieved it.

On day 5, a single 200-mg dose of quinidine was administered inadvertently (The case report failed to state why or how it was given). Shortly, she developed atrioventricular tachycardia/fibrillation. A lidocaine drip was started, along with concurrent administration of codeine, meperidine, and diazepam. The digitalis blood level on day 5 was 1.6 ng/mL. An elevated bilirubin on day 6 was noted.

Over the next few days the patient's nausea continued to worsen. She did not respond to antinauseant therapy. Theophylline toxicity was suspected on day 8, and a blood sample taken for assay. A subsequent value of 60.6 μg/mL was revealed, and the theophylline was discontinued. Subsequent theophylline concentrations on hospital days 9, 10, and 12 were 52.8, 39.8, and 16.3 μg/mL, respectfully. By day 13, all symptoms had resolved. Her chest was clear, she regained her appetite, and she was ambulatory at discharge.

A pharmacokinetic study investigated why this person reacted adversely to theophylline. It revealed that for some reason, she metabolized the drug by zero-order kinetics, rather than first-order. (See ref. 32).

Discussion

1. This case study strongly illustrates that all patients should be closely monitored for plasma theophylline concentrations when placed on the drug, regardless of dose. What about the dose this patient took? Was it within the normal therapeutic range for an adult?
2. Was the serum digoxin concentration of 1.6 ng/mL on day 5 within the normal therapeutic range?
3. What was the first clue in this case study that this person was possibly reacting adversely to theophylline?
4. Discuss the meaning of the terms first-order and second-order kinetics. What is the importance of knowing the kinetics of a drug metabolism?

CASE STUDY: FATAL THEOPHYLLINE INTOXICATION

History

An 80-year-old man with a history of congestive obstructive pulmonary disease visited his physician for routine examination. He had a history of liver disease, heavy smoking and alcoholism, and peptic ulcer disease. On a previous visit he had been prescribed cimetidine 300 mg at bedtime, and 100 mg-tablets of theophylline, taken three times a day. He was doing well. To simplify his dosing regimen, the physician changed his theophylline prescription to a 200 mg long-acting product, to be taken twice a day.

Four days later, he was admitted to an emergency facility with persistent nausea and vomiting, and headache. Examining physicians believed his gastrointestinal symptoms resulted from a worsening of his peptic ulcer disease. They increased his cimetidine to 300 mg four times daily. He was released.

Three days later he returned to the emergency facility with continued nausea and vomiting, and confusion. He experienced a seizure on arrival.

Examination showed the patient to be lethargic and confused. His pulse was rapid and irregular. Systolic blood pressure was 60 mm Hg. ECG showed atrial fibrillation with rapid ventricular response to 150 to 170 beats/min.

The patient remained confused, with tachycardia, and hypotension. Attempts were made to convert the fibrillation and he was placed on digitalis intravenously. He developed seizures and was given diazepam. Blood pressure dropped further, bradycardia developed, and he soon died. Meanwhile, a blood sample that had been taken at the time of admission, but not previously analyzed for theophylline, was assayed. It disclosed a theophylline concentration of 80 mg/L. (See ref. 1).

Discussion

1. Outline the specific events, beginning with this person's first prescriptions for cimetidine and theophylline, that led to his death.

2. Convert the theophylline blood concentration at the time of death (i.e., 80 mg/L) to μg/mL. Would this value have contributed to the adverse cardiovascular events?

CASE STUDY: STRYCHNINE POISONING

History: Case 1

The patient was a 34-year-old woman who had a medical history of personality disorders and attempted suicides. She was brought to the hospital about 30 min after ingesting a rodenticide product containing approximately 340 mg strychnine.

Upon admission the patient was alert and displayed continuous spontaneous muscular twitches. While she was being examined, she experienced a generalized tonic seizure with opisthotonos positioning. All the while she remained fully aware of her surroundings and was frightened. She maintained full voluntary respiration and showed no signs of cyanosis.

The victim's seizures were controlled with intravenous diazepam and succinylcholine. Thiopental sodium was administered to induce generalized anesthesia.

A nasogastric tube was then positioned and gastric lavage with saline performed. A slurry of activated charcoal and potassium permanganate (1:5000) was instilled through the tube.

Laboratory values are presented in Table 16.12. Treatment with diazepam was continued. Phenytoin, sodium bicarbonate, and potassium chloride were added to her drug regimen. Diuresis was forced with saline.

The patient awoke in a quiet, darkened room. She continued to display spastic contractions of the muscles of her limbs, back, and neck for the next several hours. However, by 6 hr postadmission, she had recovered fully and no further spastic activity was noted. (See ref. 31.)

History: Case 2

The patient was a 19-year-old man. He was transported to an emergency department approximately 30 min after intranasally snorting two lines of a white powder that he thought was cocaine. Within 15 to 30 min, he exhibited nervousness and uncontrollable and painful muscle twitching and spasms.

Physical examination revealed an alert and anxious man who responded to all types of stimuli with intermittent extensor spasms. These lasted from several seconds to several minutes. Vital signs included blood pressure, 150/50 mm Hg; pulse, 150 beats/min; temperature, 39.5°C; and respirations, 35/min and regular. Arterial blood had a pH value of 6.55. Twelve hours after admission, a blood specimen revealed a myoglobin level of 124 mg/dL (normal = 0).

By three hours after admission, the patient's body temperature had increased to 43°C. He was now less responsive, and became cyanotic during each spasm. He had been receiving sodium bicarbonate and 100% oxygen, but his arterial blood pH was still 6.73. He was therefore intubated, mechanically ventilated, paralyzed with pancuronium, and cooled. Muscle spasms ceased immediately.

TABLE 16.12. *Laboratory values of a victim of strychnine poisoning*[a]

Measurement	Admission to ED	Hours after arrival		
		0.5	1	3
Sodium (mmol/L)	148	139	139	142
Potassium (mm/L)	3.5	4.2	3.5	4.1
Chloride (mmol/L)	103	102	103	109
Bicarbonate (mmol/L)	9	4	18	24
Anion gap (mmol/L)	36	33	20	9
pH	—	7.02	7.33	7.41

[a] Modified from ref. 31.

By two hours of treatment, his body temperature decreased to 38°C, and arterial pH corrected to 7.37. Pancuronium was continued for 9 hr. The patient was extubated 20 hr after admission.

Convalescence was largely unremarkable, except for severe muscle weakness and myalgia. By six weeks after discharge, muscle strength had returned to normal. He experienced no further adverse sequelae. (See ref. 9.)

History: Case 3

Neighbors heard loud moans of pain coming from within a locked apartment. They called police and emergency personnel who forced entry into the apartment. There, they found a 56-year-old man lying on the floor, face down, writhing in pain. He was fully conscious and related that about 45 min earlier, he had ingested approximately one-half can of mole poison containing strychnine sulfate (calculated ingested dose was approximately 260 mg).

The victim was lifted to a couch. He was then observed to have a tonic seizure with extreme body rigidity and opisthotonos, followed by a period of total flaccidity. The patient stopped breathing and appeared cyanotic during the tonic phase of the attack. After another few moments, he experienced another attack, then lost consciousness and collapsed. Emergency personnel had not yet had a chance to take his vital signs. Cardiopulmonary resuscitation was attempted, but the patient died. An autopsy was performed 3 hr later. The body was still extremely rigid. (See ref. 37.)

Discussion

1. Cite the reason why the patient in case 1 was acidotic and had an anion gap of 33. Would a similar condition exist for other patients poisoned with (a) strychnine and (b) other convulsants? Comment on why this patient was placed in a quiet, darkened recovery room.

2. It seems that the victim in case 1 was not lavaged until after she was under generalized anesthesia. Why did the treating physicians wait so long?

3. The patient in case 2 experienced elevated body temperature, and had a blood myoglobin concentration well above normal. What was the physiologic cause of each event?

4. Discuss the type of drug that pancuronium represents. Why did the patient in case 2 need mechanical ventilation while he received this drug?

5. Patient 3 was moved from the floor onto a couch, shortly after which time he suffered a tonic convulsion. Considering all of the facts presented in this case study, would he have experienced the convulsions if he had been left to lie on the floor of the apartment? Also, what do you think about how emergency personnel entered the man's apartment. There must have been massive commotion! Would this have contributed to increase the toxicity of strychnine?

CASE STUDIES: COCAINE INTOXICATION

History: Case 1

This case involved a 38-year-old man who had a history of light cigarette smoking (40 packs per year). He did not suffer from diabetes mellitus, hypertension, or hyperlipidemia, and had never experienced a myocardial infarction. There also was no family history of any of these conditions. On routine medical examination, he was found to be slightly overweight. His pulse was 68 beats/min, and blood pressure 120/80 mm Hg. His physical condition was otherwise normal, as were all laboratory test results, chest X-ray films, and ECG recording.

Approximately one year later, he was admitted to a hospital complaining of dizziness and a feeling of "heaviness" in his left arm. On examination, a subendocardial anterolateral myocardial infarction was discovered.

Isoenzyme studies revealed an increased serum creatinine phosphokinase (CPK) level of 310 IU/L (normal: 2 to 83), with elevated MB bands.

He recovered from this infarction and was eventually able to walk 3 miles a day without difficulty. He remained symptom-free until approximately 3 years later.

At that time he experienced pain in his chest and left neck area, dyspnea, diaphoresis, and felt anxious and nervous after snorting (inhaling) approximately 500 mg cocaine. His blood pressure was 151/98 mm Hg, and pulse rate was 88 beats/min. His ECG failed to reveal any abnormalities, and the chest pain was relieved with nitroglycerin. The diagnosis was angina, and he was sent home.

He abstained from cocaine use for about 6 months, but after again snorting cocaine he experienced substernal chest pressure radiating to the left arm, as well as dyspnea and sweating.

On admission to an emergency facility, his blood pressure was 130/90 mm Hg; pulse rate, 96 beats/min; and an S_1-gallop rhythm was noted. The ECG showed an elevated ST segment and a flattened T wave. Pain was alleviated with nitrates and morphine sulfate. An inferolateral subendocardial myocardial infarction was noted on ECG examination.

The patient stopped using cocaine after that incident and has remained symptom-free. He has also returned to work full-time without apparent sequelae. (See ref. 11.)

History: Case 2

A 25-year-old man had been admitted to a hospital for psychiatric care on two previous occasions as a result of drug abuse problems. He was admitted again, this time in a psychotic state due to the use of large quantities of cocaine.

The patient believed he had special powers that could solve the current world problems, and he felt he was in constant communication with government agencies, including the FBI and CIA. He also claimed he was writing a book about his experiences that would be the salvation of mankind. Overall, he was grandiose, paranoid, and hyperactive.

Treatment consisted of neuroleptic agents, but when side effects developed, he refused further medication. Lithium therapy was therefore initiated, and when serum levels reached 0.7 mEq/L, his psychotic behavior subsided. He then started to attend group psychotherapy and was soon released from the hospital. He became productive to society without recurrence of his former psychotic episode. (See ref. 50.)

History: Case 3

A 26-year-old man boarded an airplane in Colombia that was destined for the United States. About 45 min after takeoff, he began to experience nausea. Oxygen was administered by flight attendants. However, 75 min later he experienced a generalized seizure and died.

On autopsy, 27 rubber condoms measuring about 2 cm in diameter were found in his stomach. Each contained approximately 5 g of a white powder, consisting of 35% cocaine. The bags were tied closed with string. One of these bags had ruptured.

Gross examination of the patient's tissues revealed pulmonary congestion and edema, hepatic congestion, and gastric hyperemia. (See ref. 61.)

Discussion

1. Explain the probable origin of the heart irregularities displayed by the patient in case 1.

2. Do symptoms experienced by patient 2 sound like they were caused by cocaine? Characterize cocaine symptoms.

3. Discuss the mechanism of how cocaine caused patient 3 to convulse.

CASE STUDIES: CAMPHOR INTOXICATION

History: Cases 1 and 2

Male and female twins, aged 39 months, were found by their mother at 1:45 a.m., 15 min after the family had returned home from an evening of visiting friends. The boy was on the floor, convulsing. The girl was holding an empty bottle that had contained camphorated oil. Both children smelled of camphor, so they were rushed to a hospital.

Upon admission, both children were lavaged and given diazepam and phenobarbital intravenously, to control convulsions. The boy vomited spontaneously, revealing a quantity of undigested food. He was again lavaged and the returning solution revealed a strong odor of camphor. Shortly thereafter, he experienced respiratory arrest, but his breathing was supported artificially. Over the next 24 hr, he experienced three additional seizures.

The sister was convulsing by the time she arrived at the hospital. She also vomited undigested food spontaneously. Lavage revealed a thick, yellow, oily material that smelled of camphor. She later experienced another convulsion, and after a 24-hr period of intense neuromuscular irritability, resumed normal activity.

Both children were discharged after 4 days of intensive supportive care. The quantity of poison ingested by either child was not determined. (See ref. 2.)

History: Case 3

A 3-year-old girl suffering from generalized seizures was brought to the emergency room. Two hours before, she had projectile vomiting and complained of intense gastric discomfort. Upon admission, secobarbital was given intramuscularly, and within 30 min the seizures were controlled.

Vital signs included: respiration, 28/min; pulse, 126 beats/min; temperature, 36.4°C; blood pressure, 120/90 mm Hg. The only other immediate finding was a distinct odor of camphor on her breath.

The mother revealed that she had been applying Vicks VapoRub (4.81% camphor) intranasally, twice a day for 5 months, because of the child's persistent rhinorrhea. Two hours before the convulsion, the child was found with an open jar of the product. An estimated tablespoonful (0.7 g camphor) was missing.

Previously, the child enjoyed the taste of the product, often sucking on the cotton-tipped applicator used to apply it.

All laboratory tests for pathology were negative. Serum concentration of camphor was determined to be 1.95 mg/dL. The child was discharged 24 hr after admission. A follow-up examination with an EEG 15 days later was normal. (See ref. 39.)

Discussion

1. Comment on the fact that patients 1 and 2 had food in their stomach. Did this increase or decrease absorption of the poison, and on what information do you base your answer?
2. What was stated about patient 3 that leads you to suspect she also had food in her stomach at the time of poisoning?
3. Assuming that these three patients had not responded positively to the treatment they received, what would have been the next step?

Review Questions

1. A toxic dose of amphetamine would be expected to produce which of the following symptoms of poisoning: tachypnea (I), hypertension (II), or tachycardia (III)?
   A. II only
   B. III only
   C. I and II only
   D. II and III only
   E. I, II, and III
2. All of the following are true statements *except*:

A. Cocaine causes direct stimulation of the heat-regulation center.

B. Death from camphor poisoning is caused by hemorrhaging into the GI tract.

C. Opisthotonos is a characteristic symptom of strychnine poisoning.

D. Amphetamine excretion is enhanced by forced diuresis and urine acidification.

3. Which of the following convulsants is a cause of euphoria, along with its other manifestations of CNS stimulation: strychnine (I), camphor (II), or cocaine (III)?

A. II only

B. III only

C. I and II only

D. II and III only

E. I, II, and III

4. Which of the following is a true statement?

A. The largest single cause of camphor poisoning has been camphorated oil.

B. Motor coordination is adversely affected at minimal doses of cocaine that cause euphoria.

C. Strychnine action on the CNS is restricted to the motor cortex.

D. The acute lethal adult dose for amphetamine is 5 mg/kg.

5. In which of the following situations is emesis contraindicated?

A. Ingestion of 30 amphetamine sulfate tablets.

B. Ingestion of 15 mL of camphorated oil.

C. Ingestion of five 300 mg theophylline tablets with seizures.

D. Ingestion of 12 look-alike amphetamine capsules.

6. Severe hypertension, as a result of amphetamine poisoning, is best treated with:

A. Isoproterenol

B. Propranolol

C. Nitroprusside

D. Nitroglycerin

7. The mechanism of action of theophylline may be due to:

A. Blocking catecholamine reuptake

B. Decreasing sodium conduction

C. Increasing intracellular cAMP concentration

D. Blocking alpha-adrenergic receptors

8. Sympathomimetic effects of amphetamine, cocaine, or caffeine may include all of the following except:

A. Miosis

B. Hypertension

C. Hyperthermia

D. Increased intestinal motility

9. Which of the following are recommended to control amphetamine-induced seizures?

A. Phenothiazines

B. Diazepam

C. Haloperidol

D. Phenytoin

10. Which of the following inhibits glycine competitively?

A. Cocaine

B. Theophylline

C. Strychnine

D. Camphor

11. Which of the following best describes the action of theophylline toxicity?

A. Block catecholamine reuptake

B. Enhance catecholamine release

C. Inhibit Na^+/K^+ ATPase

D. Increase cyclic nucleotides

E. Block alpha-adrenergic receptors

12. Which of the following is a symptom of amphetamine toxicity: diaphoresis (I), hypertension (II), or increased intestinal motility (III)?

A. I only

B. III only

C. I and II only

D. I and III only

E. I, II and III

13. Excessive adrenergic discharge, secondary to drugs such as cocaine or amphetamine, will cause all of the following except:

A. Hyperpyrexia

B. Hypertension

C. Hyperactive bowel sounds

D. Miosis

E. Diaphoresis

14. Overdoses with sympathetic stimulants, such as amphetamines, can be differentiated from an anticholinergic overdose by the presence of:

A. Tachycardia

B. Urinary retention

C. Dilated pupils

D. Hyperactive bowel sounds

15. To enhance the excretion of amphetamine:

A. The urine should be alkalinized with acetazolamide

B. The urine should be acidified with ascorbic acid

C. The urine should be alkalinized with NaHCO$_3$

D. The urine should be acidified with ammonium chloride

16. Toxic doses of amphetamine may cause hallucinations in certain individuals. Describe these reactions and relate their occurrence to the victim's dosing history.

17. Diazepam is the drug of first choice for controlling convulsive episodes caused by strychnine. Cite the reasons why it is preferred.

18. What is postictal depression? What causes it, and what is its toxic significance?

19. Discuss the medical significance of amphetamine-induced hyperpyrexia.

20. Explain what is meant by the following statement, "Strychnine causes a characteristic convulsive pattern, but it may differ in various people."

References

1. Anderson JR, Poklis A, Slavin RG. A fatal case of theophylline intoxication. *Arch Intern Med* 1963; 143:559–560.
2. Aronow R, Spigiel RW. Implications of camphor poisoning. *Drug Intell Clin Pharm* 1976; 10:631–634.
3. Baker MD. Theophylline toxicity in children. *J Pediatr* 1985; 109:538–542.
4. Baldessarini RJ. Pharmacology of the amphetamines. *Pediatrics* 1972; 49:694–701.
5. Beckett AH, Rowland M, Tutner P. Influence of urinary pH on excretion of amphetamine. *Lancet* 1965; 1:303.
6. Benchimol A, Bartall H, Desser KB. Accelerated ventricular rhythm and cocaine abuse. *Ann Intern Med* 1978; 88:519–520.
7. Bernheim J, Cox JN. Amphetamine overdosage in an athlete. *Br Med J* 1960; 2:590(abst).
8. Biberstein MP, Fiegler MG, Ward DM. Use of beta-blockade and hemoperfusion for acute theophylline poisoning. *West J Med* 1984; 141:485–490.
9. Boyd RE, Brennan PT, Deng J. Strychnine poisoning: recovery from profound lactic acidosis, hyperthermia, and rhabdomyolysis. *Am J Med* 1983; 74:507–512.
10. Bruner DA, Page T, Grego C, et al. Progressive neurodegenerative disorder in a patient with nonketotic hyperglycinemia. *J Pediatr* 1981; 98:272–275.
11. Coleman D, Rosse TF, Naughton JL. Myocardial ischemia and infarction related to recreational cocaine use. *West J Med* 1982; 136:444–446.
12. Curatolo PW, Robertson D. The health consequences of caffeine. *Ann Intern Med* 1983; 98:641–653.
13. Espelin DE, Done AK. Amphetamine poisoning. *N Engl J Med* 1968; 278:1361–1365.
14. *Federal Register*. 1982 Sep 21; 47:41716.
15. Franz DN. Strychnine, picrotoxin, pentylenetetrazol, and miscellaneous agents (Doxapram, Nikethamide, Methylphenidate). In: Gilman AG, Goodman LS, Rall TW, Murad F, eds. *The pharmacological basis of therapeutics.* 7th ed. New York: Macmillan; 1985:582–588.
16. Gaft HH. Camphor liniment poisoning. *JAMA* 1925; 84:1571.
17. Garriott JC, Simmons LM, Poklis A, Mackell MA. Five cases of fatal overdose from caffeine-containing "look-alike" drugs. *J Anal Toxicol* 1985; 9:141–143.
18. Gary NE. Methamphetamine intoxication: a speedy new treatment. *Am J Med* 1978; 64:537–540.
19. Gaudreault P, Guay J. Theophylline poisoning: pharmacological considerations and clinical management. *Med Toxicol* 1986; 1:169–191.
20. Ginsberg MD, Hertzman J, Schmidt-Nowara WW. Amphetamine intoxication with coagulopathy, hyperthermia, and reversible renal failure. *Ann Intern Med* 1970; 73:81–85.
21. Greenwood R, Peachey RS. Acute amphetamine poisoning, an account of 3 cases. *Br Med J* 1957; 1:742–744.
22. Heard JD, Brooks RC. Clinical and experimental investigation of the therapeutic value of camphor. *Am J Med Sci* 1913; 145:238–253.
23. Heath A, Knudsen K. Role of extracorporeal drug removal in acute theophylline poisoning: a review. *Med Toxicol* 1987; 2:294–308.
24. Hendeles L, Weinberger M. Improved efficacy and safety of theophylline in the control of airway hyperreactivity. *Pharmacol Ther* 1982; 18:91–105.
25. Jaffe JH. Drug addiction and drug abuse. In: Gilman AG, Goodman LS, Rall TW, Murad F, eds. *The pharmacological basis of therapeutics.* 7th ed. New York: Macmillan; 1985:532–581.
26. Johnston GAR. Neuropharmacology of amino acid inhibitory transmitters. *Ann Rev Pharmacol Toxicol* 1978; 18:269–289.
27. Jones DV, Work CE. Volume of a swallow. *Am J Med Child* 1961; 102:427.

28. Jonsson S, O'Meara M, Young JB. Acute cocaine poisoning: importance of treating seizures and acidosis. *Am J Med* 1983;75:1061–1064.
29. Jordan C, Lehane JR, Jones JG. Respiratory depression following diazepam: reversal with high-dose naloxone. *Anesthesiology* 1980;53:293–298.
30. Kew MC, Hopp M, Rothberg A. Fatal heat-stroke in a child taking appetite-suppressant drugs. *S Afr Med J* 1982;62:905–906.
31. Lambert JR, Byrick RJ, Hammeke MD. Management of acute strychnine poisoning. *Can Med Assoc J* 1981;124:1268–1270.
32. Legatt DF. Theophylline toxicity—a consequence of congestive heart failure. *Drug Intell Clin Pharm* 1983;17:59–60.
33. Levine B, Caplan YH, Kauffman G. Fatality resulting from methylphenidate overdose. *J Anal Toxicol* 1986;10:209–210.
34. McDowell JR, LeBlanc HJ. Phenylpropanolamine and cerebral hemorrhage. *West J Med* 1988;142:688–691.
35. McGee MB. Caffeine poisoning in a 19-year-old female. *J Forensic Sci* 1979;25:29–32.
36. Mountain RD, Neff TA. Oral theophylline intoxication. *Arch Intern Med* 1984;144:724–727.
37. Perper JA. Fatal strychnine poisoning—a case report and review of the literature. *J Forensic Sci* 1985;30:1248–1255.
38. Perry PJ, Tuhl RP. Amphetamine psychosis. *Am J Hosp Pharm* 1977;34:883–885.
39. Phelan WJ. Camphor poisoning: over-the-counter dangers. *Pediatrics* 1976;57:428–431.
40. Poklis A, Mackell MA, Graham M. Disposition of cocaine in fatal poisoning in man. *J Anal Toxicol* 1985;9:227–229.
41. Rall TW. The methylxanthines. In: Gilman AG, Goodman LS, Rall TW, Murad F, eds. *The pharmacological basis of therapeutics*. 7th ed. New York: Macmillan; 1985:589–603.
42. Rappolt RT, Gay GR, Inaba DS. Propranolol in the treatment of cardiopressor effects of cocaine. *N Engl J Med* 1976;295:448.
43. Rappolt RT, Gay GR, Inaba DS, Rappolt NR. Propranolol in cocaine toxicity. *Lancet* 1976;2:640–641.
44. Rappolt RT, Gay GR, Inaba DS, Rappolt NR. Use of Inderol (propranolol-Ayerst) in a I-a (early stimulative) and I-b (advanced stimulative) classification of cocaine and other sympathomimetic reactions. *Clin Toxicol* 1978;13:325–332.
45. Richards W, Church JA, Brent DK. Theophylline-associated seizures in children. *Ann Allergy* 1985;54:276–279.
46. Ritchie JM, Green NM. Local anesthetics. In: Gilman AG, Goodman LS, Rall TW, Murad F, eds. *The pharmacological basis of therapeutics*. 7th ed. New York: Macmillan; 1985:302–321.
47. Robertson NJ. Fatal overdose from a sustained-release theophylline preparation. *Ann Emerg Med* 1985;14:115–119.
48. Rosenberg J, Pentel P, Pond S, et al. Hyperthermia associated with drug intoxication. *Crit Care Med* 1986;14:964–969.
49. Sahney S, Abarzua J, Sessums L. Hemoperfusion in theophylline neurotoxicity. *Pediatrics* 1983;71:615.
50. Scott ME, Mullaly RW. Lithium therapy for cocaine-induced psychosis: a clinical perspective. *South Med J* 1981;74:1475–1477.
51. Sessler CN. Theophylline toxicity—clinical features of 116 consecutive cases. *Am J Med* 1990;88:567–576.
52. Shannon M, Lovejoy FH. Effect of acute versus chronic intoxication on clinical features of theophylline poisoning in children. *J Pediatr* 1992;121:125–130.
53. Siegel E, Wason S. Camphor toxicity. *Pediatr Clin North Am* 1986;33:375–379.
54. Slater IH. Strychnine, picrotoxin, pentylenetetrazol, and miscellaneous drugs. In: DiPalma JR, ed. *Pharmacology in medicine*. 4th ed. New York: McGraw-Hill; 1971:517–532.
55. Smith A, Margolis G. Camphor poisoning. *Am J Pathol* 1954;30:857.
56. Snyder SH. Catecholamines in the brain as mediators of amphetamine psychosis. *Arch Gen Psychiatry* 1972;27:169–179.
57. Teitelbaum DT, Ott JE. Acute strychnine intoxication. *Clin Toxicol* 1970;3:267–273.
58. Trestrail JH, Spartz ME. Camporated and castor oil confusion and its toxic results. *Clin Toxicol* 1977;11:151–158.
59. Tsiu SJ, Self TH, Burns R. Theophylline toxicity update. *Ann Allergy* 1990;64:241–257.
60. vonWendt L, Simila S, Saukkonen AL, et al. Prenatal brain damage in nonketotic hyperglycinemia. *Am J Dis Child* 1981;135:1072.
61. Wetli CV, Mittleman RE. The "body packer syndrome"—toxicity following ingestion of illicit drugs packaged for transportation. *J Forensic Sci* 1980;26:492–500.
62. Yamarick W, Walson P, DiTraglia J. Strychnine poisoning in an adolescent. *Clin Toxicol* 1992;30:141–148.
63. Zalis EG, Parmley LF. Fatal amphetamine poisoning. *Arch Intern Med* 1963;112:822–826.

17 ‖ Hallucinogens (Psychotomimetics) and Marijuana

TABLE 17.1. *Classification of psychotomimetic agents*

Ergot alkaloids
  Lysergic acid diethylamide (LSD-25)
Tryptamine derivatives
  DMT (*N,N*–dimethyltryptamine)
  DET (diethyltryptamine)
  Bufotenine (5-hydroxy-*N,N*-dimethyltryptamine)
  Psilocybin and psilocin
Phenethylamine derivatives
  Mescaline
  DOM (STP, 2,5-dimethoxy-4-methylamphetamine)
  MDA (3,4-methylenedioxyamphetamine)
Miscellaneous
  Phencyclidine (PCP)
  Marijuana

Hallucinogens are substances that produce changes in perception, thought, and mood. The drugs and chemicals discussed in this chapter are also referred to as psychotomimetic agents, psychedelics (*mind magnifying*), psycholytics (*mind releasing*), or psychotogens.

Bear in mind that there is a fine line of distinction in this definition. Several classes of legitimate drugs, such as the anticholinergics, opioids, and corticosteroids, also can cause perceptual changes, euphoria, and distort cognitive functions, when used in sufficient dosage.

Hallucinogens can be derived from natural products or synthesized in the laboratory. The classification used in this text is based on the chemical structure. Table 17.1 outlines major chemical categories and lists representative examples of each category.

ERGOT ALKALOID: LYSERGIC ACID DIETHYLAMIDE

In 1938, lysergic acid diethylamide (LSD-25) (Fig. 17.1) was synthesized (19). Nearly a decade later, the first report of its effects in humans was released. As little as 25 to 50 μg given orally produced marked behavioral effects. When LSD was first investigated, it appeared that it might be useful in elucidating an etiology for schizophrenia, but after several years of intensive study and misuse, the con-

clusion was that the substance had no legitimate medical use (13).

LSD is potent, odorless, colorless, and tasteless. It appears on the street in many dosage forms. Liquid LSD is sometimes placed on sugar cubes or pieces of blotter paper. Solid dosage forms consist of extremely small, colorful *micro-dot* tablets. The average dose is 100 mg, but doses as high as 1,500 mg have been reported with no major complications. There have been reports of chronic users ingesting amounts as high as 10,000 mg without suffering serious complications. The reason for an abuser of LSD to use such a high dose may be due to tachyphylaxis, or rapid production of tolerance, which occurs with repeated administration. A significant increase in dose may be necessary in 3 to 4 days after continued use, but physical dependence has not been established. An interesting element in LSD abuse is that recovery from tolerance occurs just as rapidly. Therefore, little tolerance to LSD is possible if taken only on weekends or recreationally. Cross-tolerance with both mescaline and psilocybin has occurred.

The primary actions of LSD are on the CNS, especially changes in mood and behavior. Psychologic effects can last 6 to 12 hr after an average dose. LSD affects both the pyramidal and extrapyramidal systems. Mood changes range from euphoria to dysphoria. The LSD user may feel euphoric, displaying hilarious laughter at times, with the mood swiftly changing to sadness and crying episodes. These mood swings tend to be influenced by small changes in the environment.

LSD acutely affects sensory perception. Although it acts on the auditory, tactile, olfactory, and gustatory senses, the most marked effects are on visual perception. Colors of objects become more intense. Flat surfaces as-

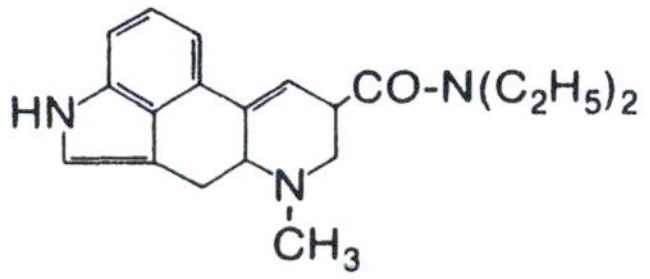

FIG. 17.1. Chemical structure of LSD (lysergic acid diethylamide).

sume depth. Fixed objects begin to undulate and flow. Since there is alteration in time perception, these visual changes seem to continue forever. LSD also causes disruption of ego function and the fear of self-destruction. Body parts may feel unnatural or foreign.

In addition to its effects on the CNS, LSD affects both sympathetic and parasympathetic nervous systems, but sympathetic activities predominate. Therefore, as a sympathomimetic agent, some of the characteristics of LSD include marked mydriasis, hyperthermia, piloerection, hyperglycemia, tachycardia, and hypertension.

Acute Lysergic Acid Diethylamide Toxicity

By extrapolation of animal data, the LD_{50} value of LSD for humans is estimated to be 0.2 mg/kg. An adult weighing 150 pounds would require a single oral dose of about 14 mg to achieve the LD_{50}. Thus, LSD has a high therapeutic index. Because large dose variations can be tolerated without significant physiologic consequences, variations in dose of street preparations of LSD are not as critical on a potential toxicity basis when compared to other street drugs, such as phencyclidine (PCP). The major concern regarding street forms of LSD, as well as any other crudely manufactured preparations, is the possibility of contaminants or impurities and, in some cases, adulterants used to dilute the drug.

When hallucinogens, such as LSD, are taken in a so-called "therapeutic" dose, a temporary psychotic state or *trip* results. Usually an experienced user is knowledgeable about adjusting the amount of drug needed to obtain this desired experience. On occasion, hallucinogens produce *bad trips* or adverse reactions. This has been attributed to first-time users' lack of experience in relating observed effects as pleasurable. Other times, adverse reactions occur from contaminants or impurities because the drug may have been synthesized in a clandestine laboratory that lacks quality control assurance measures. The mental state of the user also influences the incidence of adverse effects. Adverse effects fall into three categories: acute panic reactions, flashbacks, and prolonged psychoses.

Panic reactions are often seen at some stage of LSD usage, but rarely result in major complications. This reaction is described as a feeling of losing control. The person can no longer think rationally and feels he will not be able to come to grips with himself. It is important during these episodes that the individual be reminded that what he is experiencing is drug induced, and that the bad trip will not last forever. For the panicked hallucinogen user who may feel that his body and the chair in which he is sitting are one and the same, continued reassurance that he is a real person is helpful. Repeating the person's name and the present location and surroundings may help alleviate some of the anxiety associated with these panic reactions.

One of the more widely publicized chronic reactions to LSD use is the flashback. It is impossible to predict who will experience flashbacks, but the incidence is commonly stated as one of every 20 users. They occur more frequently in users who have previously experienced bad trips and constantly abuse this drug, but flashbacks have also been reported after a single LSD exposure. There is no set pattern of frequency or intensity. Flashbacks can be brief or last several hours. One study showed that flashbacks occur more frequently just before going to sleep and while under severe stress (28).

Three categories of flashbacks have been described: *perceptual*—seeing vivid colors, hearing sounds from previous trips; *somatic*—paresthesia, tachycardia; and *emotional*—feelings of loneliness, panic, and depression. The most serious are the emotional flashbacks, because persistent feelings of fear, loneliness, and other emotions can lead to suicide.

Treatment of flashbacks is based on the same principles as treatment for acute panic reactions. The surroundings should be quiet. The person should be reassured that the condition is temporary. If sedation is necessary, diazepam is recommended. A lighted room at bedtime may decrease the incidence of flashbacks.

TABLE 17.2. *Chemical formulas for various derivatives of tryptamine*

Chemical name	Substitutions				$R_4\!-\!\overset{R_3}{\diagdown}\!\!\diagup\!\!\diagdown_N\!\!\diagup\!-CH_2\text{-}CH_2\text{-}N\!\!\diagup^{R_1}_{\diagdown R_2}$
	R_1	R_2	R_3	R_4	
DMT (*N,N*-dimethyltryptamine)	CH_3	CH_3	—	—	
DET (diethyltryptamine)	$CH_2\text{--}CH_3$	$CH_2\text{--}CH_3$	—	—	
Bufotenin (5-hydroxy-DMT)	CH_3	CH_3	—	OH	
Psilocybin (*O*-phosphoryl-4-hydroxy-DMT)	CH_3	CH_3	OPO_3H	—	
Psilocin (4-hydroxy-DMT)	CH_3	CH_3	OH	—	
Serotonin (5-hydroxytryptamine)	H	H	—	OH	

Another danger that has plagued the hallucinogen abuser is occurrence of prolonged psychosis or neurosis. States of paranoia and schizophrenia have been reported, even after the general state of intoxication subsided (11).

TRYPTAMINE DERIVATIVES

Hallucinogenic effects are produced by a variety of tryptamine derivatives listed in Table 17.2. Chemically, these compounds do not differ greatly from one another. Their pharmacologic and toxicologic profiles are likewise similar. The major difference is in potency. Psilocybin will be used as a prototype for this group because it is the most commonly encountered hallucinogen of this category.

Psilocybin and Psilocin

Psilocybin occurs naturally in several species of mushrooms (Fig. 17.2), notably *Psilocybe mexicana*. Teonanacatl (*food of the Gods*) has been used by the Indians of Mexico and Central America for centuries (12). The custom of incorporating the sacred mushroom into a semireligious ceremony dates back to 1500 B.C. In 1958, Hoffman, the discoverer of LSD, successfully isolated two alkaloids from *Psilocybe mexicana*: psilocybin, identi-

fied as the major constituent, and psilocin, which was shown to be equally as active but present in small quantities. These alkaloids are also contained in numerous other varieties of mushrooms belonging to the genus *Psilocybe*, as well as in other mushroom species. Psilocybin is an unstable compound and is converted to psilocin in the body.

Pharmacologic Effects of Psilocybin

As a hallucinogen, psilocybin exhibits effects similar to LSD and mescaline. However,

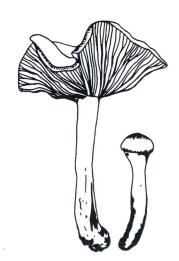

FIG. 17.2. Drawing of the psilocybe mushroom—source of psilocybin and psilocin.

the potency of LSD is considerably greater than psilocybin, which in turn is more potent than mescaline. Twenty milligrams of psilocybin is equivalent to the usual dose (100 mg) of LSD. Therefore, LSD appears to be approximately 150 to 200 times more potent than psilocybin, which is 1 to 5 times weaker than psilocin.

Oral doses of 60 to 200 mg/kg produce symptoms including weakness, nausea, anxiety, dreamy states, dizziness, blurred vision, dilated pupils, and increased deep tendon reflexes. The visual effects consist of brighter colors, longer afterimages, sharp definition of objects, and colored patterns and shapes that are generally pleasing but sometimes frightening. The duration of action is usually about 3 hr.

Psilocybin Toxicity

Toxicologic studies with psilocybin are limited. The LD_{50} in mice is 280 mg/kg. There have been few reports of toxic effects produced by psilocybin in humans when used under controlled experiments (4,34). One interesting case report is summarized at the end of this chapter. The Indians' use of the drug in its natural form provides little information as to its cumulative toxicity since the mushrooms are not ingested chronically.

However, there have been a few case reports of *Psilocybe* poisonings.

PHENETHYLAMINE DERIVATIVES

The phenethylamine compounds (Table 17.3) represent a larger group of hallucinogens found in street use. Except for mescaline, the others are synthetic analogs of amphetamine. The pharmacologic actions of these drugs are similar to those of epinephrine and norepinephrine. This group of hallucinogens does not contain the indole nucleus; therefore, they are structurally dissimilar to ergot alkaloids (LSD) and tryptamine derivatives (e.g., psilocybin).

Mescaline

One of the best documented hallucinogenic plants is the Peyote cactus, *Lophophora williamsii*, which contains mescaline as its primary active ingredient. This plant has been used by Indians in northern Mexico as an adjunct to religious ceremonies since earliest recorded history (5). Individuals have also used mescaline-containing buttons to relieve fatigue and hunger, and for treatment and prevention of various diseases. The peyote cult was largely confined to Mexico until the 19th century when a number of tribes and tribal segments migrated north into the United States, and promoted the use of the plant. Today, illicit use of mescaline is reported to be widespread (27).

Interest in peyote for nonreligious purposes began around 1890. A tincture was used in treatment of angina pectoris and pneumothorax, and as a depressant, respiratory stimulant, and cardiac tonic. The *National Standard Dispensatory* of 1905 devoted an entire page to peyote and its tinctures.

Pharmacologic Actions of Mescaline

Mescaline is a phenethylamine derivative that belongs to the structural class of tetrahydroisoquinoline alkaloids and differs structurally from LSD, psilocybin, and other hallucinogenic drugs.

Taken orally in doses of 200 to 500 mg (27), mescaline produces unusual psychic effects and sensory alterations similar to those caused by small doses of LSD or psilocybin. The hallucinogenic dose of mescaline is about 4,000 to 5,000 times higher than that of LSD. The pupil size increases, pulse rate quickens, and blood pressure is elevated. Deep tendon reflex thresholds are decreased. Hallucinations are usually visual, consisting of brightly colored lights, geometric designs, animals, and sometimes people.

Mescaline is readily absorbed from the intestine and concentrates in the kidney, liver, and spleen. In humans, 60% to 90% of the

TABLE 17.3. *Chemical formulas for various phenethylamine derivatives*

Chemical name	Substitutions	R_3 R_2 R_4—⬡—CH_2-CH-NH_2 R_5 R_1
		β-phenethylamine

Chemical name	R_1	R_2	R_3	R_4	R_5
Mescaline (3,4,5-trimethoxyphenethylamine)	H	H	OCH_3	OCH_3	OCH_3
Amphetamine	CH_3	H	H	H	H
DOM, STP (2,5-dimethoxy-4-methyl amphetamine)	CH_3	OCH_3	H	CH_3	OCH_3
MDA, XTC (3,4-methylenedioxyamphetamine)	CH_3	H	O ＼CH_2／ O		H

dose is excreted unchanged; the remainder is eliminated as inactive metabolites. Peak blood concentrations are achieved about 2 hr after ingestion, with a duration of about 12 hr. The half-life is about 6 hr.

Mescaline Toxicity

Documented deaths associated with mescaline are rare. A case study of one death is presented at the end of this chapter. Certain drugs, such as insulin, barbiturates, and physostigmine, are known to increase mescaline toxicity.

2,5-Dimethoxy-4-methylamphetamine

2,5-Dimethoxy-4-methylamphetamine (DOM) is an amphetamine derivative having psychotomimetic effects. It is sometimes referred to as STP (Serenity, Tranquility, and Peace).

Pharmacologic Actions of 2,5-Dimethoxy-4-methylamphetamine

DOM, like other hallucinogens, produces feelings of both euphoria and dysphoria at doses of 5 mg. DOM is 50 to 100 times more active than mescaline, but only one-thirtieth as potent as LSD. After oral administration, initial effects are noted within 90 min with peak effects occurring at about 3 to 4 hr, and hallucinations terminating in 6 to 24 hr. Anxiety is increased at 3 to 6 hr, and obsessive compulsive symptoms increased after 6 hr.

DOM also stimulates of the sympathetic nervous system. This produces increased blood pressure, heart rate, pupillary diameter, and sweating. The CNS effects include nausea, anorexia, increased deep tendon reflexes, altered EEG, paresthesia, tension, tremors, and fatigue.

2,5-Dimethoxy-4-methylamphetamine Toxicity

The median lethal dose (MLD) in rats is 60 mg/kg. There have been no deaths yet reported from the direct effects of DOM, but adverse reactions have been documented. These include an *acid trip*, and anticholinergic symptoms (e.g., dry mouth, blurred vision, etc.).

3,4-Methylenedioxyamphetamine

3,4-Methylenedioxyamphetamine (MDA, XTC, Ecstasy) continues to be a popular illicit drug. Chemically, MDA is related to mescaline and amphetamine. MDA is an anorexiant, but has gained acceptance as a recreational drug due to its perceptual effects. Although the suggested anorexiant dose is 8 to 50 mg, the psychotropic dose is closer to 100 mg.

On the street, MDA has been available as a liquid or powder that is often incorporated into capsules or tablets. Although MDA is commonly taken orally, it is sometimes inhaled. It is rarely injected. Adulterations and varying percentages of purported drugs can be the source of acute toxicity. As with many drugs obtained illegally, it is never certain that the drug is pure, or whether it has been combined with such items as LSD, amphetamine, atropine, or cocaine.

Pharmacologic Actions of 3,4-Methylenedioxyamphetamine

MDA has mild sympathomimetic properties, such as mydriasis, and produces stimulatory effects especially on the respiratory center. It produces a sense of physical well-being with heightened tactile sensations. Visual and auditory hallucinations characteristic of an LSD trip usually do not occur. MDA is only one-third as potent as amphetamine, and three times more potent than mescaline.

A major distinction between MDA and other psychedelics (e.g., mescaline and LSD) is that the former causes less distortion of perceptions. Hallucinations seem to manifest when the person is most relaxed. Consequently, psychic effects are reported to be more within the control of the user, than with other hallucinogens. MDA produces an "inward, talk experience" in subjects who show interest in interpersonal relationships, and an overwhelming desire or need to be with other people. For this reason, it is often referred to as the "Love Drug."

A common undesired effect of MDA is periodic tensing of the muscles in the neck, tightening of the jaw, and grinding of the teeth. Other side effects include erratic behavior, delirium, temporary amnesia, and neuropsychiatric sequelae (20). Several deaths have been associated with MDA (9). Lethal blood concentrations cited have ranged from 0.4 to 2.6 mg/dL.

MANAGEMENT OF THE ADVERSE EFFECTS OF HALLUCINOGENS

The major dilemma encountered in treating psychoactive drug toxicity is being able to accurately identify the compound. Substance abuse has taken several forms over the years. The same drug may be found on the street as a fine powder, tablet, or capsule, or it may be disguised on a sugar cube or piece of blotter paper. Moreover, the abuser or experimenter may think he is using a certain drug but, in actuality, the substance may contain an entirely different drug (33). Compounds that were popular last year may not be this year. The patient's history is often difficult to interpret. A scared young person is not always willing to admit to what he has been enjoying at the concert besides the music!

Most hallucinogens have a high therapeutic index and, therefore, toxicity due directly to their pharmacologic actions is seldom encountered. It is the psychologic manifestations that need to be addressed.

In general, the victim who experiences adverse effects to hallucinogens should be placed in a quiet environment to minimize external stimuli that could aggravate the psychotic state. He must not be left unattended, and must be given constant positive assurance.

Other treatment is largely supportive. Increased blood pressure may be severe, especially with amphetamine-like hallucinogens that have strong sympathomimetic activity. Rapid lowering of blood pressure to normal can be achieved with a vasodilator. Convulsions and anxiety are usually managed successfully with diazepam. Bad trips, panic reactions, and psychotic episodes generally respond well to treatment with chlorpromazine. After recovery, psychiatric consultation is mandated.

PHENCYCLIDINE

Phencyclidine (PCP, 1-phenylcyclohexyl piperidine) (Fig. 17.3) was developed in the late 1950s, patented in 1963, and marketed as Sernyl. Early animal studies reported the drug to have strong analgesic activity with sympathomimetic and CNS stimulant and depressant action. It did not block ganglia, or cholinergic or histamine receptors. In 1957, clinical experiments were initiated. Doses of 25 mg/kg given intravenously produced anesthesia sufficient for major surgery. It is chemically related to the dissociative anesthetic ketamine, but is much more toxic. Since in some cases the drug produced postanesthetic confusion and delirium of prolonged duration, clinical investigations were soon discontinued. All legal manufacture of PCP for human use in the United States has ceased.

PCP first appeared on the streets in 1967 and was sold on the west coast area as the "*PeaCe Pill*." Many users reported unpleasant experiences, and the drug soon developed a questionable reputation. It disappeared in 1968, only to resurface in the East as *hog*. It also received a bad reputation there and soon disappeared. At this time, its popularity has again increased and it is currently a commonly used street drug (6,14). It is sold on the street in a variety of different sizes, shapes, and colors of tablets and capsules, and as a white or off-color powder to be sprinkled on pieces of parsley, mint, and marijuana, or other plant material. It appears under a variety of exotic names including Angel Dust, Dust, Crystal, Crystal Joints, CJ, KJ, Peace, and Hog, to name a few.

Pharmacologic Actions

PCP may be used by any route of administration. The estimated amount used per epi-

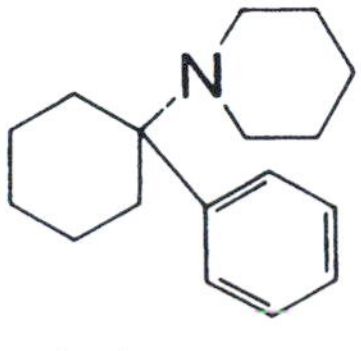

FIG. 17.3. Chemical structure of phencyclidine (1-phenylcyclohexyl piperidine).

TABLE 17.4. *Characteristics of phencyclidine intoxication*

Serum concentration	Signs and symptoms
20–30 ng/mL	Agitation and irritability, blank stare, catatonia, catalepsy, sweating, flushing, nystagmus, inability to speak, body image changes, disorganized thoughts
30–100 ng/mL	As above; and coma or stupor, vomiting, hypersalivation, repetitive muscular movements, rigidity, shivering, fever, decreased peripheral feelings (pain, touch, etc.), depression, schizophrenia
>100 ng/mL	As above, but more intense and prolonged, i.e., hypertension, opisthotonos, convulsions, absent peripheral sensations, decreased reflexes, hallucinations, disorientation, loss of memory

sode when smoked is 1.5 to 3.5 mg. The quantity per dose in powders and tablets averages 2 to 6 mg. Onset of subjective effects after smoking occurs within 1 to 5 min and may last for 4 to 6 hr. A more rapid onset of 30 sec to 1 min is observed after insufflation of the powder.

Blood concentrations of PCP as low as 10 ng/mL may be associated with behavioral effects listed in Table 17.4. Concentrations greater than 100 ng/mL are usually associated with coma, which may result in death due to secondary complications such as seizure and respiratory depression. Doses of PCP resulting in blood concentrations of 200 to 250 ng/mL and greater are probably uniformly fatal (2).

Neurologic signs of PCP at low doses or after chronic administration of doses that provide blood concentrations up to 100 ng/mL include: horizontal and vertical nystagmus, variable pupil size with depressed light reflex, and occasional blurred or double vision. Additionally, ataxia, tremors, slurred speech, muscle weakness, drowsiness, and increased respiratory rate and depth are observed (13). Sudden and dramatic mood changes are also seen along with delusion, purposeless talk, disoriented thought process, and sometimes visual hallucinations. As the state of intoxication wears off, the person gradually shifts to a state of mild depression where he is irritable, and feels isolated and sometimes paranoid.

The chronic PCP user generally requires 24 to 48 hr to return completely to normal. Most individuals who have used PCP find the subjective effects difficult to describe, but agree that the experience is distinctly different from other drug experiences they have encountered. Although many describe the experience as positive, first-time users or those who use PCP unknowingly encounter an unpleasant and often frightening experience.

Psychologic dependence and tolerance to the psychic effects of PCP, requiring increasing doses to obtain the desired effects, are reported by chronic users. Paranoia, auditory hallucinations, violent behavior, severe depression, and anxiety have followed prolonged periods of daily, regular use.

Phencyclidine Toxicity

PCP toxicity is manifested by a stuporous, comatose state in which the patient is responsive only to deep pain. Hypertension and tachycardia are present. Important diagnostic features of intoxication include the presence of vertical and horizontal nystagmus, which are associated with hypertension in a comatose individual (21).

Massive oral overdoses of up to 1 g streetgrade PCP have resulted in periods of stupor and coma of several hours to 5 days in duration. Delayed and prolonged respirations and apnea may follow. Intoxication is also marked by sustained hypertension and tachycardia, and general motor seizures preceded by muscle tremors and rigidity (15).

There are numerous reports of PCP-induced psychosis described as an initial violent, aggressive, and/or disorganized behavior with or without paranoia lasting from less than 4 hr to as long as several days (26). Restless and combative behavior and thought patterns are usually complete in one week, but severe

cases may require 12 to 18 months to return to predrug status.

Many deaths associated exclusively with PCP intoxication have been reported in the United States. The manner of death has been accidental, suicidal, and homicidal. In most cases, circumstantial evidence suggested that death was secondary to the behavioral toxicity of PCP (3,6). In other words, most victims died from trauma, drowning, or similar accidents.

Management of Acute Poisoning

PCP is a common cause of psychotic, drugrelated emergency room admissions. The most common diagnostic features for PCP intoxication include horizontal or vertical nystagmus, muscular rigidity, and hypertension. The patient may be agitated, psychotic, or comatose, but respirations are not usually compromised unless PCP was ingested with alcohol, sedatives, or opioids. Since there is no specific antidote, treatment of acute PCP intoxication is focused on supportive and symptomatic care. Complete recovery may require several weeks or longer. Also, fluctuations in symptoms are common. A victim may emerge from coma, only to worsen later (8,21,26).

There has been some success with placing the agitated, psychotic individual in an attended, quiet, and darkened room, but the *talking down* techniques commonly used for LSD and other hallucinogens usually are ineffective.

Diazepam has been used successfully to treat hyperactivity and agitation of the intoxicated patient. Phenothiazines (e.g., chlorpromazine) and butyrophenones (haloperidol) are not recommended for initial treatment of PCP intoxication because they lower the seizure threshold and may produce severe hypotension. However, they have been recommended to treat persistent phencyclidineinduced psychosis (33).

Unlike the phenethylamine hallucinogens, severe hypertensive crisis is not usually encountered. If present, however, it should be

TABLE 17.5. *Influence of urine and plasma acidification on phencyclidine distribution*

Body fluid	Before acidification[a]		After acidification	
	pH	PCP (ng/mL)	pH	PCP (ng/mL)
Serum	7.4	66	7.2	50
CSF[b]	—	140	—	8
Urine	7.5	43	5.0	3,997

From ref. 8.
[a] Acidification performed with ammonium chloride.
[b] CSF, cerebrospinal fluid.

treated with a rapidly acting vasodilator, such as diazoxide or nitroprusside.

Renal damage is sometimes a complication of PCP because of profound involuntary muscular activity, which can lead to diffuse muscle injury and myoglobinuria (7,17). To reduce the possibility of acute renal failure, diuretics, such as furosemide, have been used. Physical restraints should be used only when necessary to keep muscle injury minimized and, hence, help prevent onset of renal damage (17).

At this point, efforts should be focused on hastening elimination of PCP. It is extremely lipid soluble, and a weak base with a pKa between 8.6 and 9.4. The drug also undergoes enterohepatic circulation. As a result, when PCP enters the acidic environment of the stomach, it becomes trapped in ionized form, which may be efficiently removed by gastric suction and adding 30 to 40 g of activated charcoal every 6 to 8 hr (23). In severe PCP intoxication, urine acidification to a pH between 5.0 and 5.5 with ammonium chloride will greatly enhance elimination of this basic drug. Once urinary pH is approximately 5, furosemide can be given to promote diuresis (1). Decreases in plasma pH have also been shown to aid in removal of PCP from the CNS (2). Because of small quantities involved and because the PCP-intoxicated patient often has other drugs in his blood and urine, accurate monitoring of PCP concentrations is extremely difficult (16,29).

Table 17.5 illustrates the effect of acidification on PCP distribution. When urine pH was lowered from 7.5 to 5.0 with ammonium chloride, urinary PCP concentration increased from 43 ng/mL to nearly 4,000 ng/mL. This clearly illustrates that excretion is enhanced. Furthermore, PCP concentrations in the cerebrospinal fluid were lowered from an initial value of 140 ng/mL to 8 ng/mL. But although acidification has been shown to be effective, it is no longer recommended due to development of renal complications, including acute tubular necrosis, and urate nephropathy.

Immunotherapy may someday be used to counteract the toxic effects of PCP. Investigators have developed an antibody that is reported to have an affinity for PCP that is 130 to 750 times greater than the drug's affinity for receptors in the brain. When PCP-treated animals received the PCP-specific antibody 2 hr later, PCP shifted from peripheral body tissues into the blood; blood PCP concentration increased 17- to 56-fold within several minutes (22,23). Normally, PCP is distributed equally between erythrocytes and plasma. In the presence of the antibody, the drug was confined to plasma and could not cross cell membranes or the blood-brain barrier to cause pharmacologic effects (22,23).

These studies are preliminary, and have been conducted only in animals. There is little doubt, however, that they will eventually lead to clinical application. A specific antibody for treating digoxin intoxication is currently being used (see chapter 18).

MARIJUANA

Marijuana (marihuana, MJ) is a mixture of crushed leaves, flowers, and stems of the Indian hemp plant, *Cannabis sativa*. The principal active ingredient is delta-9-tetrahydrocannabinol (THC). The content of THC in marijuana varies broadly in the United States, ranging from 0.5 to 11%, depending on methods of cultivation. *Sinsemilla* (*without seeds*) refers to a mixture of flowering tops and leaves of cultivated, unfertilized female plants. THC content in *Sinsemilla* may range from 8% to 11%.

In the United States, the average marijuana joint contains 500 to 1000 mg of plant material, with 1% to 2% THC (5 to 20 mg). Fifty percent of the dose is available for absorption, since half is lost by pyrolysis (32). Therefore, the average dose of THC from one joint is 2.5 mg.

THC is rapidly absorbed into the blood after inhalation, producing subjective effects within seconds to minutes that last at least 2 to 3 hr. After a single usage, only 5% to 10% of an oral dose of THC is absorbed. Onset of effects may be delayed for 30 min, but last as long as 5 hr or more (18,35). THC is fat soluble, being rapidly cleared from plasma and stored in adipose tissue. Tissue half-life is approximately 7 days. Low concentrations of THC may be detected for 15 to 30 days after a single dose.

Characteristics of Marijuana

Marijuana itself does not produce significant toxicity when used only for short-term. Signs of marijuana intoxication may be difficult to quantify. Eyes are *bloodshot* and the individual appears "high." Subjective effects are dependent on personality and expectations of the user, social setting (i.e., being alone or with friends), and dose. Low doses of THC (2 mg) will generally produce a sense of relaxation, mild euphoria, and increased auditory, visual, and gustatory perceptions. Periods of hilarity may be followed by silence. With moderate doses (5 to 7 mg), a progression to disturbances in thought processes and time perception, impairment in short-term memory, and ataxia may be prominent. High doses (15 mg and greater) may induce feelings of deper-sonalization, disorientation, paranoia, and marked sensory distortion (13).

Cardiovascular effects may include dose-related sinus tachycardia, but blood pressure is usually not significantly affected. Marijuana has been shown to decrease alveolar macrophage activity after chronic use. Impaired pulmonary function is evidenced by bronchitis, pharyngitis, cough, and an asthma-like condition. Marijuana smoking may cause cancer due to its high tar content (24).

Contrary to popular belief, marijuana does not produce an aphrodisiac action. In fact, high doses decrease libido. Animal studies have demonstrated a decrease in sperm count and testosterone. Also, a decrease in lymphocytes and impairment of immune function have been proposed.

The long-term effects from chronic marijuana use are controversial and not well understood. They include flashbacks, panic reactions, and the amotivational syndrome. Physical dependence has not been demonstrated with marijuana alone. Toxic psychosis has been demonstrated in some marijuana abusers (31). Psychologic dependence and tolerance may occur with prolonged, moderate-to-high dose use.

Management of Adverse Reactions to Marijuana

Management of marijuana-induced reactions is purely supportive and symptomatic. Ingested material should be removed from the stomach with emesis, lavage, or activated charcoal. If the patient is disoriented or experiencing hallucinations or panic reactions, a prolonged *talkdown* period may be necessary. Since acute toxic reactions due to marijuana alone are rare, whenever a patient presents with serious manifestations, consideration should be given to other drugs such as PCP, LSD, or cocaine being at fault.

SUMMARY

Hallucinogens are chemicals that cause intense psychologic alterations in very small doses. Poisoning by hallucinogens is a fairly common event. Management of hallucinogenic poisoning is largely supportive and symptomatic. Intense psychotherapy will be necessary to avoid or correct long-term complications.

Case Studies

CASE STUDIES: PHENCYCLIDINE INTOXICATION

History: Case 1

The patient was a 26-year-old woman with a history of psychiatric disease. She had no history of abusing alcohol and other drugs, including PCP.

One evening at a party, she was offered a joint containing PCP and smoked approximately one-half of it. Shortly thereafter, she developed paranoia and reported visual and auditory hallucinations.

Two days later she was admitted to a psychiatric hospital for treatment. At this point, both blood and urine were negative for PCP, but symptoms persisted.

Her psychosis, which persisted for over two weeks, was treated with haloperidol. Eventually she recovered, but she continued to suffer from depression. (See ref. 30.)

History: Case 2

A chronic male abuser of PCP, age 29 years, was sitting in front of the television, smoking a PCP joint. His wife began to nag him about his habit, his laziness, and his not having a job. She told him their new baby was sick and she was going to take the child to a doctor. An argument ensued and continued for the next few minutes, at which time the man blacked out.

He awoke to a state of partial consciousness sometime later. He was next observed running naked along the street, covered with blood from self-inflicted wounds. He carried a knife in his hands, chanting, "Hallelujah, I'm Je-sus!" Some time later, he entered the house of a strange woman who was pregnant. He killed the woman, her unborn child, and her two-year-old child.

The crazed man was apprehended, and later convicted of murder. He still has no recollection of the event and cannot explain his motives for these actions. (See ref. 30.)

History: Case 3

A 25-year-old man was seen in an emergency room. He did not have a history of psychiatric illness or drug abuse. His family reported that he had been acting strangely for the past three days. The man had initially denied taking drugs, but eventually admitted to his family that he had swallowed a quantity of some powder.

On admission the patient became suspicious of the staff and feared that they were trying to kill him. He was agitated and uncooperative and therefore was bound in full body restraints. He was given 5 mg haloperidol intramuscularly.

Physical examination revealed blood pressure, 190/95 mm Hg; pulse, 100 beats/min; and temperature, 99°F. The patient had nystagmus on lateral gaze. A toxicology screen was positive for phencyclidine and benzodiazepines, and negative for alcohol. Laboratory results included creatinine, 5.3 mg/dL; BUN, 43 mg/dL; serum uric acid, 31.4 mg/dL; and serum creatinine phosphokinase (CPK), 203,000 IU (normal: 21 to 232). Arterial blood gases revealed metabolic acidosis (pH 7.32).

After the first few hours following admission, the patient complained of back pain and pain in his right knee. His nystagmus disappeared in a few hours. Over the next 24 hr urine output decreased gradually. The creatinine concentration increased to 8.1 mg/dL, and BUN to 53 mg/dL. His acute renal failure was believed possibly due to urate nephropathy. He was started on hemodialysis.

After approximately 36 hr postadmission, the patient remained disoriented to time, and lethargic. Because he was less agitated, his restraints were removed without incident.

Hemodialysis was continued each day for a week. He subsequently entered the diuretic phase of acute renal failure, and renal activity recovered without event. He remained guarded and depressed during this time. He was largely nonverbal but did admit to regularly consuming 6 cans of beer each 1 to 2 days. He refused psychiatric help, and was eventually dismissed. (See ref. 17).

Discussion

1. Outline the management steps usually used to treat PCP intoxication. Why was the patient in case 1 not subjected to these procedures?
2. Various experts in treating PCP intoxication agree there is frequently a triggering stimulus that causes these patients to react unpredictably and violently. What was the stimulus for the patient in case 2 to behave as he did?
3. What leads you to suspect that part of the symptoms experienced by patient 1 were actually due more to underlying mental illness rather than to PCP?
4. Renal failure is sometimes a complication of PCP poisoning. Can you postulate what probably caused this problem in the patient in case 3?

CASE STUDIES: LYSERGIC ACID DIETHYLAMIDE INTOXICATION

History: Case 1

A 21-year-old woman was admitted to a hospital accompanied by a male friend who was experienced in using LSD. About 30 min after he had convinced her to ingest approximately 200 μg of LSD, she began to experience the effects of the drug and said she felt that the bricks on the wall moved in and out. A panic reaction developed when she was unable to distinguish her body from the chair in which she was sitting, or from her friend's body. Her fears worsened when she felt "she would not be able to get back into herself."

On admission to the hospital she was hyperexcited and laughed inappropriately. Her talk and reactions to others were disorganized and illogical.

Two days later the panic reaction subsided; however, she was still afraid of the drug and indicated she would never again take it. (See ref. 10.)

History: Case 2

A man in his late twenties was seen at the admitting office of an emergency facility in a state of panic. He had at least 15 previous experiences with LSD and other hallucinogens. Most prior encounters with LSD were pleasurable except that he had experienced panic reactions twice. During these episodes, he stated that he was losing control and his whole body was disappearing. It had been at least two months since he had taken his last LSD dose, and the problems he experienced were now apparently resulting as a flashback to a prior encounter.

His present experience, on flashback, depicted some of the delusions, perceptual distortions, and feelings of union with things around him that mimicked the kinds of trips he previously encountered. (See ref. 10.)

Discussion

1. Why do flashbacks occur and what provokes them?
2. What is the mode of treatment for a panic reaction as seen in case 2?
3. What kinds of long-term psychologic problem might this patient experience?

CASE STUDY: PSILOCYBIN INTOXICATION

History

A 26-year-old man with no previous history of psychiatric drug abuse ate at least 30 mushrooms in a discotheque. He became excited and anxious, and was taken to a hospital. On arrival, he vomited.

He remained conscious, and his auditory perceptions were enhanced. He began to experience visual hallucinations several times each minute. These were characterized as a flashback phenomenon, in which he referred back to traumatic incidences in his past. The patient remained extremely agitated and restless, and could not be addressed.

Prominent symptoms included warm and dry skin, and a red face. He had difficulty with urination. Vital signs included: heart rate 120 beats/min, blood pressure 170/115 mm Hg, and rectal temperature 37.8°C. The most striking feature was his dilated pupils, which were unreactive to light.

The patient's clinical presentation suggested intoxication by an anticholinergic substance. Physostigmine, 4.0 mg, was given intravenously. Within 10 min the rate of hallucinations decreased, and by 25 min, all hallucinations ceased. After 40 min he was relaxed; blood pressure was 125/80 mm Hg, and pulse, 80 beats/min. He urinated one liter in 15 min. His pupils remained dilated, but were reactive to light.

Pupil diameter returned to normal over the next several hours. He experienced no further hallucinations, and required no additional therapy.

The mushrooms and urine samples were sent for analysis. The plants were identified as *Psilocybe semilanceata*, and they contained psilocybin. His urine tested negative for atropine and scopolamine. (See ref. 34.)

Discussion

1. Clinical characteristics of psilocybin intoxication are often defined as sympathomimetic. Did this patient present typically?
2. Why was physostigmine indicated in management of this patient?
3. What are some precautions follow when using physostigmine?

CASE STUDY: MESCALINE-ASSOCIATED FATALITY

History

Eyewitnesses stated that three people were standing at the bottom of a steep hill that overlooked the ocean. One of the three started running up the hill full-speed. Reaching the top, and without stopping, he jumped into midair as if he were doing a swan dive. He fell onto the rocks approximately 600 feet below, and suffered massive trauma to his head, torso, and extremities. Witnesses indicated that it appeared the jump was deliberate, rather than as the result of a drug-induced trip. A medical examiner pronounced the victim dead.

Samples of blood, urine, gastric contents, bile, liver and kidney tissues were submitted to toxicology screening. The results of analysis are shown in Table 17.6.

There was no indication of the amount of mescaline ingested or time of poisoning. The positive identification of the substance in various body tissues and fluids lends positive support to the belief that the death was drug related. (See ref. 27.)

Discussion

1. Calculate a "rough" dose of mescaline the victim may have ingested, based on information for the tissue and fluid levels listed above. Was this amount close to the dose that is reported to cause psychic effects?
2. Review the type of hallucinogen that mescaline is reported to be. How is it classed pharmacologically, and what is its natural source?

TABLE 17.6. *Laboratory findings*

Sample	Mescaline (μg/mL or μg/g)
Blood	9.7
Urine	11.63
Liver	70.8
Gastric contents	167 (total mg)
Bile	22.9

CASE STUDY: 3,4-METHYLENEDIOXYAMPHETAMINE MISUSE

History

A 24-year-old man arrived at a party around 7:30 p.m. He ingested one tablet containing 300 mg methaqualone. Approximately 15 min later he took 500 mg of a white powder that was believed to contain a mixture of LSD, morphine, and amphetamine. The powder was wrapped in a tissue and formed into a ball, which he swallowed. At 11:00 p.m. he ingested an additional 700 mg of the powder.

Within an hour he complained of being extremely "high" and needed to calm down. While resting, he was sweating profusely and speaking irrationally.

For the next hour or so, he was totally incoherent and thrashing violently. His hands were continually moving as if trying to pick up things. Finally, the victim's eyes rolled back and he swallowed his tongue.

He was attended to immediately by guests at the party. They pulled his tongue back and initiated mouth-to-mouth resuscitation, and he seemed to improve. He then became very calm and slept. At 2:30 a.m. he was found completely unresponsive and was rushed to a hospital. On admission, pupils were dilated and fixed, and his ECG showed no signs of cardiac activity. He was pronounced dead at 4:00 a.m.

Autopsy findings were unremarkable except for visceral coagulation and signs of anoxia. Toxicity screening confirmed ingestion of methaqualone by the presence of its metabolite in the urine, but failed to demonstrate the presence of amphetamine or morphine. However, thin-layer chromatographic analysis of the urine did reveal an unusual amine compound identified by using more specific analytical instruments, as 3,4-methylenedioxyamphetamine (MDA). (See ref. 25.)

Discussion

1. Explain the patient's "thrashing" about. How did MDA cause this?

2. Following an episode of apparent hyperexcitability, the victim became sedated and slept. What is the most likely explanation?
3. Comment on the probable cause of death.
4. If the patient had been sent to the emergency room, what treatment would he have been given?

Review Questions

1. Which of the following is true concerning LSD?
   A. LSD produces tachyphylaxis.
   B. LSD is metabolized to an active ergot alkaloid.
   C. LSD is stored in fat tissue for many years.
   D. LSD has a low therapeutic index.
2. Which of the following has the lowest potential for causing toxicity?
   A. LSD
   B. PCP
   C. Mescaline
   D. DOM
3. LSD-induced tachycardia and hypertension are due to:
   A. Stimulation of the sympathetic nervous system
   B. Inhibition of the sympathetic nervous system
   C. Cholinomimetic action
   D. Serotonergic action
4. A victim of DOM toxicity should receive treatment directed toward:
   A. Increasing the blood pressure
   B. Decreasing the blood pressure
5. A patient experiencing a toxic reaction to PCP should expect symptoms referable to which of the following pharmacologic actions: ganglionic blocking effect (I), sympathomimetic action (II), or anticholinergic action (III)?
   A. II only
   B. III only
   C. I and II only
   D. II and III only
   E. I, II, and III
6. Tolerance to LSD develops rapidly; recovery from this tolerance occurs slowly.

A. True
B. False

7. Phencyclidine concentrations in urine:
   A. Are generally increased by acidification
   B. Correlate well with degree of intoxication
   C. Are always greater than blood concentrations in acute overdose
   D. Are generally increased by alkalinization of urine

8. The phenethylamine derivatives mimic effects of which of the following naturally occurring endogenous neurotransmitters?
   A. Tryptamine
   B. Serotonin
   C. Norepinephrine
   D. Acetylcholine

9. In which of the following situations would the *talk-down* method be *least* effective?
   A. LSD-induced panic reaction
   B. LSD-related flashback
   C. Hyperexcitability due to MDA
   D. PCP-induced hallucinations

10. Moderate doses of marijuana may lead to all of the following *except*:
    A. Convulsions
    B. Loss of short-term memory
    C. Distortion of perception of time
    D. Loss of coordination

11. Most hallucinogens have a low therapeutic index.
    A. True
    B. False

12. Which of the following is considered to be the most potent hallucinogen?
    A. LSD
    B. Psilocybin
    C. Mescaline
    D. They are all equipotent

13. Which of the following is correct with respect to hallucinogen toxicity?
    A. In general, hallucinogens have a wide margin of safety.
    B. Toxic CNS manifestations of LSD can be usually controlled with chlorpromazine.
    C. Most hallucinogen-related overdoses

present with severe respiratory and pulmonary edema.
    D. All of the above are true.
    E. A & B only, are true.

14. All of the following are likely effects of LSD *except*:
    A. Dilated pupils
    B. Mild bradycardia
    C. Increased perception of visual color intensity
    D. Perceived "slowing" of the passage of time
    E. Elevation of blood glucose levels

15. The effects of marijuana commonly include all of the following *except*:
    A. Miosis
    B. Bloodshot eyes
    C. Mild euphoria
    D. Impaired short-term memory
    E. Mild sinus tachycardia

16. When attempting to differentiate a PCP overdose from a sedative-hypnotic overdose, a PCP overdose can be distinguished because:
    A. Only PCP can cause nystagmus
    B. PCP may cause hypertension
    C. PCP overdoses rarely present in a coma
    D. Muscle rigidity is markedly developed with PCP

17. PCP overdoses can be distinguished from amphetamine overdoses by the presence of:
    A. Miosis and nystagmus
    B. Tachycardia
    C. Hallucinations
    D. Hypertension

18. Describe the presenting symptoms that would most likely be noted in a victim of STP poisoning.

19. List the major reasons why it is often difficult to effectively treat a person who presents at the emergency room with symptoms of toxicity from an unknown psychotomimetic agent.

20. Describe the treatment protocol and objectives for PCP intoxication.

References

1. Aronow R, Done AK. Phencyclidine overdose: an emerging concept in management. *J Am Coll Emerg Physicians* 1978;7:56–59.
2. Aronow R, Miceli JN, Done AK. A therapeutic approach to the acutely overdosed PCP patient. *J Psychedelic Drugs* 1980;12:259–267.
3. Beeson HA. Intracranial hemorrhage associated with phencyclidine abuse. *JAMA* 1982;248:585–586.
4. Benjamin C. Persistent psychiatric symptoms after eating psilocybin mushrooms. *Br Med J* 1979;1:1319–1320.
5. Bergman RL. Navajo peyote use: its apparent safety. *Am J Psychiatry* 1971;128:51–60.
6. Budd RD, Lindstrom DM. Characteristics of victims of PCP-related deaths in Los Angeles county. *J Toxicol Clin Toxicol* 1983;19:997–1004.
7. Cogen FC, Regg G, Simmons JL. Phencyclidine-associated acute rhabdomyolysis. *Ann Intern Med* 1978;88:210–212.
8. Done AK, Aronow R, Miceli JN. Pharmacokinetic bases for the diagnosis and treatment of acute PCP intoxication. *J Psychedelic Drugs* 1980;12:253–258.
9. Dowling GP, McDonough ET, Bost RO. "Eve" and "Ecstasy": a report of five deaths associated with the use of MDEA and MDMA. *JAMA* 1987;257:1615–1617.
10. Frosch WA, Robbins ES, Stern M. Untoward reactions to lysergic acid diethylamide (LSD) resulting in hospitalization. *N Engl J Med* 1965;273:1235–1239.
11. Hatrick JA, Dewhurst K. Delayed psychosis due to LSD. *Lancet* 1970;2:742–744.
12. Hofmann A. Chemical, pharmacological and medical aspects of psychotomimetics. *J Exp Med Sci* 1961;5:40.
13. Jaffee JH. Drug addiction and drug use. In: Gilman AG, Goodman LS, Rall TW, Murad F, eds. *The pharmacological basis of therapeutics.* 7th ed. New York: Macmillan; 1985:532–581.
14. Karp HN, Kaufman ND, Anard SK. Phencyclidine poisoning in young children. *J Pediatr* 1980;97:1006–1009.
15. Kessler GF, Dewers IM, Berlin C, et al. Phencyclidine and fatal status epileptics. *N Engl J Med* 1979;291:979.
16. Khajawall AM, Simpson GM. Peculiarities of phencyclidine urinary excretion and monitoring. *J Toxicol Clin Toxicol* 1982–83;19:835–842.
17. Lahmeyer HW, Stock PG. Phencyclidine intoxication, physical restraint, and acute renal failure: case report. *J Clin Psychiatry* 1983;44:184–185.
18. Lieberman C, Lieberman B. Marijuana—a medical review. *N Engl J Med* 1971;284:88–91.
19. Mace S. LSD. *Clin Toxicol* 1979;15:219–224.
20. McCann MD, Ricanrte GA. Lasting neuropsychiatric sequelae of (+/−) methylene dioxy-methamphetamine ("Ecstasy") in recreational users. *J Clin Psychopharmacol* 1991;11:302–305.
21. McCarron MM, Schulze BW, Thompson GA, et al. Acute phencyclidine intoxication: incidence of clinical findings in 1,000 cases. *Ann Emerg Med* 1981;10:237–242.
22. Owens SM, Mayershon M. Modifications of phencyclidine (PCP) pharmacokinetics with PCP-specific Fab fragments. In: Clouet DH, ed. *Phencyclidine: an update.* NIDA research monograph 64. Rockville, MD: National Institute of Drug Abuse; 1986:112–126.
23. Owens SM, Mayersohn M. Phencyclidine-specific Fab fragments alter phencyclidine disposition in dogs. *Drug Metab Dispos* 1986;14:52–58.
24. Peterson RC, ed. *Marijuana research findings.* National Institute on Drug Abuse Research Monograph Series, Department of Health and Human Services publication no (ADM) 80-1001. Washington: US Government Printing Office; 1980.
25. Poklis A, Mackell MA, Drake WK. Fatal intoxication from 3,4-methylenedioxyamphetamine. *J Forensic Sci* 1979;24:70–75.
26. Rapport RT, Gay GR, Farris RD. Emergency management of acute phencyclidine intoxication. *J Am Coll Emerg Physicians* 1979;8:68–76.
27. Reynolds PC, Jindrich EJ. A mescaline associated fatality. *J Anal Toxicol* 1985;9:183–184.
28. Shick JFE, Smith DE. Analysis of the LSD flashback. *J Psychedelic Drugs* 1970;3:13–19.
29. Simpson GM, Khajawall AM, Alatorre E, Staples FR. Urinary phencyclidine excretion in chronic abusers. *J Toxicol Clin Toxicol* 1982–83;19:1051–1059.
30. Smith DE, Wesson DR. PCP abuse: Diagnostic and psychopharmacological treatment approaches. *J Psychedelic Drugs* 1980;12:293–299.
31. Solomons K, Nepps VM, Kuyl JM. Toxic cannabis psychosis is a valid entity. *S Afr Med J* 1990;78:476–481.
32. Truitt EG. Biological disposition of tetrahydrocannabinols. *Pharmacol Rev* 1971;23:273–278.
33. Unwin JR. Illicit drug use among Canadian youth. *Can Med Assoc J* 1968;98:449–454.
34. VanPoorten JF, Stienstra R, Duoracek B, et al. Physostigmine reversal of psilocybin intoxication. *Anesthesiology* 1982;56:313.
35. Weil AT, Zinberg NE, Nelson JM. Clinical and psychological effects of marijuana in man. *Science* 1968;162:1234–1242.

18 || Cardiovascular Drugs

The list of drugs that are used for therapeutic intervention of cardiovascular disease is large. There is also another sizable list of drugs that are used for noncardiac afflictions, but that can exert toxic manifestations on the cardiovascular system. Some of them, such as the tricyclic antidepressants, anticholinergics, phenothiazines, and cocaine, have been discussed in previous chapters.

In this chapter, two drug classes will be discussed: digitalis glycosides, and beta-adrenergic blockers. These drugs are commonly used. Signs and symptoms associated with poisoning are also descriptive of cardiovascular outcomes that follow toxicity of various other drugs.

DIGITALIS TOXICITY

Digitalis glycosides are life-saving drugs when they are used in therapeutic doses in the treatment of congestive heart failure, and for management of certain supraventricular rhythm disturbances. Digitalis increases the effective refractory period of atrial and ventricular cells. It also prolongs phase 3 of the cardiac action potential and increases the refractory period of the atrioventricular (AV) node and the Purkinje system. These actions account for its usefulness in protecting the ventricles during certain atrial arrhythmias.

Digoxin is one of the most widely prescribed drugs (14). Other digitalis preparations are less commonly used, and at some point in the near future may no longer be available. Prospective studies report that a digitalis glycoside is used by about 15% of all hospitalized persons (4). It is also estimated that 20% to 30% of patients taking a digitalis preparation will experience toxicity because the drugs have an extremely narrow therapeutic index (3,24). To illustrate, the serum concentration of digoxin for therapeutic activity is in the normal range of 1.2 to 1.7 ng/mL. Concentrations that cause clinically significant toxicity are usually only 2 to 3 times greater (16). The mortality rate with toxic doses is reported to be as great as 25% (3).

With increased medical awareness of the problem and availability of sensitive tests for determining serum concentrations, the incidence of poisoning may decrease in the future (2). Also, with use of the specific antidote (digoxin immune Fab) for treating toxicity, the mortality rate may also improve.

Excessive intake is a common cause of poisoning (21). Accidental overdosage usually occurs in children who ingest medication belonging to a relative. Suicide with digitalis is not common in the United States, although it is more prevalent in other countries. Concurrent administration of a diuretic that induces potassium loss is reported to be the most frequent cause of toxicity (14). Variability in bioavailability of digoxin tablets was a common cause of toxicity until recently. With adoption of strict standards for manufacture, the problem has been overcome (4).

Pharmacokinetics

The pharmacokinetic parameters for digoxin and digitoxin are summarized in Table 18.1 (10). The half-life of digoxin is about 1.5 days. Renal excretion is the major route of elimination. Digitoxin is the least polar of the digitalis glycosides. It, therefore, binds readily with serum proteins and is excreted slowly, with a half-life of 4 to 6 days. Digoxin has a large volume of distribution, which limits the usefulness of dialysis (See chapter 3).

Digitalis intoxication is influenced by the presence of other drugs. The most significant pharmacokinetic drug interaction reported has been with concomitantly administered quinidine. Combined use of quinidine and digoxin can result in a two-fold increase in serum digoxin concentration (4,11,19). The total body clearance and volume of distribution are reduced; the half-life is not prolonged (9). Though the exact mechanism of this interaction is not fully known, displacement of digoxin from tissue-binding sites appears to be a likely mechanism. A similar interaction has also been demonstrated with verapamil (17,26).

TABLE 18.1. *Digitalis preparations*

Measurement	Digoxin	Digitoxin
Onset time (oral ingestion)	1.5–6 hr	3–6 hr
Peak	4–6 hr	6–12 hr
Half-life	31–40 hr[a]	4–6 days
Protein-bound (%)	20–25%	90–97%
Volume of distribution	7–8 L/kg	0.6 L/kg
Route of elimination	Renal, 75%	Hepatic, 80%
Toxic blood levels	2.4 ng/mL	Over 30 ng/mL
Enterohepatic cycling	Small	Large (6.6%/day)

[a] For persons with normal renal function. Value will increase with renal functional impairment.

Individuals with the anaerobic microorganism *Eubacterium lentum* in their colon may require larger doses of digitalis to achieve therapeutic serum concentrations. This microorganism reduces the lactone ring of digitalis. When these patients receive antibiotics, such as tetracycline or erythromycin, which eradicate the organism, digitalis blood concentrations may become toxic (23).

Digitalis toxicity is also influenced by other pathologic findings. For example, renal disease increases the likelihood of toxicity (4). Enhanced sympathomimetic amine release during periods of stress, such as dental office visits, can provoke digitalis toxicity (4,25). One of the case studies at the end of this chapter illustrates this point. Table 18.2 summarizes many of the factors that influence individual patient sensitivity to digitalis. The numerous factors once again illustrate many of the principles of poisoning that were discussed earlier in this text.

Mechanism of Toxicity

Withering (38) clearly described the toxic manifestations of digitalis in his original treatise on the drug in 1785: "The foxglove when given in very large and quickly repeated doses, occasions sickness, vomiting, purging, giddiness, confused vision, objects appearing green or yellow; increased secretion of urine with frequent notions to part with it; slow pulse, even as low as 35 in a minute, cold sweats, convulsions, syncope and death."

Digitalis toxicity is not as common today as a decade or two ago. Nevertheless, it remains one of the most significant causes of adverse drug reactions (31). The mechanism of toxicity has not been fully explained. Toxicity is believed to result from an extension of pharmacologic actions, but effects occur more intensely (4).

A toxic dose of digitalis interferes with transport of Na^+ and Ca^{2+} (29). The glyco-

TABLE 18.2. *Factors that influence the toxicity to digitalis glycosides*

Digitalis resistance
  Apparent
    Doses taken other than as prescribed
    Inadequate bioavailability of tablets
    Inadequate intestinal absorption
    Increased metabolic degradation by gut microbials
  True end-organ resistance
    Infancy
    Elevated sympathetic tone from all causes, including uncontrolled congestive heart failure
    Hyperthyroidism
Digitalis sensitivity
  Apparent
    Unsuspected use of digitalis
    Change from tablets with poor bioavailability to tablets with high bioavailability
    Decreased renal excretion
    Drug-drug interactions (e.g., quinidine)
  True end-organ sensitivity to toxic doses
    Advanced myocardial disease
    Active myocardial ischemia
    Electrolyte imbalance (especially hypokalemia)
    Acid-base imbalance
    Concurrent drug administration (e.g., catecholamines)
    Hypothyroidism
    Hypoxemia (especially in setting of acute respiratory failure)
    Altered autonomic tone (e.g., vagotonic states)

From ref. 32.

TABLE 18.3. *Arrhythmias noted in digitalis poisoning*

Bradyarrhythmias
  Sinus bradycardia
  Sinus arrest, sinus exit block
  AV-nodal block
Tachyarrhythmias
  Supraventricular
    Atrial tachycardia with AV block
    Nonparoxysmal AV-junctional tachycardia
  Ventricular
    Premature ventricular depolarizations, especially bigeminy
    Ventricular tachycardia, especially bidirectional tachycardia
    Ventricular fibrillation

From ref. 5.

sides bind with high affinity to an inhibitory site on the portion of the NaK-ATPase structure that faces the outside of the cell. Consequently, Na^+ and K^+ transport are blocked as long as the drug molecule remains in place. Since K^+ transport back into cells is blocked, its concentration in the extracellular fluid increases. This is why serum K^+ concentration is a good indication of the extent of digitalis poisoning. The changes in Na^+ fluxes across cardiac cell membranes result in disturbed impulse conduction. Accumulation of Ca^{2+} intracellularly produces a positive inotropic action. An overdose of digitalis causes a reduction in resting membrane potentials, and cardiac pacemaker cells cannot function properly. The outcome is asystole with complete loss of all cardiac function.

The electrophysiologic changes result in a variety of cardiac arrhythmias (Table 18.3). Arrhythmias may be produced by direct ionic membrane changes, as well as autonomic neuronal effects (13).

Characteristics of Poisoning

Digitalis toxicity may appear after acute or chronic administration of therapeutic doses or massive intentional or accidental overdose. In any case, digitalis produces a wide array of signs and symptoms of toxicity that vary in frequency and severity. They involve not only

the heart, but also the GI tract, CNS, and other targets, independently or together (Table 18.4).

Early manifestations of intoxication that occur in approximately 50% of all cases generally involve the GI tract. Complaints of anorexia, nausea, vomiting, and abdominal pain are common, but not universal. Nausea and vomiting occur from direct drug action on the chemoreceptor trigger zone, rather than to irritation of the GI tract. Anorexia often precedes nausea and vomiting. Constipation, diarrhea, and abdominal cramping are uncommon. Blurred vision, loss of visual acuity, and green-yellow halos have been described as early-appearing symptoms. Intoxicated patients often report that they perceive yellows and greens more prominently. Onset of any of these complaints in a person taking digitalis should be a signal that toxicity is underway.

CNS effects include a variety of neuropsychiatric disturbances. Digitalis intoxication can provoke a large number of dysarrhythmias, as listed in Table 18.3. All portions of the cardiac conduction system are affected. These include bradyarrhythmias, tachyarrhythmias, or a combination of both. No specific arrhythmia is pathognomonic (i.e., absolutely characteristic) of digitalis poisoning. Younger persons without significant heart disease usually develop bradyarrhythmias and heart block. Older individuals and those with cardiac pathology generally present with ventricular arrhythmias with or without heart block (28). Atrioventricular block and severe

TABLE 18.4. *Clinical manifestations of digitalis toxicity*

Fatigue
Visual symptoms
Weakness
Nausea
Anorexia
Psychic complaints
Abdominal pain
Dizziness
Abnormal dreaming
Headache
Diarrhea
Vomiting

From ref. 20.

bradycardia may be mediated by increased vagal activity, whereas sympathetic stimulation may be manifested in digoxin toxicity as tachyarrhythmias. Serious arrhythmias are more likely to appear when the heart is compromised by concurrent disease states.

Management of Poisoning

Digitalis toxicity is common enough so that any new arrhythmia, generalized malaise, or gastrointestinal distress encountered during therapy should suggest that a reduction in dosage is needed. This is especially true when there are predisposing factors, such as old age or renal or pulmonary disease present.

Management of acute digitalis toxicity must be individualized since many of the therapeutic measures are toxic in their own right. Management involves removal of ingested drug, maintenance of a normal potassium concentration, reversal of arrhythmias, and increased removal of unabsorbed drug. More recently, it may include the use of a specific antidote, digoxin immune Fab.

After massive overdoses of digitalis, efforts to decontaminate the GI tract should be undertaken. The stomach should be lavaged to remove unabsorbed drug, although vomiting may already have accomplished this. Cardiac glycosides bind to activated charcoal, cholestyramine, and colestipol (7,27). Repeated administration of one of these adsorbents is, therefore, recommended to enhance elimination of the glycoside by interrupting enterohepatic cycling exhibited by digitoxin, and possibly digoxin.

Hypokalemia is more common after chronic digitalis toxicity. Massive acute overdoses often cause hyperkalemia (5.5 to 13.5 mEq/L) as discussed earlier (2,28). Hyperkalemia may require treatment with insulin, dextrose, bicarbonate, and sodium polystyrene sulfonate (Kayexalate). The latter is an ion exchange resin used to reduce elevated potassium levels. This procedure can be dangerous in that it may aggravate intracellular deficits.

The patient should be monitored continuously with frequent electrocardiogram and electrolyte determinations. Specific treatment to reverse digitalis-induced arrhythmias is chosen based on the type of arrhythmia present.

When hypokalemia is encountered with tachy- or bradyarrhythmias, continuous potassium replacement alone may be sufficient. Even in the absence of hypokalemia, potassium administration may correct arrhythmias by restoring intracellular concentrations (7). This must be undertaken very cautiously when hypokalemia has not been specifically demonstrated. Potassium administration in a person with digitalis-induced hyperkalemia can result in heart block terminating in sinus arrest (28). For atrial and ventricular arrhythmias that do not respond to potassium therapy, the treatment of choice includes phenytoin and lidocaine (7).

An advantage to using these drugs is that they depress ventricular automaticity without slowing AV nodal conduction, as seen with quinidine and procainamide. Additionally, phenytoin increases AV nodal conduction and directly reverses the toxic action of digitalis at the AV node without interfering with its inotropic action. If digitalis has produced AV block, the vagolytic action of atropine may increase the heart rate and AV conduction. Catecholamines are contraindicated for treating bradyarrhythmias resulting from digitalis toxicity (7). They can increase the risk of precipitating more serious ectopic arrhythmias.

Beta-adrenergic blockers, such as propranolol, are useful to suppress supraventricular and ventricular arrhythmias induced by digitalis toxicity. However, these drugs may further depress SA node and AV node conduction, which can be disadvantageous in a person with an already failing heart. This, therefore, limits their usefulness.

Last-resort therapy involves direct-current countershock. The greatest mortality to this procedure is associated with its use in patients intoxicated with digitalis.

Efforts to enhance elimination of digoxin by diuresis, hemoperfusion, or hemodialysis, have not been successful because of its large volume of distribution. The clinical literature is unclear on the reliability of these procedures. Hemodialysis is still sometimes required to control hyperkalemia (7).

Digoxin Immune Fab (Digibind)

One approach to successful treatment of toxicity is the use of digoxin-specific antibodies. The initial use of purified digoxin-specific Fab fragments was reported in 1976 (33). These are antibody fragments prepared by conjugation of digoxin to human or bovine serum albumin. This is then used to immunize sheep, which produce antibodies. Their sera are obtained and purified, yielding the drug. The fragments are less immunogenic than whole antibodies, and can be eliminated by glomerular filtration (8).

The antidote is reserved for life-threatening overdoses because it has not yet been thoroughly evaluated. Indications of such toxicity include ingestion of more than 10 mg digoxin by healthy adults or 4 mg by children; steady-state serum concentrations greater than 10 ng/mL; or if the blood potassium concentration exceeds 5 mEq/L. Within minutes of injecting the antidote, free serum digoxin or digitoxin levels drop to almost unmeasurable concentrations.

Dosage can be calculated from the amount of digoxin or digitoxin in the patient's body. This is estimated from the actual amount of drug ingested, or by measuring its concentration in the serum. After acute ingestion, the estimated total body concentration of digoxin is assumed to be equal to 80% of the total amount ingested; this corrects for incomplete absorption. For digitoxin, the total body load is equal to 100% of the quantity ingested.

When steady-state serum concentrations of digoxin or digitoxin are known, the total body load can be estimated as shown below:

Digoxin: Body load (mg)

$$= \frac{(SDC)(5.6)(\text{wt in kg})}{1000}$$

Digitoxin: Body load (mg)

$$= \frac{(SDC)(0.56)(\text{wt in kg})}{1000}$$

SDC is the serum digitalis concentration in ng/mL. This is multiplied by the mean volume of distribution of digoxin (5.6 L/kg) or digitoxin (0.56 L/kg), times the patient's weight in kg. The product is then divided by 1,000 to obtain the estimated amount of drug in the body in mg (34).

Each vial of antidote contains 40 mg of digoxin-specific antibody fragments. This will bind 0.6 mg digoxin or digitoxin. The total number of vials needed can be obtained by dividing the total body load of drug in mg, by 0.6 mg/vial.

Adverse effects to digoxin immune Fab have been minimal. Sensitivity, erythema at the site of injection, and rash and urticaria have been reported.

BETA-ADRENERGIC BLOCKERS

A number of drugs that block beta-adrenergic receptors are widely used for treatment of a multitude of disease states, including hypertension, cardiac arrhythmias, angina pectoris, open-angle glaucoma, and to protect against migraine headaches (22). In fact the drugs have over 50 clinical applications (1). These drugs have significant pharmacologic and pharmacokinetic differences, as outlined in Table 18.5. The three major pharmacologic considerations include differences in cardioselectivity, intrinsic sympathomimetic activity (ISA), and membrane stabilizing activity. The pharmacokinetic properties of importance include lipid solubility, route of metabolic elimination, plasma half-life, degree of protein binding, and volume of distribution. Variations in pharmacologic and pharmacokinetic properties of various beta-adrenergic blockers influence their therapeutic application, incidence of side effects, and type and severity of toxic reactions when taken in overdose. Most poisonings involve propranolol (36).

TABLE 18.5. *Beta-adrenergic blockers*

Drug	Adrenergic receptor blocking activity	Membrane stabilizing activity	Intrinsic sympathomimetic activity	Lipid solubility	Half-life (hr)	Elimination
Acebutolol	B_1	+	+	Low	3–4	Hepatic, renal, bile
Atenolol	B_1	0	0	Low	6–9	Unchanged (50%)
Betaxolol	B_1	+	0	Low	14–22	Hepatic
Bisoprolol	B_1	0	0	Low	9–12	Unchanged (50%)
Esmolol	B_1	0	0	Low	0.15	Esterases in RBCs
Metoprolol	B_1	0	0	Moderate	3–7	Hepatic, renal
Carteolol	B_1, B_2	0	+ +	Low	6	Unchanged (50–70%)
Nadolol	B_1, B_2	0	0	Low	20–24	Unchanged
Penbutolol	B_1, B_2	0	+	High	5	Hepatic
Pindolol	B_1, B_2	+	+ + +	Moderate	3–4	Renal, unchanged
Propranolol	B_1, B_2	+ +	0	High	3–5	Hepatic
Sotolol	B_1, B_2	0	0	Low	12	Unchanged
Timolol	B_1, B_2	0	0	Low to moderate	4	Hepatic
Labetalol	B_1, B_2	0	0	Moderate	5.5–8	Hepatic, unchanged

Mechanism of Toxicity

Toxic effects of acute overdose with beta-adrenergic blockers are predictable and result from the drug binding to and inhibiting beta-adrenergic receptors throughout the body. The principle manifestations of poisoning include bradycardia and hypotension. In overdose, the membrane stabilizing or quinidine-like action of some beta-adrenergic blockers predominate (Table 18.6). This is responsible for the severe myocardial depressant actions leading to heart block, and possibly CNS effects, such as sedation and seizures. High doses of beta-adrenergic blockers with ISA (e.g., acebutolol, carteolol, oxprenolol, and pindolol) can cause tachycardia and hypertension as a result of their partial agonist effect.

Oral doses of beta-adrenergic blockers are absorbed rapidly. They readily distribute throughout the body tissues and undergo a rapid first-pass metabolism. Their high lipid solubility accounts for the CNS effects seen with certain ones, especially propranolol. In overdose, pharmacokinetic parameters may change drastically due to decreased cardiac output with subsequently reduced hepatic and renal blood flow. As a result, high drug concentrations and extended plasma half-life values are expected.

Overt toxicity may be apparent as early as 20 min postingestion, but usually is not observed until 1 to 2 hr later (12). Clinical symptoms persist beyond the drugs' half-life. As a result, blood level determinations alone are unreliable for assessing possible overdose, prognosis, or predicting therapy.

Characteristics of Poisoning

The most commonly reported signs and symptoms of beta-adrenergic blocker poisoning are listed in Table 18.6. Underlying pathology may influence the toxicity of beta-adrenergic blockers significantly. Bronchospasm and pulmonary edema, for example, may be more prominent in patients with chronic obstructive pulmonary disease (12). Congestive heart failure or diminished cardiac reserve can worsen the prognosis.

The major features of beta-adrenergic blocker toxicity are related to their antagonistic action on cardiac beta receptors. An overdose causes a diminution of myocardial contractility, producing bradycardia (92%) and severe hypotension (77%) leading to cardiogenic shock. Electrocardiographic changes consist of first-degree AV block (prolonged PR interval), widening of the QRS complex,

TABLE 18.6. Clinical manifestations of beta-adrenergic blocker toxicity

Cardiac	CNS	Other
Arrhythmias	Sleepiness	Bronchospasm
Bradycardia	Dizziness	Pulmonary edema
Atrioventricular block	Unconsciousness	Hypoglycemia
Hypotension	Coma	Hyperkalemia
Tachycardia	Seizures	
Shock	Respiratory depression	

absence of P waves, and prolongation of the QT interval (30,36). There are numerous incidences of complete heart block. Cardiac changes are not reported uniformly in all beta-adrenergic blocker poisonings. They do occur most frequently with drugs that have membrane-stabilizing action. Electrocardiographic changes are more prominent at serum drug concentrations that are 50 to 100 times greater than needed for beta receptor blockade (6).

CNS effects may involve seizures. In one report they occurred in 58% of patients. These generally followed propranolol doses greater than 1,600 mg. Seizure activity results from hypoglycemia, cerebral hypoxia, or from a membrane-stabilizing effect (36).

Management of Poisoning

Since overdoses of beta-adrenergic blockers are likely to involve solid dosage forms, gastric decontamination after a large ingestion may be indicated. Gastric lavage is usually preferred over emesis because of the possibility of beta-blocker-induced seizures. Activated charcoal can be given repeatedly during the first 24 hours to minimize enterohepatic cycling. Other areas of general management include giving glucose for hypoglycemia, diazepam for convulsions, and monitoring potassium levels.

The major emphasis in management of toxicity will be to minimize cardiovascular manifestations. In the treatment of bradycardia, if the patient is stable hemodynamically, no specific therapy is required. If the patient is compromised hemodynamically, atropine may be given. If vagal blockade is unsuccessful, iso-

proterenol, a specific beta-1 agonist, can be given cautiously. The hypotensive patient may respond to fluids in the absence of pulmonary edema. Pressor agents, such as dopamine, dobutamine, or norepinephrine, may be useful. However, beta blocker-induced hypotension generally does not respond well to these agents (see the case studies at the end of this chapter). The treatment of choice in the hemodynamically compromised person appears to be glucagon.

Glucagon produces positive inotropic and chronotropic activity and improves AV conduction by binding to glucagon-specific receptors (not beta-one receptors) in the myocardium and activating the adenyl cyclase system (37). This results in increased intracellular cyclic AMP concentration. The action is similar to beta-receptor stimulation by catecholamines, except that beneficial activity continues despite the presence of beta-adrenergic blockers. The effect of glucagon in beta-adrenergic blocker poisonings is dramatic (6,18,30,36,37).

It has been suggested that inhibitors of phosphodiesterase, such as theophylline, can elevate intracellular cyclic AMP concentrations also. Given with glucagon, the two will theoretically act synergistically to elevate intracellular cyclic AMP levels thereby causing sustained elevation of cardiac tone. However, benefit from such therapy has not yet been evaluated (15).

Hemoperfusion or hemodialysis may be considered in cases involving nadolol or atenolol, especially if there are signs of renal failure. Due to their extensive protein binding and large volume of distribution, most other beta-adrenergic blockers are poor candidates for dialysis.

SUMMARY

As with other drug toxicities, patients who have taken an overdose of cardiotherapeutic agents should be treated according to the general principles of management of poisons discussed earlier in this text. Emphasis is on supportive care, efforts to remove unabsorbed drug from the GI tract, and actions, when appropriate, to clear the toxic agent from the blood.

Case Studies

CASE STUDY: STRESS-INDUCED DIGOXIN TOXICITY

History

The patient was a 48-year-old woman who was undergoing dental surgery for gingival hyperplasia. Her preoperative vital signs were normal.

She received multiple intraoral injections of 2% mepivacaine with 1:20,000 levonordefrin for local anesthetic preparation. Within 5 min of receiving the anesthetic, she became dyspneic and exhibited bilateral neck vein distention. Her heart rate was 80 beats/min. Blood pressure was 110/60 mm Hg. Using a standard lead II electrocardiogram, premature ventricular contractions at a rate of 12/min were revealed. The QRS complex was widened and ST depression observed.

After placing the patient in a sitting position, 100% oxygen was administered. A 5% dextrose in lactated Ringer's solution was given intravenously, and 75 mg of lidocaine administered. She was transported to a nearby hospital.

On admission, additional dysrhythmias such as right bundle branch block and atrial fibrillation were noted. The serum potassium level was 3.1 mEq/L. Digoxin assay revealed a serum concentration of 2.1 ng/mL. She was admitted to the cardiac care unit for further observation. (See ref. 25.)

Discussion

1. It is highly likely that the stress from impending dental surgery initiated this toxic outcome to normal doses of digoxin. Explain a probable mechanism(s) that precipitated the toxic event.
2. Of what significance to digitalis toxicity was this patient's potassium level (3.1 mEq/L)?
3. How extensive was this individual poisoned? What is the normal therapeutic dose range for digoxin?
4. After reviewing this patient's cardiac activity upon admission to the hospital, outline a treatment protocol to best treat her abnormalities.

CASE STUDY: DIGOXIN TOXICITY TREATED WITH DIGOXIN IMMUNE FAB

History

A 65-year-old woman was admitted to an emergency department after ingestion of seventy 0.0625-mg tablets of digoxin (4.375 mg total) in a suicide attempt, 5 hr previously. Her medical history revealed rheumatic fever and analgesic nephropathy. Usual therapy included digoxin 0.0625 mg/day.

She underwent lavage and received a slurry of activated charcoal via a nasogastric tube. Laboratory values included serum potassium, 4.3 mmol/L; serum creatinine, 395 μmol/L; and serum digoxin, 19.8 mmol/L. Blood pressure was 135/85 mm Hg. Heart rate was 130 beats/min and irregular.

The patient was alert. She was nauseated and vomited several times. Her vision was blurred.

An electrocardiogram revealed atrial and junctional tachycardia with intermittent 2:1 to 4:1 block, and occasional ventricular ectopic beats. After several hours, her serum potassium concentration was 5.0 mmol/L.

Treatment included phenytoin 500 mg. She did not respond to therapy. By now her serum potassium concentration had risen to 5.4 mEq/L. Vitals remained unchanged. She was then given 400 mg of digoxin immune Fab over 30 min. Her ECG remained unaltered, so another 400 mg dose of the antidote was administered 1 hr later.

One hour after the second dose, her ECG showed a sinus rhythm of 110 beats/min. Serum potassium concentration had returned to 4.5 mEq/L. She maintained a sinus rhythm and her heart rate stabilized at 90 beats/min over the next 4 hr. An assay for free digoxin in the serum revealed that none was present at 20 min after the first dose of the Fab fragments. (See ref. 16.)

Discussion

1. This patient's serum potassium concentration rose during the early part of her intoxication, then fell after administration of the Fab fragments. Explain the origin of this ion, and its later fate.
2. For what specific purpose was the dose of phenytoin given?
3. Outline the mechanism by which digoxin immune Fab treats digoxin overdoses.
4. Convert the serum potassium concentrations given as mmol/L to mEq/L.

CASE STUDIES: MONITORING SERUM DIGOXIN CONCENTRATIONS DURING DIGOXIN IMMUNE FAB THERAPY

History: Case 1

A 63-year-old white woman (55 kg) with renal insufficiency (serum creatinine 299 μmol/L) developed complete heart block with a ventricular heart rate of 30 to 40 beats/min at an outside hospital. Chronic digoxin toxicity was diagnosed and the patient received 40 mg of Fab. It was reported that the patient responded to the Fab therapy with increased heart rate (50 to 60 beats/min). However, upon arrival at the hospital 8 hr later, the patient again developed complete heart block with a

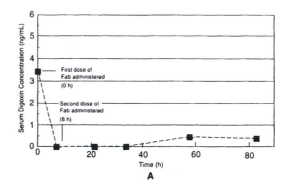

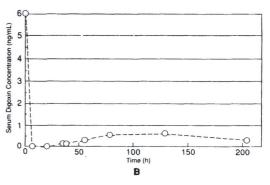

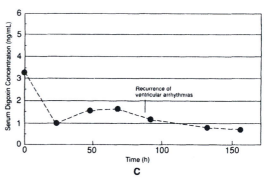

FIG. 18.1. Effect of Fab treatment of digoxin intoxication; serum digoxin concentration vs. time in 3 patients. (From ref. 35.)

ventricular heart rate of 30 to 40 beats/min. She received an additional 80 mg of Fab. When no response was evident, a temporary ventricular lead pacemaker was inserted.

Figure 18.1A depicts the free serum digoxin concentration-versus-time profile for this patient. Free serum digoxin concentrations were undetectable before the second Fab dose and for the subsequent 48 hours. This suggested that another etiology was responsible for the continuing heart block. The absence of detectable free serum digoxin concentrations correlated with the lack of response to the second dose of Fab. If free serum digoxin concentration had been monitored prospectively, digoxin intoxication could have been ruled out quickly as the cause of the second episode of heart block.

History: Case 2

A 69-year-old woman on chronic hemodialysis presented to the emergency room with signs (atrial tachycardia with block) and symptoms (severe abdominal pain, nausea, lethargy, mental status changes) of digoxin toxicity and an SDC of 7.686 nmol/L. One hundred and sixty milligrams of Fab were administered and the patient experienced prompt resolution of her arrhythmia, gastrointestinal distress, lethargy, and confusion.

Over the following three weeks serum digoxin concentrations were obtained prospectively and determined by radioimmunoassay, which is known to be adversely affected by Fab. Reported SDCs were >8,198 nmol/L during the majority of this time period, although no signs or symptoms of digoxin intoxication were evident. The internist and nephrologist refused to discharge the patient from the hospital with a "toxic" serum digoxin concentration. They were concerned about medical liability on account of the lack of data regarding the use of Fab in hemodialysis patients as well as the possibility of free serum digoxin concentration rebound and digoxin toxicity recrudescence. This resulted in two additional weeks of hospitalization for the patient although her serum digoxin concentration declined.

Figure 18.1B depicts the free serum digoxin concentration-versus-time profile for this patient. Free serum digoxin concentration determined after Fab administration never exceeded 0.769 nmol/L, which correlated well with her clinical response to Fab. If free serum digoxin concentration had been monitored prospectively, the patient could have been discharged after the expected rebound in SDC had occurred, i.e., between 129 and 204 hours after Fab administration.

History: Case 3

A 25-year-old morbidly obese man (150 kg) with renal insufficiency (serum creatinine 343 μmol/L) was admitted to the hospital for signs and symptoms of digoxin toxicity, including atrial flutter with 3:1 block, frequent premature ventricular complexes, and a serum digoxin concentration of 4.227 nmol/L. Fab 180 mg was administered with subsequent resolution of his atrial and ventricular arrhythmias. Because of the patient's obesity it was very difficult to determine the proper Fab dose. Four days after Fab administration, however, the patient again experienced digoxin intoxication characterized by frequent premature ventricular complexes and a run of nonsustained ventricular tachycardia.

Figure 18.1C depicts the free serum digoxin concentration-versus-time profile for this patient. As can be seen in his figure, the patient's free SDC 24 hours post-Fab administration was 1.281 nmol/L and progressively increased to 2.045 nmol/L over the next three days. The rebound in free serum digoxin concentration was temporally related to when the patient again experienced digoxin toxicity, manifested as ventricular arrhythmias. However, if free serum digoxin concentration had been monitored prospectively, subsequent doses of Fab could have been calculated and administered to prevent the rebound in free SDC and recrudescence of digoxin toxicity in this patient. (See ref. 35.)

Discussion

1. Why is it imperative to measure free serum digoxin concentration when assessing toxicity?
2. Explain the mechanism of action of digoxin immune Fab. What other types of

intoxication do you think would be amenable to this approach to treating?

CASE STUDIES: PROPRANOLOL POISONING

History: Case 1

The patient was a 17-year-old girl who ingested 97 of her mother's 40-mg propranolol tablets (3,880 mg). Until this time she was well; her medical history was unremarkable.

Approximately one hour after taking the overdose, she presented to an emergency facility. She was lethargic, but able to stand. Heart rate was 75 beats/min. She experienced two generalized tonic-clonic seizures in succession, each lasting 20 to 30 sec. At this point her blood pressure was unobtainable; pulse was 40 beats/min. Expirations produced diffuse wheezing. Pupils were dilated and sluggish to light.

The patient was given oxygen, sodium bicarbonate (50 mEq), glucose (25 g), epinephrine (0.5 mg), and naloxone. Chest compressions (CPR) were begun. She failed to respond to treatment.

She was then intubated and placed in an antishock garment adjusted to a pressure of 100 mm Hg. Ringer's lactate solution was started. Over the next hour she also received atropine (1 mg), dopamine (5 μg/kg/min increased to 20 μg/kg/min), and 5 mL calcium chloride (10%), all without effect. Diazepam boluses were given as needed to control intermittent seizure activity.

Forty minutes later an isoproterenol infusion (8 μg/min) was initiated. The pulse increased transiently to 80 beats/min and systolic blood pressure to 60 mm Hg. These effects persisted for several minutes.

At 50 min she underwent lavage. The return was clear and contained no tablet fragments. One hundred grams of activated charcoal and 8 ounces of magnesium citrate solution were administered via the nasogastric tube.

By 60 min (2 hr postingestion), systolic blood pressure was 50 mm Hg and pulse was 64 beats/min. The patient was then given 2 mg glucagon. Within 4 min, blood pressure increased to 100/60 mm Hg. The antishock garment was removed. Glucagon was continued by infusion. Dopamine and isoproterenol were added.

The patient remained comatose until about 10 hr when she awoke. Vital signs included: blood pressure, 108/72 mm Hg; pulse, 72/min. She was weaned from all treatment over the next 11 hr, at which time her vital signs were stabilized. Blood pressure was 110/70 mm Hg, and pulse, 89/min.

A routine toxicology examination on admission failed to detect any drug other than propranolol. Serum propranolol concentrations were 2,640 ng/mL at 1.75 hr postadmission; 3,100 ng/mL at 4 hr; 1,657 ng/mL at 10 hr; and 1,240 ng/mL at 19 hr. (See ref. 37.)

History: Case 2

An 18-year-old man was brought to the emergency department after ingesting an estimated 2.4 g propranolol. On admission (30 min postingestion) he had gasping respirations. Blood pressure was not obtainable. He had experienced a brief seizure before admission. The patient was not taking any other therapy.

Treatment was started with atropine, isoproterenol, and glucagon. Pulse rate increased from 15 to 20 to 40 beats/min. Blood pressure rose to 80/60 mm Hg.

Gastric lavage returned a few tablet fragments. Activated charcoal therapy at 100 g every 4 hr was initiated. A pacemaker was placed and adjusted to 80 beats/min.

After a brief period of stabilization, the patient developed noncardiogenic pulmonary edema, mild bronchospasm, and pulmonary infiltrates. He became progressively hypotensive. Treatment with dobutamine, dopamine, and glucagon were begun. Over the next 12 hr the mean arterial pressure remained approximately 60 mm Hg.

Despite continued administration of dopamine and glucagon, along with levarterenol, epinephrine, naloxone, and calcium chloride, the patient developed bradycardia that rapidly progressed to asystole at 9 hr postingestion. He subsequently died. At autopsy, no other substance was found on urine and serum drug testing. (See ref. 1.)

Discussion

1. Comment on the range of therapy the patients received during treatment: epinephrine, norepinephrine, dopamine, dobutamine, naloxone, atropine, glucagon, sodium bicarbonate, and calcium chloride. What was the pharmacologic rationale for each?
2. Patient 1 ingested 3,880 mg propranolol and survived. Patient 2 ingested 2,400 mg and died. Both were treated approximately the same way. Cite the factors that may have been responsible for these different outcomes.
3. Patient 1 received activated charcoal after it was shown that no tablet remnants were left in her stomach. Patient 2 received multiple doses, every 4 hr. Explain the goal of therapy with each of these dosage regimens.

Review Questions

1. The half-life for digoxin and digitoxin, respectively, are closest to which of the following?
   A. 0.5 days; 1 day
   B. 1 day; 2 days
   C. 1.5 days; 4 days
   D. 2.5 days; 6 days
   E. 3.0 days; 8 days
2. Which of the following drugs causes the most significant pharmacokinetic drug interaction when it is added to therapy of a patient stabilized on digoxin?
   A. Phenytoin
   B. Aspirin
   C. Quinidine
   D. Morphine
   E. Lidocaine

3. Which of the following is a true statement about beta-adrenergic blocker poisoning?
   A. Blood level concentrations alone are unreliable for assessing possible overdose.
   B. Electrocardiogenic changes involve a narrowed QRS complex.
   C. Most reported poisonings have involved metoprolol.
   D. Seizure activity is rare, although CNS sedation is common.
   E. Diazepam is contraindicated in a person who exhibits signs of poisoning.
4. One symptom of digitalis intoxication is vision that appears:
   A. Yellow to green
   B. Pinkish to red
   C. Blue to purple
   D. Brown to dark
5. Digitalis glycosides produce their toxic actions by binding with which of the following enzyme systems?
   A. Monoamine oxidase
   B. Pseudocholinesterase
   C. Carbonic anhydrase
   D. NaK-ATPase
6. The most common indicator of impending digitalis intoxication is:
   A. Palpitations
   B. Dizziness
   C. Headache
   D. Nausea
7. The principal manifestations of poisoning with a beta-adrenergic blocker are:
   A. Bradycardia
   B. Hypotension
   C. Both of the above
   D. Neither of the above
8. The treatment that is most likely to block enterohepatic cycling of digitoxin is:
   A. Cholestyramine
   B. Fab fragments
   C. Dobutamine
   D. Glucagon
   E. Sodium polystyrene sulfonate
9. All of the following are reasonable emergency medical approaches to management of a digitalis-intoxicated patient *except*:

A. Hemoperfusion and/or hemodialysis
B. IV administration of digoxin immune Fab (Digibind)
C. IV lidocaine or phenytoin for ventricular arrhythmias
D. Repeated p.o. doses of activated charcoal
E. Repeated p.o. administration of cholestyramine

10. All of the following are likely EKG manifestations of beta-adrenergic blocker toxicity *except*:
    A. AV block (1st, 2nd, or 3rd degree)
    B. Absence of P waves
    C. Widening of QRS complex
    D. Shortening of the PR interval
    E. Prolongation of the QT interval

11. Which of the following is/are reasonable therapeutic measures in the emergency medical management of beta-adrenergic blocker intoxication?
    A. Administration of atropine to control the excessive bradycardia
    B. Administration of glucagon to stimulate both cardiac inotropy and chronotropy
    C. Administration of dopamine, dobutamine, or norepinephrine to counteract the extreme hypotension
    D. All of the above are reasonable
    E. Only two of the above are reasonable

12. Explain the mechanism of action of glucagon in treating beta-adrenergic blocker toxicity.

13. Discuss reasons why hyperkalemia is a usual symptom of acute digoxin intoxication, although hypokalemia normally appears with chronic poisoning.

14. Cite the reason why the microorganism *Eubacterium lentum* can modify the outcome of digoxin therapy.

15. What is the reason why digoxin is a poor candidate for removal from the blood by hemodialysis?

16. Explain why it may be unwise to attempt electroshock conversion in a person intoxicated with a digitalis glycoside.

17. Suggest why theophylline may be a suitable treatment for beta-adrenergic blocker toxicity.

18. Explain how ISA activity of a beta-adrenergic blocker can significantly alter the outcome of an overdose.

References

1. Amundson DE, Brodine SK. A fatal case of propranolol poisoning. *Drug Intell Clin Pharm* 1988;22:781–782.
2. Antman EM, Smith TW. Digitalis toxicity. *Ann Rev Med* 1985;36:357–367.
3. Beller GA, Smith TW, Abelmann W, et al. Digitalis intoxication: prospective clinical study with serum level correlations. *N Engl J Med* 1971;284:989–997.
4. Bigger JT. Digitalis toxicity. *J Clin Pharmacol* 1985;25:514–521.
5. Bigger JT, Leahey EB. Quinidine and digoxin: an important interaction. *Drugs* 1982;24:229–239.
6. Buiumsohn A, Eisenberg ES, Jacob H, et al. Seizures and intraventricular conduction defect in propranolol poisoning: a report of two cases. *Ann Intern Med* 1979;91:860–862.
7. Bullock RE, Hall RJC. Digitalis toxicity and poisoning. *Adverse Drug React Acute Poisoning Rev* 1982;1:201–222.
8. Cole PL, Smith TW. Use of digoxin-specific Fab fragments in the treatment of digitalis intoxication. *Drug Intell Clin Pharm* 1986;20:267–269.
9. Doering W. Digoxin-quinidine interaction. *N Engl J Med* 1979;301:400–404.
10. Doherty JE. Digitalis glycosides: pharmacokinetics and their clinical implications. *Ann Intern Med* 1973;79:229.
11. Ejrinsson G. Effect of quinidine on plasma concentrations of digoxin. *Br Med J* 1978;1:279–280.
12. Frishman W, Harold J, Eisenberg E, Hillel R. Appraisal and reappraisal of cardiac therapy. *Am Heart J* 1979;98:798–811.
13. Gillis RA, Quest JA. The role of the nervous system in the cardiovascular effects of digitalis. *Pharmacol Rev* 1980;31:19–97.
14. Hoffman BF, Bigger JT. Digitalis and allied cardiac glycosides. In: Gilman AG, Goodman LS, Rall TW, Murad F, eds. *The pharmacological basis of therapeutics.* 7th ed. New York: Macmillan; 1985:716–747.
15. Jones B. Treatment of beta-blocker poisoning. *Lancet* 1980;1:1031.
16. Jones M, Hawker F, Duggin G, Falk M. Treatment of severe digoxin toxicity with digoxin-specific antibody fragments. *Anaesth Intensive Care* 1987;15:234–236.
17. Klein HO, Lang R, Weiss E, et al. The influence of verapamil on serum digoxin concentrations. *Circulation* 1982;65:1163–1170.
18. Kosinski EJ, Malindzak GS. Glucagon and isoproterenol in reversing propranolol toxicity. *Arch Intern Med* 1973;132:840–843.
19. Leakey EG, Reiffel JA, Drusin RE, et al. Inter-

action between digoxin and quinidine. *JAMA* 1978; 240:533–534.

20. Lely AH, VanEnter CHJ. Large-scale digitoxin intoxication. *Br Med J* 1970;3:737–740.

21. Lewander WJ, Gaudreault P, Einhorn A, et al. Acute pediatric digoxin ingestion. *Am J Dis Child* 1986;140:770–773.

22. Lewis RV, McDevitt DG. Adverse reactions and interactions with beta-adrenoceptor blocking drugs. *Med Toxicol* 1986;1:343–361.

23. Lindenbaum J, Rund DG, Butler VP, et al. Inactivation of digoxin by the gut flora: reversal by antibiotic therapy. *N Engl J Med* 1981;305:789–794.

24. Mason DT, Zelis R, Lee G, et al. Current concepts and treatment of digitalis toxicity. *Am J Cardiol* 1971;27:546–557.

25. Milam SB, Giovannitti JA. Digitalis toxicity: a case report. *J Periodontol* 1984;55:414–418.

26. Pederson KE, Dorph-Pederson A, Haidt S, et al. Digoxin verapamil interaction. *Clin Pharmacol Ther* 1981;30:311–316.

27. Pond S, Jacobs M, Marks J, et al. Treatment of digitoxin overdoses with oral activated charcoal. *Lancet* 1981;2:1177–1178.

28. Rumack BH, Lovejoy FH. Clinical toxicology. In: Klaassen CD, Amdur MO, Doull J, eds. *The basic science of poisons.* 3rd ed. New York: Macmillan; 1986:879–901.

29. Schwartz A. Is the cell membrane Na^+,K^+-ATPase enzyme system the pharmacological receptor for digitalis? *Circ Res* 1976;39:1.

30. Shore ET, Cepin D, Davidson MJ. Metoprolol overdose. *Ann Emerg Med* 1981;10:524–527.

31. Smith TW. Digitalis—mechanisms of action and clinical use. *N Engl J Med* 1988;318:358–365.

32. Smith TW, Antman EM, Friedman PL, et al. Digitalis glycosides: I. Mechanisms and manifestations of toxicity. *Prog Cardiovasc Dis* 1984;26:413–441.

33. Smith TW, Haber E, Yeatman L, Butler VP. Reversal of advanced digoxin intoxication with Fab fragments of digoxin-specific antibodies. *N Engl J Med* 1976;294:797–800.

34. Stolshek BS, Osterhout SK, Dunham G. The role of digoxin-specific antibodies in the treatment of digitalis poisoning. *Med Toxicol* 1984;3:167–171.

35. Ujhelyi MR, Colucci RD, Cummings DM, et al. Monitoring serum digoxin concentrations during digoxin immune FAB therapy. *DICP Ann Pharmacother* 1991;25:1047–1049.

36. Weinstein RS. Recognition and management of poisoning with beta-adrenergic blocking agents. *Ann Emerg Med* 1984;13:1123–1131.

37. Weinstein RS, Cole S, Kuaster HB, Dahlbert T. Beta blocker overdose with propranolol and with atenolol. *Ann Emerg Med* 1985;14:161–163.

38. Withering W. *An account of the foxglove and some of its medicinal uses with practical remarks on dropsy and other diseases.* Birmingham, England: M Sweeney; 1785.

19 || Vitamins

Accidental poisoning by vitamin products currently ranks as a major cause of poisoning in children under the age of five. Similar toxicity also occurs in adults, and reports of such poisonings have increased since the advent of the *megadose* concept of dosing vitamins (10). Fortunately, few deaths have been reported.

Consumption of vitamins (and minerals) has increased in the United States over the past several years due to heightened interest in good health and nutrition. It is also a time of interest in fad diets, and generalized belief that vitamins will prevent many major diseases from occurring, and treat others that do occur. Although this trend has contributed to the decrease in vitamin deficiency diseases, this same expanded consumption has also increased unnecessary potential toxicity to these substances. Indeed, most reported cases of toxicity result from accidental rather than intentional administration (27). Vitamins can be purchased without prescription in nonpharmacy outlets in dosage strengths that often require a prescription when purchased in pharmacies. Because of intense advertising promotions in consumer-oriented publications and direct mail announcements, excessive self-dosing is not uncommon (7,24). It is expected to increase to even greater heights. A long battle to gain control of vitamin regulation for American consumers appears to have at least temporarily ended, as the Food and Drug Administration put this issue to rest (11). With reduced governmental pressure on vitamin product manufacturers and promoters, increased use, rational and irrational, is expected. Additionally, many health professionals lack sound scientific knowledge and good judgment regarding absolute benefits of vitamins and their potential for toxicity, and may fail to adequately advise their patients about these issues.

Only rarely is an acute vitamin toxicity reaction reported. Most cases involve chronic use over months to years (7). Generally, symptoms appear slowly over a period of time so that they can be recognized early, allowing the victim to seek medical help before the event causes serious, irreversible damage.

Most cases of toxicity involve multivitamin therapy (24). In some instances, there is no doubt that many reported cases of toxicity to "vitamins" are actually due to iron-containing products, or even some other mineral. Some manufacturers have responded by reducing the amount of iron in their formulations (24).

MEGADOSING

A vitamin megadose is arbitrarily defined as a dose that is 10 or more times the recommended daily allowance (RDA) (5,41). It is estimated that 37% of Americans take these doses (18). This differs from most *therapeutic formulas,* which include vitamins at 2 to 5 times the RDA. Most people who advocate the use of megadoses report that they personally feel better when they take these large quantities. They argue strongly that, if a little is good, more is better. They continue taking these megadoses even though they are advised to the contrary (Fig. 19.1). Rarely do they take megadoses of any vitamin because of a professionally diagnosed vitamin deficiency state. In fact, controlled studies have failed to demonstrate efficacy for megadoses (31). Vitamin overdosing (megadosing) can produce toxic reactions along with confusing symptoms that lead to expensive and inappropriate laboratory tests.

Toxic manifestations of vitamin overingestion are more commonly seen with fat-soluble vitamins A and D. Fat-soluble vitamin K has been less frequently reported to induce toxicity, probably because it is not available for self-administration in OTC products. Vitamin E is practically nontoxic, at least according to current knowledge. For the most part, excessive intake of the water-soluble B complex group and vitamin C is eliminated by the kidney. Although they produce minor adverse reactions and may cause drug interactions or modify laboratory values, these are not generally life-threatening. An exception is vitamin C, which can induce serious renal toxicity in a small number of susceptible individuals. Be-

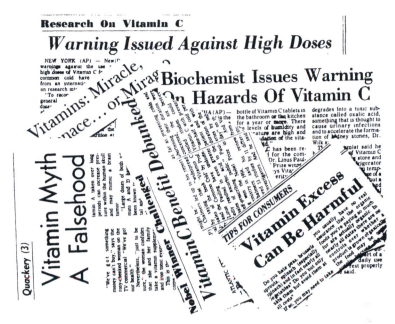

FIG. 19.1. Montage of newspaper clippings that report on vitamin toxicity.

cause of the *potential* seriousness of vitamins A, D, and C in overdoses, their toxicity is discussed in more detail than the other vitamins.

VITAMIN A

Vitamin A toxicity was first reported by Arctic explorers in 1857 when they consumed large quantities of polar bear liver. Numerous accounts of toxicity continue to appear in the literature (9). Whereas modern, sophisticated techniques and instrumentation provide detailed knowledge on the overall problem, there is little factual information concerning the exact pathogenesis of vitamin A-induced toxicity.

Vitamin A poisoning is usually due to over-ambitious prophylactic use from extended self-therapy. It has resulted from food faddism, and unfortunately from solicitous parents who have inadvertently given overdoses to children. In addition, hypervitaminosis A has occurred in patients receiving large doses of vitamin A or other vitamin A analogs such as isotretinoin and tretinoin to treat skin dis-

eases such as ichthyosis, acne, and Darier's disease (a genetically transmitted disease in which the skin becomes extremely crusty) (3). Large doses of vitamin A taken during pregnancy are teratogenic, causing a variety of fetal malformations (23,29).

Chronic renal disease may also result in a state of relative hypervitaminosis A. This is compounded in patients on hemodialysis because of the failure of this procedure to remove it from the blood. The practice of prescribing vitamins for patients undergoing hemodialysis is common, but it is suggested that these patients avoid supplementing their diets with products containing vitamin A (36).

Mechanisms of Poisoning

The mechanism of Vitamin A toxicity on the CNS is unclear. A retinol-binding protein is involved in transport of the vitamin to peripheral tissues. Clinical manifestations of hypervitaminosis A occur when this protein becomes saturated with the vitamin. Cellular membranes are then exposed to unbound vitamin, which leads to degradation of the membrane structure (29). This mechanism may be responsible for increased cerebral spinal fluid pressure and other CNS manifestations that characterize vitamin A toxicity (8,17).

The exact pathogenesis of vitamin A-induced liver damage is, likewise, not clear. Strong evidence suggests that excessive hepatic vitamin A concentrations lead to fibrosis, sclerosis of the central hepatic veins, and destruction of sinusoidal spaces with subsequent portal hypertension and ascites (12). Vitamin A is normally stored in hepatocytes. When massive doses are consumed, the Ito cells (lipocytes) take up the vitamin. It is believed that this transforms the Ito cells into fibroblasts that can produce collagen, which in turn causes subsequent hepatic pathology (17).

Vitamin A elevates serum parathyroid hormone concentrations significantly in otherwise healthy men, at doses as low as 25,000 U. Toxic symptoms resulting from hypercalcemia, bony changes, and premature epiphyseal closure are felt to be due to this action (4).

TABLE 19.1. *Signs and symptoms of vitamin A intoxication*

Gastrointestinal
  Nausea/vomiting, anorexia, diarrhea, cheilitis, gingivitis, mouth fissures, abdominal cramping, weight loss
Central nervous system
  Headache, irritability and restlessness, fatigue, nystagmus, increased intracranial pressure, hydroencephalus, neurological symptoms and psychiatric disturbances, paresthesias (arms and legs), vision changes, diplopia, papiledema, dizziness, sluggishness, bulging fontanels
Skin
  Dry, pruritic skin; rash; desquamation; alopecia; brittle nails
Muscle and joints
  Myalgia; muscle fasciculations; tender, deep, and hard swellings on extremities and occipital area of head; joint and muscle pain
Bone
  Hyperostoses
Other
  Hepatosplenomegaly, lymph node enlargement, hepatic fibrosis, bleeding, chafonic fever, hypercalcemia, sensitivity reactions, cirrhosis, anemia, conjunctivitis, dysuria, edema, epistaxis, hyperlipidemia, menstrual irregularities, teratology

Characteristics of Poisoning

Vitamin A-induced symptoms of toxicity are summarized in Table 19.1. Although these outcomes seem to be widely diverse, they are readily categorized into several subheadings. A patient intoxicated with vitamin A may not display all symptoms, and since many of them are nonspecific, early suspicion and diagnosis of toxicity may be missed.

Another problem is that detection of vitamin A toxicity is occasionally missed because many symptoms of poisoning are similar to those that characterize the underlying condition for which the vitamin was taken.

Most toxicity reports indicate that daily doses of vitamin A in the range of 300,000 to 600,000 U (given over a period of a few months to several years) are required to produce symptoms. However, lesser doses are occasionally reported to be toxic. For example, daily doses of 50,000 U or more in adults (given over several months) have caused tox-

icity symptoms (2). Ingestion of as little as 25,000 to 50,000 U of retinol daily for 30 days has induced signs of increased intracranial pressure in infants (23).

Management of Poisoning

Treatment of vitamin A intoxication includes immediate discontinuation of the substance. Most signs and symptoms will disappear within a week or two. Hyperostoses may remain evident for several months after clinical recovery. If symptoms are ignored and the vitamin is not withdrawn, irreversible hepatic damage, including cirrhosis, may result.

Vitamin E is reported occasionally to protect against hypervitaminosis A (23). Although some papers state that vitamin E offers a degree of protection against toxicity, others have shown that vitamin E may actually enhance tissue uptake of vitamin A. If significant, this could answer why earlier reports indicate that vitamin E lowers vitamin A blood concentrations.

VITAMIN D

Vitamin D is the most toxic of all vitamins. A large number of cases of toxicity have been reported in people using vitamin D to treat arthritis, muscle cramps, cold hands and feet, and a variety of other real or imagined disorders. The vitamin is used occasionally in excess to treat various nutritional disorders in persons of all ages. Because excessive and repeated doses are frequently taken, reports of toxicity have increased in recent years (9).

Vitamin D misuse in Britain and Europe, with intakes averaging 300,000 to 400,000 U daily, is believed to have been responsible for the idiopathic hypercalcemia of infancy that was frequently reported during and immediately after World War II. At that time, ambitious supplementation of food with vitamins reached a peak and was often far in excess of what was needed. The disorder was characterized clinically by hypercalcemia and skeletal abnormalities, as well as premature hardening of the arteries, irreversible mental retardation, and early death, usually before puberty. Symptoms disappeared after the dietary intake of vitamin D was reduced to less than 1,500 U daily (28).

Mechanisms of Poisoning

All of the clinically significant problems inherent in vitamin D toxicity are caused by its action to elevate the concentration of plasma calcium. Vitamin D per se does not elevate calcium. Rather, this is dependent on its conversion through a succession of steps to 1,25-dihydroxycholecalciferol as shown in Fig. 19.2. Once formed, 1,25-dihydroxycholecalciferol exerts activity at several sites, including intestinal epithelium, to promote calcium absorption (13). Vitamin D toxicity would be expected to be more severe in an individual whose thyroid has been removed since the counterhormone, calcitonin, is synthesized within the parafollicular cells of this gland. Calcitonin normally exerts a negative effect on plasma calcium concentrations. In its defi-

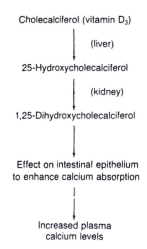

FIG. 2. Synthesis of cholecalciferol to its active form, 1,25-dihydroxycholecalciferol.

cient state, however, the control for calcium is reduced, and plasma levels rise unchecked.

Characteristics of Poisoning

Symptoms of vitamin D toxicity are largely suggestive of hypercalcemia (Table 19.2). Deaths occurring after acute toxic doses are usually attributed to this finding. Toxic effects from chronic use are due to deposition of calcium in soft tissues, especially the kidneys and heart. Aortic valvular stenosis (narrowing)

TABLE 19.2. *Signs and symptoms of vitamin D intoxication*

Hypercalcemia (weakness, fatigue, lassitude, headache, nausea/vomiting, diarrhea)
Impaired renal function (polyuria, polydipsia, nocturia, decreased urinary concentrating ability, nephrolithiasis)
Deposition of calcium salts in soft tissues (nephrolithiasis and nephrocalcinosis)
Hypertension
Osteoporosis, skeletal abnormalities
Supravalvular aortic stenosis
Premature hardening of the arteries
Irreversible mental retardation
Anorexia
Hypotonia
Constipation
Arrested growth
Obtundation
Coma

and nephrocalcinosis with calcification of other soft tissues are characteristic findings. Renal function may be severely and irreversibly impaired. Cardiac rhythm may become abnormal after prolonged deposition of calcium salts within the heart's myofibrils. X-ray examination of patients poisoned with vitamin D shows metastatic calcification and generalized osteoporosis of bone. A single episode of moderately severe hypercalcemia may completely arrest the growth of children for six months or more, and physicians often report that this deficit in height may never be fully corrected (32).

A large single dose of vitamin D_3 or D_4 generally does not cause toxicity. However, vitamin D intoxication can occur after chronic oral ingestion of large doses of vitamin D_2 or D_3 (usually 50,000 or more units daily) taken for several months (13). These excessive quantities are stored in body fat, later to be released slowly into the blood.

A study compared vitamin D consumption in patients who suffered from angina pectoris, previous myocardial infarction, or degenerative joint disease (22). It specifically correlated men with different dietary intakes of vitamin D over many years to their incidence of myocardial infarction. The result suggested that high doses of vitamin D (dietary consumption of 12,000 U or more per day) was a precipitating cause of myocardial infarction.

Management of Poisoning

Hypervitaminosis D treatment consists of immediately discontinuing vitamin intake, reducing calcium intake, administering glucocorticoids, and assuring a generous fluid intake.

If hypercalcemia occurs, it may persist for weeks to months after termination of ingestion. However, the normal effect is that cessation of the vitamin and lowering of oral calcium intake lead to rapid disappearance of symptoms. When they persist, a glucocorticoid such as prednisone (20 to 40 mg or more orally per day) can be given to reduce intesti-

nal absorption, control hypercalcemia, and prevent irreversible renal damage and ectopic calcification (40). In this manner, a dramatic lowering of calcium to normal concentrations may be accomplished within days.

VITAMIN K

Fad uses for vitamin K have not surfaced since it is not a component of over-the-counter remedies. Thus, there are few cases of toxicity reported in the literature.

Characteristics of Poisoning

The major toxicity is associated with water-soluble synthetic analogs such as menadione. These derivatives are oxidants and may cause erythrocytic membranes to rupture with resultant cell hemolysis, jaundice, and kernicterus. In animals, large doses of menadione cause anemia, polycythemia, splenomegaly, renal and hepatic damage, and death (23). Erythrocytic damage occurs more prevalently in persons with glucose-6-phosphate dehydrogenase deficiency and at doses exceeding 10 mg (42). Vitamin K_1 (phytonadione) generally does not lead to hyperbilirubinemia and for this reason, it is the preferred form.

VITAMIN E

At present, vitamin E is believed to have a low toxicity profile (23). Research is under way to determine its toxic potential. Reported undesirable side effects of megadoses of vitamin E include headaches, nausea, fatigue, dizziness, blurred vision (perhaps related to the fact that large doses may antagonize the action of vitamin A), inflammation of the mouth, chafing of the lips, gastrointestinal disturbance, muscle weakness, hypoglycemia, increased bleeding tendencies, degenerative changes, and emotional disorders (19). Also reported are disturbances in growth, thyroid function, mitochondrial respiration rate and bone calcification, and decreased hematocrit.

Adults can tolerate doses up to 1,000 IU per day without developing toxicity (41).

In humans and experimental animals, it is believed that vitamin E may interfere with vitamin K metabolism, resulting in a prolonged prothrombin time. Excessive vitamin E intake in experimental animals decreases the rate of wound healing, and in humans, induces gastrointestinal symptoms and creatinuria.

VITAMIN C

Serious toxicity to vitamin C is uncommon. However, numerous untoward effects may occur when it is taken in overdose, or by persons susceptible to larger-than-normal doses. Vitamin C toxicity is not a cause of death (25). Major symptoms are summarized in Table 19.3.

Several controversial points should be examined. It is often reported that large doses of vitamin C destroy substantial amounts of vitamin B_{12}, and therefore reduce its concentration in the blood. However, megadoses of vitamin C would be required over a period of several years before this destruction of vitamin B_{12} would be significant to produce symptoms of megaloblastic anemia (8,15).

Some reports state that vitamin C will acidify urine. Although this is not an absolute toxic effect per se, these reports must be considered because of the implication that concurrently administered drugs may be made more or less active. Current consensus is that doses up to 6 g/day (and in some studies, up to 12 g/day) will not significantly alter urine pH

TABLE 19.3. *Side effects of vitamin C administration*

Interference with urine and stool testing
  Negate occult blood tests
  Cause false-negative reaction with glucose
    oxidase tests
Decrease absorption of vitamin B_{12}
Rebound scurvy following prolonged administration
    of megadoses
Increased urinary oxalate, cysteine, and uric acid
Acidification of urine
Diarrhea; occasional nausea

(26). This opinion is contrary to earlier reports indicating that doses of 1 g or more per day will acidify the urine.

Large doses of vitamin C taken during pregnancy may cause scurvy in some newborns. The effect is reported to occur in newborns of some women who have ingested as little as 400 mg ascorbic acid daily throughout pregnancy. One suggestion is that vitamin C enhances development of fetal liver microsomal enzymes, which then causes scurvy because of enhanced destruction of the vitamin after birth (23). Another theory states that the fetus recognizes the danger of increased vitamin C concentrations and increases its own metabolic rate to destroy the excess concentration of the vitamin. After birth, this enhanced destruction rate continues, and symptoms of scurvy are seen shortly after delivery. A similar, but less dangerous rebound scurvy is reported occasionally in adults who suddenly withdraw from large doses. For these reasons, it is considered wise to taper megadoses of vitamin C by about 10% to 20% daily (14).

Kidney Stone Formation

Ascorbic acid increases renal excretion of oxalate, uric acid, and calcium. These may increase the potential for stone formation in the kidney and bladder (37). This potential seems to be governed by genetic factors, and only occurs in a small segment of the population. When it does occur, however, susceptible individuals may experience the problem at doses of 1 g or more daily. The toxicologic problems associated with oxalate on the kidney were discussed in chapters 4 and 11.

VITAMIN B_1

Numerous toxicities were reported in the 1940s and 1950s to parenterally administered vitamin B_1 (thiamine). Symptoms ranged from nervousness, convulsions, weakness, trembling, headache, and neuromuscular paralysis to cardiovascular disorders including rapid pulse, peripheral vasodilation, arrhythmia, edema, and anaphylactic shock. Hypersensitivity reactions to injectable doses of 100 times the RDA were reported. With the subsequent decline in use of thiamine in its parenteral form, there have been fewer toxicities reported and it is no longer considered to possess a major toxicologic threat (9).

NIACIN

In single doses of 50 mg niacin (nicotinic acid), intense flushing and pruritus have been reported. When the practice of giving niacin in doses ranging upward to 30 g or more a day was advocated, more serious toxicity was noted. These effects included intense flushing and unbearable pruritus, skin rash, heartburn, nausea and vomiting, diarrhea, ulcer activation, abnormal liver function, hypotension, tachycardia, fainting, hyperglycemia, hyperbilirubinemia and jaundice, dermatoses, hyperuricemia, elevated serum enzymes, and hyperkeratosis of the skin. A greater incidence of atrial fibrillation and other cardiac arrhythmias is seen in persons taking niacin (6).

The most common serious toxicities reported for niacin include abnormal liver function and jaundice. The body uses niacin for NAD and NADH formation, which serve as coenzymes for various dehydrogenase enzymes in oxidation-reduction reactions. Many of these enzymes are found in the liver, and modulation of their activity with megadoses of niacin may explain the abnormal hepatic functions.

VITAMIN B$_6$

Vitamin B$_6$ (pyridoxine)-induced reactions are rare. Convulsive disorders have occurred due to both vitamin excess as well as a deficiency state (35). Oral doses of up to 1 g daily have not shown adverse reactions, although doses of 200 mg daily followed by abrupt withdrawal have caused symptoms of dependency.

VITAMIN B$_{12}$

Vitamin B$_{12}$ (cyanocobalamin) is associated on rare occasion with allergic reactions to the injectable products. Symptoms of edema of the face, urticaria, shivering, bronchospasm, rash, dyspnea, aphonia, and anaphylaxis have appeared, but only after years of continuous vitamin administration.

Consideration has been given to preservatives and other substances contained in vitamin B$_{12}$ preparations as being the cause of toxic symptoms (1). However, patients have continued to experience such reactions when purified cyanocobalamin was injected, or when another commercial brand was substituted.

FOLIC ACID

Folic acid is relatively nontoxic, with oral doses as high as 15 mg daily showing no substantial reports of adverse effects. A few sensitivity reactions have been recorded (16). Long-term folic acid therapy increased seizure frequency in some epileptic patients and may precipitate vitamin B$_{12}$ deficiency neuropathy in some cases of megaloblastic anemia (33). It is also suspected of inducing mild psychologic disorders in normal subjects. Although not a direct toxicity, folic acid can mask symptoms of pernicious anemia. In doses exceeding 0.4 to 1 mg/day, the hematologic warning signs of pernicious anemia are masked by folic acid, but the life-threatening neurologic toxicities continue undetected until it may be too late to adequately treat the condition.

MANAGEMENT OF VITAMIN TOXICITY AND ADVERSE EFFECTS

In the majority of cases, vitamin-induced toxicities and adverse effects are best managed by discontinuing the vitamin and treating specific symptoms, if needed. With exception of vitamin D-induced hypercalcemia, rarely are other measures necessary. Treatment of vitamin D intoxication was discussed earlier in this chapter.

SUMMARY

Vitamin-induced toxicity usually manifests only after prolonged ingestion of vitamin A or D. Vitamin C taken in megadoses may also inflict toxic problems, again, usually after chronic therapy. Remember also that any product containing multiple vitamins may also contain iron, which can be extremely toxic in overdose (see chapter 9). Thus, care must always be taken when drawing a conclusion on a *vitamin product* ingestion to assure that iron is not a constituent.

Case Studies

CASE STUDY: GLUCOCORTICOID MODIFICATION OF VITAMIN D INTOXICATION

History

We are presented with a 49-year-old woman who had undergone a subtotal thyroidectomy 16 years earlier. She received thyroid replacement therapy and was directed to consume a high calcium diet.

Six years after her thyroid surgery, dihydrotachysterol was added. Two years later, vitamin D was substituted for dihydrotachysterol, and she was given calcium supplements to go along with a high calcium diet. At no time thus far was her serum calcium concentration above 9.7 mg/dL (normal, 8.5 to 10.5 mg/dL).

Two years later, the patient passed a kidney stone, and calcium supplementation was stopped. Vitamin D (100,000 U/day) was continued.

After another two years, the serum calcium concentration measured 14.2 mg/dL. The patient reported weight loss and anorexia, intense itching, back pain, and bone pain. Vitamin supplementation was discontinued, but the serum calcium concentration remained elevated. Three years before this present interview, two renal stones were discovered by intravenous pyelography.

The patient was put on prednisone therapy, 10 mg every 6 hr, and dietary calcium intake was limited. Serum calcium concentrations decreased from 12.2 mg/dL to 9.1 mg/dL. Fecal calcium excretion was only minimally affected. (See ref. 40.)

Discussion

1. The patient had a subtotal thyroidectomy years before. However, she was receiving thyroid hormone treatment. Was removal of her thyroid gland probably significant or insignificant? Explain how you arrived at your answer.
2. The fact that serum calcium concentrations decreased while fecal calcium excretion remained unchanged with prednisone therapy suggests a possible site of glucocorticoid activity. What is it?
3. What was the cause of back pain and bone pain?

CASE STUDIES: VITAMIN A INTOXICATION

History: Case 1

A 4-year-old boy was brought to the hospital by his grandmother, the proprietress of a health food store. She was concerned about his persistent fever and irritability, which had continued over the past 4 months, but recently had become more severe.

The boy had been previously examined on two different occasions for hyperkinetic activity. One physician recommended megavitamin therapy, but the grandmother denied giving her grandson any vitamins.

Physical examination revealed a febrile (39.5°C) and very irritable child. His lips were irritated, and fissures were present at the corners of his mouth. He had a slight murmur, and his liver was palpable 3 cm below the right costal margin. Neurologic examination was normal, but he refused to walk, stating that it was painful to do so.

Laboratory results were unremarkable, except for an SGOT level of 93 U/mL (normal, 15 to 35 U/mL) and LDH of 1,100 U/mL (normal, 200 to 600 U/mL). Computerized tomography of the brain showed mild enlargement of the lateral ventricles; the echocardiogram was normal. Laboratory results also showed a vitamin A concentration of 1,430 mg/dL.

The boy's grandmother continued to deny that she gave him vitamins, although his nursery schoolteacher later observed him ingesting vitamin tablets throughout the day.

His hospital stay lasted 4 weeks, during which time no more vitamins were given, and his vitamin A concentration decreased to 320 mg/dL in 1 week. Liver function tests remained abnormal and a liver biopsy revealed mild fatty infiltration. The child was released to the care of foster parents. (See ref. 38.)

History: Case 2

A female college student, age 20 years, was admitted to a neurologic institute for assessment of a possible brain tumor. Two days before, she developed emesis and diplopia. She also reported that she had a history of severe headache.

A medical history revealed that 2 years previously she began taking 50,000 IU of vitamin A per day, which was prescribed by a dermatologist for acne. After 16 months of vitamin A therapy she went on a weight-reducing diet and decreased her weight from 56 to 41 kg. Two months previously, she became anorectic. A diffuse scaling erythematous dermatitis developed. Headaches also appeared, and became increasingly severe. The patient complained of headache as a major event. She preferred to lie still without movement, because forward flexion of her neck intensified pain.

Examination revealed normal vital signs. Her liver was palpable and not tender. She had diffuse dry skin and patchy erythema over the entire body, with petechiae on the soft palate. She had bilateral hemorrhagic papilledema. Other neurologic and physical parameters were within normal limits.

Laboratory values were normal for glucose, plasma proteins, blood urea nitrogen, bilirubin, cholesterol and electrolytes. Her vitamin A concentration was 128 μg/dL (normal, 50 μg/dL); retinol, 76 μg/dL; and retinyl esters, 41 μg/dL (normal, 1.6 μg/dL). Alkaline phosphatase was 15 U (normal, 5 to 13 U); glutamic oxaloacetic transaminase, 70 U (normal, 12 to 30 U); and prothrombin time, 15 sec (normal, 13 sec). A liver scan revealed hepatomegaly with irregular uptake suggestive of parenchymal cell disease and portal hypertension.

The patient revealed that she had started taking vitamin A treatment 2 years previously as prescribed by her dermatologist. But over the years she had sporadically increased intake to 400,000 IU/day. She also admitted to consuming a diet rich in yellow and green vegetables.

Treatment consisted of dietary counseling in foods low in vitamin A. The case history did not specifically report it, but one can assume that her vitamin A medication intake was curtailed. Her symptoms disappeared, appetite improved, and weight increased to 45 kg by the time of discharge, 22 days later. At that time, the patient's vitamin A concentration was 58 μg/dL and retinyl esters, 19 μg/dL (see ref. 5).

Discussion

1. Two primary sites of vitamin A intoxication were evident in the young patient in case 1. What were they? Was this what you anticipated?
2. The child's symptoms (case 1) were those of vitamin A overdose. Assuming he took a multiple-vitamin preparation, why did symptoms of poisoning from the other vitamins not show up?
3. Fever is not usually mentioned in most vitamin A intoxication reports. What caused the fever in case 1?

4. Comment on the relationship between vitamin A intoxication in case 2 and the laboratory test results for liver function.

5. There is no mention of drug treatment being given to either patient. Is this normal?

VITAMIN A TOXICITY PRESENTING AS JAUNDICE

History

A 67-year-old man consulted a dermatologist for evaluation of generalized pruritus. On examination, jaundice was noted, and the patient was admitted to a hospital for further testing. The patient had experienced itching over the back, groin, and chest for about three weeks. One week before admission to the hospital, anorexia and mild nausea developed. The patient denied having abdominal or back pain, fever, chills, or weight loss.

Past medical history included asthma for ten years and an episode of diverticulitis. Current medications were terbutaline, 2.5 mg three times daily; theophylline, 200 mg three times daily; and albuterol aerosol as needed. The patient drank about two cans of beer a day, had been a smoker, and was retired from a career with an aluminum manufacturer. He denied exposure to known toxins, and had never had a blood transfusion.

Normal vital signs were found during physical examination. The skin and sclera were slightly jaundiced, and the skin was dry in general. There were no cutaneous signs of chronic liver disease (e.g., spider angiomas). Head, chest, and lymph nodes were normal. The abdomen was soft, with no palpable masses or ascites. The liver was not enlarged, but the right upper quadrant was mildly tender. The spleen could not be palpated.

Laboratory test results included a hemoglobin concentration of 14.1 g/dL and a white blood cell count of 6,200/mm^3, with a normal differential. Platelet count, prothrombin time, and partial thromboplastin time were within normal limits. Electrolytes, BUN, serum creatinine, and serum glucose concentrations were all normal. Liver function test results included SGOT, 118 IU/liter; lactate dehydrogenase, 250 IU/liter; serum alkaline phosphatase, 300IU/liter; total serum bilirubin, 4.0 mg/dL; conjugated serum bilirubin, 2.5 mg/dL; total serum protein, 7.0 g/dL; and serum albumin 4.4 g/dL.

X-ray films of the chest showed changes consistent with chronic obstructive pulmonary disease. An ultrasound examination of the abdomen revealed a liver of normal size and consistency but none of the following: calculi in the gallbladder, dilation of bile ducts, enlargement of the spleen or ascites. The pancreas was not well visualized.

Because a tumor in the head of the pancreas could not be excluded, an abdominal computed tomographic scan was performed, which indicated possible enlargement of the pancreatic head. Fine-needle aspiration of the pancreas yielded normal pancreatic cells. Endoscopic retrograde cholangiopancreatography was performed; the common bile duct and the main pancreatic duct were both normal.

A liver biopsy showed that the architectural pattern of the liver was intact. Neither bile duct proliferation, as is seen with long-standing extrahepatic obstruction, nor inflammation was present. A mild, fatty change was noted, as well as dramatic intercanalicular bile stasis, principally in the midzone. This histologic picture seemed most consistent with a drug reaction or toxin exposure.

The patient denied using drugs other than those prescribed for asthma. He was discharged with instructions to return in two weeks with the bottles of all his medications. On the return visit, he brought a grocery sack containing many over-the-counter vitamins.

The patient was taking about 150,000 IU of vitamin A daily and had done so for several years. He had stopped taking vitamins before admission to the hospital and had not resumed taking them since discharge. When liver function tests were repeated, results were entirely normal except for an alkaline phosphatase value of 191 IU/liter. The patient's serum vitamin A concentration was 1,681 μg/dL (normal, 20 to 60) more than a month after his last admitted dose. A month later, all liver enzyme values were normal, as was the vitamin A concentration. The patient was instructed to limit his ingestion of vitamins, and laboratory tests results have remained normal for one year. (See ref. 39)

Discussion

1. Which symptom or altered laboratory value discussed in this case study was/were probably caused by vitamin A ingestion, and which ones were not?

CASE STUDY: VITAMINS A AND D INTOXICATION

History

A male farmer, age 62 years, ingested 8 mL of a veterinary preparation containing vitamins A and D (500,000 U/mL vitamin A, and 50,000 U/mL vitamin D). The contents of the vial was intended for parenteral use at a dose of 1 mL/600 pounds. He reported no immediate ill effects, but developed severe headache, became nauseous, and vomited over the next several hours.

During the night he continued to suffer from a severe generalized headache as well as blurred vision and scotomas (areas of absent vision within the usual visual area). When the headaches became increasingly severe, he went to the hospital.

On admission, his physical examination was generally unremarkable. Laboratory results consisted of Hct 37%, WBC 4,500/mm^3, and serum Ca^{2+} 9.0 mg/dL. Electrolytes, glucose, and creatinine concentrations were all normal.

During his 5-day hospital stay, the patient continued to experience photophobia, scotomas, nausea, and headache. These symptoms subsided on the fourth hospital day, but at that time exfoliation of skin on the face and hands occurred. Also during his hospital stay, vitamin A concentrations (normal, 15 to 60 μg/dL) were determined and are listed as follows:

Day 1	340 μg/dL
Day 3	126 μg/dL
Day 4	101 μg/dL
Day 5	106 μg/dL

Results of liver-function tests were within normal limits, but thyroid function studies underwent some complex changes during his hospital stay. The patient had an uneventful recovery over several months. (See ref. 20.)

Discussion

1. Does the patient in this case study manifest the typical signs and symptoms of vitamin A toxicity?
2. What is the major mode of toxicity for vitamin D? Was vitamin D toxicity clinically significant in this patient?

CASE STUDY: VITAMIN D-INDUCED BLADDER STONE

History

A 2-year-old girl had received excessive calcium and vitamin D since the age of 9 months because she refused to eat the quantity of meat her mother felt was necessary for normal body growth. She was therefore given large quantities of cheese and a minimum of 36 ounces of vitamin D-fortified milk each day, as well as daily vitamin supplements. It was estimated that her daily intake for calcium was 2 g, and for vitamin D, 400 to 600 U.

She was hospitalized for treatment of a urinary tract infection when an abdominal X-ray film revealed calcification in the bladder. Urinalysis for electrolytes and other excreted compounds was normal except for excessive elimination of the amino acids cystine, lysine, and ornithine. The calculus, composed of calcium and cystine, was surgically removed and the child had an uneventful recovery. (See ref. 30.)

Discussion

1. This patient experienced a classical vitamin D intoxication that was caused by

well-meaning parents. What particular food substance do you suppose actually contributed most to this reaction?

CASE STUDY: CHRONIC VITAMIN D OVERDOSE—A REMINDER

History

A 6-month-old Indian boy was admitted with a six day history of vomiting, constipation, and increasing apathy. Examination revealed a drowsy, listless child with signs of 5% to 10% dehydration. Plasma electrolyte concentrations on admission showed a urea of 7.4 mmol/L, sodium 148 mmol/L, potassium 2.9 mmol/L, and a grossly raised calcium concentration of 5.86 mmol/L.

Subsequent investigations showed an appreciably increased vitamin D concentration (25-hydroxycholecalciferol) at 2226 nmol/L (normal 10 to 120 nmol/L) and undetectable parathyroid hormone. On close questioning, his parents admitted to administering a compound preparation of vitamins A, C, and D since the age of 4 months, and as he had refused to take these from the dropper, they poured the vitamin into his mouth directly from the bottle instead! They had obtained their vitamin supply from a chemist privately and had received no professional supervision of administration.

The baby was given intravenous fluids for five days and also commenced on a low calcium, low vitamin D diet. He was discharged home on day 12. His calcium concentration returned to normal by day 19 but his vitamin D concentration remained raised for over six months. Follow up at one year showed moderate global developmental delay. (See ref. 21.)

Discussion

1. This case illustrates the dangers of unsupervised vitamin supplementation. To prevent further incidents, what precautions need to be implemented?
2. Comment on what was right or wrong

about the low calcium diet this infant was placed on.

CASE STUDY: VITAMIN C INGESTION AND RENAL STONES

History

A 21-year-old man had a calcium oxalate kidney stone removed after it was discovered by a urologist. The man had complained of flank pain. Physical examination was unremarkable and his family history did not show previous renal disease.

Laboratory results showed that serum and 24-hr urine concentrations of calcium, phosphorus, and uric acid were normal, but urine oxalate concentration was 126 mg/24 hr (normal, less than 40 mg/24 hr).

When it was revealed that he had been taking 1 g vitamin C each day for many months to prevent colds, he was advised to discontinue the vitamin. He did so, and his urinary oxalate level decreased to 56 mg/24 hr 18 days later. (See ref. 34.)

Discussion

1. Outline the mechanism of formation of a calcium oxalate renal stone. How could vitamin C cause its appearance?
2. What advice should a patient who is contemplating taking large doses of vitamin C be given?

Review Questions

1. All of the following are true statements about vitamin A intoxication *except*:
   A. Its occurrence is usually due to over-ambitious prophylactic use.
   B. Chronic renal disease is more likely to result in its occurrence than when kidney function is normal.
   C. Hepatic damage occurs from destruction of sinusoidal spaces.
   D. Brain damage occurs when the vita-

min binds to the retinal-binding protein.

2. Most *therapeutic formulas* of vitamin
   product mixtures contain these substances
   at 10 times their RDA.
   A. True
   B. False

3. Which of the following would be contra-
   indicated in a patient who ingested an
   acute vitamin D overdose?
   A. Forced fluids
   B. Calcium lactate
   C. Ascorbic acid
   D. Prednisone

4. All of the following are symptoms of vita-
   min A intoxication *except*:
   A. Myalgia
   B. Headache
   C. Muscle pain
   D. Weight gain

5. Ascorbic acid increases renal excretion of
   which of the following: oxalate (I), uric
   acid (II), or calcium (III)?
   A. II only
   B. III only
   C. I and II only
   D. II and III only
   E. I, II, and III

6. Which of the following is a prominent
   toxic effect associated with excessive vi-
   tamin A ingestion including all of the fol-
   lowing *except*:
   A. Elevated intracranial pressure
   B. Nausea
   C. Headache
   D. Oxalate production
   E. Generalized peeling of the skin

7. Which of the following is associated with
   animal and/or human teratogenicity?
   A. Vitamin A
   B. Vitamin E
   C. Isotretinoin
   D. All of the above
   E. Only two of the above

8. Which of the following is a clinically significant problem associated with hypervitaminosis D?
   A. CNS depression
   B. Cholinergic stimulation

C. Hypokalemia
D. Erythrocyte hemolysis
E. Hypercalcemia

9. Which of the following is the most toxic
   vitamin?
   A. Vitamin A
   B. Vitamin B complex
   C. Vitamin C
   D. Vitamin D
   E. Vitamin E

10. State the reasons why vitamin D intoxica-
    tion could be expected to be more severe
    in a person with a previous complete thy-
    roidectomy.

11. Give a plausible explanation why a neo-
    nate, whose mother took large doses of
    vitamin C during pregnancy, may develop
    scurvy after birth.

12. A symptom of vitamin A intoxication is
    hyperostosis. What is this, and why do
    you think it occurs?

13. After ingestion of a toxic dose of many
    poisons, the event may be missed, or the
    presenting symptoms misdiagnosed. This
    also may occur with vitamin A. Why does
    it occur with the vitamin?

14. Vitamin K shares an important feature
    with vitamins A and D (i.e., all are fat
    soluble). Still, vitamin K toxicity is only
    rarely seen. Why?

15. In toxic ingested amounts, vitamin A
    causes hypercalcemia. What is the most
    significant mechanism through which this
    effect occurs?

References

1. Avery GS, Heel RC, Speight TM. Guide to adverse
   drug reactions. In: Avery GS, ed. *Drug treatment:
   principles and practice of clinical pharmacology and
   therapeutics.* 2nd ed. Littleton MA: Publishing Sciences Group; 1980:1225–1251.
2. Baxi SC, Dailey GA. Hypervitaminosis A: a cause
   of hypercalcemia. *West J Med* 1982;137:429–431.
3. Benke PJ. The isotretinoin teratogen syndrome.
   JAMA 1984;251:3267–3269.
4. Chertow BS, Williams GA, Kiani R. The interactions
   between vitamin A, vinblastine, and cytochalasin B
   in parathyroid hormone secretion. *Proc Soc Exp Biol
   Med* 1974;147:16–27.
5. Clinical Nutrition Cases. The pathophysiological ba-

sis of vitamin A toxicity. *Nutr Rev* 1982;40:272–274.

6. Coronary Drug Project Research Group. Clofibrate and niacin in coronary heart disease. *JAMA* 1975;231:360–381.

7. Davidson RA. Complications of megavitamin therapy. *South Med J* 1984;77:200–203.

8. DiPalma J. Vitamin toxicity. *Am Fam Physician* 1978;10:106.

9. DiPalma JR, Ritchie DM. Vitamin toxicity. *Am Rev Pharmacol Toxicol* 1977;17:133–148.

10. Evans CDH, Lacey IH. Toxicity of vitamins: complications of a health movement. *Br Med J* 1986;292:509–510.

11. *FDA Consumer* 1981;15:2.

12. Forouhar F, Nadel MS, Gondos B. Hepatic pathology in vitamin A toxicity. *Ann Clin Lab Sci* 1984;14:304–310.

13. Haynes RC, Murad F. Agents affecting calcification: calcium, parathyroid hormone, calcitonin, vitamin D, and other compounds. In: Gilman AG, Goodman LS, Rall TW, Gilman A, eds. *The pharmacological basis of therapeutics.* 7th ed. New York: Macmillan; 1985:1517–1543.

14. Herbert VD. Megavitamin therapy. *NY J Med* 1979 Feb;278.

15. Herbert VD, Jacob E. Destruction of vitamin B_{12} by ascorbic acid. *JAMA* 1974;230:241–242.

16. Hillman RS. Vitamin B_{12}, folic acid, and the treatment of megaloblastic anemias. In: Gilman AG, Goodman LS, Rall TW, Gilman A, eds. *The pharmacological basis of therapeutics.* 7th ed. New York: Macmillan; 1985:1323–1337.

17. Inkeles SB, Connor WE, Illingworth DR. Hepatic and dermatologic manifestations of chronic hypervitaminosis A in adults. *Am J Med* 1986;80:491–496.

18. Jarvis WT. Vitamin use and abuse. *Bol Asoc Med P R* 1985;77:168–170.

19. Kingman AM. Vitamin E toxicity. *Arch Dermatol* 1982;118:280.

20. LaMantia RS, Andrews CE. Acute vitamin A intoxication. *South Med J* 1981;74:1012–1014.

21. Liberman MM, Salzmann M. Chronic vitamin D overdosage: a reminder. *Arch Dis Child* 1991;66:1002.

22. Linden V. Vitamin D and myocardial infarction. *Br Med J* 1974;3:647–649.

23. Mandel HG, Cohn VH. Fat-soluble vitamins. In: Gilman AG, Goodman LS, Rall TW, Gilman A, eds. *The pharmacological basis of therapeutics.* 7th ed. New York: Macmillan; 1985:1573–1591.

24. Manners S. Children and vitamins: too much of a good thing? *Can Pharm J* 1985;118:63–66.

25. Marcus R, Coulston AM. Water-soluble vitamins. In: Gilman AG, Goodman LS, Rall TW, Gilman A, eds. *The pharmacological basis of therapeutics.* 7th ed. New York: Macmillan; 1985:1551–1572.

26. Nahata MC, Shimp L, Lampman T, McLeod DC. Effect of ascorbic acid on urine pH in man. *Am J Hosp Pharm* 1977;34:1234.

27. National Clearinghouse for Poison Control Centers Bulletin. Rockville, MD: US Department of Health Services; 1980;24:3.

28. National Research Council, Food and Nutrition Board. Hazards of overuse of vitamin D. *Am J Clin Nutr* 1975;28:512–513.

29. Olson JA. Adverse effects of large doses of vitamin A and retinoids. *Semin Oncol* 1983;10:290–293.

30. O'Regan S, Robitaille P, Mongeau JC, Homsy Y. Cystine calcium bladder calculus in a 2-year-old child. *J Urol* 1980;123:770.

31. Ovesen L. Vitamin therapy in the absence of obvious therapy. What is the evidence? *Drugs* 1984;27:148–170.

32. Parfitt AM. Hypophosphatemic vitamin D refractory rickets and osteomalacia. *Orthop Clin North Am* 1972;3:653–680.

33. Reynolds EH. Anticonvulsants, folic acid, and epilepsy. *Lancet* 1973;1:1376–1378.

34. Roth DA, Breitenfield RV. Vitamin C and oxalate stones. *JAMA* 1977;237:768.

35. Schaumburg H, Kaplan J, Windebank A, et al. Sensory neuropathy from pyridoxine abuse. *N Engl J Med* 1983;309:445–448.

36. Schmunes E. Hypervitaminosis A in a patient with alopecia receiving renal dialysis. *Arch Dermatol* 1979;115:882–883.

37. Sestili MA. Adverse health effects of vitamin C and ascorbic acid. *Semin Oncol* 1983;10:299–304.

38. Shaywitz BA, Siegel NJ, Pearson HA. Megavitamins for minimal brain dysfunction. *JAMA* 1977;238:1749–1750.

39. Smith JW. Vitamin A toxicity presenting as jaundice. *Postgrad Med* 1989;85:53–55.

40. Streck WF, Waterhouse C, Haddad JC. Glucocorticoid effects in vitamin D intoxication. *Arch Intern Med* 1979;139:974–977.

41. Woolliscrift JA. Megavitamins: Fact and fancy. *DM* 1983;29:1–56.

42. Zinkham WH, Childs B. Effect of vitamin K and naphthalene metabolites of glutathione metabolism of erythrocytes from normal newborns and patients with naphthalene hemolytic anemia. *Am J Dis Child* 1957;94:420–423.

Appendix

The figures listed in the following tables are not absolute values. Many are dependent on intralaboratory variations and the sensitivity of analytical methods used in their determination. The values are to be used only for reference when comparing data present in the text or in the case studies that follow the chapters.

TABLE 1. *Vital signs*

Respiration	
Adult	12–18/min
Child	20–50/min
Pulse	
Adult	60–90 beats/min
Child	80–160 beats/min
Blood pressure	
Adult	
Systolic	100–140 mm Hg
Diastolic	60–90 mm Hg
Child	80 (+ 2 × age in
Systolic	years)
Diastolic	2/3 of systolic
Temperature	98.6°F (96.8–99.3°F)
	37°C (36–37.4°C)

419

TABLE 2. *Normal clinical laboratory values: blood*

Test	Normal value
δ-Aminolevulinic acid	0.01−0.03 mg/dL
Base, total	145−160 mEq/L
Bicarbonate	24−28 mEq/L (24−28 mM/L)
Bilirubin, serum	
Total	0.1−1.2 mg/dL
Direct	0.1−0.3 mg/dL
Indirect	0.1−1.0 mg/dL
Blood gases	
pH	7.35−7.45 (arterial)
	7.36−7.41 (venous)
pCO_2	35−45 mm Hg (arterial)
pO_2	95−100 mm Hg (arterial)
BUN—see urea nitrogen	
Calcium	
Serum	8.5−10.5 mg/dL
Total	4.2−5.2 mEq/L
Carbon dioxide, serum	
Content	24−29 mEq/L (24−29 mM/L)
Combining power	24−30 mEq/L (24−30 mM/L)
Tension, pCO_2	35−45 mm Hg
Chloride	95−106 mEq/L (95−106 mM/L)
Creatinine	0.8−1.2 mg/dL
Glucose (fasting)	65−110 mg/dL
Hemoglobin—whole blood	
Female	12.0−16.0 gm/dL
Male	13.5−18.0 gm/dL
Iron	
Total	50−175 μg/dL (9−31.3 μM/L)
Binding capacity	250−450 μg/dL
Percent saturation	20−55/dL
Lactate dehydrogenase (LDH)	110−250 IU/mL
Osmolality, serum	275−295 mOsm/kg water
Oxygen	
Capacity	16−24 vol/dL (varies with Hb)
Content	15−23 vol/dL (arterial)
Saturation	94−100/dL of capacity
Tension, pO_2	95−100 mm Hg (arterial)
pCO_2	35−45 mm Hg (arterial)
pH	7.35−7.45 (arterial)
Phosphatase, alkaline	5−13 units/dL (King-Armstrong)
Potassium	3.5−5.0 mEq/L
Sodium	136−145 mEq/L
Transaminases	
SGOT (aspartate aminotransferase)	8−40 units/mL
SGPT (alanine aminotransferase)	1−36 units/mL
Urea nitrogen (BUN)	8−25 mg/dL (2.9−8.9 mM/L)
Vitamin A	15−60 μg/dL
Vitamin B_{12}	200−1,025 pg/mL
Vitamin D	
25-hydroxycholecalciferol	10−80 ng/mL
1,25-dihydroxycholecalciferol	21−45 pg/mL

TABLE 3. *Therapeutic, toxic, and lethal blood concentrations*

Substance	Therapeutic or normal	Toxic	Lethal
Alcohols			
Ethanol	—	100 mg/dL (legal intoxication)	>350 mg/dL
Ethylene glycol	—	150 mg/dL	200−400 mg/dL
Isopropranol	—	150 mg/dL	—
Methanol	—	20−80 mg/dL	>80 mg/dL
Antidepressants			
Amitriptyline	5−20 μg/dL	>50 μg/dL	1−2 mg/dL
Desipramine	15−30 μg/dL	>50 μg/dL	1−2 mg/dL
Doxepin	10−25 μg/dL	50−200 μg/dL	1−2 mg/dL
Imipramine	15−25 μg/dL	50−150 μg/dL	>200 μg/dL
CNS depressants			
Barbiturates			
Short-acting	0.01−0.1 mg/dL	0.7−1.0 mg/dL	>1.0 mg/dL
Intermediate-acting	0.1−0.5 mg/dL	1.0−3.0 mg/dL	>3.0 mg/dL
Long-acting	1.5−5.0 mg/dL	4.0−6.0 mg/dL	8−15 mg/dL
Benzodiazepines	0.01−0.3 mg/dL	0.5−2.0 mg/dL	—
Chloral hydrate	0.2−1.0 mg/dL	10 mg/dL	25 mg/dL
Ethchlorvynol	0.05−0.5 mg/dL	2−10 mg/dL	15 mg/dL
Glutethimide	0.02−0.08 mg/dL	1−8 mg/dL	3−10 mg/dL
Meprobamate	0.8−2.4 mg/dL	6−10 mg/dL	14−35 mg/dL
Methaqualone	0.3−0.6 mg/dL	1−3 mg/dL	>3.0 mg/dL
Methyprylon	0.5−1.5 mg/dL	3−6 mg/dL	10 mg/dL
CNS stimulants			
Amphetamine	2−3 μg/dL	50 μg/dL	200 μg/dL
Caffeine	0.5−1.0 mg/dL	—	>10 mg/dL
Cocaine	5−15 μg/dL	90 μg/dL	0.1−2.0 mg/dL
Diethylproprion	0.7−20 μg/dL	—	—
Methamphetamine	20−60 μg/dL	60−500 μg/dL	1−4 mg/dL
Methylphenidate	1−6 μg/dL	80 μg/dL	230 μg/dL
Strychnine	—	0.2 mg/dL	0.9−1.2 mg/dL
Theophylline	1−2 mg/dL	2−4 mg/dL	—
Metals			
Arsenic	0.0−2.0 μg/dL	100 μg/dL	1.5 mg/dL
Cadmium	0.01−0.02 μg/dL	5 μg/dL	—
Copper	100−150 μg/dL	540 μg/dL	—
Iron	65−175 μg/dL	500−600 μg/dL	2−5 mg/dL
Lead	0−30 μg/dL	2.5 μg/dL	>200 μg/dL
Mercury	0−8 μg/dL	100 μg/dL	>600 μg/dL
Opiates			
Codeine	1−12 μg/dL	20−50 μg/dL	>60 μg/dL
Diphenoxylate	1 μg/dL	—	—
Hydromorphone	0.1−3 μg/dL	10−200 μg/dL	>300 μg/dL
Meperidine	30−100 μg/dL	500 μg/dL	1−3 mg/dL
Methadone	30−110 μg/dL	200 μg/dL	>400 μg/dL
Morphine	1−7 μg/dL	10−100 μg/dL	>400 μg/dL
Oxycodone	1−10 μg/dL	20−500 μg/dL	—
Pentazocine	10−60 μg/dL	200−500 μg/dL	1−2 mg/dL
Propoxyphene	5−20 μg/dL	30−60 μg/dL	80−200 μg/dL
Nonopiate analgesics			
Acetaminophen	0.5−2.0 mg/dL	12−30 mg/aL	150 mg/dL
Acetylsalicylic acid	2−10 mg/dL	15−30 mg/dL	>55 mg/dL
Ibuprofen	50−420 μg/dL	—	—

continued

TABLE 3. *Continued*

Substance	Therapeutic or normal	Toxic	Lethal
Ibuprofen	50–420 μg/dL	—	—
Phenothiazines			
Chlorpromazine	50 μg/dL	100–200 μg/dL	0.3–1.2 mg/dL
Haloperidol	0.05–0.9 μg/dL	100–400 μg/dL	—
Perphenazine	0.5 μg/dL	100 μg/dL	—
Promazine	—	100 μg/dL	—
Prochlorperazine	—	100 μg/dL	—
Thioridazine	100–150 μg/dL	1.0 mg/dL	2–8 mg/dL
Thiothixene	1.0 μg/dL	—	—
Trifluoperazine	80 μg/dL	120–300 μg/dL	0.3–0.8 mg/dL
Psychotomimetics			
LSD	—	0.1–0.4 μg/dL	—
MDA	—	—	0.4–1.0 mg/dL
Phencyclidine	—	0.7–24 μg/dL	100–500 μg/dL

Bibliography

Baselt RC, Cravey RH. A compendium of therapeutic and toxic concentrations of toxicologically significant drugs in human biofluids. *J Anal Toxicol* 1977;1:81–103.

Hansted PD. Laboratory indices. In: Knoben JE, Anderson PO, eds. *Handbook of clinical drug data.* 5th ed. Hamilton, IL: Drug Intelligence Publications; 1983:187–193.

Henry JB. *Clinical diagnosis and management by laboratory methods.* 16th ed. Philadelphia: WB Saunders; 1981.

Krupp MA, Tierney LM, Jaweta E, et al. *Physicians handbook.* 21st ed. Los Altos, CA: Lange Medical Publications; 1985:117–229.

Lauwerys RR. Occupational toxicology. In: Klaassen CD, Amdur MO, Doull J, eds. *Toxicology—the basic science of poisoning.* 3rd ed. New York: Macmillan; 1986:902–916.

McBay AT. Toxicology findings in fatal poisonings. *Clin Chem* 1973;19:361–365.

Scully RE. Normal reference laboratory values: case records of the Massachusetts General Hospital. *N Engl J Med* 1978;298:34.

Swinyard EA. Principles of prescription order writing and patient compliance instruction (Table A-II-1). In: Gilman AS, Goodman LS, Rall TW, Murad F, eds. *The pharmacological basis of therapeutics.* New York: Macmillan; 1985:1651–1713.

Winek CL. Tabulations of therapeutic, toxic, and lethal concentrations of drugs and chemicals in the blood. *Clin Chem* 1976;22:832–836.

Winek CL. Drug and chemical blood level data (tabulation). Distributed by Fisher Scientific Co, Pittsburgh.

Subject Index